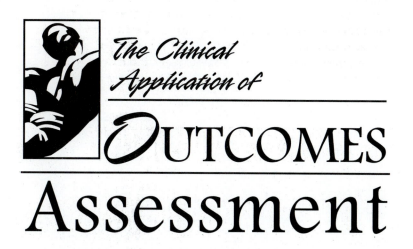

The Clinical Application of

OUTCOMES

Assessment

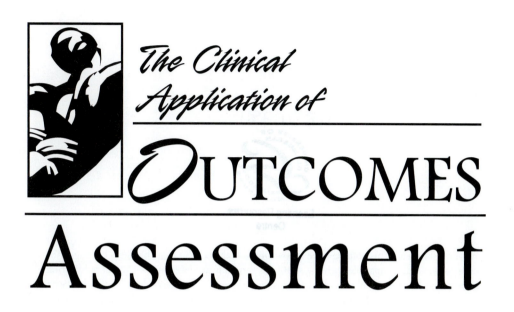

The Clinical Application of OUTCOMES Assessment

Steven G. Yeomans, DC, FACO
Director, Yeomans Chiropractic Center
Ripon, Wisconsin
Postgraduate Faculty Appointments
National College of Chiropractic
Lombard, Illinois
Los Angeles College of Chiropractic
Los Angeles, California
Northwestern College of Chiropractic
Bloomington, Minnesota
Canadian Memorial College of Chiropractic
Toronto, Ontario, Canada

APPLETON & LANGE
Stamford, Connecticut

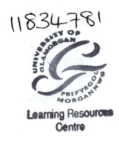
Notice: The authors and the publisher of this volume have taken care to make certain that the doses of drugs and schedules of treatment are correct and compatible with the standards generally accepted at the time of publication. Nevertheless, as new information becomes available, changes in treatment and in the use of drugs become necessary. The reader is advised to carefully consult the instruction and information material included in the package insert of each drug or therapeutic agent before administration. This advice is especially important when using, administering, or recommending new or infrequently used drugs. The authors and publisher disclaim all responsibility for any liability, loss, injury, or damage incurred as a consequence, directly or indirectly, of the use and application of any of the contents of this volume.

Copyright © 2000 by Appleton & Lange

www.appletonlange.com

00 01 02 03 / 10 9 8 7 6 5 4 3 2 1

Prentice Hall International (UK) Limited, *London*
Prentice Hall of Australia Pty. Limited, *Sydney*
Prentice Hall Canada, Inc., *Toronto*
Prentice Hall Hispanoamericana, S.A., *Mexico*
Prentice Hall of India Private Limited, *New Delhi*
Prentice Hall of Japan, Inc., *Tokyo*
Simon & Schuster Asia Pte. Ltd., *Singapore*
Editora Prentice Hall do Brasil Ltda., *Rio de Janeiro*
Prentice Hall, *Upper Saddle River, New Jersey*

ISBN 0-8385-1528-2
Library of Congress Catalog
Card Number: 99-073500

Acquisitions Editor: Robin Lazrus
Production Service: Andover Publishing Services
Illustrations: Wendy Jackelow
Cover Designer: Janice Bielawa

ISBN 0-8385-1528-2

9 780838 515280   90000

PRINTED IN THE UNITED STATES OF AMERICA

To my family, Brigid, Adam, Rachel, and Abigail.
Without your love, patience, and understanding,
this project would still only be a dream.

Contents

Contributors

Hannu Alaranta, MD, PhD
The Rehabilitation Unit of The Invalid Foundation
Helsinki, Finland

Gunnar Andersson, MD, PhD
Rush University Medical School
Chicago, Illinois

William D. Defoyd, DC
The Spine Center
Austin, Texas

Ed Dobrzykowski, MHS, PT, ATC
Director of Development
Focus On Therapeutic Outcomes, Inc.
Knoxville, Tennessee

Michael Feuerstein, PhD
Department of Medical and Clinical Psychology
Uniformed Services University of the Health Sciences
Bethesda, Maryland

Jeffery E. Fitzthum, DC, MD
Department of Rehabilitation Medicine
University of Wisconsin Hospital and Clinics
Madison, Wisconsin

Jeff Gullickson, DC
Private Practice
Apple Valley, Minnesota

Carol Hagino, BSc, MBA
Canadian Memorial College of Chiropractic
Toronto, Ontario, Canada

Daniel T. Hansen, DC
Chiropractic Provider
Coordinator of Quality Improvement
Texas Back Institute
Plano, Texas

Bruce Hoffmann, DC, CCSP
Private Practice
Apple Valley, Minnesota

Craig Liebenson, DC
Postgraduate Faculty
Los Angeles College of Chiropractic
Los Angeles, California

Silvano A. Mior, DC, FCCS(C)
Dean of Research and Postgraduate Education
Canadian Memorial Chiropractic College
Toronto, Ontario, Canada

Robert D. Mootz, DC, DABCO, FICC
Associate Medical Director for Chiropractic
Department of Labor & Industries
State of Washington
Olympia, Washington

David Stude, DC, FACO
Northwestern College of Chiropractic
Bloomington, Minnesota

Howard Vernon, DC, FCCS(C)
Canadian Memorial Chiropractic College
Toronto, Ontario, Canada

Jeffrey M. Wilder, DC, FACO
Private Practice
Madison, Wisconsin

David A. Williams, PhD
Department of Psychiatry
Georgetown University Medical Center
Washington, D.C.

Thomas R. Zastowny, PhD
Departments of Psychiatry and Occupational Medicine
University of Rochester
Rochester, New York

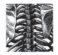

Preface

In the mid-1980s, I found myself frustrated with the challenge of tracking patient progress in the care I provided. Typically, patients appreciated the efforts provided through treatment but were not very helpful when I tried to establish firm endpoints of care, particularly for those with chronic, permanent conditions. I had been exposed to a few outcome assessment tools and found the data derived from these tools quite meaningful, especially when the results were compared to previously completed tools. My interest soon after turned to objective tools that could guide me in a similar manner, but on a more functional level rather than only through subjective measures.

In the late 1980s, I was asked to present a course on the use of outcome assessment tools to a group of health care providers (HCPs) in a postgraduate program. When I performed a literature search, it became apparent that while many tools were available, how to implement them into a clinical setting was far from clear. In fact, so many of the tools seemed to gather the same or similar information that it became very confusing as to which were considered "the best" or the "gold standard."

I noticed that many of the studies that introduced a new outcome-gathering tool compared the new tool to previously published and validated instruments. A consistent pattern emerged from the literature review, allowing me to identify what seemed to be considered the "gold standards"—tools that were being used as the standard to which a new tool was compared. In this text, I have tried to relay this information, while realizing full well that the "gold standard" of today may not remain the gold standard in years to come. Therefore, I must caution the reader that a particular instrument may fit much better into a certain type of clinical practice—better, perhaps, than one of the identified "gold standards." In that scenario, I recommend using the instrument(s) that best apply to your needs in your specific clinical setting.

This project was further stimulated by the obvious lack of a resource in which to access various tools that might be applied in a clinical setting. During interviews that I conducted with staff at over 25 rehabilitation facilities throughout the midwestern United States in 1996, it became apparent that few centers were using outcomes assessments with their patient population. When I asked the directors if they would find value in determining baseline functional deficits, implementing the rehabilitation approaches, and then following up with the same functional assessment to determine the success of the program, I received a unanimous affirmative response. No one, however, knew where to find such a protocol, and interest in locating and utilizing this type of program was significant.

In today's increasingly competitive healthcare market, it is often difficult to obtain insurance preauthorization for rehabilitation services. The use of specific protocols to track the changes that occur over time before and after treatment and rehabilitation has proven to be an essential part of securing the economic return for this service. The subjective tools quantify the patient's disability, while the objective tools or tests quantify the patient's functional losses or impairment. Quantifying this information initially allows the HCP to provide third-party payers with information that supports "medical necessity" or the need for the service. In addition, by readministering the same tests, for example, a month later, the successes or failures in remedying the abnormal disabilities and functional impairment can be easily identified and, if available, alternative rehabilitation approaches can be implemented or discharge from the program can be supported.

As a bonus of utilizing objective physical performance tests, specific rehabilitation prescriptions or goals can be identified based on the subnormal test results and the rehabilitation program established can then be tailored specifically to address those deficiencies. When this information is shared with the patient, compliance in performing the rehabilitation protocols is greatly enchanced. In addition, the clinical information gained from the assessment gives the HCP a heightened level of confidence in promoting the rehabilitation concept to both the patient and third-party payers. The preponderance of today's literature shows that rehabilitation of the locomotor system is an essential part of the long-term success of patient management and patient satisfaction. Applying outcomes management to that process benefits the patient, the HCP, and the third-party payer; thus, everyone wins.

This text is divided into five sections, each of which is designed to introduce the HCP to a practical approach to the use of outcome measures and the implementation of outcomes management in a clinical setting. The popular SOAP-note form of reporting is used to divide the text into sections. Thus, the text begins with an initial introduction and overview of outcomes assessment, followed by a discussion of the outcomes measures in the respective categories of subjective and objective tools. The process of how to apply the tools in the clinical setting is next addressed, followed by the practical aspects of outcomes management. The closing chapter describes how outcomes data can be utilized to enhance patient satisfaction as well as to secure a niche in the managed health care system in the future.

On a personal note, since implementing an outcomes-based model into my practice, I have observed many benefits of this approach. Most notable is my ability to identify *with confidence* endpoints of care. As a result, prompt decision making to change my treatment approach, obtain additional tests or consults, or discharge the patient—sometimes with residuals—occurs on a much more timely manner. Patient education has also been enhanced, because sharing the outcomes data with the patient as a portion of the report of findings puts us both on track with realistic goals and allows for an appreciation of what has transpired as the result of care (ie, what goals have been met). In addition, when submitting records to third-party payers, it is much easier to communicate whether an end of healing or a plateau has been reached; hence, the ability to prove "medical necessity" has been greatly enhanced. Another benefit of outcomes management involves medical–legal enhancement. I have served as an expert witness in many malpractice claims, and those providers who utilized outcomes management were the most successful in proving benefit from care, which usually resulted in a determination of no award and no court appearance. In other words, it was much easier to defend the actions of the HCP when outcomes management was followed.

My objective in compiling the information in this text is to offer to all HCPs a singular location in which to obtain methods to enhance confidence when making clinical decisions. As presented in the last section of the text, the step after collecting the data—or the "big picture" and goal of outcomes management—is to take the outcomes information and, from it, identify the most efficacious way in which treatment can be implemented. More specifically, for a given diagnosis, outcomes management can facilitate a determination of the "value" (sometimes expressed as the ratio between cost divided by the number of visits *and* patient satisfaction, equaling outcome) of a treatment protocol. Using this approach, a "best-practice" assessment can be performed and the information disseminated to HCPs, which can then stimulate the HCP to implement the new approach into practice. To this end, however, data must be collected in order to fulfill the ultimate goal of establishing best-practice protocols. Therefore, a second major focus of this text is to provide the HCP with the necessary tools for data collection. Once collected, data can be pooled, decisions can be derived from the results, and improvements can be made in how we approach patient care.

Steven G. Yeomans

Acknowledgments

In my 20 years of practice, I have had the great fortune to have been guided by many gifted and talented people. In this educational journey, my first and finest educational experience has been with my father, a man who provided me with 15 years of guidance and from whom I still learn; a man who continues to be a reassuring source of information. He combines the skill of a great manual practitioner with the wisdom that only his 50 years of practice experience could teach. Since my initial exposure to manipulation at the age of 14, I have continued to utilize some of the key concepts my father taught me at that time. I have also had the honor to learn from as well as lecture with Dr Joseph Janse, who was president of National College at the time of my attendance in the late 1970s. This chiropractic father and pioneer taught me to extend myself to the fullest and to pass nothing by. My appreciation and deepest respect next turns to Dr Dennis Skogsbergh, who guided me during my orthopedic residency. The growth and maturation that resulted during this period made me aware of how little I truly know, opening many doors to continue the never-ending process of investigation. I owe my formal exposure to rehabilitation concepts to perhaps the greatest catalyst of self-motivation I have known, Dr Craig Liebenson, who continues to prod me to further my love of research and who was instrumental in making this project a reality. During professionally based learning experiences in France, the People's Republic of China, and the Czech Republic, I have been further humbled by the great healers and health facilitators with whom I have come in contact. In part, these individuals have included Vladimir Janda, MD, Chief of the Department of Rehabilitation Medicine in Prague, and Karel Lewitt, MD, DSc, Professor, Charles University, Prague, whose invaluable information will forever be a significant part of my daily practice. Perhaps most importantly, my deepest and most sincere thanks go to all of my colleagues who gave of their valuable time to contribute to this project. Without their participation, this text would not have become a reality. I also want to recognize the chapter reviewers who offered their perspective and guidance. This book also would never have been possible without the support, encouragement, and trust of my editors at Appleton & Lange, especially Lin Marshall, who originally conceived this entire project. I also wish to thank my righthand woman, Elena Mauceri, for the many hours spent making this text readable, and Sharon Rounds, for her perseverance in locating authors and publishers while securing the many permissions that were needed to complete this practical guide.

Foreword

The priests of Asklepios took an oath to put their patients' needs before their own and provide the best recommendations to their patients and colleagues. They did so to avoid the fate of Asklepios, slain by Zeus for becoming greedy and presumptuous. This became the basis for the Hippocratic oath, which physicians today take to protect themselves from the wrath of society or the gods in the event of bad results. The present-day oath is defined further by the 1910 medical report of Abraham Flexner, which urged that medical recommendations be based upon science rather than a "mysterious process." Both of these historical issues still define the modern health care provider (HCP) and his or her link to being protected by being a good Samaritan.

Unfortunately, today's professional faces a great challenge to balance the many aspects of what is considered appropriate care. The HCP must provide care that enhances the patient's self-reliance, while maintaining quality in a cost-conscious way. This dual goal not only opens the door but makes imperative the need for evidence-based practice to become a reality. Health care delivery and financing, not to mention the expectations of the HCP by both patients and health purchasers, seem to be in an overwhelming, continuous state of flux. As the administrative side of practice requires more resources than ever before, the HCP sees reimbursement shrinking. Consumers demand the latest and greatest in care. HCPs desire to be as accurate as possible in diagnosis while anxiety over professional liability can often be at odds with the current state of the literature, payer policies, or government regulation.

Traditionally, HCPs have relied upon assumption-based science, which provides so-called "objective" indicators of physiology and function, only to learn that many of these tests and examination findings have limited value, are not reproducible, and at times even fail to accomplish what is expected. Our understanding is further complicated by new, more expensive medical technologies that are evolving at breakneck speed, based on either intuitive thinking or assumptions that require great leaps of faith to be applicable to our patients. According to our oath, however, we must continue to try to guard against the possibility that our fascination with technology will lead us to further mysterious processes.

Only outcomes management can provide particular attention to patient response in innovative and meaningful ways. Paying attention to a patient's health status, changes in his or her functional ability and physiological indicators, as well as the patient's satisfaction, are becoming second nature to being a modern professional. However, in the state of today's health care system, it can be difficult to systematically balance all of these components. A reasonable use of outcomes assessment appears to be the only way to live within our oath and the expectations of our patients and society.

Outcomes can provide needed tools to more effectively focus patients on meaningful treatment goals. Moreover, outcomes tracking can be integral to assuring the quality and relevance of the work we do with our patients. Outcomes management is essentially a toolbox that helps HCPs focus on what is important to the patient's life, rather than just the indirect clinical indicators we have been trained to rely upon for making many of our treatment decisions.

I hope you will find this book helpful in your professional practice. A section on pain-driven (self-report) outcomes is complemented by a section on provider-driven (including examination) outcomes, and pulled together with a section on applying outcomes management in the real world of practice. This book is timely and brings the issue of outcomes management into focus within a single resource that has utility for any HCP who works with musculoskeletal disorders.

The information comes from a multidisciplinary cast of contributors who have been developing outcomes management in real-world situations. There are clinical, academic, and policy perspectives to consider, and while scholarly, the book remains relevant and practical. Its principal aim is to help newcomer and experienced HCP alike to enhance clinical efficiency. There is an emphasis on simple and economic tracking mechanisms, with the goal of returning patients to self-reliance as quickly as possible (something that is important to both patients and "the system" in general) being underscored.

Although outcomes management has a learning curve, it is not a steep one. I think you will find this book a resource that helps ease the transition from business-as-usual to getting-ahead-of-the-curve by providing an appropriate context for gathering information from your patients. Since the AHCPR Guidelines on acute low back problems came out in 1994, I have often been accused of chiding my professional colleagues about specific interventions that might not really matter, or might even make a patient worse. We must begin to focus on function and results while avoiding the deconditioning that results from inactivity. Overresting can physically and emotionally devastate the lives of our patients and their families. By sensibly incorporating meaningful outcomes tracking in practice, we as professionals may just be able to find out what we are really doing and what we can do better. Otherwise, we may provoke the return to the days before the Asklepion oath,

exemplified by Hammurabi's Code of 1700 BC, which states: "Should a physician drain an abscess and the patient dies, cut off the hands of the physician." Only through outcomes research will we be able to stand on firm ground to meet the many challenges facing today's HCP. Outcomes research not only keeps us in compliance with our oath but also can help us avoid the temptations of shiny new technology, blinding us from what is real and returning us to the "mysterious processes" begun in the dark ages.

Stanley J. Bigos, MD
Professor of Orthopaedics and Environmental Health
University of Washington
Seattle, Washington

SECTION

I

Outcomes Assessment Overview

This first section serves as an introduction to the concepts of outcomes assessment (OA) and outcomes management (OM). The objective of this section is to lay the foundation necessary to facilitate the reader's understanding and appreciation of terminology commonly utilized when addressing the subject of OM. The first chapter discusses the utility of OA and brings into perspective the concepts surrounding the reasons why OA is important. The second and third chapters address terminology commonly utilized in outcomes-oriented literature, which will help the reader more fully appreciate the information being reviewed. This section concludes with Chapter 4, which offers a practical classification system for categorizing the various outcome tools. This classification approach also serves as the foundation for the next several sections.

CHAPTER 1

Why Outcomes? Why Now?

DANIEL T. HANSEN, SILVANO MIOR, & ROBERT D. MOOTZ

▶ INTRODUCTION

▶ THE ERA OF OUTCOMES ASSESSMENT

▶ SO, WHAT HAPPENED AND WHY OUTCOMES?

▶ THE "VALUE" EQUATION
Quality Measures: Patient Satisfaction and Clinical Outcomes
Value of Health Care: Favorable and Unfavorable Attributes

▶ INFORMATION AGE: CONSUMER NEEDS FOR MAKING DECISIONS

▶ HOW CAN OUTCOMES ASSESSMENT MEET THE NEEDS OF THE CUSTOMER?

▶ SCIENTIFIC SCRUTINY OF OUTCOMES MEASUREMENTS
Defining Utility
Reliability and Validity
Sensitivity and Specificity
Discriminability and Responsivity
Clinical Usefulness

▶ OUTCOMES ASSESSMENT MEASURES

▶ SELECTING THE APPROPRIATE OUTCOME ASSESSMENT TOOL

▶ CONCLUSION

INTRODUCTION

Consumerism is in the midst of change all over the world. At the heart of that change is the new relationship between the "consumer" and the supplier. Some observers swiftly reduce this phenomenon to the basic theories of economics, such as supply and demand. But even economists and trend analysts are quick to remind us that the more important factors driving this change have to do with the recognition of, and response to, customer needs and expectations. Competition in the manufacturing and service industries focuses on this very issue. Automobiles, airplanes, homes, furniture, entertainment systems, and telecommunication systems are now being built in response to needs and expectations of their ultimate customer, the consumer.

Service companies and manufacturers are touting that they are the industry leaders in "quality" and "customer satisfaction." And how do they know that? Very simply, they measure it. They measure it through telephone surveys or mail-in surveys usually using recognized public survey vendors. They also operationally measure and track customer complaints, flaws in product quality, employee productivity, and system productivity, often referred to as throughput. After collecting data, they compare their results against recognized industry benchmarks and the results of their competition. They then respond to those quality appraisals by improving their internal systems and customer service. Awareness of quality and value in products and services is now at the forefront of the consumer-centered transaction.

The health care industry has also recognized this recent phenomenon of consumerism. A consumer-centered philosophy is what created and continues to drive *outcomes assessment* and *outcomes management* strategies and initiatives in the increasingly competitive health care arena. Gone are the days when physicians would dictate what they felt patients needed for health care without any consumer scrutiny. Gone are the days when we could merely say "this is what our patients need" without actually doing the measurements and displaying the data for public consumption and analysis. And gone are the days when the supplier–customer interaction was just between the physician and the patient.

CLINICAL TIP 1–1
Outcomes Definitions

For the clinical setting to become outcomes-based, it is essential that the following two elements take place:

- **Outcomes Assessment**—collection and recording of information relative to health processes.
- **Outcomes Management**—using information in a way that enhances patient care.

THE ERA
OF OUTCOMES ASSESSMENT

There is now a social challenge to the importance of outcomes assessment as the fundamental supportive framework for monitoring an effective clinical practice. **Outcomes in clinical practice provide the mechanism by which the health care provider (HCP), the patient, the public, and the payer are able to assess the end results of care and its effect upon the health of the patient and society.** Assessment of various patient health outcomes is achieved by developing and utilizing tools that measure health status and analyze the effectiveness of specific treatment procedures (Andersson and Weinstein, 1994).

Outcomes assessment has emerged from economic and therapeutic concerns to become a practical reality in today's clinical practice. Federal, state, provincial, and private third-party payers; patients; and consumer organizations are requiring that HCPs provide objective evidence of the outcomes of therapeutic interventions (Hinderer and Hinderer, 1993). To respond to these new times of accountability, processes must be implemented that will allow for the evaluation and assessment of all procedures in the delivery of health care. However, outcome assessment strategies are not merely reactions to the needs of accountability. As this book conveys, outcomes management can be a pro-active tool, enabling the HCP to stay on top of patient progress, identify the needs of a patient, and obtain a larger view of his or her practice that can help the provider remain competitive.

An increasing number of existing diagnostic and treatment procedures are coming under scrutiny, as are nearly all new technologies. This trend seems likely to continue and it

can be expected that convincing scientific evidence of validity, reliability, and clinical utility will have to be available. Routine incorporation of clinical and administrative measures of quality will be another expectation of all HCPs. The health care system is positioned and poised to assess the efficiency of individual practitioners and their ability to deliver efficient, cost-effective, quality health care. **To survive, in fact to flourish, in this era of accountability HCPs must be prepared to maintain and be able to provide appropriate documentation and patient records in a clinically efficient and economical manner** (Hansen, 1994).

SO, WHAT HAPPENED
AND WHY OUTCOMES?

By the end of the 1960s and well into the 1970s, the health care industry was in a boom era. Medical schools were graduating increasing numbers of physicians, the medical specialties grew at alarming rates, hospitals grew and flourished, and even with all that growth the demand continued to be stronger than the supply. Health insurance payments replaced more and more of the family's health expenditure and at the same time health benefits became part of the worker's earnings. Health care reimbursement was essentially a "retail" transaction (Fig. 1–1). There were no discounts to speak of, nor volume purchasing agreements. Hospitals and physicians got paid what they billed for. The health care industry's sovereignty relied on restricted competition, limited government regulation, and the authority to define and interpret standards of medical care (Enzmann, 1997).

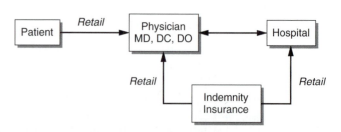

Figure 1–1. Retail health transactions. The protected fee-for-service market in which physicians largely controlled the distribution channel.

(Adapted from Enzmann, 1997. Used with permission.)

Since the mid-1980s there has been increasing study and awareness of what occurred in that era of "retail" health care. Investigators found significant differences in how patients were cared for between communities and even within the same community (eg, Shekelle and Brook, 1991). Expensive technologies found their way into health care communities, resulting in utilization with no clear medical necessity. Additionally, hospital length of stay has been, and continues to be, scrutinized.

The success realized in the decades of the 1970s and 1980s was indeed dangerous for the industry. Increased health care costs resulted from the public's ravenous appetite for health care and the profession's eagerness to feed it. Individuals and families could no longer bear their portion of the costs, which required more involvement by third-party payers. At the same time, health care facilities, institutions, and academic centers of excellence were expanding, requiring increasingly higher levels of capital. Add to that the increasing importance of broad health care coverage for employees to U.S. business and industry, and health care finally was pulled into the capitalistic orbit. Medicine's ability to stand apart from business ended (Enzmann, 1997).

Since the mid-1980s, changes in society, customer expectations, and health care markets have weakened medicine's control of its competition, government regulation, and its "cultural authority" over health care. The key manifestations of this shift are: (1) movement away from "physician-centeredness" to "customer centeredness"; and (2) movement away from "retail" purchase of health care to the "wholesale" systems we have seen in the 1990s (Fig. 1–2). Presently, volume purchasing, discounted prices, true competition in the market, and outside scrutiny over many medical necessity decisions are the norm. Health care futurist Dieter Enzmann defines this "cultural authority" as empowering the medical professions to define truth and fact in medicine. He suggests that cultural authority grants HCPs the right to define illness and health (Enzmann, 1997).

In those old days, training and licensing were sufficient to demonstrate a level of competence that validated physicians' cultural authority over health care. This is no longer true. Validation now requires credible data. And competence in the eyes of the consuming public will be verified by the very same credible data. **With the dawning of the "era of accountability," there are new social mandates directed toward HCPs and health-related facilities. Measurements of quality, satisfaction, efficacy, and effectiveness now serve as essential elements for health care decisions and matters of health policy.**

The interface between the patient/employer and health plan in Figure 1–2 is manifested by agreements and acknowledgments that the health care purchased will be as economical as possible, even as a retail transaction. To meet that need, the health plan warrants that the health care consumed will be "necessary," by eliminating wastes in health resource consumption. The other way the health plan can enhance its value is to purchase health care at discounted or "wholesale" prices. Thus, there is some recognition of quality and cost controls at the customer interfaces on each side of the health plan. Mature health care systems in several markets are working toward eliminating the "middle man" health plan by establishing direct relationships between employer coalitions and accountable HCP networks (including hospitals). Incumbent on this arrangement is the need to assure controls on quality and resource consumption.

Enzmann opines that "the current emphasis on outcome assessment and analysis is not only warranted but crucial for the health professions. Physicians must base their practice on science and evince its impact on outcome. Markedly different practice patterns for the same disease process in various parts of the country weakens competence" (Enzmann, 1997). This professional flaw is now displayed in vivid color maps, such as the Dartmouth Atlas of Health Care in the United States, and in numerous discipline-specific studies (Wennberg and Gittelsohn, 1973; Shekelle and Brook, 1997). Even our language is inconsistent. A recent study revealed 49 spine surgeons used 53 different terms to describe 8 conditions causing low back pain (Fardon et al, 1993). Enzmann further states, "Believe it or not, standardization is to the benefit of the

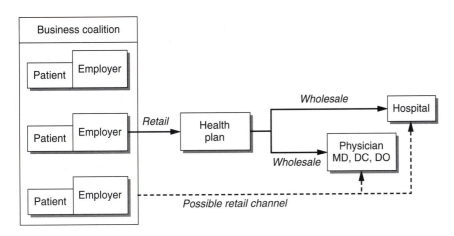

Figure 1–2. Wholesale health transactions. The distribution channel is now controlled by the health plan. The insurance entity now resides between patients and physicians and hospitals. A possible direct relationship exists between physicians or hospitals and business coalitions.

(Adapted from Enzmann, 1997. Used with permission.)

doctors. Rather than interpreting this as cookbook medicine, it should be seen as living up to peer validation of competence. To the extent that medicine is an art, the artistic component will also be measured by outcome. Bad art will not survive" (Enzmann, 1997).

There is growing evidence, very persuasive evidence, that health care has now shifted to a customer-driven market. What is important is what matters to the "customer." Customers in the health transaction can now be patients, employers, governments, managed care organizations, insurance companies, other HCPs, or society as a whole (Enzmann, 1997; Hansen and Vernon, 1997). This evidence also shows that customers want choice and value and they tend to seek data to calculate those equations (Magnusson and Hammonds, 1996; Enzmann, 1997). With advancing information technologies, extensive health-related data can be collected and warehoused to later be collapsed and analyzed. Currently, sophisticated systems that collect and synthesize data in "real time" and then generate useful systems reports are being beta-tested in large and small health care facilities alike. Future competencies of HCPs likely will depend on their ability to work with these new information systems. **The methods of outcomes assessment, even in their currently evolving form may help provide tools HCPs can use to learn to focus on important attributes of care that not only meet accountability demands, but enhance efficiency, quality, and patient satisfaction.**

THE "VALUE" EQUATION

Society assesses value by considering quality and costs. In the past, quality was recognized as minimizing mistakes and excesses. Currently, quality in health care is taking on a multifaceted look ranging from the credentials and competencies of the providers to comparison of clinical behaviors and facility attributes against recognized benchmarks. **Determining the price of health care services now involves complicated formulas that factor cost issues such as provider work, including cognitive value, practice overhead, professional liability, and time spent.** The *value* of the health care transaction is directly proportional to the *quality*, whereas the *cost* (price) has an inverse relationship to value. Currently, quality of health care is best assessed by total outcomes, not just favorable clinical components (Fig. 1–3).

$$\text{Value} = \frac{\text{Quality}}{\text{Cost}}$$

$$\text{Health care value} = \frac{\text{Change in patient health status} + \text{satisfaction measure}}{\text{Costs (indirect + direct)}}$$

Figure 1–3. The "value" equation.

Although the formula is simple, it highlights the parameters that define market interactions. Costs of care are allowed to be the driving force in health care market decisions in the absence of outcome measurements. Value requires an outcome measure. For HCPs to regain some power in the marketplace, they must quickly develop and incorporate outcome measures to demonstrate value.

Many segments of health care have generated little in the way of outcome measures. Historically, the pharmaceutical industry has led the way in clinically based outcomes research, and outcomes assessment for certain integrated disease management systems is maturing at a rapid pace. But for care of neuromusculoskeletal conditions such as back pain, few measures have been reported. More can be expected to evolve. This is particularly true in the management of nonmusculoskeletal conditions by alternative and complementary medicine practitioners. The process of outcomes measurement and management may be the single most useful tool to address these issues in a timely manner.

QUALITY MEASURES: PATIENT SATISFACTION AND CLINICAL OUTCOMES

Perhaps the easiest customer-oriented outcome HCPs can collect is *patient satisfaction*. Such measures are relatively straightforward to obtain using survey instruments and have provided reliable data in other service industries (Ware et al, 1978; Coulter et al, 1994). **Measures of this kind are essential to any service industry, but they do not reflect health outcomes.**

The second key measure is *medical or clinical outcome*. It is the other factor in the numerator of the value equation and **is measured as a change in health status after exposure to a health care delivery system.** It can easily be seen by the *value equation*, that the numerator can largely be driven by the customer's perception—not the HCP's. Much of the current application of outcomes assessment is based on patient self-assessment of clinically related measures and assessment of the various domains of patient satisfaction.

Much of health care is aimed at reducing disability, disfigurement, and discomfort. As described in this text, several useful outcome instruments are available to assess and monitor the response of those *three-D's* to the care provided. Some success has been attained on those fronts, yet many benefits have been difficult to measure so their value is not easily gauged or understood. Measurement must be made, however, because only then will society be able to properly allocate resources for this social service. Unmeasurable health benefits run the risk of being lumped together with other unmeasurable social services that suffer fluctuating, politically driven support. Mental health faces this risk (Starr, 1982). There are areas where chiropractors now have increased legitimacy. Results of recent critical study into the appropriateness of spinal manipulation and mobilization have elevated public support of chiropractic management at least for acute and chronic neck and back pain. The other clinical dimensions of the chiropractic scope of practice will likely be held in the same "risk" or politically driven categories until data of measurable health benefits is produced.

VALUE OF HEALTH CARE: FAVORABLE AND UNFAVORABLE ATTRIBUTES

Value of health care is currently being evaluated through processes of public policy according to four dimensions: safety, efficacy, effectiveness, and efficiency. These are the fundamental components of formal technology assessment in health care (Woolf, 1990; Hansen and Mootz, 1996). Very simply, answering the following simple questions that may beg for complex answers can address each of those dimensions.

Safety:	*Are side effects acceptable?*
Efficacy:	*Can it work?*
Effectiveness:	*Does it work?*
Efficiency:	*Does it provide sufficient value?*

Obviously all of these assessments imply that some measure of outcome is required. Assessment for safety implies that there is a comparative tolerance against either no side effects or the side effects that are already tolerated. But even if such side effects are rare and not life threatening, if there is no evidence to support the effectiveness or efficacy of a treatment in managing a specific condition, then the treatment is inefficient. Useless treatment, regardless of its safety, is still useless treatment.

Those issues that increase the numerator and/or decrease the denominator of the *value equation* are recognized as *favorable* attributes for a health care system and the caregiving processes utilized within the respective health care community. Each of the favorable attributes listed in Table 1–1 is highly dependent on favorable outcome measures and/or evidence of cost-effectiveness. For each of those attributes, there are mature outcome assessment tools available for clinical application or research investigation.

The health care issues that tend to diminish the numerator or increase the denominator of the value equation are the *less-than-favorable* attributes to the health care com-

munity. Formal studies of those health care procedures and systems that have been found to be wasteful, unnecessary, unsafe, excessive, and/or costly continue to be exposed in the technical health care literature, popular press, and news media. Or, those procedures have not been subject to the rigor of today's technology assessment (Hansen and Mootz, 1996). As a result, payers of health care are not reimbursing for those procedures as a matter of policy, and the public is growing less tolerant of purchasing such practices with discretionary family money. Mature quality management programs found in payer systems and provider networks now have formalized quality improvement initiatives to identify and correct for variations in practice and use of inappropriate procedures and devices. Those same initiatives also employ use of protocols and guidelines to control for ill-defined treatment thresholds and clinical endpoints (Hansen and Vernon, 1997; JCAHO, 1997; O'Kane, 1997).

INFORMATION AGE: CUSTOMER NEEDS FOR MAKING DECISIONS

The release of medical information, including outcomes data, physician profiling data and reports of professional consensus exercises has historically been controversial. HCPs, including chiropractors, have sought to contain and restrict such dissemination claiming that it would be misunderstood or misused. These self-serving exclamations usually follow attempts to use such data to measure the quality of their own health care practices. Enzmann proclaims, "Now is the time to discard this cloistered reluctance. Physicians must come to the realization that preserving their role in health care depends on a fully informed consumer (patient). Medical consumerism is now their ally. An informed consumer understands the difference between someone who provides health care and a financial intermediary who does not" (Enzmann, 1997).

A most important variable in the health care market, as previously stated about other markets, **is specific, comparative information about health care services**—information that has been missing. We are witnesses to an un-

Table 1–1: Favorable and Unfavorable Attributes in Health Services

FAVORABLE ATTRIBUTES	UNFAVORABLE ATTRIBUTES
• Better health, quality of life	• Variations in practice
• Clinically effective methods and devices	• Inappropriate or ineffective procedures
• Appropriate care for given conditions	• Ill-defined treatment thresholds and endpoints
• Safety of procedures	• Barriers to obtaining appropriate care
• Cost efficiency and effectiveness	• Discretionary spending for health care
• Predictable and auditable outcomes	
• Competency of practitioners	

derlying, inexorable drive to improve the availability, access, and accuracy of such information. Some of it will be based on health outcome measures but most will not. Both types will define quality. This kind of information will likely be the great equalizer in health care.

Recalling the earlier discussion about patient-centered care, exchange of information is the most essential feature of that customer-centered interface. Typically, HCPs point out that patients do not recognize essential features of quality of care or understand all aspects of determining the need for health care services. This can be true if the patient does not have the relevant information with which to make an informed judgment. In this age of advancing information technologies and enhanced opportunities for lay education, it is becoming contemptuous to many to think that only HCPs are capable of such judgments and action.

Use of outcomes data and related information for management of clinical conditions is the easy part, and should not generate professional controversy. However, use of outcomes data for measurement of quality by third parties will likely result in resistance. Such resistance will probably be both futile and counterproductive. **By helping shape quality measures, HCPs have a major opportunity to influence buying decisions.** It is in the long-term interest of the health care professions for all "consumers" (not just the patient) to be knowledgeable and to have necessary information to make a judgment of value. Despite the usual disclaimers from HCPs and professional guilds about how their quality cannot be measured, it will be (Hansen and Triano, 1993; Enzmann, 1997).

At a simple level, people want results. All aspects of the health care system will now be driven by results.

HOW CAN OUTCOMES ASSESSMENT MEET THE NEEDS OF THE CUSTOMER?

With different parties putting their fingers in the health care "pie," there has to be some sensitivity to the context from which the diversified interests spring. It is important to understand what benefits should be achieved from accountable health systems using outcomes assessment, as perceived by each constituent (Table 1–2).

Expectations from outcome measurements are consistent with accountability initiatives such as cost containment, compliance, and efficiencies. For outcomes experts and research scientists, the outcome measures are used in exercises testing for validation of a premise. And for HCPs, they are used to assist in monitoring progress of a clinical condition or overall health status of a patient, not to mention staying on top of one's own clinical performance.

Implicit with the recognition of the various players in health care delivery and policy is understanding how results of outcome measures and outcomes assessment are reported back to the various customer groups. A community clinic or specialty center proclaiming, "We have outcomes," has no impact other than self-gratification unless it can communicate the effect of those outcomes to meet the expectations or needs of that customer. "We have outcomes demonstrating decreased episode duration and lower direct medical costs in the management of uncomplicated back pain," will play well to those customers seeking solutions for cost and efficiency. "We have data that correlates functional measures to anchored pain scales for neck pain," will impact researchers and outcomes experts, and probably affect the way practitioners manage neck pain cases.

Each customer group is searching for some tangible benefit through the use of accountability measures such as outcomes assessments. At the same time, those customers need to be assured that outcome measurements meet all general expectations of scientific rigor and utility. The competitive market advantage that is evidenced has not gone unnoticed by major players. Outcomes assessment, and the use of that information to shape how services are delivered is becoming common in large clinics, hospitals, and medical centers. Even managed care plans and provider networks seeking contracts from group health and industrial insurance are finding the strategies of quality improvement and customer service are tools they need to stay in business.

Table 1–2: Meaning of Outcomes

HEALTH CARE CUSTOMER	MEANING OF "OUTCOMES"
For payers and purchasers	• Cost containment
For regulators	• HCP compliance
For administrators	• Efficiency and lower utilization
For clinical researchers	• Proof of a premise
For outcomes experts	• Benefit perceived by patients
For HCPs	• Clinical/health status

SCIENTIFIC SCRUTINY OF OUTCOMES MEASUREMENTS

Do the outcome measurements employed in your clinical system demonstrate *utility*, *reliability*, *validity*, *sensitivity*, *specificity*, and *responsiveness*? Should I, as an HCP, be concerned about this technical jargon? The answers to these questions should be "yes." It is essential to realize the importance of these characteristics of measurement, especially in the clinical setting. **The introduction of new or novel measurements in the clinical setting should be preceded by formal investigation into the "meaningfulness" of the test or measure.** An HCP would do well to expect to see evidence of scientific investigation before engaging in the use of a measuring method. Society is expecting to see that evidence.

DEFINING UTILITY

Measurements are used in clinical practice to provide the HCP with an understanding and evaluation of attributes specific to patients and their presenting complaint. They can also be used to differentiate between conditions; for example, a straight leg raise of 60 degrees has a different meaning than one of 10 degrees with positive cross leg sign. Thus, measurements provide the HCP with objective definitions of physical and behavioral characteristics in terms of measurable qualitative and quantitative entities. **By objectifying such measures, the HCP can communicate information in "real" terms as opposed to those that are more abstract and ambiguous, such as "the patient is feeling better"** (Portney and Watkins, 1993). Further, the HCP can make decisions about the progress of the patient's condition based upon the objective outcomes of the measures selected. However, the outcome chosen must be meaningful (valid), dependable (reliable), useful (clinical utility), and be able to measure differences (discriminability and responsiveness). If the HCP is to rely upon out-

comes to determine patient's health status or clinical disposition, the measures must be meaningful (Hansen, 1994).

RELIABILITY AND VALIDITY

For outcomes to be meaningful, they must adhere to the principles of measurement and be properly applied. The starting point for any measure is understanding its reliability and validity (Hinderer and Hinderer, 1993). Measures that are not reliable and valid will not provide meaningful information, but rather will provide "numbers or categories that give a false impression of meaningfulness" (Rothstein, 1985). **Reliability refers to the consistency of measurement.** Consistency may be affected by numerous factors, including instrument error, operator proficiency and skill, operator judgement and dexterity, patient compliance, and the environment in which the test is conducted (Triano et al, 1992). In fact, measurements are rarely perfectly reliable. "All instruments are fallible to some extent, and all humans respond with some inconsistency" (Portney and Watkins, 1993). Therefore, the reality is that some degree of discrepancy in measurements within and between patients is expected. The HCP, however, must be aware of the dimension of this discrepancy and make a clinical judgment regarding the usefulness of the test and the extent to which the observed changes, compared to the baseline measures (ie, the initial measures), are "real." If reliability is important, than validity is indispensable.

Validity refers to the extent to which an instrument accurately measures what it is intended to measure. There are various attributes to the assessment of the validity of a measure, ranging from "face" to "discriminant" validity (Vernon, 1995). These various attributes reflect how an instrument is to be used, the nature of the data collected and the objectivity of response variables. Portney and Watkins (1993) point out that the issues of reliability and validity must be separated because an instrument that measures something consistently does not mean that it is measuring what we want it to measure. **The HCP must remember that "although reliability is a prerequisite to validity, this relationship is unidirectional; that is, reliability states the limits of validity, but it is no guarantee of it"** (Portney and Watkins, 1993). Figure 1–4 (A–C) graphically represents this relationship. Figure 1–4A illustrates that the target hits are clustered nicely around one area, but they are distant from the central point; this represents consistent or reliable hits, but accuracy or validity is poor. Figure 1–4B shows that the hits are clustered around the central point of the target, depicting an accurate or valid and reliable hit. In Figure 1–4C the hits are all over the target illustrating that the hits were neither valid nor reliable.

SENSITIVITY AND SPECIFICITY

In addition to the test's reliability and validity, the HCP must also be aware of its sensitivity and specificity. **Sensitivity refers to the test's ability to detect whether some-**

CLINICAL TIP 1–2
Outcomes Criteria

The following are criteria that are important when choosing an outcome measure:

Utility:	*Is it useful?*
Reliability:	*Is it dependable?*
Validity:	*Does it do what it is supposed to?*
Sensitivity:	*Can it identify patients with a condition?*
Specificity:	*Can it identify those that do not have the condition?*
Responsiveness:	*Can it measure differences over time?*

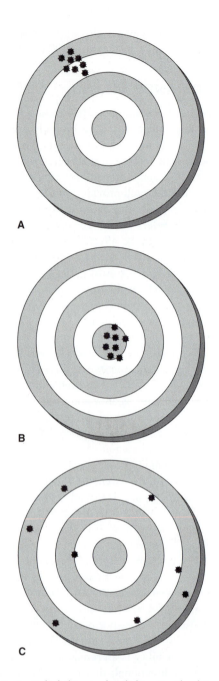

Figure 1–4. Reliability and validity. **A.** The hits are in the same area, representing a consistent or reliable shot. **B.** The hits are all located at the center of the target, indicating accuracy, and are consistent, representing a valid and reliable finding. **C.** The hits on the target are scattered everywhere, reflecting the lack of accuracy and consistency, representing neither a reliable nor valid shot.

of the test. The sensitivity and specificity of a test is important if it is to be used as a diagnostic tool. The discrepancy found with instruments that measure strength and mobility to differentiate between patients with symptoms, functional ability, or psychological disorders impacts upon the ability of such instruments to aid in making a diagnosis (Deyo, 1990; Dainty et al, 1998). In contrast, laboratory and physical measures tend to be better at differentiating between patients who have the disorder and those who do not (Deyo, 1990).

DISCRIMINABILITY AND RESPONSIVITY

The chosen test must also be *discriminating*; **that is, tests assessing different patient attributes should have different results.** For example, assessing deep tendon reflexes may not correlate with range of motion testing of that limb. HCPs must understand the purpose of the selected measure and not extrapolate the findings so as to make conclusions that are inconsistent with the inherent properties of the test. Understanding the measurement properties of a test will enable the HCP to determine the test's responsivity.

Responsivity or response stability of a test **refers to the test's ability to provide consistent measurements with repeated use, over time.** If a test does not provide consistent measures over time, then it is difficult to conclude whether the changes noted from intervention to intervention were a function of the intervention or the inherent error in the test's measure. Response stability is determined using specific statistical tests that basically measure the amount of error found with repeated measures (Portney and Watkins, 1993). This measure can be used to assess whether the degree of change recorded is, in fact, the degree of change that actually occurred (Vernon, 1995). For example, Dainty et al (1998) assessed the reliability of an isometric dynamometer and found that the average differences in back flexion strength measured over 2 days ranged from −7.78 to 7.18 lb. If an HCP were to introduce a rehabilitation program, he or she must be aware of this inherent measurement difference of about 15 lb when making decisions on the effectiveness of his or her program on increasing the patient's back flexion strength (Dainty et al, 1998). Assessing the Neck Disability Index (NDI) responsiveness to care, Vernon and Mior (1991) reported that the NDI scores correlated with improvements reported by the patient, thus providing preliminary evidence that this instrument can measure change over time.

CLINICAL USEFULNESS

The final item to consider is the clinical usefulness of the selected test. **The most important criterion an HCP should use in selecting an outcome measure is that it is clinically sensible.** In addressing this item, the HCP must determine if the test is able to: (1) provide an accurate diagnosis; (2) provide evidence for supporting the use of a

one has the condition or disease being tested or the "**proportion of patients with the target disorder who have a positive test result**" (Sackett et al, 1991). Sensitivity is the *true positive rate of the test*. **Specificity on the other hand, refers to the ability of the test to detect those that do not have the condition or disease;** *the true negative rate*

specific treatment; or (3) enable the HCP to determine the true outcome or effectiveness of the treatment (Sackett et al, 1991).

Understanding the measurement properties of the test will enable the HCP to make educated decisions about which tests to use, in the appropriate clinical situation. Only when this is done will the test results be meaningful and contribute to patient care.

OUTCOME ASSESSMENT MEASURES

HCPs are expected to record and report patient progress (Haldeman et al, 1992; Henderson et al, 1994; Ebrall et al, 1998). Such recording typically focuses upon specific patient entrance data (ie, presenting complaint and health history) and treatment progress (ie, progress notes or SOAP notes) (McElheran and Sollecito, 1994). However, in order to assess the effectiveness of the treatment plan, both objective and subjective data on patient results or outcomes must be collected and documented. These data typically focus upon the physical changes noted at the time of consultation and in subsequent visits (eg, range of motion, neurological tests, x-ray findings). **But what matters most to patients and payers is the change in functional health status (eg, quality of life, activities of daily living, return to work, and economic efficiency)** (Hansen, 1994; Mootz, 1994). Table 1–3 provides a list of outcome assessment measures that can be used in clinical practice. The reliability and validity of each of these outcomes have been documented. The table divides the measures into four categories: (1) questionnaires (general

Table 1–3: Outcome Measures Appropriate for Clinical Use

PURPOSE	QUESTIONNAIRE/INSTRUMENT
1. Questionnaires	
General health status	• Sickness Impact Profile
	• SF-36/SF-12
	• Dartmouth COOP Charts
Pain	• Visual analog scales/numeric rating scale
	• McGill Pain Questionnaire
	• Pain drawing
Functional status	• Neck Disability Index
	• Roland-Morris Disability Questionnaire
	• Oswestry Disability Questionnaire
	• Waddell Disability Index
	• Pain Disability Index
	• Million Scale
Patient satisfaction	• Chiropractic Satisfaction Questionnaire
	• Patient satisfaction (Ware)
2. Physiological outcomes	• Ranges of motion (inclinometer)
	• Straight leg raising
	• Dynamometer measures (strength)
	• Physical tests
	• Electromyography
	• Mobility by x-ray
3. Utilization measures	• Number services per occurrence
	• Treatment days (weeks) per occurrence
	• Utilization of technology
	• Episode duration
4. Cost measures	• Charges per occurrence
	• Charges per service
	• Disability compensation
	• Return-to-work

health status, pain, functional status, patient satisfaction); (2) physiological outcomes; (3) utilization measures; and (4) cost measures. Each measure has its specific purpose and must be chosen in the correct situation in order to provide clinically useful information. Detailed analysis of the psychometric properties of these instruments can be found elsewhere (Deyo, 1990; Sackett et al, 1991; McDowell and Newell, 1997).

The outcome assessments outlined in Table 1–3 can be used to measure change in patients who present with musculoskeletal complaints and who may undergo rehabilitation. The general health status self-administered questionnaires have been shown to take relatively little time to complete by the patient and provide the HCP with information about the various aspects of the patient's general health and ability to cope with his or her pain; that is, physical functioning, social functioning, limitations of activities due to pain or emotional distress, vitality, and general mental health (Millard, 1991). The pain diagrams are very useful guides in helping to identify the intensity, quality, and location of the patient's pain (Vernon, 1995).

The functional status self-administered questionnaires listed in Table 1–3 have been designed to assess the impact of certain types of painful musculoskeletal conditions on certain patient functions. These include the neck (Neck Disability Index), the low back (Roland-Morris Disability Questionnaire, Oswestry Disability Questionnaire, Million Scale), and more general body involvement (Waddell Disability Index and Pain Disability Index). The patient satisfaction questionnaire (Chiropractic Satisfaction Questionnaire) was developed to measure patient visit specific satisfaction with chiropractic care.

The physiological outcomes, however, tend to suffer from a lack of correlation between what they measure and the patient's presenting symptoms, functional ability, or psychological status (Deyo, 1990). For example, static plain radiographs may have an important role to play in the diagnosis of certain pathologies, but their interpretation may be more variable than the questionnaires (Deyo et al, 1985), let alone that they correlate poorly with the absence or presence of back pain (Phillips et al, 1986). Even the more sophisticated measures of spinal function have not been shown to correlate highly with patient's pain (Liebenson and Oslance, 1995). **The HCP must remember that the "principal value of instrumentation lies in its ability to focus on the patient's functional capacity and not on the symptoms"** (Triano et al, 1992).

Measures of utilization are also important in helping to provide information about various attributes of a clinical practice. Information on utilization together with cost analysis of care are important outcome measures that can be used to assess the quality of care (Hansen, 1994). This information can be used to determine the costs of managing certain conditions, including the frequency of patient visits, duration of care, type of care rendered, length of time on compensation, and return to work. **The resultant information can be used to compare performances within** and between HCPs, and, ultimately, to improve the quality of patient care.

Each of the listed outcomes can be helpful in determining what influences are present and should be considered when creating a patient plan of management. They can also be used to measure how effective the plan was in modifying the identified patient dysfunctions.

SELECTING THE APPROPRIATE OUTCOME ASSESSMENT TOOL

When selecting the appropriate outcome assessment tool the first question to answer is "why am I gathering this data?" Sackett et al (1991) provide four different purposes for why data should be gathered:

1. To judge severity of the condition or disorder, in addition to its cause.
2. To predict the prognosis or the course of the condition.
3. To estimate the likelihood of responsiveness to treatment.
4. To determine the actual responsiveness of the treatment plan.

Therefore, the HCP must assess the usefulness of the selected test and determine if the information that it generates will facilitate the improvement of the delivery of health care. The HCP should evaluate each instrument and determine if it is first clinically sensible. Can the measurement be made within the confines of the clinical practice? Does the measure require elaborate instrumentation and skilled operators? Is the measure appropriate for what is being evaluated? Can the selected instrument measure change in a patient's symptoms or functions? In order to answer some of these questions, the HCP will have to carefully assess the various attributes defining the utility of the instrument selected. If a search of the literature fails to provide evidence of the reliability and validity of the instrument, then the manufacturer should be contacted. If the manufacturer cannot provide normative and reliability data, then the HCP should reconsider the decision to use the instrument. **Using or purchasing instruments that do not have adequate evidence of clinical utility may appear impressive but will nevertheless render useless information.**

If the selected instrument is clinically sensible, then determine if it suitable to be used with the patient population in your clinic environment. Ensure that patients who will be asked to complete a self-administered questionnaire can read and interpret the instructions and answer the questions. If functional capacity evaluations are to be performed, ensure that patients meet the selection criteria for the test and can provide the necessary information to the operator to ensure test accuracy.

Finally, assess the feasibility of administering the selected outcome assessment tool. Care must be taken to administer the assessment tool as instructed by the manual or literature. Assessments must be administered according to test protocol, and distributed or conducted in a timely fash-ion. The HCP must then correctly interpret and report the results. **Most importantly, the results should be integrated and used to make any necessary modifications to the patient's clinical plan of management.**

Conclusion

The health care market now has informed consumers who have become skilled buyers of health services; and they vote with their money and with their feet. With increased access to health-related data, health care consumers demand to know how their HCPs and managed care organizations compare to established or emerging benefit standards for common health problems. Quality initiatives, such as protocols, clinical guidelines, and outcomes assessment, are becoming the vehicle for consumers and suppliers of health care to meet each other's expectations, since the market has less ability to dictate standards based on cost alone.

Outcomes data is required to facilitate the quality initiatives. Thus, there is increasing demand for coordinated collection and synthesis of outcomes data from clinical practice, and for prospective outcomes studies in research centers. Currently, studies affecting chiropractic are being done in health care centers of excellence (ie, RAND), private sector companies (ie, Group Health Cooperative of Puget Sound, Texas Back Institute), and academic centers (ie, University of North Carolina, University of Washington, UCLA, and several chiropractic colleges). And as more and more of these programs mature and generate results, there will be a stronger attraction for academic chiropractic HCPs, from inside and outside our colleges, to move into these growing health policy research centers. This feature contributes strongly toward expanding the profession's research infrastructure (Mootz et al, 1997). Additionally, it amplifies the suggestion that the expected competencies of modern practitioners include outcomes assessment and outcomes-based clinical management.

There is a growing body of knowledge describing the clinical utility of outcome assessment instruments. Understanding how this knowledge can be used in deciding which instrument to use, when, and why, will lead to their more efficient use. HCPs must continue to demand that evidence be provided to support the clinical utility of instruments. They must not fall victim to the high-pressured salesmanship of those anxious to sell the latest flashy, sophisticated widget, only to find that it generates useless information. Collecting useless information, regardless of the cost of the instrument, is still useless. HCPs must be cognizant of Palmer and Cochshott's Law, which states, "clinical investigations, like filing cabinets, tend to proliferate" (Palmer and Cochshott, 1984).

When outcome measures are appropriately used and integrated into an evidence-based, patient-centered model of practice, there is accountability and quality assurance. HCPs who evolve toward this model of health care delivery will be able to deal with the demands and expectations of the present era of health care delivery.

REFERENCES

Andersson GBJ, Weinstein JN. Introduction: Health outcomes related to low back pain. *Spine.* 1994; 19(18S):2026S–2027S.

Coulter ID, Hays RD, Danielson CD. The chiropractic satisfaction questionnaire. *Top Clin Chiro.* 1994; 1(4):40–43.

Dainty D, Mior SA, Bereznick D. Validity and reliability of an isometric dynamometer as an evaluative tool in a rehabilitative clinic. *J Sports Chirop Rehab.* 1998;12(3):109–117.

Deyo RA. Measuring the functional status of patients with low back pain. *Chiro Tech.* 1990;2(3):127–137.

Deyo RA, McNiesh, Cone RO. Observer variability in interpretation of lumbar spine radiographs. *Arthritis Rheum.* 1985;28:1066–1070.

Ebrall P, Chance M, Crean S, Searle R, Hansen D. *Clinical Parameters of Australian Chiropractic Practice.* Sydney, Australia: Chiropractic Association of Australia; 1998: in press.

Enzmann, DR. *Surviving in Health Care.* St. Louis, Mo: Mosby-Year Book; 1997.

Fardon D, Pinkerton S, Balderston R, Garfin S, Nasca R, Salib R. Terms used for diagnosis by English speaking spine surgeons. *Spine*. 1993;18(2):274–277.

Haldeman S, Chapman-Smith D, Petersen D, eds. *Guidelines for Chiropractic Quality Assurance and Practice Parameters*. Gaithersburg, Md: Aspen; 1992.

Hansen DT. Determining how much care to give and reporting patient progress. *Top Clin Chiro*. 1994;1(4):1–8.

Hansen DT, Mootz RD. Formal processes in technology assessment: A primer for the chiropractic profession. *Top Clin Chiro*. 1996;3(1):71–83.

Hansen DT, Triano JJ. Applications of quality assurance in chiropractic practice. In: Lawrence D, ed. *Advances in Chiropractic*. Vol 2. St. Louis, Mo: Mosby-Year Book; 1993.

Hansen DT, Vernon H. Applications of quality improvement to the chiropractic profession. In: Lawrence D, ed. *Advances in Chiropractic*. Vol 4. St. Louis, Mo: Mosby-Year Book; 1997.

Henderson D, Chapman-Smith D, Mior S, Vernon H. Clinical guidelines for chiropractic practice in Canada. *J Can Chiro Assoc*. 1994(suppl);38(1):1–203.

Hinderer SR, Hinderer KA. Quantitative methods of evaluation. In: DeLisa J, ed. *Rehabilitation Medicine: Principles and Practice*. 2nd ed. Philadelphia, Pa: JB Lippincott; 1993:96–121.

JCAHO. *1997 Accreditation Manual for Health Care Networks*. Oakbrook Terrace, Ill: Joint Commission on Accreditation of Healthcare Organizations; 1997.

Liebenson C, Oslance J. Outcomes assessment in the small private practice. In: Liebenson C, ed. *Rehabilitation of the Spine: A Practitioner's Manual*. Baltimore, Md: Williams & Wilkins; 1995:73–93.

McDowell I, Newell C. *Measuring Health: A Guide to Rating Scales and Questionnaires*. New York, NY: Oxford University Press; 1987.

McElheran LJ, Sollecito PC. Delivering quality chiropractic care in a managed care setting. *Top Clin Chiro*. 1994;1(4):30–39.

Magnusson P, Hammonds K. Health care: The quest for quality. *Business Week*. 8 April 1996;108.

Millard RW. A critical review of questionnaires for assessing pain-related disability. *J Occup Rehab*. 1991;1(4):289–302.

Mootz RD. Maximizing the effectiveness of clinical documentation. *Top Clin Chiro*. 1994;1(1):60–65.

Mootz RD, Hansen DT, Coulter ID. Health services research related to chiropractic: Review and recommendations for research prioritization by the chiropractic profession. *J Manipulative Physiol Ther*. 1997;20(3):201–217.

O'Kane M. *1997 Standards for the Accreditation of Managed Care Organizations*. Washington, DC: National Commission on Quality Assurance; 1997.

Palmer PES, Cochshott WP. The appropriate use of diagnostic imaging: Avoidance of the red goggle syndrome. *JAMA*. 1984;252:2753–2754.

Phillips RB, Frymoyer J, MacPherson B, Newburg A. Low back pain: A radiographic enigma. *J Manipulative Physiol Ther*. 1986;9(3):183–187.

Portney LG, Watkins MP. *Foundations of Clinical Research. Applications to Practice*. Norwalk, Conn.: Appleton & Lange; 1993:41–86.

Rothstein JM, ed. *Measurement in Physical Therapy*. New York, NY: Churchill-Livingstone; 1985:1–46.

Sackett DL, Hayne RB, Guyatt GH, Tugwell P. *Clinical epidemiology: A Basic Science for Clinical Medicine*. 2nd ed. Toronto, Canada: Little, Brown; 1991:51–52.

Shekelle PG, Brook RH. A community-based study of the use of chiropractic services. *Am J Public Health*. 1991;81:439–442.

Starr P. *The Social Transformation of American Medicine*. New York, NY: Basic Books; 1982.

Triano JJ, Skogsbergh DR, Kowalski MH. Use of instrumentation and laboratory examination procedures by the chiropractor. In: Haldeman S, ed. *Principles and Practice of Chiropractic*. 2nd ed. Norwalk, Conn.: Appleton & Lange; 1992:319–360.

Vernon H. Pain and disability questionnaires in chiropractic rehabilitation. In: Liebensen C, ed. *Rehabilitation of the Spine: A Practitioner's Manual*. Baltimore, Md: Williams & Wilkins; 1995:57–71.

Vernon HT, Mior SA. The neck disability index: A study of reliability and validity. *J Manipulative Physiol Ther*. 1991;14:409.

Ware JE, Davies-Avery A, Stewart AL. The measurement and meaning of patient satisfaction: A review of recent literature. *Health Mental Care Serv Rev*. 1978;1:1–15.

Wennberg J, Gittelsohn A. Small area variations in health care delivery. *Science*. 1973;182:11102–11108.

Woolf SH. Practice guidelines: A new reality in medicine—I. Recent developments. *Arch Intern Med*. 1990;150:1811–1818.

CHAPTER 2

Attributes to Look for in Outcome Measures

HOWARD VERNON & CAROL HAGINO

INTRODUCTION

This chapter provides a review of the important properties of the tests typically used in chiropractic practice for measuring the outcome of care; that is, **outcome measures.** The objective of this chapter is to enable the health care provider (HCP) to make good decisions about which treatment outcome measures to use in practice. The most important criterion to remember about outcome measures is that their primary purpose is to measure change, particularly change in the clinical status of patients. Above all else, which will be discussed, **outcome measures must be good at measuring change.** What it means to be "good at measuring change" will be the major focus of this chapter.

Clinical tests are performed in chiropractic practice for a variety of reasons. **Diagnostic tests** are conducted to identify an abnormality, which provides the most likely explanation for the patient's symptoms. Some diagnostic tests are used to rule in or out a certain possible abnormality. For example, in the case of a worker with a lifting injury to his low back with some radiation of pain into the right lower limb, a positive straight leg raising sign of less than 45 degrees with back and leg pain may help to rule in the presence of nerve root tension, the ultimate cause of which may be a lumbar disc herniation. This would even be more the case if Braggard's sign were also positive on that side. However, if a third test were performed whereby the patient was asked if his back and leg pain were worsened when the foot was *plantar-flexed*, a positive response might help to rule out the very same diagnoses and lead the HCP to consider some form of pain amplification.

Another category of tests is for **prognostic** purposes. The whole area of genetic testing to predict future health status, for example, is exploding in this decade. In chiropractic practice, a crossed straight leg raising sign, indicative of a sequestered, more central disc, typically provides a poor prognosis. The search for prognostic signs of chronicity resulting from neck and back injuries has occupied the time of many researchers. In some areas, psychosocial factors predominate (Deyo and Diehl, 1983; Waddell et al, 1984; Waddell et al, 1993; Burton et al, 1995), in other areas, injury mechanisms predominate (Triano and Schultz, 1987; Alaranta et al, 1994; Yeomans and Liebenson, 1996; Gronblad et al, 1997).

A third category of tests involves the topic of this text, **outcome measures.** Outcome measures can encompass any of the previously described tests so long as they can validly *measure change in the patient's clinical status.* In recent years, with respect to spinal pain, it has become clear that tests of various patient-oriented attributes, completed by the patient (and therefore described as "self-report" and "subjective") can be equally if not better suited to measuring a patient's current status and the magnitude of change in his or her condition (Deyo and Diehl, 1983; Vernon, 1990).

PROPERTIES OF MEASUREMENTS

Measurements are ideally designed to minimize error and to reduce variability. In the clinical setting, the involvement of the patient in the process of measurement of pain often compromises the ideal level of rigor in the measuring process. By its very definition as an experience and not an objectifiable state, pain eludes such rigorous analysis. Often, the best the HCP can do is to systematically manage the high degree of variability arising from the use of outcome assessments in practice. **These sources of variability include recall bias, in which patients can under- or over-inflate their answers due to poor recall, the emotional overlay associated with pain, difficulties in understanding and completing the questionnaires (ie, literacy, numeracy, and linguistic difficulties), and, finally, the great "bugbear" in clinical practice, secondary gain or pain amplification.** This discussion is not meant to be technically exhaustive; readers are referred to such classic texts as that by McDowell and Newell (1996) and Norman and Streiner (1991) for more in-depth treatment of these topics.

MEASUREMENT SCALES

All instruments use a scale to measure a specific **construct, parameter, or dimension.** Typically, the scale is only representative of the construct itself. For example, the increase of temperature is really measured in linear units of increase in a column of mercury—a thermometer. Similarly, the Visual Analogue Scale (VAS) uses a 100-mm line to represent pain severity. In this instance, the anchors or endpoints of the scale are both absolute and arbitrary. They are absolute because they are intended to measure the phenomenon from its lowest to its highest level. On the other hand, they are arbitrary because the numbers assigned to these and any intermediate states are purely a matter of the choice of the designer of the scale. In fact, many pain scales use the numbers 0–5, 0–10, or even 0–101, when, all the while, there is no more pain with one scale than with the next!

NOMINAL SCALES

The manner in which numbers or units are used in a scale is organized according to the degree to which the scale actually represents the quality or quantity being measured. The first level of a scale uses a numeric code to represent the response category. **If only two answers—yes or no—are possible on a certain scale, and numbers such as 1 or 2 are assigned to represent these answers, then these data are said to be nominal data.** In this respect, the numbers actually represent a code for the construct under consideration. Nominal data are said to be the lowest order of data in that little of the actual parameter measured is revealed by the data. All the qualities of the construct that are measurable are reduced to one or two states—present or absent, yes or no, male or female, and so on. As such, this type of data is also referred to as "dichotomous data" (Table 2–1).

ORDINAL SCALES

On the ordinal scale, numbers are still used as codes for other characteristics, but the numbers are used to rank the level of the characteristic and, therefore, bear some (if only indirect) relationship to the measured value. On an ordinal scale, the number 2 represents a greater value than 1; however, the true intervals of such a scale are really unknown. In other words, whether 2 really represents twice as much of the value as 1, or, on a scale from 1 to 5, whether each interval really represents 25% of the total value is, at best, uncertain. Nonetheless, this relationship of an ordinal scale to the value measured is often assumed by users, prompting some inappropriate conclusions (Vernon, 1996). The precision of an ordinal scale may be improved by clearly describing the anchor and intermediate points. This is best seen in the Oswestry Low Back Pain Disability Questionnaire (Fairbank et al, 1980).

INTERVAL SCALES

In the interval scale, numbers do not merely represent units of value, they constitute the units of value. This

Table 2–1: Scaling in Pain and Disability

Questionnaires

Nominal Scale:

"Do you have pain?"   Yes/No

                                            1 2

Ordinal Scale:

"How severe is your pain?"   0   2   4   6   8   10

                                           none   awful

Testing

Interval Scale:

Determine the thermal pain threshold in a pain patient (Range: 40 to 55 degrees)

Ratio Scale:

Determine the pressure pain threshold in a pain patient (Range: 0 to 10 kg/cm^2)

scale is synonymous with a type of data known as "continuous data." On the interval scale, data points are true numerical representations of the value of the parameter in question. These data points can be subdivided (at least theoretically) into infinitely smaller units, each of which would still represent a true unit of measurement of the parameter. For example, temperature is measured on a continuous scale, whereby a measurement of 10° is hotter than 9°, and colder than 11°, and the difference between 10° and 10.5° is real. On an interval scale, however, there may not be a true zero point; there are three different temperature scales, each with their own zero point. As such, at least on the Fahrenheit and Celsius scales, there may not be an absolute representation of the measured value by the scale, in that 20° may not be twice as hot as 10°.

CLINICAL TIP 2–1
Ratio Scale Example

As an example of an appropriate ratio scale comparison, consider a patient with low back pain who scores 30 out of 50 on an ordinal scale disability questionnaire, and whose straight leg raising signs, bilaterally, are limited to 45 degrees. If, after a course of treatment and rehabilitation, the disability score drops to 15 out of 50 and the straight leg raising signs increase to 90 degrees, it is reasonable to say that an increase of 100% has occurred. Because the disability scale uses ordinal data, however, we are advised to conclude that a substantial decrease in score has occurred, but not one that really represents 50% less disability.

RATIO SCALES

The latter aspect is the feature of scales known as ratio scales, where data are continuous and ratios can be formed such that 20 degrees of angle is, indeed, twice as much as 10 degrees. When measuring the angle of the straight leg raising test, the angular scale from 0 degrees to (typically) 90 to 100 degrees is used. This scale allows the observer to make true comparisons between measured results of a test under a variety of conditions.

ATTRIBUTES OF OUTCOMES ASSESSMENT

RELIABILITY

Reliability may be defined most technically as the degree to which random error in a test is reduced. What this really means is that reliability is characterized by the *degree of consistency* in the results obtained with repeated testing (when in fact the results really *have not* changed). The data obtained from only one application of a test can reflect results from anywhere in the typical range of the test. With repeated applications of the test, the variability of the test narrows. In fact, in classic measurement theory, the reliability of a statistic increases in proportion to the square root of the number of additional data (or test applications). As an example, the mean of 16 data points is four times more reliable than that of a single data point.

Test–Retest Reliability

Test–retest reliability measures stability over time in repeated applications of the test. Some assumptions must be made when considering this form of reliability. In determining if the test itself is a source of error, all other factors that can contribute to variability in the test result must remain constant and controlled. It is generally assumed that the attribute being measured is remaining unchanged over the time interval during which the test–retest is performed—an assumption that cannot always be defended. In clinical settings, the natural history of the condition under investigation is variable. Changes in the course of the condition will naturally introduce variability with repeated applications of the test, making it difficult to determine the reliability of the test itself.

Typically, at least two applications of the test are made in an interval of time that is suitable for the natural history of the condition itself (typically within hours to 1 or 2 days—sometimes even 1 or 2 weeks). The agreement between these two tests is calculated using some form of reliability statistic, such as the **kappa index of concordance (k) or the intraclass correlation coefficient (ICC).** Acceptable levels of reliability typically range from .70 to 1.00, whereby "1.00" indicates perfect agreement. The term *"intra-examiner reliability"* refers to a specific type of test–retest reliability, which **quantifies the degree of consistency of one human examiner with himself or herself.** It should be noted, however, that the actual term "test–retest reliability" is usually used in connection with self-report questionnaires that measure such constructs as pain, disability, and other outcomes.

Internal Consistency

Another important aspect of the reliability of scales such as questionnaires for pain, disability, and health status is **"internal consistency."** This term refers to the degree to which answers to individual items in a questionnaire are correlated with the total score or with each of the other items. This correlation indicates: (1) the degree to which the items measure the same (Vogt, 1993) or related constructs; and (2) the degree to which the item response anchors and the item wording are aligned in a consistent direction.

The **reliability coefficient,** which depicts the degree of internal consistency, should be approximately .60 to .85. For example, **Cronbach's alpha** (Cronback, 1951) is used for ordinal data; the **Kuder-Richardson tests** are used for binary data. When this coefficient is higher than .85, it may be indicative of item redundancy (Norman and Streiner, 1991).

Inter-examiner Reliability

Another important type of reliability is the consistency of findings *between* different raters (inter-examiner reliability). Depending on the type of data comprising the outcome measure, reliability statistics, such as the **ICC** or the **k Index,** can be used to quantify the strength of the agreement between examiners. As previously stated, acceptable levels of reliability typically range from .70 to 1.00, whereby "1.00" indicates perfect agreement. Tables 2–2 and 2–3 list numerous attributes of measures that are important when discussing the use of outcomes assessment.

VALIDITY

The concept of validity pertains to the accuracy of any outcome measure test, or the degree to which it truly measures the attribute under investigation. McDowell and Newell (1996) propose a somewhat broader definition of validity to include the context in which the measurement occurs, "the range of interpretations that may be placed upon the test"; that is, what do the results mean? This definition also has the advantage of connecting results (data) of the outcome measure/diagnostic test to the theoretical constructs underlying the measurement's use. In this way, data plus meaning becomes something useful; that is, *information.* There are several forms of validity (Vernon, 1996).

Face Validity

Face validity, or content validity, refers to the degree to which a measurement fits with accepted theory (ie, an accepted "theoretical construct"). As an example, lift strength testing has a high degree of construct validity when used in assessing an injured worker with low back pain whose job involves significant manual handling and carrying. Assessing small differences in the length of the legs in such a worker has poor construct validity given that no evidence suggests that a small leg length difference equates with work impairment.

Content Validity

Content validity refers to the degree to which the measurement tool (typically a questionnaire) includes all items that are relevant and useful to measure. More specifically, each question of a questionnaire is weighted for the construct being measured and some questions are

---

> ### CLINICAL TIP 2–2
> ### Biovariability
>
> A good example of the biovariability that results in difficulty in obtaining consistent and, therefore, reliable data, is range of motion (ROM) mensuration. For example, when attempting to measure lumbar ROM, diurnal differences, subject position, instrument error, test administrator error, human-device error, and others compete with the objective of obtaining reliable results (refer to Chapter 14 for a more complete discussion of this topic). Because inherent problems associated with biovariability exist, HCPs must first recognize the existence of these problems, and the resulting "imperfections" that occur with objective clinical testing. Second, HCPs must accept these inadequacies and, as a result, follow strict protocol when performing physical tests such as range of motion.

Table 2–2: Attributes to Look for in Diagnostic Tests in Clinical Rehabilitation

---

Acceptable Reliability (ICC, k ≥ .70)
  Test–retest or intra-examiner reliability
  Inter-examiner reliability
Acceptable Validity
  Face validity
  Construct validity
  Concurrent validity (ICC, k ≥ .7)
            or
  Convergent validity (r_p, r_s, r_c ≥ .7)
  Discriminant validity
    Sensitivity
    Specificity
    Positive predictive value
    Negative predictive value
    Likelihood ratio
Feasibility
  Implementation time
  Availability
  Assessor skills required
  Costs
Acceptability to Patients

ICC, intraclass correlation coefficient; r_c, "C" coefficient for frequency counts; r_p, Pearson's rho; r_s, Spearman's rho.

weighted more heavily than others are. A question regarding neck pain in a low back questionnaire has no place in the instrument or, has poor content validity.

Convergent Validity

One way of determining the validity of a measurement is to correlate it with another measurement that is different, but related, and performed at the same time. In some cases, different measurements have been designed to measure the same attributes. For example, a VAS for pain intensity can be validated by comparison to a verbal rating scale for pain intensity. In this context, relatively higher correlations are expected between tests of the same attribute. On the other hand, a measurement of one attribute can be correlated with a measurement of another attribute that is related, at least theoretically if not empirically; for example, reduction in levels of activities of daily living with levels of pain severity. In such a circumstance, the levels of expected correlation are usually lower than when the same attributes are compared.

Concurrent/Criterion Validity

This form of validity is particularly robust in that it **compares one measurement with the best alternative available at the time—known as the "gold standard."** If the

new measurement is acceptably similar, then it can be said to have good criterion validity.

Discriminant Validity

A measurement with good discriminant validity has the ability to correctly discriminate the findings into categories such as "normal or abnormal," "positive or negative," "symptomatic or asymptomatic." This may be useful in screening procedures or in categorizing patients as either recovered or not. Sensitivity and specificity (with regard to diagnostic tests), are a form of discriminant validity for diagnostic tests. *Sensitivity* is the attribute of a test whereby a positive test result is highly correlated with the true diseased or abnormal state; that is, a high true positive rate with a low false-negative rate. In short, a sensitive diagnostic test is very good at detecting the disorder when it is in fact present in the patient. *Specificity* is the opposite, wherein test negatives equate highly with true negatives (with low false positives) (Vernon, 1996). In short, a diagnostic test with good specificity is very good at detecting "when the disorder is *not* present" in the patient.

RESPONSIVENESS

Responsiveness involves the performance of an outcome measurement over time and is (1) the ability of the outcome measure instrument to detect clinically important changes (Bolton, 1997; Bolton and Fish, 1997), and (2) the sensitivity of the instrument to real change. In other words, an outcome measurement with good responsiveness will accurately measure the amount of change in a condition when such change truly occurs. In the development of the Neck Disability Index (NDI) (Vernon and Mior, 1991), we studied ten subjects with neck pain who had undergone chiropractic treatment for 3 or 4 weeks. All ten individuals reported improvement. They were asked to complete two instruments—the NDI and a visual analogue pain scale (VAS)—at the beginning of treatment and again at the end of the treatment period. We correlated the change in VAS scores (as a percentage) with the change in the NDI scores. The average change in VAS scores was approximately 75% whereas the change in NDI scores averaged only about 50%. These outcome measures correlated at r_p = .62, which is a relatively good level of correlation. Which test result reflected the true level of improvement? Which was the more responsive? There are several ways to measure and describe the responsiveness of outcome measures, remembering that the magnitude of change and the reliability of measuring that change (in a clinical setting) are the key issues.

Percentage Change

The simplest method of evaluating responsiveness is to express the mean change score as a percentage of the baseline score. If a patient (or a group of subjects) had an initial score (or a mean score) on a pain VAS of 8/10 and, after a treatment program, the score reduced to 4/10, then the change score would be 50%. Unfortunately, such stan-

Table 2–3: Attributes to Look for in Prescriptive Outcome Measures[a] in Clinical Rehabilitation

Acceptable Reliability

  Test–retest/intra-examiner reliability (ICC, k ≥ .070)

  Inter-examiner reliability (ICC, k ≥ .07)

  For questionnaires: Internal consistency (Cronbach's alpha = .60–.85)

Acceptable Validity

  Face validity

  Construct validity

  Convergent validity (r_p, r_s, r_c ≥ .7)
    or (better yet)

  Concurrent validity (ICC, k ≥ .70)

  Discriminant validity

  Responsiveness/sensitivity to real change

  Predictive validity

  For questionnaires: Comprehension/ambiguity testing (accurate paraphrasing of the items)

Feasibility

  Implementation time

  Availability of the instrument

  Assessor skills required

  Costs

Acceptability to Patients/Patient Compliance

ICC, intraclass correlation coefficient; r_c, "C" coefficient for frequency counts; r_p, Pearson's rho; r_s, Spearman's rho.
[a] Measures for assessing effect/change in response to a clinical intervention.

dardization (to a percent scale) is not sensitive to low initial scores, so that a change from 2/10 to 1/10 would still be a 50% improvement, but would only involve one unit on the VAS scale (ie, one out of ten, or 10%). This makes it difficult to compare change across the full spectrum of the scale. On the other hand, most people (including HCPs and patients) intuitively understand the percentage scale, so it is helpful to measure change in that way. In our work on the NDI, pain scores improved by an average of 71%, while disability scores improved by only 57%. Which value represented the true level of change? Which value gives the best depiction of change?

T-test and ANOVA

In group studies, the baseline data can be compared to the post-treatment data using a t-test. If the average baseline Oswestry Questionnaire score of a group of low back pain patients was 20 ± 4 (this is the standard deviation) and after treatment it was 18 ± 4, then a t-test would determine that this difference was not statistically significant. If the scores dropped to 10 ± 4, then the t-test would be significant. The value of the t-statistic can be used as a measure of the magnitude of change or as a ratio between "signal" and "noise" in the test. **The t-value must be greater than 1.00 in order for the magnitude of the change (the signal) to be meaningfully greater than the standard deviation (the noise).**

With more than one measurement interval, such as with a second post-treatment measurement, **an even stronger test of differences (ie, a measure of the magnitude of change) would be to conduct an analysis of variance (ANOVA).** Hsieh et al (1992) did just that in comparing the Oswestry Questionnaire to the Roland-Morris Questionnaire (RMQ) (Roland and Morris, 1983) and found that, in their sample of low back pain patients, the RMQ was more sensitive or responsive to change.

Effect Size

This measure is a standardized means of determining the magnitude of change in outcome measures (Guyatt et al, 1987; Bolton, 1997; Bolton and Fish, 1997). One of the formulas for calculating effect sizes involves subtracting the mean value at post-treatment (post-Tx) from the mean value at baseline (pre-Tx) and dividing that figure by the pooled standard deviation (SD), as shown here:

$$\frac{\text{Mean pre-Tx} - \text{Mean post-Tx}}{\text{Pooled SD}}$$

This measure is then calculated in standard deviation units against the original mean. **Effect sizes of .1 to .4 are small, .5 to .7 medium, and above .8 are large.** In most studies of the benefit of spinal manipulation for low back pain, the "effect sizes" have been in the medium range.

Correlation Analysis

The change in scores of one outcome measure can be compared or correlated with those of another measure,

typically a "gold standard" measure. In our study of the NDI, we correlated NDI change scores with pain VAS improvement scores, with an r = .62 (Vernon and Mior, 1991). This was highly significant, indicating a strong trend in NDI scores toward measuring improvement.

Minimal Clinically Important Difference

Several investigators have drawn attention to the issue of how much change is clinically important in the first place (ie, meaningful to the patient, and possibly to researchers and health policy analysts). Through some sophisticated statistics, Stratford et al (1996) have determined that the minimally clinically important difference (MCID) of the RMQ is about 4 points (out of 24 or about 17%). **Any change of less than 4 points is both too small to matter and too small to be reliable.** Do not forget that there is an error factor in every measurement and reliability is a measure of the random error. **The lower the error factor, the higher the reliability.** Scores below 3/24 are within the typical error margin of low back pain sufferers completing a RMQ, and changes this small are too unreliable to accept as valid.

Conclusion

This chapter has provided a number of basic parameters concerning the nature of outcome measures in clinical practice with an emphasis in neuromusculoskeletal category. First, the measurement scales of such instruments were reviewed, followed by the properties of reliability and validity. Finally, since outcome measures are fundamentally used to measure clinical change (improvement, we hope!), the issue of responsiveness was reviewed in greater depth. The reader is urged to give all these issues due consideration when selecting the appropriate outcome measures in the clinical setting.

REFERENCES

Alaranta H, Hurri H, Heliovaara M, Soukka A, Harju R. Non-dynamometric trunk performance tests: Reliability and normative data. *Scand J Rehab Med.* 1994;26:211–215.

Bolton JE. On the responsiveness of evaluative measures. *Eur J Chiro.* 1997;45:5–8.

Bolton JE, Fish RG. Responsiveness of the Revised Oswestry Disability Questionnaire. *Eur J Chiro.* 1997;4:9–14.

Burton AK, Tillotson KM, Main CJ, Hollis S. Psychosocial predictors of outcome in acute and subacute low back trouble. *Spine.* 1995;20:722–728.

Cronbach LJ. Coefficient alpha and the internal structure of tests. *Psychometrika.* 1951;16:297–340.

Deyo RA, Diehl AK. Measuring physical and psychosocial function in patients with low-back pain. *Spine.* 1983;8:635–642.

Fairbank JC, Park WM, McCall IW, O'Brien JP. Apophyseal injection of local anesthetic as a diagnostic aid in primary low-back pain syndromes. *Spine.* 1981;6(6):598–605.

Gronblad M, Hurri H, Kouri J-P. Relationships between spinal mobility, physical performance tests, pain intensity and disability assessments in chronic low back pain patients. *Scand J Rehab Med.* 1997;19:17–24.

Guyatt G, Walter S, Norman G. Measuring change over time: Assessing the usefulness of evaluative instruments. *J Chron Dis.* 1987;40:171–178.

Hsieh C-Y, Phillips RB, Adams AH, Pope MH. Functional outcomes of low back pain: Comparison of four treatment groups in a randomized clinical trial. *J Manipulative Physiol Ther.* 1992;15:4–9.

McDowell I, Newell C. *Measuring Health: A Guide to Rating Scales and Questionnaires.* New York, NY: Oxford Press; 1996.

Norman G, Streiner D. *Health Measurement Scales: A Practical Guide to Their Development and Use.* New York, NY: Oxford Press; 1991.

Roland M, Morris R. A study of the natural history of back pain. Part 1: Development of a reliable and sensitive measure of disability in low-back pain. *Spine.* 1983;2:141–144.

Stratford PW, Finch E, Solomon P, Binkley J, Gill C, Moreland J. Using the Roland-Morris Questionnaire to make decisions about individual patients. *Physiother Can.* 1996;48:107–110.

Triano JJ, Schultz AB. Correlation of objective trunk motion and muscle function with low-back disability ratings. *Spine.* 1987;12:561–565.

Vernon HT. Applying research-based assessments of pain and loss of function to the issue of developing standards of care in chiropractic. *Chiro Tech.* 1990;2:121–126.

Vernon HT. Pain and disability questionnaires in chiropractic rehabilitation. In: Liebenson C, ed. *Rehabilitation of the Spine: A Practitioner's Manual.* Baltimore, Md.: Williams & Wilkins; 1996:57–72.

Vernon HT, Mior S. The Neck Disability Index: A study of reliability and validity. *J Manipulative Physiol Ther.* 1991;14:409–415.

Vogt WP. *Dictionary of Statistics and Methodology.* Newbury: Sage Publications; 1993.

Waddell G, Main CJ, Morris EW, DiPaolo M, Gray ICM. Chronic low-back pain, psychological distress and illness behavior. *Spine.* 1984;9:209–213.

Waddell G, Newton M, Henderson I, Somerville D, Main CJ. A Fear-Avoidance Beliefs Questionnaire (FABQ) and the role of fear-avoidance beliefs in chronic low back pain and disability. *Pain.* 1993;52:157–168.

Yeomans SG, Liebenson C. Quantitative functional capacity evaluation: The missing link in outcomes assessment. *Top Clin Chiro.* 1996;3:32–43.

CHAPTER 3

Subjective versus Objective, Qualitative versus Quantitative Tests, and Provocative Tests: What Does It All Mean?

STEVEN G. YEOMANS

INTRODUCTION

The field of testing protocols has advanced greatly over the past decade. For years, there was very little reliance on testing protocols that utilized "subjective" criteria, or criteria that were patient-driven. In addition, many standard "objective" provocative tests were not considered reliable if a verbal response from the patient was required. As a result, few tests—with the exceptions of electromyography/nerve conduction velocity (EMG/NCV), radiology, and the like—met this rigid criterion of objectivity. This concept of omitting the use of subjective data was further reinforced by insurance companies, reimbursement review companies and claims reviewers. Until recently, this trend has been the standard. However, with the increase in research utilizing subjective information gathered by patient-driven, self-administered forms and questionnaires, the measurement of outcomes has gained a new level of respect (Their, 1992). In addition, the use of reliable, valid, safe, and practical functional tests is becoming popular, and is redefining the objective standards. More tests are also being found to carry criteria that define them as "good" tests (see Chap. 2) (Yeomans and Liebenson, 1996).

As managed care becomes increasingly more popular, more and more pressure is being placed on the health care provider (HCP) to prove outcomes. Hence, the outcomes-based management approach is beginning to gain the attention of those who are on the cutting edge of case management and record keeping trends. This evolution has been further catalyzed by the pressures felt by managed care companies to meet or exceed the minimum standards dictated by government or accrediting agencies such as the National Commission for Quality Assurance

(NCQA). As a result, independent provider associations (IPAs), preferred provider organizations (PPOs), and health maintenance organizations (HMOs) are beginning to require the use of the various outcome assessment methods available to capture outcomes.

Due to the numerous additional pressures that are now placed on the HCP in the managed care setting, many HCPs may feel that they are being forced to do twice as much for half the reimbursement. This issue has been at the heart of many heated debates between HCPs and third-party payer administrators. It is now even more important for the outcomes-based HCP to not waste time doing the "soft," less informative tests, but rather to concentrate on the "hard," more clinically useful information. Since many of the recognized methods of tracking outcomes are based on patient-driven information (subjective), they are ideal in the managed care environment where HCPs are constantly in search of methods to trim back services but not quality. Because many of these outcomes assessment methods are "patient-driven," the HCP is left free to care for others while the patient gathers and reports his or her own information. The HCP can then review the information, compare the data to the same forms completed in the past, and formulate a rational clinical decision based on the results, rather than relying on gut instinct, or some other method.

DEFINITION OF TERMS

The terms "subjective" and "objective," "qualitative" and "quantitative," and "provocative" must be defined in order to be fully appreciated.

SUBJECTIVE

The term **"subjective"** is defined as: "of or resulting from the feelings of the person thinking; not objective; personal" (*Webster's*, 1990). A thesaurus provides a list of synonyms that illustrate the negative connotation that is associated with the term (Table 3–1). However, without a subjective description of a patient's complaint, an HCP would have a difficult time determining what aspects of physical examination should be applied to that patient. Moreover, as Deyo noted, when comparing the reliability of subjective (history) to objective (physical examination) data in cancer patients, only the historical information was found to be discriminatory in differentiating between healthy subjects and cancer patients (Deyo & Diehl, 1988; Deyo, 1991).

> ### CLINICAL TIP 3–1
> ### Importance of Subjective Information in Diagnosis
>
> The importance of the history or subjective information can be vital in determining a diagnosis, since ruling out "red flags" is the first order of business when applying "triage" to a case (Bigos et al, 1994; Rosen et al, 1994).

OBJECTIVE

The term **"objective"** is defined as: "1. Existing as an object or fact, independent of the mind; real. 2. Concerned with the realities of the thing dealt with rather than the thoughts of the artist, writer, etc. 3. Without bias or prejudice" (Their, 1992). A thesaurus again provides several synonyms that illustrate the positive connotation of these terms and support the reasons why objective items are preferred over subjective items (Table 3–2).

QUALITATIVE

Similarly, **"qualitative"** is defined as: "1. That which makes something what it is; characteristic element. 2. Basic nature; kind. 3. The degree of excellence of a thing" (Their, 1992). Although a thesaurus does not provide synonyms

Table 3–1: Synonyms for the Term "Subjective"

Deceptive
Emotional
Fanciful
Ideal
Illusionary
Imaginary
Misleading
Partial
Unreal

Table 3–2: Synonyms for the Term "Objective"

Detached
Fair
Impartial
Impersonal
Unbiased
Unprejudiced

for this term, it offers synonyms for the term "quality" (Table 3–3). The term "qualitative" implies a positive connotation and, when applied to outcomes, includes instruments or tests that are reliable, but not quantifiable. Therefore, tests that are qualitative can only be compared to the level of function tested at a prior time period if the same test was previously utilized and performed similarly. **A qualitative test can drive a prescription or treatment method if the clinical information gathered relates to functional testing or physical examination.** Therefore, qualitative tests have been—and always will be—considered important in clinical decision making.

QUANTITATIVE

The term **"quantitative"** is defined as: "1. An amount; portion. 2. That property by which a thing can be measured" (Their, 1992). Again, the thesaurus does not provide synonyms for this term, but it lists the following synonyms of "quantity": characteristic, attribute, affection, mark, peculiarity, etc. (Table 3–4). The application of the term "quantitative" to the measurement of outcomes is vital to the ability to measure disability or activity intolerance (through questionnaires) and/or impairment or loss of function (through physical exam). **Because of the ability to quantify the patient's results, a "score" can be obtained at baseline and compared at future reassessment dates.** Therefore, quantitative testing protocols are favored by HCPs over qualitative tests as outcome assessment instruments because a numerical, quantitative result is obtained.

PROVOCATIVE

The term **"provocative"** means: "provoking or tending to provoke; incitement." The root word, "provoke," means "1. To excite to some action or feeling 2. To anger or irritate 3. To stir up (action or feeling) 4. To evoke" (*Webster's*, 1990). The thesaurus reveals synonyms to the term provoke to be as follows: vex, affront, aggravate, anger, annoy, and so forth (Table 3–5). **It is generally considered appropriate to provoke a pain response during the orthopedic exam in order to isolate the tissue involved in the injury.** When doing so, a pain "grade" can be assigned for

use in gathering baseline and follow-up information. This information then becomes the basic elements of outcomes assessment. However, only a few of the standard orthopedic tests include a means of measuring or quantifying the result. In other words, most provocative tests are qualitative.

APPLICATION OF THESE TERMS IN A CLINICAL CONTEXT: THE SOAP NOTE

Documentation of patient-driven data can be accomplished in many different ways. There is one method, however, that appears to be well accepted across the various healing art disciplines. This particular approach uses the acronym SOAP (*s*ubjective, *o*bjective, *a*ssessment, and *p*lan). By using this approach, an HCP, when documenting the patient encounter, is less likely to leave out potentially vital information that might otherwise be forgotten. The "S" of the SOAP note stands for "*subjective*" a term that has typically been applied to the process of gathering a history from the presenting patient. This information is gathered initially to determine the location of complaint, duration of symptoms, mechanism of injury, past and present treatment(s), and the response to the care. **For each current complaint, further historical gathering includes information about onset, factors that provoke and relieve pain and/or symptoms, symptom quality, radiation fea-**

Table 3–4: Synonyms for the Term "Quantity" (Quantitative)

Characteristic
Attribute
Affection
Mark
Peculiarity
Feature
Property
Trait

Table 3–3: Synonyms for the Term "Quality" (Qualitative)

Capability
Character
Essence
Material
Matter
Substance
Stuff

Table 3–5: Synonyms for the Term "Provoke"

Affront
Aggravate
Anger
Annoy
Chafe
Enrage
Exacerbate
Vex

tures, severity levels, and timing issues. In addition, past history, family history, psychosocial history, review of systems, and the determination of risk factors for chronicity are included in the initial clinical evaluation. Pertinent information of the current complaint(s) are then gathered on a visit by visit basis in order to follow progress or the lack thereof. This information is covered in greater detail in Chapters 19, 20, and 22.

Subjective outcomes assessment information is gathered by the patient in self-administered questionnaires and scored by either staff members or by a computer with appropriate software. In spite of the definition and synonyms associated with the term "subjective," these "pen-and-paper tools" have been described as very valid and reliable—in many cases more so than many of the "objective" tests that HCPs have relied upon for years (Chapman-Smith, 1992; Hansen, 1994; Mootz, 1994). Moreover, since it is patients' complaints that ultimately drive them to seek the services of an HCP, it seems only appropriate that they play a large role in setting goals and tracking outcomes. In addition, since the treatment goals generally follow the activity intolerance of a patient, the use of questionnaires is ideal since they can be scored and are, therefore, quantitative. A "score" can be derived at the onset, or baseline, and at periodic intervals over the course of the treatment plan. Because of their scoring capability, subjective tests make excellent prognosticators when trying to determine endpoints of care. Subjective tests comprise the heart of the outcomes-based practice, as critical clinical decision making can be accomplished through this information. These tests or instruments will be categorized and further discussed in Chapter 4 and in Section II of this text, respectively.

The term *"objective"* has traditionally been synonymous with the physical examination, which has been predominantly a "physician-driven" service. Objective information is reported in the "O" portion of the SOAP note and, in general, qualifies and/or quantifies the patient's complaints described in the "S" portion. The objective information has historically been viewed as an essential part of a SOAP note; the absence of this information is the reason for many insurance claim denials. It has been published and accepted by most that periodic re-examinations are needed in order to determine the case management plan of a patient. (Haldeman and Chapman-Smith, 1992) Special tests such as radiology, laboratory findings, and any other high- or low-tech methods of assessment are also reported in the objective portion of the file.

The information gathered in the "S" and the "O" portions of the SOAP note should then logically lead to an as-sessment, or "A," in which the diagnosis in listed. Treatment goals are also defined, including risk factors of chronicity or complicating aspects of a specific case. If desired, a problem list can also be included in this portion of the SOAP note. A comment regarding the status of a patient, such as "improved," "not changed," or "worse," is usually reported in this section on a periodic basis.

The plan (or "P") portion of the SOAP note lists treatment frequency, passive care approaches (such as physical therapies, manipulation, and other therapeutic procedures), test orders, exercise prescriptions, activities of daily living (ADLs) training, ergonomic training, work restrictions, and/or work site modifications, referral or consult orders, discharge summary, and other pertinent information. The point that is most critical is to support the prior information obtained in the S, O, and A portions of the SOAP note with therapeutic protocol, to quantify it as often as possible, and then to apply it so that it becomes "outcomes-based." Specific documentation information will be addressed in Chapter 21 of this text.

Conclusion

The objective of this chapter was to introduce various terms in context with their value in case management. It is often difficult to focus on the forest rather than the trees, especially when information so vitally important to clinical decision making is often degraded, typically by insurers who are disputing a claim. This often is handed down to the HCP with the phrase, "there are no objective findings to support the ongoing subjective complaints." It is vitally important for HCPs, allied health professionals, and third-party payers to understand that subjective data is at least on an equal level of importance as objective findings since the subjective data reflects the patient's disability (activity intolerance) while the objective findings support the presence or absence of impairment (loss of function). Though both are important, the patient-generated history is especially important as it identifies disabilities and these intolerant activities immediately become viable or "real" treatment goals.

The popular SOAP note documentation format was discussed with emphasis made to correlate the information between each item of the S-O-A-P. The use of a designated system such as this provides, in a sense, protection against failing to remember to ask a question. Each complaint receives its own SOAP note and is typically reported in the order of importance.

REFERENCES

Bigos S, Bowyer O, Braen G, et al. Acute low back problems in adults. Clinical practice guideline No. 14. Rockville, Md: Agency for Health Care Policy and Research, Public Health Service, US Department of Health and Human Services; 1994. AHCPR Publication No. 95-0642.

Chapman-Smith D. Measuring results—The new importance of patient questionnaires. *Chiro Report*. 1992; 7(1):1–6.

Deyo RA. Early detection of cancer, infection, and inflammatory disease of the spine. *J Back Musculoskeletal Rehabil*. 1991;1:69–81.

Deyo RA, Diehl AK. Cancer as a cause of back pain: Frequency, clinical presentation, and diagnostic strategies. *J Gen Intern Med*. 1988;3:230–238.

Goertz CMH. Measuring functional health status in the chiropractic office using self-report questionnaires. *Top Clin Chiro*. 1994;1(1):51–59.

Haldeman S, Chapman-Smith D, Petersen D, eds. *Guidelines for Chiropractic Quality Assurance and Practice Parameters*. Gaithersburg, Md: Aspen, 1992.

Hansen DT. Back to basics . . . Determining how much care to give and reporting patient progress. *Top Clin Chiro*. 1994;1(4):1–8.

Mootz RD. Maximizing the effectiveness of clinical documentation. *Top Clin Chiro*. 1994;1(1):60–65.

Rosen M, Breen A, et al. Management guidelines for back pain. Appendix B in: *Report of a Clinical Standards Advisory Group Committee on Back Pain*. London, England: Her Majesty's Stationery Office (HMSO); 1994.

Their SO. Forces motivating the use of health status assessment measures in clinical settings and related clinical research. *Med Care*. 1992;30(5)(suppl):15–22.

Webster's New World Dictionary. 3rd ed. New York, NY: Simon & Schuster; 1990:587.

Yeomans SG, Liebenson C. Quantitative functional capacity evaluation: The missing link to outcomes assessment. *Top Clin Chiro*. 1996;3:32–43.

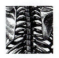

CHAPTER 4

Classification of Outcome Assessment Instruments

STEVEN G. YEOMANS

▶ INTRODUCTION

▶ CLASSIFICATIONS
Subjective Outcome Assessment Tools
Objective Outcome Assessment Tools

▶ CONCLUSION

INTRODUCTION

The number of different varieties of outcome assessment (OA) tools available can make the application of OA instruments confusing, to say the least. To add to the confusion, many OA tools measure the same thing, such as low back pain and/or disability. The health care provider (HCP), therefore, must not only have an understanding of *which* OA tool to use, but also *when* to use it. Before the question of when to apply an OA tool is addressed, each instrument must first be introduced categorically. This presentation will also reduce the difficulty in deciding which tool to utilize.

Classifications of OA tools have been developed to simplify the chore of selecting the instruments to track outcomes. However, since there are often several options of OA tools in each classification, the question of "which tool to use" is not answered completely as only the classification is addressed. In overview, Sections II and III of the text will help you to determine *how* to use each of the many tools described and classified in this chapter. Section IV will address the question of "when to use which tool." Finally, using various tools included in this classification system will prompt you to make somewhat of a paradigm shift. More specifically, after you learn how to employ and interpret the results derived from the tools, outcomes-based clinical decision making and documenting and/or report writing should reflect those decisions. An outcomes-based practice approach is adopted when decision making based on the information gathered from the various OA tools takes place. The chapters in Section V facilitate this last step.

CLASSIFICATIONS

OA tools can be classified into two broad camps: those that are subjective or patient-driven (typically pen-and-paper methods), and those that are objective or HCP-driven (typically through functional tests or physical examination procedures). Table 4–1 summarizes various OA tools into subjective and objective categories. Each is then discussed briefly in the text that follows with reference to later chapters that will address each category in greater detail.

Table 4–1: Classification of Outcome Assessment Tools into Subjective (Patient-driven) or Objective (HCP-driven)

SUBJECTIVE OA TOOLS (PATIENT-DRIVEN) (COMPRISED OF PEN-AND-PAPER TOOLS)	OBJECTIVE OA TOOLS (HCP-DRIVEN) (COMPRISED OF FUNCTIONAL TESTS)
General Health	Flexibility and Range of Motion
Pain Perception	Strength and Endurance
Condition- or Disease-Specific	Nonorganic
Psychometric	Proprioception
Disability Prediction	Cardiopulmonary
Patient Satisfaction	Developmental (pediatric–adolescent)

SUBJECTIVE OUTCOME ASSESSMENT TOOLS

It must be emphasized that although the term "subjective" carries negative connotations (see Chap. 3), the reliability/validity data published regarding these methods of collecting outcomes is exceptional, typically out-performing the test–retest reliability and validity of most physical performance tests (which are "objective") (Chapman-Smith, 1992). Also, as stated earlier, **there is little information that is more important than gaining an insight into a patient's activity intolerance, pain level, general health status, and psychometric barriers to recovery, all of which can be gathered by "subjective" methods.** This discussion is not meant to minimize the importance of objective outcomes tracking, but rather, it is meant to erase the misconception that is still present regarding the importance of tracking outcomes through subjective measures.

General Health Outcome Assessment Tools

The first group of OA tools under the subjective category are those described as **"general health."** The fact that this group of OA tools is *general,* is both its strength as well as its weakness (Deyo et al, 1990). More specifically, **its strength rests in the fact that this group of tools can be used for all patients, regardless of their ailment.** This is because these tools encompass quality of life issues and, therefore, can be applied to individuals with an ingrown toenail or gastritis, as the score of the instrument will generally parallel the individual's level of disability. For example, if the subject is nonambulatory because of a badly infected ingrown toenail, aspects of general health instruments will reflect the degree of the disability. Since no condition-specific questionnaire exists that isolates the disabilities associated with an ingrown toenail, the collection of general health information can be looked at as a universally practical OA measure. However, **its weakness also rests in the fact that this type of tool is not condition- or disease-specific, as other co-existing problems or conditions may "cloud" the ingrown toenail results.** It is, therefore, appropriate, when available, to combine the general health tool with a specific outcomes measure such

as a pain scale, balance test (one leg balance test and/or Berg Balance Scale), or some other measure with which to compare and contrast. It is not the intent to discuss in detail, at this point in the text, the different tools that belong to this category. Instead, Table 4–2 presents examples of some of the tools worth considering in the general health category. Refer to Chapter 5 for more detailed discussion of this category of outcome tools.

Pain Perception Outcome Assessment Tools

The second group of subjective OA tools is that of the *pain perception* group. There are many different ways to track pain through the use of outcome tools, of which four methods are listed in Table 4–3. These are discussed in greater detail in Chapter 6.

Condition-specific Outcome Assessment Tools

The third group of subjective outcome assessment tools is the **condition-** or **disease-specific** group. These tests can be broken down into spinal and nonspinal subcategories. Spinal condition-specific instruments are listed in Table 4–4 and the nonspinal instruments in Table 4–5, although, again, these lists are not all-inclusive. Refer to Chapter 7 for a more detailed description of several of these tests. In addition, Chapter 15 includes many upper and lower extremity-related subjective OA tools.

Psychometric Outcome Assessment Tools

The fourth group in the subjective OA instrument category is the *psychometric* group. Various tools included in this group are listed in Table 4–6. Refer to Chapter 9 for a more detailed discussion of this subject.

Disability Prediction Outcome Assessment Tools

The fifth group in this subjective classification approach is the **disability prediction** group (Table 4–7). Disability prediction questionnaires can help predict those patients who may prove "difficult to manage" due to chronic pain, work dissatisfaction, fear avoidance, or combinations thereof. Various authors have presented different perspectives of this topic (Millard, 1989; Bigos et al, 1991; Cats-Baril and Frymoyer, 1991; Waddell et al, 1993; Hazard et al, 1996; and others). Refer to Chapters 9, 10, and 21 for a more detailed discussion of this subject.

Table 4–2: Selected General Health Information Tools

TEST	CONDITIONS TESTED
Health Status Questionnaire (HSQ 2.0) (also called SF-36,[a] Rand-36, MOS-36) (Deyo et al, 1991; Brazier et al, 1992; Goertz, 1994)	Eight scales relating to general health
Dartmouth COOP Health Charts[b] (Nelson et al, 1990; Goertz, 1994)	Nine general health issues are collected using both verbal as well as pictured charts
Sickness Index Profile (SIP) (Bergner et al, 1981)	Used primarily in research due to its length and complexity
Quality of Well-Being Scale (Kaplan and Anderson, 1982)	Used in research for similar reasons as SIP

[a] Available: (SF-36) Health Outcomes Trust, 20 Park Plaza, Suite 1014, Boston, MA 02116. For order form: (617) 426-4046 (fax: -4131)
[b] Available: (Dartmouth COOP Health Charts) Deborah Johnson; Dartmouth COOP Project; Dartmouth Medical School; Hanover, NH 03755-3862; 603/650-1974. (Copyright 1989).

Patient Satisfaction Outcome Assessment Tools

A sixth category is that of **patient satisfaction,** which is frequently used as an important outcomes assessment approach, especially by managed care companies when assessing quality assurance issues (Ware et al, 1978; Deyo, 1986). Table 4–8 lists some of the available patient satisfaction questionnaires. These instruments yield important information about the quality of the health care service as perceived by the patient by assessing the following (Cherkin and MacCormack, 1989; Ware et al, 1992; Ware and Davies, 1983; Coulter et al, 1994):

- Acceptance of care
- Perception of the technical competence of the HCP
- The setting where care was provided
- The effectiveness of the HCP

Refer to Chapter 9 for a more detailed discussion regarding the clinical utilization of patient satisfaction questionnaires.

OBJECTIVE OUTCOME ASSESSMENT TOOLS

This category is comprised of physical performance tests that satisfy the criteria described in Chapter 2, and include normative data. The normative data can then be compared to the patient's test results and a percentage of normal calculated and tracked. In doing so, the outcomes of treatment can be assessed pretreatment, during treatment, and following treatment. Six categories are listed with respect to the physical performance tests. These include:

1. Flexibility and range of motion
2. Strength and endurance
3. Nonorganic/Psychometric
4. Proprioception
5. Cardiopulmonary
6. Developmental (pediatrics)

With respect to the first four categories, there are eight tests in the flexibility and range of motion category, five

Table 4–3: Selected Pain Perception Tools

TEST	CONDITIONS TESTED
Visual Analogue Scale (Dixon et al, 1981; Dworkin et al, 1990; Chapman-Smith, 1992; Von Korff et al, 1992, 1993)	Pain arising from any condition
Numerical Pain Scale (Downie et al, 1978; McDowell and Newell, 1987; Chapman-Smith, 1992)	Pain arising from any condition
McGill Pain Scale (Melzack, 1975, 1982)	Pain arising from any condition
Pain Drawing (Ransford et al, 1976; Kirkaldy-Willis, 1983; Parker et al, 1995; Ohlund et al, 1996)	Pain arising from any condition

Table 4–4: Selected Spine-related Condition-specific Questionnaires

TEST	CONDITIONS TESTED
Oswestry Low Back Pain Disability Questionnaire (original and revised) (Fairbanks et al, 1980; Hudson-Cook and Tomes-Nicholson, 1988)	Low back pain (LBP): acute, subacute, chronic
Roland-Morris Questionnaire (Roland and Morris, 1983; Deyo, 1986)	LBP: acute, subacute, chronic
NASS (North American Spine Society) (Daltroy et al, 1996)	LBP: acute, subacute, chronic
Low Back Pain TyPE (Technology of Patient Experience specification) (Deyo et al, 1992)[a]	LBP: acute, subacute, chronic
Dallas Pain Questionnaire (Lawlis et al, 1989)	LBP: acute, subacute, chronic
Low Back Outcome Score (Ruta et al, 1994)	LBP: acute, subacute, chronic
Quebec Back Pain Disability Scale (Kopec et al, 1995)	LBP: acute, subacute, chronic
Neck Disability Index (NDI) (Vernon and Mior, 1991)	Neck: acute, subacute, chronic
Headache Disability Index (HDI) (Jacobson et al, 1994)	Headaches
Dizziness Handicap Inventory (Jacobson and Newman, 1990)	Dizziness
Tinnitus Handicap Inventory (Newman et al, 1996)	Tinnitus auris
Hearing Handicap Inventory for Adults (Newman et al, 1990)	Hearing
TMD Disability Index (Steigerwald and Maher, 1997)	Temporomandibular dysfunction

LBP, low back pain.
[a] Personal correspondence: (No scoring method intended) reply letter 2-10-95.

Table 4–5: Selected Nonspinal or Extremity Condition-specific Instruments

TEST	CONDITIONS TESTED
Shoulder Self-Assessment of Function (Hawkins and Dunlap, 1995)	Shoulder pain and dysfunction
American Shoulder and Elbow Surgeons Shoulder Evaluation Form (Barrett et al, 1987)	Shoulder pain and dysfunction
Upper Extremity Pain Questionnaire (Feuerstein, 1995)	Any upper extremity joint dysfunction
CTS Questionnaire (Levine et al, 1993)	Carpal tunnel syndrome
Knee: Functional Index Questionnaire (FIQ) (Harrison et al, 1995)	Patellofemoral knee pain/dysfunction
Condition Specific TyPEs (Technology of Patient Experience specification) (Deyo et al, 1992)	CTS, asthma, COPD, depression, hypertension, osteoarthritis, rheumatoid arthritis, allergic rhinitis, smoking cessation

COPD, chronic obstructive pulmonary disease; CTS, carpal tunnel syndrome.

Table 4–6: Selected Psychometric Instruments

TEST	CONDITIONS TESTED
Health Status Questionnaire (last three questions and the mental health scale) (Deyo et al, 1991; Brazier et al, 1992; Goertz, 1994)	Depression
SCL-90-R (Bernstein et al, 1994)	Anxiety and depression (two scales)
Modified Zung Depression Index (Zung, 1965)	Depression
Modified Somatic Perception Questionnaire (MSPQ) (Main, 1983)	Perceived depression
Beck's Depression Inventory (Beck, 1967)	Depression
Waddell's Non-organic LBP Signs (Waddell et al, 1980)[a]	Nonorganic LBP
Somatic Amplification Rating Scale (SARS) (Korbon et al, 1987)[a]	Nonorganic LBP
Fear Avoidance Beliefs Questionnaire (FABQ) (Waddell et al, 1993)	Chronic pain behavior/fear avoidance behavior
Distress and Risk Assessment Method (DRAM) (Main et al, 1992)	Depression, anxiety

LBP, low back pain; SCL, symptom checklist.
[a] Tests that are "objective," as they are provider driven.

Table 4–7: Selected Disability Prediction Instruments

TEST	CONDITIONS TESTED
Vermont Disability Prediction Questionnaire (Cats-Baril and Frymoyer, 1991; Hazard et al, 1996)	Disability predictive
Work APGAR (Bigos et al, 1991)	Disability predictive
Fear Avoidance Beliefs Questionnaire (FABQ) (Wadell et al, 1993)	Chronic pain behavior, fear avoidance behavior
Functional Assessment Screen Questionnaire (FASQ) (Millard, 1989)	Disability associated with chronic pain

Table 4–8: Selected Patient Satisfaction Questionnaires

TEST	CONDITIONS TESTED
Client Experience Survey	Patient satisfaction
Client Satisfaction Questionnaire	Patient satisfaction
Patient Experience Survey (PES)	Patient satisfaction
Chiropractic Satisfaction Questionnaire (Coulter et al, 1994)	Patient satisfaction

tests in the strength and endurance category, five signs and eight tests in the nonorganic category, and one test in the proprioception category, as noted in Table 4–9. These tests, when combined, make up the Quantitative Functional Capacity Evaluation (QFCE). Refer to Chapter 16 for a more detailed summary of physical performance testing.

There are several different methods of classifying outcomes measures (Chapman-Smith, 1992; Cole et al, 1995). Basmajian, for example, segregated outcome measures into four main groupings based on the following (Cole et al, 1995):

1. Adult motor and functional activity measures (21 tests)
2. Back and/or pain measures (14 tests)
3. Cardiopulmonary measures (13 tests)
4. Developmental measures (12 tests)

The first category, the adult motor and functional activity measures (21 tests), is primarily for patients who have suffered upper motor neuron (UMN) disease such as a cerebrovascular accident (CVA) or stroke. Some of the tests, however, may be applicable to a more general population. For example, the Timed "Up and Go" test was designed to be applied to the frail elderly population affected by stroke, Parkinson's disease, rheumatoid arthritis, osteoarthritis, multiple sclerosis (MS), hip fracture, cerebellar disease, and general deconditioning (Podsiadlo and Richardson, 1991). Another example is the Modified Sphyg test, which was designed for measuring isometric muscle strength and is useful in both UMN and lower motor neuron (LMN) disease (Helewa et al, 1981). Table 4–10 lists the adult motor and functional activity measures along with the sources and a corresponding list of the conditions tested by each tool (Cole et al, 1995). Although some overlap exists with the classification system previously discussed, tests that make up the second category, back and/or pain measures, are presented in Table 4–11.

The third category, cardiopulmonary measures, include the tests that assess heart and lung function. A sample of these tests is described in Table 4–12. Refer to Chapter 18 for a more detailed discussion regarding the clinical application of cardiovascular and aerobic testing.

The fourth and last category, described as developmental measures, includes tests in which many are applicable to the pediatric patient. Several of the instruments are aimed at older child populations; for example, the Test of Motor Impairment is for children with an intelligence quotient (IQ) greater than 50, aged 5 to 14 years. The Basic Gross Motor Assessment (BGMA) is another example with population recommendations to include children with mild motor dysfunction, aged 5.5 to 12.5 years. A sample of these tests is found in Table 4–13.

Table 4–9: Physical Performance Tests

STRENGTH AND ENDURANCE TESTS

Repetitive Squat
(Alaranta et al, 1994)

Repetitive Sit-up
(Alaranta et al, 1994)

Repetitive Arch-up
(Alaranta et al, 1994)

Static Back Endurance
(Alaranta et al, 1994)

Grip Strength
(Swanson et al, 1970)

PSYCHOSOCIAL TESTS

Waddell Non-organic LBP Test (five signs/eight tests)
(Waddell et al, 1980)
- Superficial/deep pain
- Simulation
- Distraction
- Sensory/motor
- Exaggeration

FLEXIBILITY AND RANGE OF MOTION TESTS

Lumbar Spine Inclinometer Examination
(Mayer et al, 1994)

Cervical Spine Inclinometer Examination
(Mayer et al, 1994)

Gastrocnemius/Ankle Dorsiflexion Test
(Ekstrand, 1993)

Soleus/Ankle Dorsiflexion Test
(Ekstrand, 1982)

Modified Thomas Test (Iliopsoas)
(Ekstrand, 1982)

Straight Leg Raise (Hamstring)
(Ekstrand, 1982)

Knee Flexion Test (Quadriceps femoris)
(Ekstrand, 1982; Wang, 1993)

Hip Rotation (Internal and External)
(Chesworth et al, 1994)

PROPRIOCEPTION TEST

One-Leg Standing Test
(Bly and Sinnot, 1991)

LBP, low back pain.

Table 4–10: Adult Motor and Functional Activity Measures

TEST	CONDITIONS TESTED
Timed "Up and Go" (Podsiadlo et al, 1991)	Frail elderly; UMN, LMN, degenerative conditions
Modified Sphygmomanometer for Measuring Muscle Strength ("Modified Sphyg") (Helewa et al, 1981)	Rheumatoid arthritis, back injured patients
Activity Index (Stott et al, 1972)	Adult stroke (CVA) patients
Motor Assessment Scale (MAS) (Carr et al, 1985)	CVA—adult population
Chedoke-McMaster Stroke Assessment (Gowland et al, 1993)	Stroke (CVA)—adult population
Action Research Arm Test (Carroll, 1965)	Hemiplegia, CVA, cortical surgery, closed head injury
Berg Balance Scale (Berg et al, 1989)	Elderly with CVA, Parkinson's disease, and other balance impairment
Barthel Index (Mahoney and Barthel, 1965)	Adult population—spinal cord; all UMN diagnoses
Functional Independence Measure (FIM) (Granger et al, 1990)	MS, all UMN lesion patients
Fugl-Meyer Assessment of Sensorimotor Recovery after Stroke (Fugl-Meyer, 1980)	Adult stroke (CVA)
Katz Index of Activities of Daily Living (Staff of Benjamin Rose Hospital, 1959)	All adults, children: Hip fractures, CVA, MS, arthritis, malignancy, amputations, spinal cord, and others.
Kenny Self-Care Evaluation (Grodeon et al, 1978)	Adult with any disability (primarily UMN)
Klein-Bell Activities of Daily Living Scale (Klein and Bell, 1982)	Adult with any disability (primarily UMN)
Level of Rehabilitation Scale (LORS-II) (Carey and Posavac, 1980)	Primarily UMN patients
PULSES Profile (Moskowitz and McCann, 1957)	Primarily UMN patients
Rivermead Motor Assessment (RMA) (Lincoln and Ledbitter, 1979)	Stroke (CVA)
Rivermead ADL Assessment (Whiting and Lincoln, 1980)	ADL in stroke patients
Functional Autonomy Measurement System (SMAF) (Hegert et al, 1980)	Designed as a global evaluative instrument according to the WHO classification of impairment, disability, and handicap; for the disabled elderly.
Patient Evaluation Conference System (PECS) (Harvey and Jellinek, 1993)	All rehabilitation diagnostic groups (primarily UMN)
Canadian Neurological Scale (CNS) (Cote et al, 1989)	Acute phase of stroke, all ages
Clinical Outcome Variable Scale (COVS) (Harvey and Jellinek, 1993)	Modification of the PECS (see above)

ADL, activities of daily living; CVA, cerebrovascular accident; LMN, lower motor neuron disease; MS, multiple sclerosis; UMN, upper motor neuron; WHO, World Health Organization.

Table 4–11: Back and/or Pain Measures

TEST	CONDITIONS TESTED
Visual Analogue Scale (Dixon and Bird, 1981)	Back pain, cancer, rheumatoid arthritis, chronic pain
Numerical Pain Scale (Jensen et al, 1986)	LBP, rheumatoid arthritis, cancer
Pain Drawing (Ransford et al, 1976)	Acute and chronic LBP
Sickness Impact Profile (SIP) (Bergner et al, 1981)	LBP
Roland-Morris Disability Questionnaire (Roland and Morris, 1983a, 1983b)	LBP
Oswestry Low Back Pain Disability Questionnaire (Fairbanks et al, 1980)	Normal population with LBP
Partial Sit-up/Curl-up as a Test of Abdominal Muscle Strength/Endurance (Faulkner et al, 1989)	Normal population with LBP
Sorensen Test for Endurance of the Back Musculature (Biering-Sorensen, 1984)	Normal population with LBP
Pressure Biofeedback (PBF) for Measuring Muscular Endurance of the Transverse Abdominal and Abdominal Oblique Musculature (Jull and Richardson, 1992)	Normal population with LBP
Modified Schober Method of Measuring Spinal Mobility (Macrae and Wright, 1969)	Chronic LBP, ankylosing spondylitis, other arthritides
Leighton Flexometer for Measuring Spinal Mobility (Leighton, 1958)	Normal population and high-performance athletes
Inclinometer Method of Measuring Spinal Mobility (Loebl, 1967)	LBP, ankylosing spondylitis, rheumatoid arthritis
Lifting Dynamometers (Mayer and Gatchel, 1988)	Normal population with LBP
Isokinetic Dynamometers (Hasue et al, 1980)	Normal population with LBP

Table 4–12: Cardiopulmonary Measures

TEST	CONDITIONS TESTED
Heart Rate (Hurst et al, 1990)	Adults, children: normals and patients
Blood Pressure (Eilertsen and Humerfelt, 1968)	Adults, children: normals and patients
Respiration Rate (Simoes et al, 1991)	Adults, children: normals and patients
Percussion (Parrino, 1987)	Adults, children (not neonates): normals and patients
Auscultation of Lung Sounds (Mikami et al, 1987)	Adults, children: normals and patients
Chronic Respiratory Disease Questionnaire (Guyatt et al, 1987)	Adults with disability/handicap from chronic lung disease
Visual Analogue Scale for Dyspnea (VAS) (Aitken, 1969)	Pediatric (with fully developed communications, and adult cardiorespiratory patients
Six-Minute Walking Test (Cooper, 1968)	Adults, children: with cardiorespiratory problems
Self-Paced Walking Test to Predict VO_2 Max (Astrand and Roland, 1977)	Normals, those with chronic respiratory disease, back disabilities
Vital Capacity (Slow VC or Forced VC) (American Thoracic Society, 1987)	Children > age 7 and adults with respiratory problems
Peak Expiratory Flow Rate (PEFR) (American Thoracic Society, 1987)	Children > age 7 and adults with respiratory problems
Maximum Inspiratory and Expiratory Pressure (MIPs/MEPs or MIF/MEF or Pimax/Pemax) (Rahn et al, 1946)	Adults and children who can cooperate and comprehend
Oxygen Saturation (Technology Subcommittee of the Working Group on Critical Care OMH, 1992)	Adults, children: with cardiorespiratory problems

Table 4–13: Developmental Measures

TEST	CONDITIONS TESTED
Alberta Infant Motor Scale (AIMS) (Piper et al, 1992)	Infants term to age of independent walking—those at risk for developing motor problems
Bayley Scales of Infant Development (Bayley, 1969)	Children birth–36 months (motor and mental development)
Peabody Developmental Motor Scales (Folio and Fewell, 1983)	Children birth–83 months with none to severe motor impairment
Test of Motor and Neurological Functions (TMNF) (DeGangi et al, 1983)	Infants 3–12 months with known or suspected abnormal motor and neurological function
Test of Motor Impairment (Stott et al, 1972)	All children with IQ > 50, aged 5–14 years
Posture and Fine Motor Assessment of Infants (PFMAI) (Case-Smith, 1989)	All infants aged 2–6 months
Basic Gross Motor Assessment (BGMA) (Hughes, 1979)	Children aged 5.5–12.5 years with minor motor dysfunction
Bruininks-Oseretsky Test of Motor Proficiency (Bruininks, 1978)	Children aged 4.5–14.5 years with minor motor dysfunction
Gross Motor Function Measure (GMFM) (Rosenbaum et al, 1990)	Cerebral palsy < 20 years old (motor range up to age 5 years)
Gross Motor Performance Measure (GMPM) (Boyce et al, 1990)	Children with cerebral palsy
Movement Assessment of Infants (MAI) (Chandler et al, 1980)	Children birth–12 months (adjusted) at high risk for motor dysfunction
Pediatric Evaluation of Disability Inventory (PEDI) (Haley et al, 1992)	Children with disability with functional performance level under age 7 years

Conclusion

By categorizing the OA tools, one can then more easily decide which instrument(s) will best match the complaints or presentation of the patient. Once an instrument is chosen, it is important to remember to **utilize the same instrument through the course of case management with that patient,** as using different instruments at different times will not allow for comparative analysis. Although there are many options for some of the categories described above, the "gold standards" will be emphasized. For specific information such as scoring, application, and recommended utilization regarding the examples included in this chapter, refer to Sections II through IV of this text. **The use of physical performance tests allows the HCP to track outcomes objectively. In addition, a functional diagnosis can be established that can be therapeutically addressed by specific active and passive care approaches.** Refer to Section III of the text for details regarding the objective outcomes assessment tools.

REFERENCES

Aitken RCB. Measurement of feelings using visual analogue scales. *Proc R Soc Med.* 1969;62:989–993.

Alaranta H, Hurri H, Heliövaara M, Soukka A, Harju R. Non-dynamometric trunk performance tests: Reliability and normative data. *Scand J Rehab Med.* 1994b;26:211–215.

American Thoracic Society. Standardization of Spirometry—1987 Update. *Am Rev Respir Dis.* 1987;136:1285–1298.

Astrand PO, Rodahl K. *Textbook of Work Physiology: Physiological Bases of Exercise.* 2nd ed. New York, NY: McGraw-Hill; 1977.

Barrett WP, Frankin JL, Jackins SE, et al. Total shoulder arthroplasty. *J Bone Joint Surg.* 1987;69A:865–872.

Bayley N. *Manual for the Bayley Scales of Infant Development.* New York, NY: Psychological Corp; 1969.

Beck A: *Depression: Clinical, Experimental and Theoretical Aspects.* New York, NY: Harper & Row; 1967.

Berg KO, Wood-Dauphinee SL, Williams JI, Gayton D. Measuring balance in the elderly: Preliminary development of an instrument. *Physiother Can.* 1989;41(6):304–311.

Bergner M, Bobbitt RA, Carter WB, Gilson BS. The Sickness Index Profile: Development and final revision of a health status measure. *Med Care.* 1981;19:787–805.

Bernstein IH, Jaremko ME, Hinkley BS. On the utility of the SCL-90-R with low-back pain patients. *Spine.* 1994;19:42–48.

Biering-Sorensen F. Physical measurements as risk indicators for low-back trouble over a one-year period. *Spine.* 1984;9(2):106–119.

Bigos S, Battie MC, Spenglere DM, et al. A prospective study of work perceptions and psychosocial factors affecting the report of back injury. *Spine.* 1991;16:1–6.

Boyce W, Gowland C, Hardy S, et al. Reliability of the gross motor performance measure of cerebral palsy. *Physiother Can.* 1990;42(suppl):1.

Brazier J, Harper R, Jones SN. Validating the SF-36 health survey questionnaire: new outcome measure for primary care. *Br Med J.* 1992;305:160–164.

Bruininks RH. *Bruininks-Oseretsky Test of Motor Proficiency: Examiner's Manual.* United States of America: American Guidance Services; 1978.

Bly NN, Sinnot PL. Variations in balance and body sway in middle-aged adults: Subjects with healthy backs compared with subjects with low-back dysfunction. *Spine.* 1991:16:325–330.

Carey RG, Posavac EJ. *Manual for the Level of Rehabilitation Scale II.* Park Ridge, Ill: Lutheran General Hospital; 1980.

Carr JH, Shepherd RB, Nordholm L, Lynn D. Investigation of a new motor assessment scale for stroke patients. *Phys Ther.* 1985;65:175–178.

Carroll D. A quantitative test of upper extremity function. *J Chron Disabil.* 1965;18:479–491.

Case-Smith J. Reliability and validity of the posture and fine motor assessment of infants. *Occup Ther J Res.* 1989;9(5):259–272.

Cats-Baril WL, Frymoyer JW. Identifying patients at risk of becoming disabled because of low-back pain: The Vermont rehabilitation engineering center predictive model. *Spine.* 1991;16:605–607.

Chandler LS, Andrew MS, Swanson MW. *Movement Assessment of Infants—A Manual.* 1980. Available PO Box 4631, Rolling Bay, WA 98061.

Chapman-Smith D. Measuring results—The new importance of patient questionnaires. *Chiro Report.* 1992;7(1):1–6.

Cherkin D, MacCormack F. Patient evaluations of low-back pain are from family physicians and chiropractors. *West J Med.* 1989;150:351–355.

Chesworth BM, Padfield BJ, Helewa A, Stitt LW. A comparison of hip mobility in patients with low back pain and matched healthy subjects. *Physiother Can.* 1994;46:267–274.

Cole B, Finch F, Gowland C, Mayo N. In: Basmajian J, ed. *Physical Rehabilitation Outcome Measures.* Baltimore, Md: Williams & Wilkins; 1995:xi–xiii.

Cooper KH. A means of assessing maximal oxygen intake. *JAMA.* 1968;203(3):135–138.

Cote R, Battista RN, Wolfson C, Boucher J. The Canadian neurological scale: Validation and reliability assessment. *Neurology.* 1989; (A20).

Coulter ID, Hays RD, Danielson CD. The chiropractic satisfaction questionnaire. *Top Clin Chiro.* 1994; 1(4):40–43.

Dainty D, Mior SA, Bereznick D. Validity and reliability of an isometric dynamometer as an evaluative tool in a rehabilitation clinic. *J Sports Chiro Rehabil.* 1998;12:109–117.

Daltroy LH, Cats-Baril WL, Katz JN, Fossel AH, Liang MH. The North American Spine Society lumbar spine outcome assessment instrument: Reliability and validity tests. *Spine*. 1996;21:741–749.

DeGangi GA, Berk RA, Valvano J. Test of motor and neurological functions in high risk infants: Preliminary findings. Developmental and behavioral pediatrics 1983;4(3):182–189.

Deyo RA. Comparative validity of the Sickness Impact Profile Short Scales for functional assessment in low back pain. *Spine*. 1986;11(9):951–954.

Deyo RA, Cherkin DC, Franklin G, Nichols JC. Low Back Pain (forms 6.1 to 6.4), October 12, 1992. Available: HOI, 2001 Killebrew Drive, Suite 122, Bloomington, MN 55425.

Deyo RA, Diehl AK. Measuring physical and psychosocial function in patients with low-back pain. *Spine*. 1983;8:635–642.

Deyo RA, Diehl AK. Patient satisfaction with medical care for low back pain. *Spine*. 1986;11:28–30.

Deyo R, Diehl P, et al. Reproducibility and responsiveness of health status measures. *Control Clin Trials*. 1991;12:142S.

Dixon JS, Bird HA. Reproducibility along a 10 cm vertical visual analogue scale. *Ann Rheum Dis*. 1981;40(1):87–89.

Downie WW, Leatham PA, Rhind VA, et al. Studies with pain rating scales. *Anal Rheum Dis*. 1978;37:378–381.

Dworkin SF, Von Korff M, Whitney WC, et al. Measurement of characteristic pain intensity in field research. *Pain*. 1990(suppl);5:S290.

Ekstrand J, Wiktorsson M, Oberg B, Gillquist J. Lower extremity goniometric measurements: A study to determine their reliability. *Arch Phys Med Rehab*. 1982;63:171–175.

Eilertsen E, Humerfelt S. The observer variation in the measurement of arterial blood pressure. *Acta Med Scand*. 1968;184:145–157.

Fairbanks JCT, Davies JB, Couper J, O'Brien JP. The Oswestry low-back pain disability questionnaire. *Physiotherapy*. 1980;66(8):271–273.

Faulkner RA, Sprigings EJ, McQuarrie A, Bell RD. A partial curl-up protocol for adults based on an analysis of two procedures. *Can J Sport Sci*. 1989;14(3):135–141.

Feuerstein M. Multidisciplinary rehabilitation of occupational musculoskeletal disorders: Rationale, assessment strategies and clinical interventions. LACC Post-graduate program notes, session I of the 2nd 100 hours course, class notes, Chicago, Ill, September 22–24, 1995. Available: LACC Postgraduate Division, 16200 East Amber Drive, P.O. Box 1166, Whittier, CA 90609-1166.

Folio R, Fewell RR. *Peabody Developmental Motor Scales and Activity Cards*. Hingham, Mass: DLM Teaching Resources; 1983.

Fugl-Meyer AR. Post-strike hemiplegia assessment of physical properties. *Scan J Rehabil Med*. 1980;85–93.

Goertz CMH. Measuring functional health status in the chiropractic office using self-report questionnaires. *Top Clin Chiro*. 1994;1(1):51–59.

Gowland C, Stratford P, Ward M, et al. Measuring physical impairment and disability with the Chedoke-McMaster stroke assessment. *Stroke*. 1993;24(1):58–63.

Granger CV, Cotter A, Hamilton BB, Fiedler R, Hens MM. Functional assessment scales: a study of persons with multiple sclerosis. *Arch Phys Med Rehabil*. 1990;71:870–875.

Grodeon E, Drenth V, Jarvis L, Johnson J, Wright V. Neurophysiologic syndromes in stroke as predictors of outcomes. *Arch Phys Med Rehabil*. 1978;59:399–409.

Guyatt G, Berman LB, Townsend M, Pugsley SO, Chambers LW. A measure of quality of life for clinical trials in chronic lung disease. *Thorax*. 1987;42:773–778.

Haley SM, Coster WJ, Lublow LH, Haltiwanger JT, Andrellos PJ. *Pediatric Evaluation of Disability Inventory (PEDI). Development, Standardization and Administration Manual*. 1992.

Harrison E, Quinney H, Magee D, Sheppard MS, McQuarrie A. Analysis of outcome measures used in the study of patellofemoral pain syndrome. *Physiother Can*. 1995;47:264–272.

Harvey RF, Jellinek HM. *TW3 Medical Resources Group*. Madison, Wis: University of Wisconsin–Madison; 1993.

Hasue M, Masatoshi F, Kikchi S. A new method of quantitative measurement of abdominal and back muscle strength. *Spine*. 1980;2(5):143–147.

Hawkins RH, Dunlop R. Non-operative treatment of rotator cuff tears. *Clin Ortho Rel Res*. 1995; Dec(321):178–188.

Hazard RG, Haugh LD, Reid S, Preble JB, MacDonald L. Early prediction of chronic disability after occupational low back injury. *Spine*. 1996;21:945–951.

Hegert R, Carrier R, Bilodeau A. Elaboration d'un instrument de mesure des handicaps: Le systeme de measure de l'automonie fonctionelle (SMAF). In: Tilquin C, ed. Montreal, Canada: Editions Sciences des Systems; 1980.

Helewa A, Goldsmith C, Smythe H. The modified sphygmomanometer: An instrument to measure muscle strength: A validation study. *J Chronic Dis.* 1981;34:353–361.

Hudson-Cook N, Tomes-Nicholson K. *The Revised Oswestry Low Back Pain Disability Questionnaire.* England: Anglo-European College of Chiropractic; 1988. Thesis.

Hughes JE. *Basic Gross Motor Assessment.* Golden, Colo: Jeanne E. Hughes; 1979.

Hurst JW, Shlant RC. *The Heart.* 7th ed. Toronto, Canada: McGraw-Hill Information Services; 1990.

Jacobson GP, Newman CW. The development of the dizziness handicap inventory. *Arch Otolaryngol Head Neck Surg.* 1990;116:424–427.

Jacobson GP, Ramadan NM, et al. The Henry Ford Hospital Headache Disability Inventory (HDI). *Neurology.* 1994;44:837–842.

Jensen MP, Karoly P, Braver S. The measurement of clinical pain intensity: A comparison of six methods. *Pain.* 1986;27:117–126.

Jull GA, Richardson CA. The muscular protection of the lumbar spine. In: *Proceedings of National Orthopaedic Symposium.* Toronto, Canada: Orthopaedic Division, CPA; 1992:77–83.

Kaplan RM, Anderson JP. A general health policy model: Update and applications. *Health Service Res.* 1982;23:203–235.

Kirkaldy-Willis WH. *Managing Low Back Pain.* New York, NY: Churchill Livingstone; 1983.

Klein RM, Bell B. Self-care skills: Behavioral measurement with Klein-Bell ADL Scale. *Arch Phys Med Rehabil.* 1982;63:335–338.

Kopec JA, Esdaile JM, Abrahamowicz M, et al. The Quebec back pain disability scale: Measurement properties. *Spine.* 1995;20:341–352.

Korbon GA, DeGood DE, Schroeder ME, Schwartz DP, Shutty MS. The development of a somatic amplification rating scale for low-back pain. *Spine.* 1987;12(8):787–791.

Lawlis GF, Cuencas R, Selby D, McCoy CE. The development of the Dallas pain questionnaire: An assessment of the impact of spinal pain on behavior. *Spine.* 1989;14:511–516.

Leighton JR. The Leighton flexometer and flexibility test. *J Assoc Phys Mental Rehabil.* 1958;20:127–130.

Levine DW, Simmons HP, Doris MJ, et al. A self-administered questionnaire for the assessment of severity of symptoms and functional status in carpal tunnel syndrome. *J Bone Joint Surg.* 1993;75-A:1585–1592.

Lincoln N, Leadbitter D. Assessment of motor function in stroke patients. *Phys Ther.* 1979;65(2):48–51.

Loebl WY. Measurement of spinal posture and range of spinal movement. *Ann Phys Med.* 1967;9:104–110.

Macrae IF, Wright V. Measurement of back movement. *Ann Rheum Dis.* 1969;36(1):6–11.

Mahoney FI, Barthel DW. Functional evaluation: The Barthel Index. *Md Med J.* 1965;14:61–65.

Main CJ. Modified somatic perception questionnaire. *J Psychosom Res.* 1983;27:503–514.

Main CJ, Wood PL, Hollis S, et al. The distress and risk assessment method: A simple patient classification to identify distress and evaluate the risk of poor outcome. *Spine.* 1992;7:42.

Mayer T, Gatchel RJ. *Functional Restoration for Spinal Disorders: A Sports Medicine Approach.* Philadelphia, Penn: Lea and Febiger; 1988.

Mayer T, Gatchel RJ, Keeley J, Mayer H, Richling D. A male incumbent worker industrial database. *Spine.* 1994;19:762–764.

McDowell I, Newell C. *Measuring Health: A Guide to Rating Scales and Questionnaires.* New York, NY: Oxford University Press; 1987.

Melzack R. The McGill Pain Questionnaire: Major properties and scoring methods. *Pain.* 1975;1:277–279.

Melzack P. *Pain Measurement and Assessment.* New York, NY: Raven Press; 1982.

Mikami R, et al. International symposium of lung sounds. Synopsis of proceedings. *Chest.* 1987;92(2):342–345.

Millard RW. The functional assessment screening questionnaire: Application for evaluating pain-related disability. *Arch Phys Med Rehabil.* 1989;70:303–307.

Moskowitz RW, McCann CB. Classification of disability in the chronically ill and aging. *J Chronic Dis.* 1957;5:342–346.

Nelson EC, Landgraf JM, Hays RD, Wasson JH, Kirk JW. The functional status of patients: How can it be measured in physicians' offices? *Med Care.* 1990;28(12):1111–1126.

Newman CW, Jacobson GP, Spitzer JB. Development of the tinnitus handicap inventory. *Arch Otolaryngol Head Neck Surg.* 1996;122:143–148.

Newman CW, Weinstein BE, Jacobson GP, Hug GA. Test–retest reliability of the Hearing Handicap Inventory for Adults. *Arch Otolaryngol Head Neck Surg.* 1990;12:355–357.

Ohlund C, Eek C, Palmblad S, Areskoug B, Nachemson A. Quantified pain drawing in subacute low back pain: Validation in a nonselected outpatient industrial sample. *Spine*. 1996;21:1021–1031.

Parker H, Wood PLR, Main CJ. The use of the pain drawing as a screening measure to predict psychological distress in chronic low back pain. *Spine*. 1995;20:236–243.

Parrino TA. The art and science of percussion. *Hosp Prac*. 1987;22:25–36.

Piper MC, Pinnell LE, Darrah J, Maguire T, Byrne PJ. Construction and validation of the Alberta Infant Motor Scale (AIMES). *Can J Public Health*. 1992;83:46–52.

Podsiadlo D, Richardson S. The timed "up and go": A test of basic functional mobility for frail elderly persons. *J Amer Geriatr Soc*. 1991;39:142–148.

Rahn H, Otis AB, Chadwick LE, Fenn WO. The pressure-volume diagram of the thorax and lung. *Am J Physiol*. 1946;146:161–178.

Ransford AO, Cairns D, Mooney V. The pain drawing as an aid to the psychologic evaluation of patients with low-back pain. *Spine*. 1976;1(2):127–134.

Roland M, Morris R. A study of the natural history of back pain. Part 1: Development of a reliable and sensitive measure of disability in low-back pain. *Spine*. 1983a;8(2):141–144.

Roland M, Morris R. A study of the natural history of back pain. Part 2: Development of guidelines for trials of treatment in primary care. *Spine*. 1983b;8(2):145–150.

Rosenbaum P, Cadman D, Russell D, Gowland C, Hardy S, Jarvis S. Issues in measuring change in motor function in children with cerebral palsy. A special communication. *Phys Ther*. 1990;70:125–131.

Ruta DA, Garratt AM, Wardlaw D, Russell IT. Developing a valid and reliable measure of health outcome for patients with low back pain. *Spine*. 1994;19:1887–1896.

Simoes EAF, et al. Respiratory rate: measurement of variability over time and accuracy at different counting periods. *Arch Dis Child*. 1991;66(10):1199–1203.

Staff of the Benjamin Rose Hospital. Multidisciplinary studies of illness in aged persons: II. A new classification of functional status in activities of daily living. *J Chronic Dis*. 1959;9(1):55–62.

Steigerwald DP, Maher JH. The Steigerwald/Maher TMD disability questionnaire. *Today's Chiro*. 1997; 26:86–91.

Stott DH, Moyes FA, Henderson SE. *Test of Motor Impairment*. Guelph, Canada: Brook Educational Publishing; 1972.

Swanson AB, Matev IB, de Groot Swanson G. The strength of the hand. *Bull Prosthet Res*. 1970;145–53.

Technology Subcommittee of the Working Group on Critical Care OMH. Noninvasive blood gas monitoring: A review for use in the adult critical care unit. *Can Med Assoc*. 1992;146(5):703–712.

Vernon H, Mior S. The Neck Disability Index: A study of reliability and validity. *J Manip Phys Ther*. 1991;14(7):409.

Von Korff M, Deyo RA, Cherkin D, Barlow SF. Back pain in primary care: Outcomes at 1 year. *Spine*. 1993;18:855–862.

Von Korff M, Ormel J, Keefe F, Dworkin SF. Grading the severity of chronic pain. *Pain*. 1992;50:133–149.

Waddell G, McCulloch JA, Kimmel E, Venner RM. Nonorganic physical signs in low back pain. *Spine*. 1980;5:117–125.

Waddell G, Newton M, Henderson I, et al. A fear-avoidance beliefs questionnaire (FABQ) and the role of fear-avoidance beliefs in chronic low back pain and disability. *Pain*. 1993;52:157–168.

Wang S, Whitney SL, Burdett RG, et al. Lower extremity muscular flexibility in long distance runners. *J Orthop Sports Phys Ther*. 1993;2:102–107.

Ware J, Davies AR. Defining and measuring patient satisfaction with medical care. *Eval Program Plan*. 1983:6:247–263.

Ware JE, Davies-Avery A, Stewart AL. The measuring and meaning of patient satisfaction. *Health Med Care Serv Rev*. 1978;1:1–15.

Ware J, Snyder M, et al. Defining and measuring patient satisfaction with medical care. *Eval Program Plan*. 1992;6:247.

Whiting S, Lincoln N. An ADL assessment for stroke patients. *Br J Occ Ther*. 1980;43:44–46.

Zung WWK. A self-rating depression scale. *Arch Gen Psychiatry*. 1965;32:63–70. Available: (HSQ 2.0) Health Outcomes Institute, 2001 Killebrew Drive, Suite 122, Bloomington, MN 55425; 612-858-9188 (O); 612-858-9189 (Fax) (HSQ designed: 4-1-93).

SECTION

II

Subjective Outcome Assessment Tools

This section utilizes patient-driven information generated by the use of pen-and-paper questionnaires, inventories, and/or scales when classifying outcome measures. Many of the tools discussed in this section are reproduced in the appendix; the specific questionnaire or outcome tool can be accessed and photocopied for immediate implementation into practice. These outcome tools are further classified into the following domains: general health (Chap. 5), pain perception (Chap. 6), disease or condition-specific (Chap. 7), psychometric (Chap. 8), patient satisfaction (Chap. 9), and disability prediction (Chap. 10). Several guest authors bring a unique viewpoint to the topics discussed in Chapters 8, 9, and 10.

CHAPTER 5

General Health Questionnaires

STEVEN G. YEOMANS

INTRODUCTION

As described in Chapter 4, use of a category system helps in identifying the goals one wishes to achieve through the use of an outcome assessment (OA) tool. One of the goals of a general health instrument is to provide a means by which a health care provider (HCP) can track outcomes of virtually any condition, as these instruments tend not to be condition-specific in their application. For example, if a patient presents with a limp arising from an ingrown toenail, tracking the outcome of a treatment approach without an OA tool specific for the presenting condition proves difficult. To the extent of my research, there are no condition-specific questionnaires that address ingrown toenails; hence, the use of a "broad spectrum" OA tool such as a general health questionnaire (GHQ) may prove very helpful. **One can benefit from the use of a GHQ because it is not condition-specific and, therefore, can be applied to virtually any complaint.** As noted above, the importance of this is evident as many conditions do not have the luxury of having a specific OA tool. In addition, any condition has an adverse effect on quality of life. Having a measure for assessing the impact a condition is having on the patient's life quality is important as problems can then be identified and the specific treatment decisions assigned to address those problems can be implemented and tracked.

USE OF GENERAL HEALTH QUESTIONNAIRES

In practice, HCPs typically raise three questions regarding the use of GHQs:

1. Why bother measuring functional status (why take the time)?
2. How is the instrument implemented into a busy practice without disrupting the flow of the practice?
3. What is done with the information derived from the assessment?

WHY MEASURE FUNCTIONAL STATUS?

To address the first question of "why bother," the American College of Physicians (1988) lists five possible benefits of measuring health status:

1. Detecting, quantifying and identifying the sources of decreased functional capability
2. Guiding management decisions
3. Guiding the efficient use of health care resources
4. Improving the prediction of the course of chronic conditions
5. Improving patient outcomes: symptoms (morbidity), mortality, and satisfaction regarding care, function, and quality of life.

In essence, the same reasons apply to justify any outcome assessment tool, which are:

1. To improve the ability of the HCP to implement needed services by identifying the functional disabilities.
2. To improve the communication between the HCP, patient, and third-party payer.
3. To improve the ability of the HCP to identify barriers to recovery or risk factors of chronicity and then implement the appropriate treatment or referral.

The use of GHQs improves the quality of the service an HCP offers and, as a result, helps buffer the HCP from a possible liability suit. This is an important consideration; in our litigious society, malpractice issues are becoming increasingly more common.

IMPLEMENTING THE GENERAL HEALTH QUESTIONNAIRE IN A BUSY PRACTICE

The second issue of "how" to fit the instrument into the busy practice can be addressed in two ways. The first is through an HCP-assisted method, in which the HCP, nurse, medical assistant, or other office staff administer the instrument to the patient. The second method, in which the patient self-administers the instrument, is the most practical since it does not consume any staff time, especially that of the HCP. In this method, patients read the instrument and complete the questionnaire themselves. Most of the general health questions reviewed in this chapter are available in multiple languages. One includes a picture with a short verbal description of the general health variable or scale.

MAKING USE OF THE ACQUIRED INFORMATION

The third issue of "what to do" with the acquired information is fourfold:

1. Identify the problem areas.
2. Verify the problem with the patient (so that he or she knows that you are aware of it and to determine its current importance in that specific case).
3. Make a specific functional diagnosis and determine if special resources to manage the problem are needed (referral, consultation, etc).
4. Determine endpoints of care and base future management decisions on the readministration results (discharge, referral, disability/impairment evaluation, etc).

By using a GHQ, the HCP can efficiently identify the care the patient needs and by the readministration of the questionnaire, can evaluate the patient's progress or determine the outcome. Also, the report of findings or patient education needs is enhanced by identifying problem areas and sharing the results with the patient. GHQs can also measure the patient's opinion of the quality of care he or she has received. This "paradigm shift"—from depending primarily on objective measures of patient function (range of motion, orthopedic or medical tests) to the more subjective "patient-based information" derived in part, from GHQs—allows the patient's treatment goals to be identified and managed. In essence, the patient is treated, not just a test result. Objective testing such as x-ray is important for identifying a "red flag" or pathological condition as soon as possible. But once the "red flag" has been ruled out, addressing the patient's needs and goals leads to optimum patient satisfaction and reduces the likelihood of difficult patient management for the HCP.

WHEN TO USE GENERAL HEALTH QUESTIONNAIRES

My conversations with various researchers and providers who utilize GHQ have revealed an apparent division into two "camps" with respect to *when* to administer the GHQ. In the first, somewhat "conservative" camp, the use of a general health instrument is utilized simply to assess quality of life at infrequent time intervals. These time intervals are generally spread quite far apart and are not used for assessing outcomes. This group may apply the use of a GHQ at onset and at 12- to 24-month intervals. This application may be most appropriate for chronic, protracted conditions. For example, a patient with diabetes mellitus may be best served by the infrequent use of a GHQ if his or her condition is stable or not too "brittle." In a healthy population, utilizing a GHQ at 2-year intervals was suggested. The "liberal" camp, on the other hand, may advocate the use of these tools at the initial presentation and at regular intervals of time or at least at discharge to track the outcome of a treatment regimen.

This division in perception of when to use a GHQ has support on both sides and, in practice, I have noted several of the scales of a GHQ (some more than others) to be quite sensitive to the changes in health and, therefore, to serve well as outcomes gathering tools. The application of a GHQ should, at minimum, be used at the following intervals:

- At the time of the initial presentation for baseline establishment of outcomes assessment
- To identify problems for prompt management
- At a plateau in care or discharge for outcomes assessment of the treatment benefits or lack thereof
- Six months after discharge in order to evaluate the long-term benefits of treatment

If, however, there are no other OA tools—such as a condition-specific questionnaire—to compliment the OA process, increasing the use of the GHQ to each point of reexamination makes sense. Treatment modifications can then be considered along the way if the GHQ continues to identify failure to improve.

RESEARCH SUMMARY

Outcomes-based research has also embraced the use of general health tools in a variety of conditions (Wong-Chung et al, 1991; Hays and Shapiro, 1992; Bruusgaard et al, 1993; de Haan et al, 1993; Froom et al, 1993; Krousel-Wood et al, 1994; Albert et al, 1996) in a variety of disciplines (Nelson et al, 1987; Nelson et al, 1990a, 1990b; Bass, 1992; McHorney et al, 1992; Goertz, 1994), in different cultures (Shigemoto, 1990; Westbury, 1990; Hickey et al, 1994), by age groups (Wasson et al, 1992; Siu et al, 1993a, 1993b; Wasson et al, 1994), for assessing function (Landgraf et al, 1990; Meyboom-de Jong and Smith, 1992; Scholten and Van Weel, 1992; Ware et al, 1992b), and for various other research applications (Ware et al, 1980; American College of Physicians, 1988; Landgraf and Nelson, 1992; Bruusgaard et al, 1993). The utility of the GHQs is vast, as they can be applied to every patient in every conceivable form of health care presentation, regardless of condition, discipline, culture, or other factor. Such a wide range of application suggests that there is a use for a GHQ in every practice setting and, hence, they should be included in the HCP's battery of tools.

GENERAL HEALTH QUESTIONNAIRE PROS AND CONS

It seems obvious that the strength of a GHQ lies in its wide range of application. Conversely, one can also criticize the use of a GHQ for the same reason—that it is not condition specific and is, therefore, **less sensitive in the assessment of change over time** in specific conditions or situations. In addition, the manner in which the questions are presented can further support the argument that the GHQ does not serve as a sensitive OA tool. For example, the second question on the standard version of the SF-36 or HSQ-2.0 reads, "Compared to one year ago, how would you rate your health in general now?" The remaining questions of the SF-36/HSQ-2.0 as well as the questions of the Dartmouth COOP health charts, ask the patient to compare his or her current health status to that 1 month or 4 weeks ago, which may be too long a time interval to accurately track

outcomes. There is an acute version of the SF-36 available that utilizes a 1-month rather than 1-year time interval for the second question, and a 1-week rather than 1-month time interval for the remaining questions. This version may be the better choice for tracking care in an ambulatory care center, where a higher percentage of patients present with acute rather than chronic conditions.

The use of a GHQ as an OA tool is also challenged by the point that the health status score of a GHQ can change for reasons other than a change in function; for example, psychosocial factors. Suffice it to say that there is a division in the field as to the use of the GHQ as an OA instrument. However, not applying a GHQ tool in a patient population may result in difficulty in assessing outcomes, or at least quality of life issues. This is especially true in conditions for which a condition-specific instrument does not exist.

GENERAL HEALTH QUESTIONNAIRE OPTIONS

Several different instruments are readily available to choose from within the general health category. Some of these instruments include the SF-36 (Brazier et al, 1992; Goertz, 1994), the HSQ-2.0; Dartmouth COOP Charts (Nelson et al, 1990a; Goertz, 1994), the Sickness Index Profile (SIP) (Bergner et al, 1981), and the Quality of Well-Being Scale (Kaplan and Anderson, 1982). Though similarities exist between these instruments, the titles of the scales vary. Table 5–1 represents three popular general health tools and the corresponding scale titles.

SHORT HEALTH SURVEY

Interest in developing short health surveys increased when some study participants in the Health Insurance Experiment (HIE) refused to complete lengthy health surveys (Ware et al, 1980). Consequently, several short-form scales were developed and used successfully (Davies and Ware, 1981; Nelson et al, 1983; Lurie et al, 1984; Brook et al, 1987; Read et al, 1987; Fowler et al, 1988; Spiegel et al, 1988). A trade-off between practicality and validity is described when comparing the short-form surveys versus the longer scales (Manning et al, 1982). The first attempt at a comprehensive short-form survey was an 18 item form developed in 1984 (Montgomery and Paranjpe, 1985). In 1986, two more items were added to create a 20-item measure (SF-20) (Ware et al, 1992b). Considerable experience is described by Ware regarding the trade-off between the formation of short-form versus long-form surveys (Ware et al, 1993). Many full-length scales were studied for measuring limitations in physical, social, role functioning (Donald and Ware, 1984), and general health perceptions (Stewart et al, 1978; Davies and Ware, 1981; Stewart et al, 1981). Selected items that make up the current SF-36 have their roots in the long surveys that have been in use for over 20

Table 5–1: Corresponding Scale Titles of Three Popular General Health Questionnaires

SF-36	HSQ-2.0	DARTMOUTH COOP HEALTH CHARTS[a]
1. Physical functioning	Physical functioning	Physical
2. Role—physical	Role—physical	Daily activities
3. Bodily pain	Bodily pain	Pain
4. General health	Health perceptions	Overall health
5. Vitality	Energy/fatigue	NA
6. Social functioning	Social functioning	Social activities
7. Role—emotional	Role—emotional	Daily activities
8. Mental health	Mental health	Feelings

NA, not available.

[a] Available: Dartmouth COOP Project, c/o Deborah Johnson, Dartmouth Medical School, Hanover, NH 03755-3862; (603) 650-1974. Copyright 1989.

years (Ware, 1976; Ware and Karmos, 1976). Ware states that the most difficult task in developing the SF-36 was choosing the eight health concepts from the more than 40 concepts and scales reviewed in the Medical Outcomes Study (MOS). Examples of scales that were seriously considered but not chosen include health distress, sexual functioning, family functioning, and sleep adequacy (Ware and Karmos, 1976).

SF-36 and HSQ-2.0 Short-form Surveys

The SF-36 and HSQ-2.0 are very similar and, therefore, will be discussed together. These short-form surveys were constructed to measure eight health attributes or scales. Each attribute is scored using a Likert scale (Likert, 1932). This scoring method assumes that the distribution of responses to items within the same scale and item variances is near equal. The method also assumes that each item has a substantial linear relationship with the score for its scale (ie, item internal consistency). Scoring is accomplished by the completion of 2 to 10 items or questions per health attribute or scale, adding the decoded scores of the items and dividing by the number of items that make up the scale. For example, the mental health scale is made up of 5 items (questions 24, 25, 26, 28, and 30). Table 5–2 shows the section of the SF-36/HSQ-2.0 that includes questions 24 to 30 with the decoded values written in the right-hand margin. Note that questions 24, 25, 26, 28, and 30 comprise the mental health scale. The value of 1 through 6 decodes into a score of 0 to 100 or, 100 to 0, where 100 represents excellent health and 0 represents the lowest health score. The decoded value order is reversed in questions that are positively presented (eg, questions 26 and 30) and vice versa. The purpose of combining questions that make up other scales as well as positively and negatively presented questions that reverse the decoded values is to make it difficult for the patient to falsify the answers.

Calculating the Scores

The decoded values that make up the mental health scale are added together and divided by 5 to result in one score that represents the final value for the mental health scale (Fig. 5–1).

Each of the eight attributes or scales is calculated in a similar manner. More specifically, Table 5–3 includes the information needed to calculate the scores for all eight scales. The number of items that make up each scale, the scale items, and the minimum number of responses required to be completed in order to calculate a valid score are presented in the right-hand column of Table 5–3. If a question is left unanswered, it is recommended that the HCP assist the patient in arriving at an answer prior to calculating the results. If this attempt proves unsuccessful, the other items that make up the scale are averaged and that average is inserted in place of the missing item followed by a final calculation.

Making Use of the Scores

The final scores calculated in the SF-36/HSQ-2.0 can be used in different ways. The first way involves simply using the result as an outcome measure by comparing it to future scores after repeating the instrument at a later date. In this way, the response to treatment intervention can be determined by the change in the scores between the baseline score and the follow-up result.

The second way the initial score can be used is by comparing the patient's score with age- and gender-specific normative data that has been calculated. Normative data in disease populations, including hypertension, congestive heart failure, type II diabetes, recent acute myocardial infarction, and clinical depression, can also be compared with the patient's score. More specifically, the use of normative data allows for scale score interpretation for an individual respondent or the average score for a group of respondents by comparing the scores for other individuals.

Table 5–2: Portion of the SF-36/HSQ-2.0 That Includes the Mental Health Scale[a]

These questions are about how you feel and how things have been with you during the past 4 weeks. For each question, please give the one answer that comes closest to the way you have been feeling.

How much of the time during the past 4 weeks . . .   (circle one number on each line)

	ALL OF THE TIME	MOST OF THE TIME	A GOOD BIT OF THE TIME	SOME OF THE TIME	LITTLE OF THE TIME	NONE OF THE TIME	DECODING
23. Did you feel full of pep?	1	2	3	4	5	6	100, 80, 60, 40, 20, 0
24. Have you been a very nervous person?	1	2	<u>3</u>	4	5	6	0, 20, <u>40</u>, 60, 80, 100
25. Have you felt so down in the dumps that nothing could cheer you up?	1	2	3	<u>4</u>	5	6	0, 20, 40, <u>60</u>, 80, 100
26. Have you felt calm and peaceful?	1	2	3	4	5	<u>6</u>	100, 80, 60, 40, 20, <u>0</u>
27. Did you have a lot of energy?	1	2	3	4	5	6	100, 80, 60, 40, 20, 0
28. Have you felt downhearted and blue?	1	2	<u>3</u>	4	5	6	0, 20, <u>40</u>, 60, 80, 100
29. Did you feel worn out?	1	2	3	4	5	6	0, 20, 40, 60, 80, 100
30. Have you been a happy person?	1	2	3	<u>4</u>	5	6	100, 80, 60, <u>40</u>, 20, 0
31. Did you feel tired?	1	2	3	4	5	6	0, 20, 40, 60, 80, 100

[a] The items or questions that make up the mental health scale include numbers 24, 25, 26, 28, and 30. The decoding of the Likert scale (1–6) is reversed where 1 = 100 and 6 = 0 in questions that are positively asked (numbers 26 and 30) and the mixing in of questions from other health scales 23, 27, 29, and 31 make it difficult to falsify responses.

For example, one can determine that a change from a score of 46 to 66 on the health perception scale, where 72 represents the mean, is a change from the 64th percentile to the 92nd percentile in the general U.S. population (see Table 5–4 as an example). If the normative data for the patient is at a higher number than the patient's score, and the pa-

Formula:

$$\frac{24 + 25 + 26 + 28 + 30}{5} = \text{Mental health score}$$

Example from Table 5–2:

$$\frac{40 + 60 + 0 + 40 + 40}{5} \text{ or } \frac{180}{5} = 36 \text{ (Mental health score)}$$

Figure 5–1. The formula for scoring the SF-36/HSQ-2.0. The example is taken from Table 5–2.

tient's condition has not reached a plateau, additional care may be indicated. This could be useful to HCPs, patients, and insurance company case managers as additional care is needed ("medically necessary") to return the patient to a "mean" level of function if a plateau in the condition is not supported by the remaining documentation. This "mean" level of function is obtained from normative data tables, as discussed previously (Ware et al, 1993). If a plateau is present, this may indicate that residuals from a condition may be permanent. It is important to emphasize that correlation of the SF-36/HSQ-2.0 results with other clinical information such as history, physical examination findings, functional testing, and results from other OA tools (such as visual analogue pain scales and condition-specific questionnaires) is needed to firmly establish a plateau in a condition.

Table 5–4 represents an example of correlating a patient's result to prior scores and to normative data. **Correlating this information to the patient's specific clinical**

Table 5–3: Information Needed to Calculate Scores for All Eight Scales of the HSQ-2.0/SF-36

SCALE[a]	NUMBER OF ITEMS	SCALE ITEMS	MINIMUM NUMBER OF ITEMS NEEDED TO COMPUTE A SCORE
Health perception (general health)	5	1, 33, 34, 35, 36	3
Physical functioning	10	3, 4, 5, 6, 7, 8, 9, 10, 11, 12	5
Role limitations due to physical health	4	13, 14, 15, 16	2
Role limitations due to emotional problems	3	17, 18, 19	2
Social functioning	2	20, 32	1
Bodily pain	2	21, 22	1
Mental health	5	24, 25, 26, 28, 30	3
Energy/fatigue (vitality)	4	23, 27, 29, 31	2

[a] SF-36 scale titles are in parentheses, when different.

data and then making a clinical decision based on the results represents a difficult but important step in making the "paradigm shift" into becoming an "outcomes-based" practice.

Advantages and Other Uses of the SF-36/HSQ-2.0
The SF-36/HSQ-2.0 take about 15 minutes to complete, have been found to be sensitive in detecting low levels of ill health (Brazier et al, 1992), and have been utilized as OA tools in studies (Bronfort, 1992). Another indication of their broad applicability is that more than 260 clinical trials using the SF-36 to assess general health outcomes were reported and over 158 topics were registered with the Medical Outcomes Trust as of June 1993 (Ware et al, 1994).

Another optional use of the SF-36 is available: the MOS projects have developed Physical and Mental Health Summary Indexes for the SF-36 (Ware et al, 1993). The indexes are based on two components: the Physical and Mental Health Summary Indexes. A number of advantages of combining the SF-36 information into two, rather than eight, scales are discussed. They include:

- A reduction in the number of statistical comparisons necessary to capture differences in health status or health outcome
- Adjustment for substantial correlations among the eight scales
- More straightforward interpretation of the differences in physical and mental health scores
- Substantially greater precision for general physical and mental health outcomes

SF-12 Physical and Mental Health Summary Scales

In March 1995, the SF-12 Physical and Mental Health Summary Scales was introduced (Ware et al, 1995). This is a 12-item questionnaire developed from the SF-36 Health Survey and is used to monitor outcomes in general and specific populations. This questionnaire takes only about 2 to 5 minutes to complete. Like the SF-36, there is a standard and an acute version, and the scales that are derived from the SF-12 include the physical and mental health summary scales. A summary of scale construction methods and the data of preliminary evaluations of norms and empirical validity are included in the manual as well as a computer diskette for scoring (Ware et al, 1995). The *SF-36 Physical & Mental Health Summary Scales: A User's Manual* (Ware et al, 1994) is a supplement to the original *SF-36 Health Survey: Manual and Interpretation Guide* (Ware et al, 1993). The latter is also recommended for interpreting the new SF-12 Health Survey.

The Health Outcomes Institute also offers a 12-item general health questionnaire, which is also patterned after

---

CLINICAL TIP 5–1
Additional Source of Normative Data Information

The normative data is vast. Therefore, if access to a significant volume of normative data is desired, request an order form and obtain the *SF-36 Health Survey: Manual & Interpretation Guide* from: Health Outcomes Trust, 20 Park Plaza, Suite 1014, Boston, MA 02116; by phone: (617) 426-4046 or by fax: (617) 426-4131. A copy of the SF-12, SF-36, and other data are also available.

To obtain a copy of the HSQ-12, Version 2.0, and instructions on how to score the instrument, obtain an order form from Stratis Health, 2901 Metro Drive, Suite 400, Bloomington, MN 55425-1525; by phone: (612) 858-9188 or by fax: (612) 858-9189.

Table 5–4: Example of Use of SF-36/HSQ-2.0 Scores to Compare a Patient's Results with Normative Data[a]

SCALE	NORMATIVE DATA MEAN[b]	BASELINE (DATE:_____)	PERCENTILE OF NORMAL	EXAM 2 (DATE: _____)	PERCENTILE OF NORMAL
1. Health perception	72	46	64%	66	92%
2. Physical functioning	84	42	50%	78	93%
3. Role—Physical	81	0	0%	48	59%
4. Role—Emotional	81	22	27%	68	84%
5. Social functioning	83	46	55%	70	84%
6. Bodily pain	75	0	0%	68	91%
7. Mental health	75	42	56%	72	96%
8. Energy/fatigue	61	22	36%	48	79%
9. Major depression[c]	NA	NA	NA	NA	NA
10. Dysthymia[c]	NA	NA	NA	NA	NA
11. Both 9 and 10[c]	NA	NA	NA	NA	NA

NA, not available.

[a] This chart serves as a convenient summary of the scale scores of the SF-36/HSQ-2.0 and/or Dartmouth COOP Health Charts. This can serve as a very practical reference tool to use for patient report of findings, to insurers to justify "medical necessity" for additional care, and to the health care provider to facilitate the decision making process of case management (referral, discharge).

[b] The above "mean" values represent those taken from the "total sample," which includes both males and females of all ages (Ware et al, 1993).

[c] The depression items (9–11) included in the chart were taken from the HSQ-2.0.

its longer parent questionnaire, the HSQ-2.0, 36-item questionnaire. The primary difference between the SF-12 and the HSQ-12, version 2.0, is that the former is set up to drive two scales whereas the HSQ-12 maintains all eight scales of the original longer version. It should also be mentioned that the longer 36-item SF-36 can be scored to drive the same two summary scales, the physical and mental health scales, as the SF-12. The advantage of the 36-item questionnaire over the 12-item questionnaire is having a greater number of questions drive the two scales, as this is more accurate statistically. The primary disadvantage of this method of scoring, in which only two scales are included, is not having the information derived from the remaining six scales. The primary advantage of the 12-item questionnaire over the 36-item questionnaire is the improved practicality of the shorter questionnaire, as it takes less time for patients to complete, and it is easier and takes less time to score. Other subtle differences existing between the SF-12 and SF-36 are summarized in Table 5–5.

Calculating the Scores
Calculating the score of the HSQ-12, version 2.0, is identical to that of the longer HSQ-2.0, 36-item questionnaire except that the number of items belonging to each of the eight scales is fewer. Hence, the same three steps are used, as follows:

1. Decode the value of each response to each question.
2. Refer to Table 5–6 for the items that relate to each of the eight scales.
3. In the multiple item questions, add together and

average the responses to calculate the score; in the single response scales, the one score of the single question *is* the final score for the scale.

When a response is left out in the mental health or physical function scale, the score is calculated by averaging 2 of the 3 items. At least 2 items have to be completed in order to include the scale score. If any question is left unanswered that belongs to a 1-item scale, the scale cannot be calculated. Any scale that cannot be calculated should be recorded as "missing." Refer to Figure 5–1 and Tables 5–3 and 5–4 for examples of how to score the multiple-item scales (physical function and mental health). Appendix Form A–4 includes a decoded version of the HSQ-12, with scoring instructions located at the end of the questionnaire. Appendix Form A–5 is a clean/reproducible copy of the HSQ-12 (Ware, 1995), and Appendix Form A–6 is a chart for inserting the scores calculated at multiple dates so that future comparisons can be easily made.

The majority of the scales (six of eight) are scored by the use of only 1 item. Two scales contain multiple items in which the average is taken to represent the score. These are the physical function scale and the mental health scale. Table 5–6 includes the item number(s) that relate to each scale.

COOP CHART SYSTEM

The Dartmouth Primary Care Cooperative Information Project (COOP) was founded in 1978 and the COOP chart system (Nelson et al, 1990a, 1990b; Goertz, 1994)

Table 5–5: Differences Between the SF-12 and HSQ-12, Version 2.0[a]

SCALE	HSQ-12	SF-12[b]	SF-36 ITEM HSQ-12	SF-12	SF-36 (NO. OF ITEMS)	
Health perception	1	1	1	1	1, 33–36	(5)
Physical functioning	2, 3, 4	2, 3	2, 3, 4	4, 6	3–12	(10)
Role—Physical	5	4, 5	c	14, 15	13–16	(4)
Role—Mental (old: Role—Emotional)	6	6, 7	c	18, 19	17–19	(3)
Social functioning	7	12	20	32	20, 32	(2)
Bodily pain	8	8	21	22	21, 22	(2)
Mental health (MH)	9, 11, 12	9, 11	26, 28, 30	26, 28	24–26, 28, 30	(5)
Energy/fatigue	10	10	27	27	23, 27, 29, 31	(4)

[a] The first two columns to the right of the scale name column include the items that make up each of the eight scales of the 12-item questionnaires. The next two columns to the right indicate the question number of the longer 36-item questionnaire that corresponds to the shorter versions. The right-hand column indicates the item number of the SF-36 (and HSQ-2.0) that corresponds to each of the eight scales. This table allows for easy comparison among the three tools.
[b] Only includes two scales—mental health and physical functioning.
[c] Question rewritten with a different scoring approach.

was developed in 1989. It has been developed and refined over the past 10 years with the goal of producing a valid, reliable, brief, and practical method to assess functional status of adults and adolescents. The charts are similar to the Snellen eye charts. Each chart consists of a title and a question pertaining to the patient's status over the past 2 to 4 weeks, rated on a 1- to 5-point ordinal scale (1 equals normal, 5 the most abnormal). Each number is accompanied by a short written description of the severity level and is illustrated by a drawing depicting a level of function or well-being (Nelson et al, 1987, 1990a, 1990b) (Appendix Form A–7). The illustrations depicted in the charts simplify completion while not affecting the bias of the response (Larson et al, 1992). High scores of 4 or 5 represent unfavorable levels of health (life quality or social support) and a score of 1 represents no problems (Nelson et al, 1996). The score for the scale is simply the response that is circled. There are a total of nine charts and, therefore, nine total scales make up the Dartmouth COOP Chart system. **The charts represent a very simple, easily administered and scored general health screen used to assess, monitor, and maintain patient function.**

There are two sets of charts. The World Organization of National Colleges and Academies and Academic Association of General Practice/Family Physicians (WONCA) version for adults has been developed as the international standard for classifying adult patients in a primary care setting (Scholten and Van Weel, 1992). The primary differ-

Table 5–6: Information Needed to Calculate a Score for the HSQ-12, Version 2.0[a]

SCALE	NUMBER OF ITEMS	SCALE ITEMS
Physical functioning	3	2, 3, 4
Role limitations attributable to: physical health (role—physical)	1	5
Bodily pain	1	8
Health perception	1	1
Energy/fatigue	1	10
Social functioning	1	7
Role limitations attributable to: mental health (role—mental)	1	6
Mental health	3	9, 11, 12

[a] The scale and the corresponding items that make up each scale are reported. In the two multiple-item scales, the final score is taken as the average of the 3-item scores if at least 2 items are completed.
Modified from the instructions that accompanied the HSQ-12, version 2.0 obtained from Stratis Health, 2901 Metro Drive, Suite 400, Bloomington, MN 55425-1525; (612) 858-9188 (phone); (612) 858-9189 (fax)

ence between the original COOP health charts and the WONCA version is that functional status is measured for the past 2 weeks in the WONCA version, rather than 4 weeks in the original version. Health status is measured in the following areas: physical, emotional, daily activities, social activities, pain, and overall health. The adult charts are widely utilized and have been internationally tested, proving reliability, validity, and acceptability in different forms of practices (Meyboom-de Jong and Smith, 1990; Nelson et al, 1990a; Shigemoto, 1990; Westbury, 1990; Wong-Chung et al, 1991; Bass, 1992; Hays and Shapiro, 1992; Landgraf and Nelson, 1992; Meyboom-de Jong and Smith, 1992; Bruusgaard et al, 1993; de Haan et al, 1993; Froom et al, 1993; Siu et al, 1993a, 1993b; Goertz, 1994; Hickey et al, 1994; Krousel-Wood et al, 1994).

The nine charts included in the Dartmouth COOP Chart system may be used together or individually selected to better fulfill the needs of a certain patient population and/or of a certain discipline of health care provision. More specifically, in a neuromusculoskeletal type of practice, four of the nine charts track outcomes quite well while the others tend to change more slowly. These four include:

- Daily activities
- Pain
- Feelings
- Social activities

These four charts tend to be more sensitive to change over time than the other charts in an orthopedic injury type of practice. However, this may not be true in all instances. For example, those who manage a geriatric population may find benefit by including the **social support chart,** as this often becomes an issue when treating the widowed or childless population. Similarly, the **physical fitness chart** may be practical when assessing sedentary individuals such as in a work hardening or rehabilitation center, as a change in this scale would verify improved activity level if compliance with exercise prescription is being practiced. The

quality of life chart does not change in a short amount of time, and, therefore, is perhaps best used at baseline and at discharge or 1 year. The **overall health chart** is, in a sense, a summary of all the charts and may be used as such if desired. The **change in health chart** may be a practical outcome device for the internist or surgeon as this tool may provide documentation that supports "medical necessity" of a treatment for an acute or chronic illness. In essence, there are no specific "rules" or boundaries for the HCP to abide by. Rather, choosing the charts to match the type of practice of the individual HCP or of a specific patient type may yield the most valid and practical results (Wasson, personal communication, 1998).

The COOP charts were validated and found reliable using comparable methods to other studied instruments, including the RAND heath status measures (Ware et al, 1980), the Sickness Index Profile (Pollard et al, 1976; Bergner et al, 1981), and the Duke–UNC Health Profile (Parkerson et al, 1981). The results of the COOP compared to these instruments are similar (Nelson et al, 1996). Moreover, when comparing the COOP to the MOS or SF-36, very similar scores are also observed (Table 5–7). Table 5–8 offers a formula for translating the COOP chart average scores to an estimated SF-36 score.

The COOP health charts have been used in a study in which telephone care was used as a substitute for routine clinic follow-up visits (Wasson et al, 1992a). More specifically, in this 2 year study, 497 men aged 54 years or older were studied with the hypothesis that telephone calls for some clinic visits would reduce medical care utilization without adversely affecting patient health. Several interesting findings were noted in the telephone care group. Telephone calls averaged less than 10 minutes per call and resulted in:

- 19% fewer total clinic visits
- 14% less medication use
- 28% fewer total hospital days with 41% fewer intensive care unit days
- 28% less total expenditures for the 2 years with sav-

Table 5–7: Comparison of MOS SF-36 Multi-item Scale Score with COOP Chart Scores for Patients with Hypertension, Diabetes, and Depression

DOMAIN	HYPERTENSION		DIABETES		DEPRESSIVE SYMPTOMS	
	COOP	MOS	COOP	MOS	COOP	MOS
Physical	49	49	48	48	49	50
Emotional	52	52	52	53	42	43
Daily activities	51	50	51	50	47	46
Social activities	52	52	51	50	44	45
Pain	50	50	51	50	47	47
Overall health	51	51	51	48	47	45

Modified from Nelson et al, 1990a.

Table 5–8: Formula for Translation of COOP Chart Average Scores to an Estimated SF-36 Score

MOS SCORE TO BE PREDICTED	TRANSLATION	COOP CHART ITEM
Physical	105.6 minus (Physical times 13.5)	Physical
Mental health	96.2 minus (Emotional times 12.1)	Feelings
Social activities	104.1 minus (Social times 14.4)	Social activities
Pain	98.5 minus (Pain times 11.4)	Pain
Role—Physical	88.7 minus (Daily activities times 18.5)	Daily activities
Role—Emotional	94.6 minus (Daily activities times 14.3)	Daily activities
Overall health	105.6 minus (Overall times 11.6)	Overall health

Modified from Nelson et al, 1990a.

ings of $1,656 and a somewhat greater savings of $1,976 with patients who scored fair or poor overall health at the beginning of the study. In the latter subgroup, improvement in physical function from baseline and a possible reduction in mortality ($p = .06$) were also noted.

A method of tabulating the scores of the Dartmouth COOP Health Charts at multiple examination dates is located in Appendix Form A–8.

SICKNESS INDEX PROFILE

The Sickness Index Profile (SIP) (Pollard et al, 1976; Bergner et al, 1981) consists of 136 questions that are grouped into 12 categories, as follows: sleep and rest, eating, work, home management, recreation and pastimes, ambulation, mobility, body care and movement, social interaction, alertness behavior, emotional behavior, and communication. Unlike the SF-36, which takes approximately 15 minutes to complete, the SIP takes approximately 30 minutes. The SIP includes the tracking of issues that range from simple activities of daily living (ADL) scales to those belonging to the abnormal illness behavior category. The reliability of the SIP was reported with test–retest coefficients between .88 and .92 (Pollard et al, 1976). Also, higher reliability was found with interview-administration versus the self-administered approach. Deyo (1986) evaluated a shorter version of the SIP and reported that its reliability was equal to that of the full-length SIP. Due to its length and other documentation demands that are necessary for completion, the SIP has been used primarily in research settings. Similar to the SIP, the Quality of Well-Being Scale (QWBS) (Kaplan and Anderson, 1982), although valid and reliable, is complex and lengthy, and therefore, is also used primarily in research settings. Aspects of these instruments have been utilized in the formation of newer, briefer instruments such as the HSQ/SF-36.

NOTTINGHAM HEALTH PROFILE

The Nottingham Health Profile (NHP), on a 0–100 scale, measures six aspects of perceived health: pain during daily activities, reduced mobility, fatigue, disturbed sleep, emotional problems, and social isolation. This instrument was used in a low back pain study conducted in the Netherlands which categorized patients into an acute, subacute, or chronic category and was found reliable and sensitive to measure change over time (van den Hoogen et al, 1997).

Conclusion

One of the objectives of this chapter was to introduce the HCP to various methods of collecting general health information. The instruments discussed in this chapter are by no means representative of all the tools currently available to capture general health issues. Although I have had no experience with the SIP, QWBS, and NHP instruments, I have found the COOP and the SF-36/HSQ-2.0 to be practical and clinically helpful. Some authors feel other instruments, such as condition-specific tools (eg, the Oswestry Low Back Disability Questionnaire), may make better OA devices; however, I have found at least some of the scales—such as physical function, pain, and role (physical) of the SF-36 (MOS-36, HSQ-2.0, RAND-36, etc)—to be sensitive to change over time and parallel the patient's symptomatology quite well. In addition, outcomes-based research is becoming more and more prevalent as authors are becoming more reliant on patient-based information and less fixated on "objective" HCP- or test-based information. Also, by making use of the three depression screening questions located at the end of the HSQ-2.0, the HCP can address depression clinically, an important risk factor of chronicity. The GHQ should be completed at least at baseline (initial visit) and at discharge. If, however, there are no condition-specific questionnaires for the patient's specific condition, it is my opinion that the GHQ should be done on a monthly basis or at times of re-examination.

REFERENCES

Albert TJ, Mesa JJ, Eng K, McIntosh TC, Balderston RA. Health outcome assessment before and after lumbar laminectomy for radiculopathy. *Spine*. 1996;21:960–963.

American College of Physicians, Health and Public Policy Committee. Comprehensive functional assessment for elderly patients. *Ann Intern Med*. 1988;10:1111.

Bass MJ. Assessing functional status in family practice. *Fam Med*. 1992;24(2):134–135.

Bergner M, Bobbitt RA, Carter WB, Gilson BS. The Sickness Index Profile: Development and final revision of a health status measure. *Med Care*. 1981;19:787–809.

Brazier J, Harper R, Jones SN. Validating the SF-36 health survey questionnaire: New outcome measure for primary care. *Br Med J*. 1992;305:160–164.

Bronfort G. Chiropractic spinal adjustive therapy and exercise versus pharmacological treatment and exercise for chronic low back pain. In: *Proceedings of the 1992 International Conference on Spinal Manipulation*. Arlington, Va: Foundation for Chiropractic Education and Research; 1992.

Brook RH, Fink A, Kosecoff J, et al. Educating physicians and treating patients in the ambulatory setting: Where are we going and how will we know when we arrive? *Ann Intern Med*. 1987;107:392–398.

Bruusgaard D, Nessloy I, Rutle O, et al. Measuring functional status in a population survey. The Dartmouth COOP functional health assessment charts/WONCA used in an epidemiological study. *Fam Pract*. 1993: 10(2):212–218.

Davies AR, Ware JE. *Measuring Health Perceptions in the Health Insurance Experiment*. Santa Monica, Calif: RAND Corporation; 1981 (Publication no. R-2711-HHS).

de Haan R, Aaronson N, Limburg M, et al. Measuring quality of life in stroke. *Stroke*. 1993;24(2):320–327.

Deyo RA. Comparative validity of the Sickness Impact Profile. *Spine*. 1986;11:951–954.

Donald CA, Ware JE. The measurement of social support. In: Greenley JR, ed. *Research in Community and Mental Health*. Greenwich, Conn: JAI Press; 1984:325–370.

Fowler FJ, Wennberg JE, Timothy RP, Barry MJ, Mulley AG, Henley D. Symptom status and quality of life following prostatectomy. *JAMA*. 1988;259:3018–3022.

Froom J, Schlager DS, Steneker S, Jaffe A. Detection of major depressive disorder in primary care patients. *J Am Board Fam Pract*. 1993;6(1):5–11.

Goertz CMH. Measuring functional health status in the chiropractic office using self-report questionnaires. *Top Clin Chiro*. 1994;1(1):51–59.

Hays RD, Shapiro MF. An overview of generic health-related quality of life measures for HIV research. *Qual Life Res*. 1992;1(2):91–97.

Hickey ME, Carter JS, Davis SM. Adaptation of Dartmouth COOP charts for a Pueblo Native American population. *J Gen Intern Med*. 1994;9(2):105.

Kaplan RM, Anderson JP. A general health policy model: Update and applications. *Health Serv Res.* 1982; 23:203–235.

Krousel-Wood MA, McCune TW, Abdoh A. Predicting work status for patients in an occupational medicine setting who report back pain. *Arch Fam Med.* 1994;3(4):349–355.

Landgraf JM, Nelson EC. Summary of the WONCA/COOP international health assessment field trial. *Aust Fam Physician.* 1992;21(3):255–257,260–262,266–269.

Landgraf JM, Nelson EC, Hays RD, et al. Assessing function: Does it really make a difference? A preliminary evaluation of the acceptability and utility of the COOP function charts. In: Lipkin M Jr, ed. *Functional Status Measurement in Primary Care: Frontiers of Primary Care.* New York, NY: Springer-Verlag; 1990:150–165.

Larson CO, Hays RD, Nelson EC. Do the pictures influence scores on the Dartmouth COOP charts? *Qual Life Res.* 1992;1:247–249.

Likert, R. A technique for the measurement of attitudes. *Arch Psych.* 1932;140:5–55.

Lurie N, Ward NB, Shapiro KF, Brook RH. Termination from Medi-Cal: Does it affect health? *N Engl J Med.* 1984;311:480–484.

Manning WG, Newhouse JP, Ware JE. The status of health in demand estimation: Beyond excellent, good, fair, and poor. In: Fuchs VR, ed. *Economic Aspects of Health.* Chicago, Ill: University of Chicago Press; 1982. (Also RAND publication no. R-2696-HHS.)

McHorney CA, Ware JE, Rogers W, et al. The validity and relative precision of MOS short and long-form Health Status Scales and Dartmouth COOP charts: Results from the Medical Outcomes Study. *Med Care.* 1992;30(5):MS253–MS265.

Meyboom-de Jong B, Smith RJA. Studies with the Dartmouth COOP charts in general practice: Comparison with the Nottingham Health Profile and the General Health Questionnaire. In: Lipkin M Jr, ed. *Functional Status Measurement in Primary Care: Frontiers of Primary Care.* New York, NY: Springer-Verlag; 1990:132–149.

Meyboom-de Jong BM, Smith RJ. How do we classify functional status? *Fam Med.* 1992;24(2):128–133.

Montgomery EA, Paranjpe AV. *A Report Card on HMOs 1980–1984.* Menlo Park, Calif: Henry J. Kaiser Family Foundation; 1985.

Nelson EC, Conger B, Douglass R, et al. Functional health status level of primary care patients. *JAMA.* 1983;249:3331–3338.

Nelson EC, Landgraf JM, Hays RD, et al. The COOP function charts: A system to measure patient function in physicians' offices. In: Lipkin M Jr, ed. *Functional Status Measurement in Primary Care: Frontiers of Primary Care.* New York, NY: Springer-Verlag; 1990a:97–131.

Nelson EC, Landgraf JM, Hays RD, Wasson JH, Kirk JW. The functional status of patients: How can it be measured in physicians' offices? *Med Care.* 1990b;28(12):1111–1126.

Nelson EC, Wasson JH, Johnson DJ, Hays RD. Dartmouth COOP functional health assessment charts: Brief measures for clinical practice. In: Spilker B, ed. *Quality of Life and Pharmacoeconomics in Clinical Trials.* 2nd ed. Philadelphia, Pa: Lippincott-Raven; 1996:161–168.

Nelson EC, Wasson JH, Kirk J, et al. Assessment of function in routine clinical practice: Description of the COOP chart method and preliminary findings. *J Chronic Dis.* 1987;40(S1):55S–63S.

Parkerson GR, Gehlbach SH, Wagner EH, et al. The Duke–UNC health profile: An adult health status instrument for primary care. *Med Care.* 1981;19:806.

Pollard WE, Bobbitt RA, Carter WB, et al. The Sickness Impact Profile: Development and final revision of a health status measure. *Health Care.* 1976;19:787.

Read JL, Quinn RJ, Hoefer MA. Measuring overall health: An evaluation of three important approaches. *J Chron Dis.* 1987;40:7S–22S.

Scholten JHG, Van Weel C. *Functional Status Assessment in Family Practice: The Dartmouth COOP Functional Health Assessment Charts/WONCA.* Lelystad, Netherlands: MEDITekst; 1992.

Shigemoto H. A trial of the Dartmouth COOP Charts in Japan. In: Lipkin M Jr, ed. *Functional Status Measurement in Primary Care: Frontiers of Primary Care.* New York, NY: Springer-Verlag; 1990:181–187.

Siu AL, Ouslander JG, Osterweil D, et al. Change in self-reported functioning in older persons entering a residential care facility. *J Clin Epidemiol.* 1993a;46(10):1093–1101.

Siu AL, Reuben DB, Ouslander JG, Osterweil D. Using multidimensional health measures in older persons to identify risk of hospitalization and skilled nursing placement. *Qual Life Res.* 1993b;2(4):253–261.

Spiegel JS, Leake B, Spiegel TM, et al. What are we measuring? An examination of self-reported functional status measures. *Arthritis Rheum.* 1988;31:721–728.

Stewart AL, Ware JE, Brook RH. Advances in the measurement of functional status: Construction of aggregate indexes. *Med Care.* 1981;19:473–488.

Stewart AL, Ware JE, Brook RH, Davies-Avery A. *Conceptualization and Measurement of Health for Adults in the Health Insurance Study. Volume II: Physical Health in Terms of Functioning.* Santa Monica, Calif: RAND Corporation; 1978. (Publication no. R-1987/2-HEW.)

van den Hoogen HJM, Koes BW, van Eijk JTM, et al. Pain and health status of primary care patients with low back pain. *J Fam Pract.* 1997;44(2):187–192.

Ware JE. Scales for measuring general health perceptions. *Health Serv Res.* 1976;11:396–415.

Ware JE, Brook RH, Davies-Avery A, et al. *Conceptualization and Measurement of Health for Adults in the Health Insurance Study. Volume I: Model of Health and Methodology.* Santa Monica, Calif: RAND Corporation; 1980. (Publication no. R-1987/1-HEW.)

Ware JE, Karmos A. *Development and Validation of Scales to Measure Perceived Health and Patient Role Propensity. Volume II: Final Report.* Springfield, Va: National Technical Information Service; 1976. (Publication no. 288–331.)

Ware JE Jr, Kosinski M, Keller SD. *SF-12: How to Score the SF-12 Physical and Mental Health Summary Scales.* 2nd ed. Boston, Mass: Health Institute, New England Medical Center; March 1995.

Ware JE Jr, Kosinski M, Keller SD. *SF-36 Physical and Mental Health Summary Scales: A User's Manual.* Boston, Mass: Health Institute, New England Medical Center; December 1995.

Ware JE, Nelson EC, Sherbourne CD, et al. Preliminary tests of a 6-item general health survey: A patient application. In: Stewart A, Ware JE, eds. *Measuring Functioning and Well-being: The Medical Outcomes Study Approach.* Durham, NC: Duke University Press; 1992a:291–303.

Ware JE, Sherbourne CD, Davies AR. Developing and testing the MOS 20-Item Short-Form Health Survey: A general population application. In: Stewart AL, Ware JE, eds. *Measuring Functioning and Well-being: The Medical Outcomes Study Approach.* Durham, NC: Duke University Press; 1992b:277–290.

Ware JE Jr, Snow KK, Kosinski M, Bandek B. *SF-36 Health Survey: Manual and Interpretation Guide.* Boston, Mass: The Health Institute, New England Medical Center; July 1993.

Wasson J, Gaudette C, Whaley F, Sauvigne A, Baribeau P, Welch G. Telephone care as a substitute for routine clinic follow-up. *JAMA.* 1992a;267:1788–1793

Wasson JH, Kairys SW, Nelson EC, et al. A short survey for assessing health and social problems of adolescents. *J Fam Pract.* 1994;38:489–494.

Wasson J, Keller A, Rubenstein L, Hays R, Nelson E, Johnson D, and the Dartmouth Primary Care COOP Project. Benefits and obstacles of health status assessment in ambulatory settings: The clinician's point of view. *Med Care.* 1992b;30:MS42–MS49.

Westbury RC. Use of the Dartmouth COOP charts in a Calgary practice. In: Lipkin M Jr, ed. *Functional Status Measurement in Primary Care: Frontiers of Primary Care.* New York, NY: Springer-Verlag; 1990:166–180.

Wong-Chung D, Mateijsen N, West R. et al. Assessing the functional status during an asthma attack with Dartmouth COOP charts. Validity with respect to change in asthma. *Fam Pract.* 1991;8(4):404–408.

CHAPTER 6

Assessment of Pain

STEVEN G. YEOMANS

INTRODUCTION

It seems appropriate in the discussion of pain assessment to first address the definition of pain. Pain can be defined as "an unpleasant sensory and emotional experience associated with actual or potential tissue damage, or described in terms of such damage" (Merskey et al, 1994). *Stedman's Medical Dictionary* (1982) defines pain as "an unpleasant sensory and emotional experience." *Webster's New Collegiate Dictionary* (1980) defines pain as "a basic bodily sensation induced by a noxious stimulus, received by naked nerve endings, characterized by physical discomfort (as pricking, throbbing, or aching), and typically leading to evasive action." A complete listing of pain-related terms can be found in Table 6–1.

Pain is always subjective, as each individual learns through experiences related to injury. Stimuli that cause pain are considered by biologists as being indicative of tissue damage. Hence, pain is the experience associated with actual or potential tissue damage. Because pain is always unpleasant, it is, therefore, also an emotional experience. **Sensations that resemble pain but are not unpleasant, such as numbness or tingling, should not be called pain** (Merskey, 1994). Refer to Table 6–1 where pain terminology is defined (Merskey, 1994).

Many textbooks have been devoted to the topic of pain and its many mechanisms. It is beyond the scope of this text to discuss the many important related topics such as the peripheral mechanisms and central processing of pain transmission. For additional information regarding this subject, refer to Chapter 8 regarding chronic pain behavior and to Chapters 10 and 21 regarding disability prediction. The goal of this chapter is to offer the health care provider (HCP) a practical means by which pain can be measured and documented. With this in mind, several instruments that have been previously studied and found to meet reliability and validity criteria are discussed. It is important to stress that this chapter is not intended as an exhaustive literature search of pain measuring instruments. Rather, highlights of some very practical tools that can easily be adapted into a busy clinical setting are discussed.

Table 6–1: Pain Terms

Pain

An unpleasant sensory and emotional experience associated with actual or potential tissue damage, or described in terms of such damage.

Note: Pain is always subjective. Each individual learns the application of the word through experiences related to injury in early life. Biologists recognize that those stimuli which cause pain are liable to damage tissue. Accordingly, pain is that experience we associate with actual or potential tissue damage. It is unquestionably a sensation in a part or parts of the body, but it is also always unpleasant and therefore also an emotional experience. Experiences which resemble pain but are not unpleasant (eg, pricking) should not be called pain. Unpleasant abnormal experiences (dysesthesias) may also be pain but are not necessarily so because, subjectively, they may not have the usual sensory qualities of pain.

Many people report pain in the absence of tissue damage or any likely pathophysiological cause; usually this happens for psychological reasons. There is usually no way to distinguish their experience from that due to tissue damage if we take the subjective report. If they regard their experience as pain and if they report it in the same ways as pain caused by tissue damage, it should be accepted as pain. This definition avoids tying pain to the stimulus. Activity induced in the nociceptive pathways by a noxious stimulus is not pain, which is always a psychological state, even though we may well appreciate that pain most often has a proximate physical cause.

Allodynia

Pain due to a stimulus that does not normally provoke pain.

Note: The term *allodynia* was originally introduced to separate from hyperalgesia and hyperesthesia, the conditions seen in patients with lesions of the nervous system where touch, light pressure, or moderate cold or warmth evoke pain when applied to apparently normal skin. *Allo* means "other" in Greek and is a common prefix for medical conditions that diverge from the expected. *Odynia* is derived from the Greek word "odune" or "odyne," which is used in "pleurodynia" and "coccydynia" and is similar in meaning to the root from which we derive words with -algia or -algesia in them. Allodynia was suggested following discussions with Professor Paul Potter of the Department of the History of Medicine and Science at the University of Western Ontario.

The words "to normal skin" were used in the original definition but later were omitted in order to remove any suggestion that allodynia applied only to referred pain. Originally, also, the pain-provoking stimulus was described as "non-noxious." However, a stimulus may be noxious at some times and not at others, for example, with intact skin and sunburned skin, and also, the boundaries of noxious stimulation may be hard to delimit. Since the Committee (International Association for the Study of Pain [IASP]) aimed at providing terms for clinical use, it did not wish to define them by reference to the specific physical characteristics of the stimulation (eg, pressure in kilopascals per square centimeter). Moreover, even in intact skin there is little evidence one way or the other that a strong painful pinch to a normal person does not damage tissue. Accordingly, it was considered to be preferable to define allodynia in terms of the response to clinical stimuli and to point out that the normal response to the stimulus could almost always be tested elsewhere in the body, usually in a corresponding part. Further, allodynia is taken to apply to conditions which may give rise to sensitization of the skin (eg, sunburn, inflammation, trauma).

It is important to recognize that allodynia involves a change in the quality of a sensation, whether tactile, thermal, or of any other sort. The original modality is normally nonpainful, but the response is painful. There is thus a loss of specificity of a sensory modality. By contrast, hyperalgesia (qv) represents an augmented response in a specific mode, namely, pain. With other cutaneous modalities, hyperesthesia is the term which corresponds to hyperalgesia, and as with hyperalgesia, the quality is not altered. In allodynia the stimulus mode and the response mode differ, unlike the situation with hyperalgesia. This distinction should not be confused by the fact that allodynia and hyperalgesia can be plotted with overlap along the same continuum of physical intensity in certain circumstances; for example, with pressure or temperature.

See also the notes on *hyperalgesia* and *hyperpathia*.

Analgesia

Absence of pain in response to stimulation that would normally be painful.

Note: As with allodynia (qv), the stimulus is defined by its usual subjective effects.

Anesthesia dolorosa

Pain in an area or region which is anesthetic.

Causalgia

A syndrome of sustained burning pain, allodynia, and hyperpathia after a traumatic nerve lesion, often combined with vasomotor and sudomotor dysfunction and later trophic changes.

Table 6–1: (cont.)

Central pain

Pain initiated or caused by a primary lesion or dysfunction in the central nervous system.

Dysesthesia

An unpleasant abnormal sensation, whether spontaneous or evoked.

Note: Compare with pain and with paresthesia. Special cases of dysesthesia include hyperalgesia and allodynia. A dysesthesia should always be unpleasant and a paresthesia should not be unpleasant, although it is recognized that the borderline may present some difficulties when it comes to deciding as to whether a sensation is pleasant or unpleasant. It should always be specified whether the sensations are spontaneous or evoked.

Hyperalgesia

An increased response to a stimulus that is normally painful.

Note: Hyperalgesia reflects increased pain on suprathreshold stimulation. For pain evoked by stimuli that usually are not painful, the term allodynia is preferred, while hyperalgesia is more appropriately used for cases with an increased response at a normal threshold, or at an increased threshold (eg, in patients with neuropathy). It should also be recognized that with allodynia the stimulus and the response are in different modes, whereas with hyperalgesia they are in the same mode. Current evidence suggests that hyperalgesia is a consequence of perturbation of the nociceptive system with peripheral or central sensitization, or both, but it is important to distinguish between the clinical phenomena, which this definition emphasizes, and the interpretation, which may well change as knowledge advances.

Hyperesthesia

Increased sensitivity to stimulation, excluding the special senses.

Note: The stimulus and locus should be specified. Hyperesthesia may refer to various modes of cutaneous sensibility including touch and thermal sensation without pain, as well as to pain. The word is used to indicate both diminished threshold to any stimulus and an increased response to stimuli that are normally recognized.

Allodynia is suggested for pain after stimulation that is not normally painful. Hyperesthesia includes both allodynia and hyperalgesia, but the more specific terms should be used wherever they are applicable.

Hyperpathia

A painful syndrome characterized by an abnormally painful reaction to a stimulus, especially a repetitive stimulus, as well as an increased threshold.

Note: It may occur with allodynia, hyperesthesia, hyperalgesia, or dysesthesia. Faulty identification and localization of the stimulus, delay, radiating sensation, and after-sensation may be present, and the pain is often explosive in character. The changes in this note are the specification of allodynia and the inclusion of hyperalgesia explicitly. Previously hyperalgesia was implied, since hyperesthesia was mentioned in the previous note and the hyperalgesia is a special case of hyperesthesia.

Hypoalgesia

Diminished pain in response to a normally painful stimulus.

Note: Hypoalgesia was formerly defined as diminished sensitivity to noxious stimulation, making it a particular case of hypoesthesia (qv). However, it now refers only to the occurrence of relatively less pain in response to stimulation that produces pain. Hypoesthesia covers the case of diminished sensitivity to stimulation that is normally painful.

The implications of some of the above definitions may be summarized for convenience as follows:

Allodynia	Lowered threshold	Stimulus and response mode differ
Hyperalgesia	Increased response	Stimulus and response mode are the same
Hyperpathia	Raised threshold; increased response	Stimulus and response mode may be the same or different
Hypoalgesia	Raised threshold; lowered response	Stimulus and response mode are the same

The above essentials of the definitions do not have to be symmetrical and are not symmetrical at present. Lowered threshold may occur with allodynia but is not required. Also, there is no category for lowered threshold and lowered response—if it ever occurs.

(Continued)

Table 6–1: (cont.)

Hypoesthesia

Decreased sensitivity to stimulation, excluding the special senses.

Note: Stimulation and locus to be specified.

Neuralgia

Pain in the distribution of a nerve or nerves.

Note: Common usage, especially in Europe, often implies a paroxysmal quality, but neuralgia should not be reserved for paroxysmal pains.

Neuritis

Inflammation of a nerve or nerves.

Note: Not to be used unless inflammation is thought to be present.

Neurogenic pain

Pain initiated or caused by a primary lesion, dysfunction, or transitory perturbation in the peripheral or central nervous system.

Neuropathic pain

Pain initiated or caused by a primary lesion or dysfunction in the nervous system.

Note: See also *neurogenic pain* and *central pain*. Peripheral neuropathic pain occurs when the lesion or dysfunction affects the peripheral nervous system. Central pain may be retained as the term when the lesion or dysfunction affects the central nervous system.

Neuropathy

A disturbance of function or pathological change in a nerve: in one nerve, mononeuropathy; in several nerves, mononeuropathy multiplex; if diffuse and bilateral, polyneuropathy.

Note: Neuritis (qv) is a special case of neuropathy and is now reserved for inflammatory processes affecting nerves. Neuropathy is not intended to cover cases such as neurapraxia, neurotmesis, section of a nerve, or transitory impact like a blow, stretching, or an epileptic discharge. The term *neurogenic* applies to pain due to such temporary perturbations.

Nociceptor

A receptor preferentially sensitive to a noxious stimulus or to a stimulus that would become noxious if prolonged.

Note: Avoid use of terms such as pain receptor, pain pathway, and so on.

Noxious stimulus

A noxious stimulus is one that is damaging to normal tissues.

Note: Although the definition of a noxious stimulus has been retained, the term is not used in this list to define other terms.

Pain threshold

The least experience of pain that a subject can recognize.

Note: Traditionally the threshold has often been defined, as we defined it formerly, as the least stimulus intensity at which a subject perceives pain. Properly defined, the threshold is really the experience of the patient, whereas the intensity measured is an external event. It has been common usage for most pain research workers to define the threshold in terms of the stimulus, and that should be avoided. However, the threshold stimulus can be recognized as such and measured. In psychophysics, thresholds are defined as the level at which 50% of stimuli are recognized. In that case, the pain threshold would be the level at which 50% of stimuli would be recognized as painful. The stimulus is not pain (qv) and cannot be a measure of pain.

Pain tolerance level

The greatest level of pain that a subject is prepared to tolerate.

Note: As with pain threshold, the pain tolerance level is the subjective experience of the individual. The stimuli that are normally measured in relation to its production are the pain tolerance level stimuli and not the level itself. Thus, the same argument applies to pain tolerance level as to pain threshold, and it is not defined in terms of the external stimulation as such.

Table 6–1: (cont.)

Paresthesia

An abnormal sensation, whether spontaneous or evoked.

Note: Compare with dysesthesia. After much discussion, it has been agreed to recommend that paresthesia be used to describe an abnormal sensation that is not unpleasant while dysesthesia be used preferentially for an abnormal sensation that is considered to be unpleasant. The use of one term (paresthesia) to indicate spontaneous sensations and the other to refer to evoked sensations is not favored. There is a sense in which, since paresthesia refers to abnormal sensations in general, it might included dysesthesia, but the reverse is not true. Dysesthesia does not include all abnormal sensations, but only those which are unpleasant.

Peripheral neurogenic pain

Pain initiated or caused by a primary lesion or dysfunction or transitory perturbation in the peripheral nervous system.

Peripheral neuropathic pain

Pain initiated or caused by a primary lesion or dysfunction in the peripheral nervous system.

From Merskey et al, 1994, 207–213.

MEASUREMENT OF PAIN SEVERITY

The measurement of pain severity, like the optometrist's assessment of visual acuity, is dependent on the person experiencing the pain. Typically, a scale is used whereby the person who is experiencing the pain matches numbers or words to pain intensity. Both the HCP and the person experiencing the pain have critical roles in the pain assessment process. The HCP must choose a valid and reliable scaling method, record the reported values, and utilize the information in concert with the other historical data. Other pertinent information about the pain experience, such as the relative intensity of the painful sensation, its spatial distribution, and its qualities, are also appropriate to gather. **The measurement of pain is similar to the assessment of vision, audition, taste, and smell, in that the accuracy of the assessment is dependent on the efforts of the HCP and the person experiencing pain** (Price, 1994).

PAIN SCALES

Two basic approaches can be utilized regarding direct scaling methods for pain measurement (Guilford, 1954). The first is the rating scale method, in which subjects rate their pain intensity on scales with clearly defined numerical intervals or on a verbal rating scale, where words directly indicate a length rank order. The second is the direct magnitude scaling procedure, which utilizes continuous scales of sensation intensity without the constraints of categories or whole numbers. Direct magnitude scaling is reliant on the subject's ability to report the perceived intensity of one type of sensation by responses on another physical continuum. For example, patients can adjust the volume or sound intensity to represent the perceived pain intensity where an unlimited number of sound intensities exist. Similarly, patients can use an unlimited number of line lengths or distances along a visual analogue scale (VAS) to quickly represent their pain intensity.

Visual Analogue Scales

Visual analogue scales have become very popular in pain research and in the clinical assessment of pain. Reliability and validity have been reported (Jensen and Karoly, 1993) and several distinct advantages over other measurement methods have been published (Scott and Huskisson, 1976; Price et al, 1986a, 1986b; Price and Harkins, 1987; Price et al, 1994). For example, some VASs provide accurate measurements of ratios of pain intensity and include information regarding percent changes (Price and Harkins, 1987; Price, 1988). Another advantage is the ability to use a specific type of visual analogue scale in a very consistent manner to rate distinct types of pain such as low back, myofascial pain, jaw pain, as well as **experimental pain** (pain purposefully induced in a laboratory) (Price and Harkins, 1987). A psychophysical procedure using a VAS in a psychological setting to rate clinical versus experimental pain has also been reported (Gracely, 1979; Price et al, 1983). The VAS can also be adopted to measure pain sensation intensity and pain unpleasantness, or pain-related emotional disturbance, separately (Price et al, 1983, 1986a, 1986b, 1994).

Quadruple Visual Analogue Scale

Another specific application of the VAS is called the quadruple VAS (Von Korff et al, 1992). The quadruple VAS is based on four specific factors:

1. Pain level at the time of the current office visit
2. Usual or average pain since the last visit (or since the initial visit or, since the onset of the condition, depending on the chronicity of the condition)
3. Peak or maximum pain level since the last visit, time of intake, or since the onset of the condition.
4. Pain level at best. (See Appendix Form B–1.)

For the chronic patient, the HCP should request the patient's "average pain grade" as it relates to the last 6 months. The ratings are averaged and then multiplied by 10 to yield a score from 0 to 100 (Von Korff et al, 1992). The final score can then be categorized as "low intensity" (pain < 50); or "high intensity" (pain > 50). Instructions given to the patient regarding the usual or average pain level should be as simple as possible as complex questions such as "changes in lifestyle caused by pain" carry a higher failure rate (Ogan et al, 1996). There is also evidence that current pain may be routinely reported as less intense compared to average pain due to a memory artifact. Therefore, small improvements in pain intensity levels should be interpreted with caution. There is also evidence that patients with chronic pain may have more accurate recall regarding the "least pain" than "usual" or "worst" pain level. Furthermore, the most valid approach regarding the calculation of usual or average pain may be the mean between the least and usual pain level (Erskin et al, 1990; Jensen et al, 1996). Because symptoms other than pain, such as numbness, may be predominant, using appropriate anchor terms such as "unpleasantness" may yield a more accurate report. The VAS can also be given to the patient to take home to record changes in pain or unpleasantness over time. A parent can also track a child's symptoms utilizing the VAS. The VAS, like other measures of a patient's progress, should be performed every 2 weeks, since a patient's failure to progress over a 2-week period may indicate a need for a change in management approaches (Haldeman et al, 1993).

Numerical Pain Scale

The *Numerical Pain Scale (NPS)* (Chapman-Smith, 1992) or numerical rating scale (NRS) contains 11 numbers (0–10); the patient circles the appropriate number to represent his or her pain level. Various reports suggest that the VAS is more reliable than the NPS because a patient cannot memorize the numbers in a VAS. However, one study found the VAS and NPS instruments to be comparable (McDowell and Newell, 1987) while two found the NPS to be superior (Downie et al, 1978; Bolton and Wilkinson, 1998). More specifically, Bolton and Wilkinson (1998) compared the VAS to the verbal rating scale (VRS) and the 0 to 10, 11-point NRS in 79 first-time-presenting patients who were administered the instruments in an outpatient clinic setting. The first questionnaire was completed prior to initiating treatment and the second questionnaire was administered 6 weeks after initiating care. Of the three methods, the NRS proved to be the most responsive of the measures (effect size = .86) compared to the VAS (effect size = .77) and the VRS (effect size = .76). Interestingly, when patients were asked to report their *usual* level of pain, the responsiveness of all three methods was enhanced (effect size = 1.34, 1.34, and 1.12 for the NRS, VAS, and VRS, respectively). The authors concluded that the improved ease of completing and scoring of the 11-point NRS and the method of asking patients to report their usual pain levels versus their current pain levels, enhances the responsiveness of the measures and is a more representative perspective of their pain experience. The utility of the NPS appears to favor its utilization in a clinical setting, although arguments have been presented regarding the ability of the patient to memorize prior pain levels and, hence, to skew the results. In practice, both NPSs and VASs are commonly used to track outcomes of treatment and/or rehabilitation programs addressing changes in pain levels as well as activities of daily living (ADL) levels or changes (Vernon, 1995). The Mercy Center Conference document regarding quality assurance includes severe pain intensity (> 6/10) as one of four factors that can be used to document that the patient is more complicated than usual and that case management of acute low back pain may be appropriate for 12 to 16 weeks rather than 6 to 8 weeks (Haldeman et al, 1993). Subsequently, this category may function as an important factor in assessing the prognosis of a case.

Similarly, ordinal (numerical) scales can be applied to fear of pain, fear of reinjury, coping strategies regarding pain, as well as estimating the likeliness of the patient returning to work (see Appendix Form B–2) (Vernon, 1996).

OTHER METHODS OF PAIN MEASUREMENT: McGILL/MELZACK PAIN QUESTIONNAIRE

In addition to the VAS (Dworkin et al, 1990; Von Korff et al, 1992; Chapman-Smith, 1992; Von Korff et al, 1993), there are other methods of pain oriented outcome measuring. More specifically, the McGill/Melzack Pain Questionnaire (Melzack, 1975, 1982; Chapman-Smith, 1992), and the pain diagram (Ransford et al, 1976; Kirkaldy-Willis, 1983), are examples of instruments used to measure outcomes from a pain assessment approach.

The *McGill/Melzack Pain Questionnaire (MPQ)* (Melzack, 1982) is an option for measuring pain outcomes with respect to pain quality. Introduced in 1975, it has been widely utilized and can be considered a "gold standard" as a pain assessment tool (Vernon, 1996). There are 20 category scales of verbal descriptors of pain, which are categorized in order of severity and clustered into four subscales:

1. Sensory discrimination
2. Affective
3. Evaluative
4. Miscellaneous

In addition, a 5-point pain rating index representing present pain is included. A total score or separate scores for each subscale can be calculated. **The McGill/Melzack Pain Questionnaire is unique in that it can discriminate between the sensory and the affective domains of the pain experience.** Test–retest reliability was first reported at 70% response consistency for three trials applied over a 3-day period (Melzack, 1975). Similar results have been reported in a study that conducted four trials within 1 week (Allen and Weinmann, 1982). Patients suffering from headaches were studied utilizing the MPQ, revealing the following correlation coefficients:

Present Pain Index:
Total score	$r = .94$
Sensory scale	$r = .83$
Affective scale	$r = .95$

These findings support the ability of the patient to remember, in a relatively short time period, his or her pain state between two measurement time intervals. Numerous studies regarding the validity of the MPQ, especially the sensory and affective scales, have been reported (Reading, 1979; Byrne et al, 1982; Prieto and Geisinger, 1983; Pearse and Morley, 1989). Vernon (1996) reports that concurrent validity has been confirmed between the MPQ and the Minnesota Multiphasic Personality Inventory (MMPI), as well as many other instruments that measure pain intensity, mood associated with pain, and psychosocial disturbance. Discriminant validity was reported utilizing only the MPQ score in a study in which 77% of 95 patients were correctly categorized into diagnostic groups (Dubuisson and Melzack, 1976). Those suffering from acute disorders were found to utilize more sensory words compared to patients with chronic disorders, who used more affective and evaluative words (Reading, 1979). The MPQ has also been used and found to be sensitive in many treatment trials (Burkhardt, 1984).

A short form of the McGill has also been validated and found reliable (see Appendix Form B–3) (Melzack, 1987; Feuerstein, 1995). In this form, the descriptors 1 to 11 represent the sensory dimension of pain while descriptors 12 to 15 represent the affective dimension. Each descriptor is ranked on an intensity scale (0 = none, 1 = mild, 2 = moderate, 3 = severe). The Present Pain Intensity (PPI) of the standard long-form MPQ and the VAS are also included to provide overall pain intensity scores (Melzack, 1987).

MEASUREMENT OF PAIN LOCATION: PAIN DIAGRAM

As previously discussed, pain intensity, quality, duration, and location must be reported in a clinical file. The pain diagram is a very useful tool for recording location of pain. It is a patient-reported document that measures the location and, to some extent, quality of pain which the HCP can quickly scan to determine the location, radiation, and quality of a presenting patient's complaint.

The pain diagram consists of front and back outlines of a body onto which the patient draws, using different symbols to represent different qualities of pain (such as ache, pain, pins and needles, and numbness). **The intent of a pain diagram is to capture a pictorial representation of a patient's verbal pain report.** The pain diagram also reveals

---

information regarding a patient's interpretation of his or her pain as well as mood or psychological state. As a result, the pain diagram may demonstrate whether the patient's pain behavior is appropriate (consistent with the verbal complaint and objective findings) or not (Tait et al, 1990).

Although pain diagrams are used primarily as a qualitative tool, several scoring methods have described pain (Ransford et al, 1976; Kirkaldy-Willis, 1983; Uden et al, 1988; Tait et al, 1990; Parker et al, 1995; Ohlund et al, 1996). A score can be derived from points totaled from the number of body regions marked as painful, and the number of different pain qualities. These marks may be made within the pain diagram outer boundaries or outside the figure. The higher the score, the greater the likelihood of inappropriate pain behavior (Uden et al, 1988; Dworkin et al, 1990; Tait et al, 1990; Von Korff et al, 1993; Parker et al, 1995; Ohlund et al, 1996). The size of the painful area can also be measured; this measurement can serve as a quantitative outcomes tool that is clinically useful, especially when compared to future or past pain diagrams (Feuerstein, 1995). A high degree of reliability has been reported with test–retest correlations for body area ranging between .83 and .93, and a 76% test–retest agreement regarding pain location was reported (Ransford et al, 1976). More recently, the pain diagram was scored by two methods and compared (Ohlund et al, 1996). The **area raw extent assessment (AREA) score** was analyzed concurrently against the penalty point system, and its ability to predict return to work and absenteeism over a 2-year time period. Both content and construct validity (see Chap. 2) was assessed as to the relative influence of medical, psychological, and subjective disability, as well as psychosocial factors. The authors reported criterion validation of the AREA score correlated concurrently against the penalty point score and predictively against occupational handicap. In construct validation, the highest explained variance was shown for medical and psychological factors, and for subjective disability. In addition, variance in the AREA score could also be explained by psychosocial factors. The authors concluded that quantification of the extent of pain depicted on the diagram shows high criterion and construct validity for the AREA score. In addition, content validity was reported for aspects of clinical disability.

However, other studies following the Ransford et al 1976 study have failed to reproduce such results (Baeyer et al, 1983; Hildebrandt et al, 1986; Parker et al, 1995). More specifically, Parker et al compared three popular methods

---

CLINICAL TIP 6–2
Measuring Psychological Distress

The pain diagram is one of the most clinically useful tools due to its utility and practicality as it allows the HCP to be able to quickly triage the presenting patient "at first-glance." However, studies such as that by Parker et al (1995), revealed that three popular scoring methods failed to reliably measure psychological distress from pain drawings. As a result, scoring the pain diagram may not be necessary until more convincing evidence is published that the pain diagram truly can measure this domain.

---

of scoring pain diagrams, all of which were found to be highly reliable but none of which were able to identify distressed patients with sufficient sensitivity or specificity. Also, none were able to differentiate between organic and nonorganic pain patterns. These authors concluded that **the pain diagram has major limitations when used as a screen for psychological distress or to differentiate between organic and nonorganic patterns of pain.** However, they noted a high level of face validity of the pain diagram when used as an introduction to further psychometric assessment. Though it can confirm a presenting clinical picture with reliability, further investigation was recommended to establish what the pain diagram actually measures (Parker et al, 1995).

MEASUREMENT OF PAIN DURATION AND FREQUENCY

The duration and course of a condition can be followed by the use of a pain diary. This patient-reported instrument allows for the monitoring of the duration of painful episodes as well as the pain intensity during the episode, the frequency of painful episodes, medication utilization, and activities of daily living that are affected by the condition (Vernon, 1996). **The pain diary allows for a summary of the pain experience and, therefore, serves as a useful report of find-** ings for patients, insurers, and/or other HCPs. The various categories are often presented in an ordinal or continuous scale with frequency counts, and data regarding time, course, and duration of the complaint. One study that reported on the stability of the pain diary data in a headache population determined that an average of 2 weeks is a sufficient time period to establish a baseline from the diary (Andrassik et al, 1981). In pain syndromes that are constant, stable values can be obtained within days of initial use (Vernon, 1996). The downside of the pain diary includes the bias and Hawthorne effects that can occur, as well as the rare occurrence of completely false and misleading reporting such as in a malingerer. The Hawthorne effect was first described out of an experience that occurred where worker performance was significantly enhanced after management showed interest in their workers' welfare (Chapman-Smith, 1989; Dixon, 1989). Therefore, it is recommended that the pain diary be cross-checked with comparable observer-based data and patient records regarding the clinical status and pain behavior of the patient (Vernon, 1996).

When pain is reported to be intermittent rather than constant, there are two practical questions the HCP can ask the patient: (1) "In a typical 16-hour or wakeful day [assuming the patient obtains 8 hours of sleep], how many hours a day is your pain at a 0/10 pain level?"; (2) "How many hours a day are you at your worst pain level?" The patient's responses allow the HCP to determine the percentage of a day (or a week or a month, if pain is not daily) a patient is at the best or least and at the worst or most pain level (see Appendix Form B–1). By comparing the responses to similar questions at different time intervals, an HCP may better appreciate changes in the frequency and duration of pain.

 CLINICAL ALERT 6–3

Defining the Boundaries of Noxious Stimulation

A stimulus may be noxious at some times and not at others, for example, with intact skin and sunburned skin. Furthermore, the boundaries of noxious stimulation may be hard to define.

Conclusion

The use of pain questionnaire measurement results must be assessed in concert with other outcome assessing tools, the clinical history and examination, and all other pertinent information. By doing so, outcomes-based decision making can be accomplished. Refer to Section V of this text, which discusses in further detail the many uses of outcomes-driven information.

Regardless of the definition and tracking methods, pain is perceived differently by each person. More specifically, a stimulus that greatly affects one person may not provoke any pain response in another. Even though pain is interpreted differently by different people, the common denominator is suffering—which is both a physical as well as a mental process. Moreover, since pain is what typically motivates a person to seek treatment from an HCP, the success of the treatment is usually determined by the degree of pain relief, regardless of whether it is actual (organic) or imagined (nonorganic).

REFERENCES

Allen RA, Weinmann RL. The MPQ in the diagnosis of pain. *Headache*. 1982;22:20–57.

Andrassik F, Blanchard EB, Ahles T, et al. Assessing the reactive as well as the sensory component of headache pain. *Headache*. 1981;21:218.

Baeyer CLV, Berstrom KJ, Brodwin MG, Brodwin SK. Invalid use of pain drawings in psychological screening of back pain patients. *Pain*. 1983;16:103–107.

Bolton JE, Wilkinson RC. Responsiveness of pain scales: A comparison of three pain intensity measures in chiropractic patients. *J Manipulative Physiol Ther*. 1998;21:1–7.

Burkhardt CS. The use of the McGill pain questionnaire in assessing arthritis pain. *Pain*. 1984;19:305.

Byrne M, Troy A, Bradley LA, et al. Cross-validation of the factor structure of the MPQ. *Pain*. 1982;13:193.

Chapman-Smith D. Reflections on the Hawthorne effect. *Chiro Report*. 1989;4:1. Editorial.

Chapman-Smith D. Measuring results—The new importance of patient questionnaires. *Chiro Report*. 1992;7(1):1–6.

Dixon T. In praise of the Hawthorne effect and the philosophies of family medicine. *Can Fam Physician*. 1989;35:703–704 and 743–745. Editorial.

Downie WW, Leatham PA, Rhind VM, Wright V, Branco JA, Anderson JA. Studies with pain rating scales. *Anal Rheum Dis*. 1978;37:378–381.

Dubuisson D, Melzack R. Classification of clinical pain descriptions by multiple group discriminant analysis. *Exp Neurol*. 1976;51:480.

Dworkin SF, Von Korff M, Whitney WC, et al. Measurement of characteristic pain intensity in field research. *Pain Suppl*. 1990;5:S290.

Erskin A, et al. Memory for pain: A review. *Pain*. 1990;41:255–265.

Feuerstein M. Multidisciplinary rehabilitation of occupational musculoskeletal disorders: Rationale, assessment strategies and clinical interventions. LACC Chiropractic Rehabilitation, Session 1; September 23/24, 1995; class notes: 87; Chicago, Ill.

Gracely RH. Psychophysical assessment of human pain. In: Bonica JJ, Liebeskind JC, Albe-Fessard D, eds. *Proceedings of the Second World Congress on Pain. Advances in Pain Research and Therapy*. Vol. 3. New York, NY: Raven Press; 1979:805–824.

Guilford JP. *Psychometric Methods*. New York, NY: McGraw-Hill; 1954:597.

Haldeman S, Chapman-Smith D, Peterson DM Jr. *Guidelines for Chiropractic Quality Assurance and Practice Parameters*. Gaithersburg, Md: Aspen; 1993.

Hildebrandt J, Franz CE, Choroba-Mehnen B, Temme M. The use of pain drawings in screening for psychological involvement in complaints of low back pain. *Spine*. 1986;13:681–685.

Illustrated Stedman's Medical Dictionary. 24th ed. Baltimore, Md: Williams & Wilkins; 1982:1015.

Jensen MP, Karoly P. Self-report scales and procedures for assessing pain in adults. In: Turk DC, Melzack R, eds. *Handbook of Pain Assessment*. New York, NY: Guilford Press; 1993.

Jensen M, Turner L, Turner J, Romano J. The use of multiple-item scales for pain intensity measurement in chronic pain patients. *Pain*. 1996;67:35–40.

Kirkaldy-Willis WH. *Managing Low Back Pain*. New York, NY: Churchill Livingstone; 1983:635.

McDowell I, Newell C. *Measuring Health: A Guide to Rating Scales and Questionnaires*. New York, NY: Oxford University Press; 1987.

Melzack R. The McGill Pain Questionnaire: Major properties and scoring methods. *Pain*. 1975;1:277–279.

Melzack R. *Pain Measurement and Assessment*. New York, NY: Raven Press; 1982.

Melzack R. The short-form McGill Pain Questionnaire. *Pain*. 1987;30:191–197.

Merskey H, Bogduk N, International Association for the Study of Pain Task Force on Taxonomy, eds. *Classification of Chronic Pain: Descriptions of Chronic Pain Syndromes and Definitions of Pain Terms*. Seattle, Wash: IASP Press; 1994:207–213.

Ogon M, Krismer M, Sollner W, Kantner-Rumplmair W, Lampe A. Chronic low back pain measurement with visual analog scales in different settings. *Pain*. 1996;64:425–428.

Ohlund C, Eek C, Palmblad S, Areskoug B, Nachemson A. Quantified pain drawing in subacute low back pain: Validation in a non-selected outpatient industrial sample. *Spine*. 1996;21:1021–1031.

Parker H, Wood PLR, Main CJ. The uses of the pain drawing as a screening measure to predict psychological distress in chronic low back pain. *Spine*. 1995;20:236–243.

Pearse J, Morley S. An experimental investigation of the construct validity of the McGill Pain Questionnaire. *Pain*. 1989;39:115.

Price DD. *Psychological and Neural Mechanisms of Pain.* New York, NY: Raven Press; 1988.

Price DD, Bush FM, Long S, Harkins SW. A comparison of pain measurement characteristics of mechanical visual analogue and simple numerical rating scales. *Pain.* 1994;56:216–226.

Price DD, Harkins SW. The combined use of experimental pain and visual analogue scales in providing standardized measurement of clinical pain. *Clin J Pain.* 1987;3:1–8.

Price DD, Harkins SW, Baker C. Sensory-affective relationships among different types of clinical and experimental pain. *Pain.* 1986a;28:297–307.

Price DD, Harkins SW, Rafii A, Price C. A simultaneous comparison of fentanyl's analgesic effects on experimental and clinical pain. *Pain.* 1986b;24:197–203.

Price DD, Mao J, Mayer DJ. Central neural mechanisms of normal and abnormal pain states. In: Fields HL, Liebeskind JC, eds. *Pharmacological Approaches to the Treatment of Chronic Pain: New Concepts and Critical Issues. Progress in Pain Research and Management.* Vol. 1. Seattle, Wash: IASP Press; 1994:61–84.

Price DD, McGrath PA, Rafii A, Buckingham B. The validation of visual analogue scales as ratio scale measures for chronic and experimental pain. *Pain.* 1983;17:45–46.

Price DD. Psychophysical measurement of normal and abnormal pain processing. In: Boivie J, Hansson P, Lindblom U, eds. *Touch, Temperature, and Pain in Health and Disease: Mechanisms and Assessments. Progress in Pain Research and Management;* vol. 3. Seattle, Wash: IASP Press; 1994:3–25.

Prieto EJ, Geisinger KF. Factor-analytic studies of the McGill pain questionnaire. In: Melzack R, ed. *Pain Measurement and Assessment.* New York, NY: Raven Press; 1983:63–70.

Ransford HV, Cairns D, Mooney V. The pain drawing as an aid to psychological evaluation of patients with low back pain. *Spine.* 1976;1:127.

Reading AE. The internal structure of the McGill pain questionnaire in dysmenorrhea patients. *Pain.* 1979;7:353–358.

Scott J, Huskisson EC. Graphic representation of pain. *Pain.* 1976;2:175–184.

Tait RC, Chibnall JT, Margolis RB. Pain extent: Relations with psychological state, pain severity, pain history and disability. *Pain.* 1990;41:295–301.

Uden A, Astrom M, Bergenudd H. Pain drawings in chronic low back pain. *Spine.* 1988;13:389–392.

Vernon H. Information management in rehabilitation programs: Tools for quality management. LACC Chiropractic Rehabilitation, Session 9; August 26/27, 1995; class notes: 106; Philadelphia, Pa.

Vernon H. Pain and disability questionnaires in chiropractic rehabilitation. In: Liebenson C, ed. *Rehabilitation of the Spine: A Practitioner's Manual.* Philadelphia, Pa: Williams & Wilkins; 1996:61.

Von Korff M, Deyo RA, Cherkin D, Barlow SF. Back pain in primary care: Outcomes at 1 year. *Spine.* 1993; 18:855–862.

Von Korff M, Ormel J, Keefe F, Dworkin SF. Grading the severity of chronic pain. *Pain.* 1992;50:133–149.

Webster's New Collegiate Dictionary. Springfield, Mass: G & C Merriam; 1980:817.

CHAPTER 7

Condition-specific Outcome Assessment Tools

STEVEN G. YEOMANS

The clinical use of condition-specific questionnaires for outcomes assessment has been well established, due to their ability to measure and track outcomes of specific conditions. As discussed earlier in this text, the ability to track change over time is best accomplished by the use of instruments that specifically address the patient's specific complaint(s). However, one problem has been that the patient often presents with a condition for which no questionnaire or outcome assessment (OA) tool yet exists. As time passes, this problem is becoming more rare, as a significant number of condition-specific tools have been introduced in the past few years to fill at least a portion of this need. However, when no specific tool is available, the general health questionnaire will have to suffice as well as the pain gathering outcomes tool such as a visual analogue scale (VAS).

To keep in perspective the use of condition-specific questionnaires within the larger "outcomes-based" picture, these valid, reliable, practical, and responsive "subjective" tools should be completed at baseline or at the time of the initial encounter with the patient. The condition-specific questionnaire along with a pain measuring tool (such as VAS, pain drawing, etc), and a general health tool (SF-36, COOP, etc) comprise the initial "battery" of instruments that are used to track patient progress over the initial treatment time period.

CLINICAL APPLICATION

Just as the VAS measures the intensity or quantity of pain, **condition-specific tools measure loss of activity tolerance or the inability to perform activities of daily living (ADLs).** Tracking this area is vitally important as disability, or "an activity or task the individual cannot accomplish" (Luck and Florence, 1988), as well as pain, are two common reasons why patients present to health care providers (HCPs). Therefore, when used in concert with a pain intensity OA tool, two treatment goals common to most patients can be tracked to determine if the patient's goals are being met. When documenting a patient's historical data by using a condition-specific questionnaire such as the Oswestry Low Back Pain Disability Questionnaire, more specific subjective information can be obtained. For example, the patient's generalized subjective statement of "I hurt when I lift" can then be replaced with a "grade" of lifting difficulty. At re-examination time, if lifting still increases pain, a change in the patient's lifting intolerance can be ascertained by using the same OA tool, and comparing the new "grade" or score to the initial score.

This feature may have far reaching reimbursement or medico-legal consequences when compared to only reporting the generalized, subjective information. More specifically, it may appear that the patient has not improved if the patient still reports "I hurt when I lift" at re-examination time. However, if the score or grade of lifting intolerance improves from a 4 to a 2 out of 5 score (where 0 = no disability and 5 = severe disability), the records now obviously reflect patient improvement. Moreover, since the use of a goal-oriented treatment plan is a recommended patient management approach, each question of a condition-specific questionnaire can be used as a specific treatment goal. Thus, the HCP, the patient, and the insurer will know when an endpoint in care has been reached. The task of determining an endpoint in care can be very difficult without the use of a quantitative method of documentation. Condition-specific questionnaires manage this task very effectively. More details regarding turning a "soft" SOAP note into an improved "hard" SOAP note can be reviewed in Chapter 20 of this text.

OUTCOMES DATA COLLECTION METHODS AND TOOLS

LUMBAR SPINE ASSESSMENT TOOLS: THE "GOLD STANDARDS"

Many lumbar spine OA tools have been introduced, but only a few have qualified as "gold standards." This may be due, in part, to the more recent introduction of several tools that simply have not been utilized enough as of yet to determine their quality or value. Deyo (1988) has classified assessment devices and procedures that measure functional outcomes in low back pain patients as having the following characteristics:

- Functional questionnaires
- Global ratings (eg, excellent, good, fair, poor)
- Timed activities and obstacle courses
- Employment status
- Disability days (work loss, bed days, limited activity days)
- Patient diaries
- Electronic monitors

In 1995, a two-decade search reported that over 40 low back functional questionnaires existed in the literature (Kopec and Esdaile, 1995a). However, these authors reported that the majority of the questionnaires were developed for a single study and had not been properly validated. They described five established scales as being identified by researchers between 1980 and 1984. These "gold standards" include:

1. Sickness Impact Profile (SIP) (Bergner et al, 1981)
2. Roland-Morris Disability Questionnaire (Roland and Morris, 1983a, 1983b) (derived from the SIP)
3. Oswestry Low Back Pain Disability Questionnaire (Fairbank et al, 1980)
4. Million Visual Analogue Scale (Million et al, 1982)
5. Waddell Disability Index (Waddell, 1984).

Kopec reported that the Roland-Morris Questionnaire was the most frequently cited back pain scale, followed by the Oswestry, Waddell, Million, and SIP, respectively. The SIP was found to be used the most in randomized clinical studies while the Oswestry and Million scales were often found to be utilized in "pre–post" studies. New scales reported by Kopec include the Dallas Pain Questionnaire (Lawlis et al, 1989), the Functional Assessment Screening Questionnaire (FASQ) (Seltzer et al, 1982; Millard, 1989), the Pain and Impairment Relationship Scale of Riley (PIRSR) (Riley et al, 1988; Slater et al, 1991), the Low Back Outcome Score (LBOS) (Greenough and Fraser, 1992), and the Chronic Illness Problem Inventory (CIPI) (Kames et al, 1984). Table 7–1 summarizes the various attributes of each of these scales.

Roland-Morris Questionnaire

A commonly utilized instrument for measuring spinal disability is the Roland Morris Disability Questionnaire (Roland and Morris, 1983a, 1983b). **The Roland-Morris Questionnaire was derived from Bergner et al's (1981) Sickness Index Profile (SIP).** The SIP is a lengthy questionnaire from which Roland and Morris, in an attempt to improve its utility and practicality, extracted 24 items (from its 136 items) that they believed would be most relevant for low back pain. The reliability of this shorter scale was established but the validity was tested initially only by comparing it to a small number of clinical observations rather than to the entire SIP or its major subscales. Deyo (1986) also compared reliability of the Roland-Morris Questionnaire (RMQ) to the SIP and its major subscales, which include Physical Dimension (45 items) and Psychosocial Dimension (48 items). Deyo reported that the RMQ correlates better (.89) than the overall SIP (.85) to the Physical Dimension but substantially weaker to the Psychosocial Dimension (.59) than the SIP (.88). In addition, reliability (reproducibility) was found when studying two patient groups. Among the group with no "clinically rated change," the test–retest correlations were all above .80 with the RMQ being comparable to the other scales. The correlations were somewhat lower for both instruments when test–retest scores were correlated for patients who stated they had not resumed full activities, with the RMQ actually showing the best correlation (.76 compared to .73 for the SIP, and .69 for both Physical and Psychosocial Dimensions). Validity was also very strong, with the

Table 7–1: Content and Format of Five "New" Questionnaires

SCALE	NUMBER OF SECTIONS/ ITEMS; STYLE	MINUTES TO COMPLETE	MEASUREMENT ATTRIBUTES
Dallas PQ (Lawlis et al, 1989)	4/16; VAS	3–5 min	Impact of spinal pain on behavior; four areas assessed: (1) ADLs, (2) work-leisure activities, (3) anxiety-depression, (4) social interest
FASQ (Millard, 1989)	5/15; 5 options	< 5 min	Five sections: (1) personal care, (2) instrumental, (3) transportation, (4) leisure, (5) occupational
PIRSR (Riley et al, 1988)	0/15; 7 options	"Brief"	Assesses the extent to which patients with chronic pain believe that pain prevents them from functioning normally
LBOS (Greenough and Fraser, 1992)	13; 3–4 options	Not included	Eight areas assessed: (1) current pain, (2) employment, (3) domestic, (4) sport activities, (5) use of drugs and medical care, (6) rest, (7) sex life, (8) five daily activities
CIPI (Kames et al, 1984)	18/65; 5 options	"less time than the SIP"	Eighteen scales assessing problems in physical limitations, psychosocial functioning, health care behaviors, and marital adjustment

CIPI, Chronic Illness Problem Inventory; FASQ, Functional Assessment Screening Questionnaire; LBOS, Low Back Outcome Score; PIRSR, Pain and Impairment Relationship Scale of Riley.
Reprinted with permission from Kopec JA and Esdaile JM, 1995a.

RMQ showing the strongest or equal to the highest correlation of all the scales. Again, only the Psychosocial Dimension correlated with the three measures of psychological distress. **Deyo (1986) concluded that the RMQ appears at least as valid as the lengthier scales (SIP).** Similarly, the RMQ appeared to perform at least as well or better as the SIP and its subscales regarding sensitivity to change. The advantages of the RMQ over the SIP were discussed in this study of conservatively treated mechanical low back pain patients. The advantages included: (1) a shorter instrument (24 vs 136 questions); (2) similar correlation to the Physical Dimension portion of the SIP; and (3) psychosocial function that was less susceptible to change than physical function. Additional advantages, including differences in sentence structure (the RMQ changed the wording from the 24 SIP items using ". . . because of my back"), and its brevity, favor the use of the RMQ in a low back pain population as it is condition-specific for low back pain, unlike the generic or general health SIP.

Because the RMQ is comprised of 24 questions, it allows for easy scoring. One simply totals the sum of the circled items (maximum score = 24) which represents the final score. Von Korff and Saunders (1996) discuss the RMQ citing a cut-off score of 14 or greater as representing significant disability associated with an unfavorable outcome, which they felt was too high to identify all patients functioning poorly. A pain rating scale accompanies the RMQ 24 activity limitation–oriented questions. The scale differentiates the following categories: no pain at all, little pain, moderate pain, bad pain, very bad pain, or almost unbearable pain. A pain rating of moderate was described as being

sufficient to be associated with significant activity limitation in many patients. The Roland and Morris study was referred to as the best single study of assessing short-term outcomes of primary care patients with low back pain (Von Korff and Saunders, 1996). More specifically, in the population of 230 initial patients, 212 were reassessed at 1 week and 193 at 4 weeks (Roland and Morris, 1983a, 1983b). Study results are summarized in Table 7–2.

Recently, a revised version of the RMQ, the RM-18, has been introduced. This revised version met reliability and validity criteria in a pretest–post-test design. (Stratford and Binkley, 1997). An item analysis suggested that 6 items could be deleted from the 24-item tool without changing the measurement property when compared to the longer version. The true-positive rate (sensitivity) was 62% and the true-negative rate (specificity) was 87%, identical to the 24-item version (see Appendix Form C–1).

Oswestry Low Back Pain Disability Questionnaire

Another popular low back pain and associated disability OA tool is the Oswestry Low Back Pain Disability Questionnaire (Fairbank et al, 1980). The Oswestry is made up of ten categories, in which one of six responses is chosen to represent the level of low back disability for each category. A score of 0 to 5 is possible for each of the ten categories, which provides a total possible score of 50 (if all responses were fives). This score is then doubled to define the answer on a 100% scale where 100 represents the highest disability score possible. A formula for scoring is necessary if the patient does not complete any of the ten categories. In addition, a chart can be utilized to ascertain an interpretation of the disability

Table 7–2: Summary of the Roland-Morris Study

	INITIAL (n = 230 patients)	1 WEEK (n = 212)	4 WEEKS (n = 193)
Pain-free status ("no pain at all")	NA	20%	33%
Moderate or worse pain	90%	54%	34%
Bad or worse pain	54%	22%	15%
Activity limitations (a score of 14 or greater)	43%	28%	20%
Activity limitations (at least 1 or more positive responses answered)	NA	NA	75%

NA, not available.
Modified from Low Back Pain and Disability Questionnaire, from Roland and Morris, 1983a.

severity level, although the importance of using this tool is in assessing change over time or outcomes (see Table 7–3). A "revised" version measures both impairment (function) and disability (limited ADLs) (Hudson-Cook and Tomes-Nicholson, 1988). Erhard et al (1994) reported that a score of 11% may be used as an appropriate cut-off score for HCPs to consider for discharge and/or return to work in an uncomplicated LBP case (see Appendix Form C–2).

Leclaire and colleagues (1997) studied the ability of the Oswestry and the Roland-Morris questionnaires to discriminate between two very different groups of patients: one without nerve root signs or mechanical low back pain, and the other with nerve root signs and electromyographic evidence of radiculopathy. The authors concluded that both scales were able to accurately discriminate between the two groups of patients with respect to functional disability and diagnosis. Another study reported that the Roland-Morris questionnaire was found to be more sensitive than the Oswestry in measuring functional status changes in patients with minor disability. However, the opposite was found in severely disabled patient groups for whom the Oswestry was more sensitive (Baker et al, 1989). In 162 low back pain patients, moderate correlation between the two scales was also reported (Yang et al, 1983). However, differing severity of the patients' low back pain was not taken into account.

A revised Oswestry questionnaire was introduced with a retitled section 8. Now identified as "Social Life," this section was originally entitled "sex life" and was left blank quite often by respondents. In the revised version, all ten sections are completed more often than in the original 1980 version. The revised Oswestry Low Back Pain Questionnaire (ROLBPQ) and RMQ were also compared in a randomized controlled trial including chiropractic manipulation, stroking massage, corset, and transcutaneous muscular stimulation (Hsieh et al, 1992). The inclusion and exclusion criteria included 18-to-55-year-old subjects with nonspecific low back pain for a duration of 3 weeks to 6 months. Sixty-three of 85 patients completed the initial and final evaluations. Both questionnaires showed good internal consistency, with alpha coefficients ranging from .77 to .93. In addition, both instruments showed a significant difference between chiropractic manipulation and massage

groups (< .05) but only the RMQ was able to discriminate between the chiropractic manipulation and transcutaneous muscular stimulation groups and between the corset and massage groups. The authors concluded that both instruments are reliable for measuring low back pain disability, and chiropractic manipulation has a superior short-term benefit when compared to stroking massage and transcutaneous muscular stimulation in subacute low back pain patients. The RMQ was preferred in clinical trials for subacute low back pain as it was found to be more sensitive than the ROLBPQ to detect changes (Hsieh et al, 1992). Haas et al (1995) reported that the ROLBPQ and the ADL (activity of daily living) and work/leisure scales from the Dallas Pain Questionnaire (DPQ) were both appropriate for monitoring low back pain patients returning for care to chiropractic teaching clinics. The social and anxiety/depression portions of the DPQ were not responsive in this 1-year study of 663 consecutive low back pain patients.

Stratford (1998) administered the RMQ to a group of 226 patients with low back pain of less than six weeks duration during an initial visit for physical therapy and follow-up 3 to 6 weeks later. The objective was to determine the score change the best classified patients as having achieved an important change. The results indicate that the patient's intitial score determines the estimate of important change because less change is required for those who score low initially, and conversely, a greater change is required to qualify as important when initial scores are higher. The initial scores were broken down into five groups that included 0 to 8, 5 to 12, 9 to 16, 13 to 20, and 17 to 24. The estimate of important change was 2, 4, 5, 8, and 8, respectively. Please refer to Chapter 2 for further information regarding the use of a t-test or an ANOVA, the effect size, and minimal clinically important difference (MCID) to better appreciate the amount of change that is necessary to be statistically significant.

OTHER LUMBAR SPINE ASSESSMENT TOOLS

There have been additional low back–specific questionnaires published more recently. Many have significant and

Table 7–3: Scoring Technique for the Oswestry Low Back Disability Questionnaire and Neck Disability Index

1. Each of the 10 sections is scored separately (0 to 5 points each) and then added up (max. total = 50).

   Example:

Section 1. Pain Intensity	Point Value
A. ___ I have no pain at the moment	0
B. ___ The pain is very mild at the moment	1
C. ___ The pain is moderate at the moment	2
D. ___ The pain is fairly severe at the moment	3
E. ___ The pain is very severe at the moment	4
F. ___ The pain is the worst imaginable	5

2. If all 10 sections are completed, simply double the patient's score.

3. If a section is omitted, divide the patient's total score by the number of sections completed times 5.

   Formula:

   $$\frac{\text{Patient's score}}{\text{No. of sections completed} \times 5} \times 100 = \underline{\hspace{1cm}} \% \text{ DISABILITY}$$

   Example:

   If 9 of 10 sections are completed, divide the patient's score by $9 \times 5 = 45$.

Patient's Score:	22
Number of sections completed:	9 ($9 \times 5 = 45$)
	$22/45 \times 100 = 48\%$ disability

4. Interpretation of disability scores (from original article):

SCORE INTERPRETATION OF THE OSWESTRY LBP DISABILITY QUESTIONNAIRE	
0–20% Minimal disability	Can cope with most ADLs. Usually no treatment is needed, apart from advice on lifting, sitting, posture, physical fitness, and diet. In this group, some patients have particular difficulty with sitting and this may be important if their occupation is sedentary (typist, driver, etc).
20–40% Moderate disability	This group experiences more pain and problems with sitting, lifting, and standing. Travel and social life are more difficult and they may well be off work. Personal care, sexual activity, and sleeping are not grossly affected, and the back condition can usually be managed by conservative means.
40–60% Severe disability	Pain remains the main problem in this group of patients, but travel, personal care, social life, sexual activity, and sleep are also affected. These patients require detailed investigation.
60–80% Crippled	Back pain impinges on all aspects of these patients' lives both at home and at work. *Positive intervention is required.*
80–100%	These patients are either bed-bound or exaggerating their symptoms. This can be evaluated by careful observation of the patient during the medical examination.
Data compiled from Fairbanks et al, 1980.	

new attributes, but more than likely have simply not been around long enough to replace the "gold standards" such as the Oswestry and Roland-Morris. Most of these newer tools include validating information that includes using many of the "gold standards" previously mentioned. Some of the low back outcome tools more recently published include the following:

- Quebec Back Pain Disability Scale (Kopec et al, 1995b)
- North American Spine Society Instrument (NASS) (Deyo et al, 1994)
- Curtin Back Screening Questionnaire (CBSQ) (Harper et al, 1995)
- Activities Discomfort Scale (Turner et al, 1983)

- Low Back Outcome Score (Greenough and Fraser, 1992)
- Low Back Pain TyPE (Deyo, 1990)
- Clinical Back Pain Questionnaire (Ruta et al, 1994)
- Spinal Stenosis Questionnaire (Stucki et al, 1996)

Quebec Back Pain Disability Scale

The Quebec Back Pain Disability Scale is a 20-item self-administered instrument designed to evaluate functional disability in individuals with back pain (Kopec et al, 1995b). The questionnaire was studied for reliability, validity, and responsiveness in a group of 242 back pain patients. Follow-up data was obtained after several days and after 2 to 6 months. The responsiveness was tested against a global index of change and direct comparisons to the Roland-Morris, Oswestry, and SF-36 scales were carried out. This testing found the instrument to be reliable (test–retest was .92) and responsive to changes in disability over time; its Cronbach's alpha coefficient was .96 (see Appendix Form C–3).

North American Spine Society

The North American Spine Society (NASS) developed an instrument that incorporates selected items from various previously validated instruments, including measures of symptoms, functional status, and role function. Other items are drawn from the medical history, comorbidity, and satisfaction (Deyo et al, 1994). The final version requires about 20 minutes to complete. An eighth grade reading level and patient acceptance was also reported (see Appendix Form C–4).

The self-report measures were grouped into five categories, of which questions about pain and current behavior referenced the previous week. Categories included in this instrument are:

- Demographics: Age, gender, race, education, and insurance information.
- Medical history: Diagnosis, date of surgery, onset and relative painfulness of back and leg pain, past surgeries and use of other HCPs; comorbidities, use of assistive devices, and the consumption of cigarettes, alcohol, narcotic, and nonnarcotic medications. The SF-36 general health question (no. 1) and the five mental health subscale questions (questions 24 to 26, 28, and 30) are used, as well as satisfaction with respect to the current back condition.
- Pain, neurogenic symptoms, and function: nine of the ten questions are derived from the Oswestry Disability Questionnaire (Fairbank et al, 1980). Job characteristics and demands as well as satisfaction are also included.

Table 7–4 summarizes many of the different tools from which the NASS was derived and to which it is compared.

Curtin Back Screening Questionnaire

The Curtin Back Screening Questionnaire (CBSQ) was developed as a discriminative screening instrument to as-sist in both the early recognition of disability and in the management planning for patients with disabling occupational low back pain (Harper et al, 1995). This instrument was validated in a population of 74 moderately disabled low back pain patients, using questions taken from previously published studies. These included the Million Visual Analogue Scale (no. 39) (Million, 1982), the Pain Disability Index (no. 36) (Pollard, 1984), the General Health Questionnaire (no. 22) (Goldberg and Hillier, 1979), Beck's Depression Inventory (no. 14) (Beck, 1961), and the SIP (no. 49) (Bergner, 1981). The initial 253 items were reduced to 73 functional health status items that were used to identify 14 and eventually 11 categories of problems. From the 11 categories, eight questions were extracted in order to make the screening process easy and quick to administrate. The eight questions were derived from the categories listed in Table 7–5.

Test–retest stability, internal consistency, criterion construct validity (Pearson correlations), means, and 95% confidence intervals were determined using three patient groups. These groups consisted of normal, mild to moderate, and severe low back pain patients. The calculation of the CBSQ screening score is performed by choosing the response option, which is arranged on a 4-point Likert scale, that best applies to the patient's clinical status. Each option is weighted and the weighted responses for each of the eight questions are added, yielding a total score (see Appendix Forms C–5a and C–5b).

The CBSQ can be either self-administered or completed by an interview. The total screening score is utilized to categorize the patient into one of three categories: type A (screening score 143–234), type B (screening score 235–282), or type C (screening score 283–416). One consistent distinguishing demographical feature was its ability to consistently distinguish time off work between the three types. Among those classified as type A, 17% had lost time from work, versus 53% in type B, and 100% in type C. The authors state that the CBSQ 8-item screening score can be used clinically or epidemiologically and they present a "prototype clinical description of the disability" for each type (A, B, and C) (Table 7–6) (Harper et al, 1995).

The CBSQ can be calculated and interpreted in 3 minutes, but the full 11 categories of 79 items typically takes 20 to 30 minutes to complete. The 8-item screen yields a single number that represents the severity of disability whereas a single unweighted score of severity by employing all questions of each of the 11 categories of disability, summarizes the patient's functional health status. This score can also be used clinically or epidemiologically. This screening tool was tested on a population in which 50% of subjects were severely disabled. Therefore, the screen was recommended to be employed not prior to a 4 week post-injury point to avoid false positives. The authors conclude that prospective evaluation will be necessary to demonstrate whether it can function as a prognostic tool (Harper et al, 1995). Also, its ability to detect change over time had not yet been evaluated.

Table 7–4: Selected Low Back Pain Outcome Tools

CATEGORY	INSTRUMENT	NO. OF ITEMS	APPROXIMATE TIME TO COMPLETE	DIMENSIONS
Symptoms	McGill Pain Questionnaire	26	15 minutes	Pain severity, affective response
	Visual Analogue Scale	Variable	1 minute	Pain severity, frequency
	Chronic Pain Grade	7	5 minutes	Pain intensity, perceived impact
	NASS[a] Questionnaire	12	3 minutes (for pain questions only)	Back pain, leg pain, numbness, weakness; frequency, severity, duration
Disease-specific functional status	Roland-Morris Disability Questionnaire	24	5 minutes	Various daily functions
	Oswestry LBP Disability Questionnaire	10	5 minutes	ADLs: Stand, sit, lift, walk, etc
	Million Scale	15	10 minutes	Various ADLs
	NASS[a] Questionnaire	9	5 minutes	Adapted from the Oswestry Questionnaire
Generic functional status (sometimes referred to as General Health)	SF-36	36	10 minutes	Eight scales: physical function, pain, vitality, mental health, etc
	Sickness Impact Profile	136	20 minutes	Ambulation, emotional status, social functions, work, sleep, others
	Nottingham Health Profile	38	5 minutes	Physical mobility, pain, sleep, energy, social emotions
	Duke Health Profile	17	5 minutes	Social, psychological, physical function
Role function	Health Interview Survey	3	1 minute	Days of work absenteeism, days in bed, days of limited activity
	NASS[a] Questionnaire	9	5 minutes	Work status, compensation status, job description

[a] The NASS questionnaire includes items related to symptoms (see also generic functional status measures) functional status, and role function, as well as medical history, comorbidity, and satisfaction (Daltroy, 1996).
Reprinted with permission from Lippincott-Raven Publishers. Deyo et al, 1994.

Activities Discomfort Scale

Another tool, called the Activities Discomfort Scale (ADS), was found to be reliable in predicting chronic low back pain patients' response to conservative treatment (Turner et al, 1983). This questionnaire is comprised of 18 common activities of daily living, such as walking, bending, sitting, standing, driving, and so on. Pain was graded on a 5-point scale. A high internal consistency and ability to discriminate between patients with low back pain and those without was reported (Yellen, 1978). The ADS was the single predictor most highly correlated with pain intensity upon follow-up. The HCP's ability to predict pain relief and activity return, the ADS, and the hypochondriasis scale of a Minnesota Multiphasic Personality Inventory (MMPI) were associated significantly with return to activities to a similar degree. Such factors as abnormality found on radiographs, on physical examinations, whether the patient was receiving disability income, age, and sex were not significantly associated with any of the outcome measures (Table 7–7) (see Appendix Form C–6).

Table 7–5: Eight Categories Comprising the Curtin Back Screening Questionnaire

Pain (two questions)

Self-care and mobility

Thinking and problem solving

Hobbies and pastimes

Social life

Home management

Emotions

CLINICAL TIP 7–1
Using the Eight-item Screening Tool

"The use of the 8-item screening tool can easily be administered in the primary care center but its longer, 79-item counterpart may be best saved for the pain center due to its poor utility and practicality in a primary care center. A totally disabled patient who scores in the Type C category may require special/multidisciplinary intervention" (Harper et al, 1995).

Table 7–6: Curtin Back Screening Questionnaire

TYPE	DESCRIPTION[a]
Type A (143–234)	Subjects in this group have clinical problems that are mainly limited to physical function. These include difficulty and pain production with activities that involve bending, turning, and twisting as well as sitting. The subject will be more fatigued than usual and will find it necessary to change positions frequently. These limitations will mean that work restrictions are necessary and commonly, subjects will be anxious about maintaining their work. In addition, subjects will be experiencing difficulty with normal activities around the house and with physical activities involving family and friends. Outdoor activities, hobbies, and pastimes will be restricted and it will take longer to do almost all activities.
Type B (235–282)	Subjects experience physical, emotional, and social problems with daily life functions. Pain is often reported as unbearable with fewer than 3 good days per week. Similar ADL intolerance is reported with turning, twisting, sitting, standing, and bending and fatigue is significant. Modifications in ADLs and work are necessary but difficult to accomplish, often resulting in anxiety over workplace demands. Other stressors often include problematic sexual activity, financial distress, and altered sleep patterns, which result in poor self-esteem, and feeling helpless and useless. Medical management is typically of little benefit, resulting in subject dissatisfaction and frustration. Difficulty in cooperating with family and friends is common, disrupting the subject's social life. Coping skills are suffering.
Type C (283–416)	Most aspects of subjects' lives have major problems. Pain related to movement results in significant disability, making most ADLs as well as even light duty at work difficult to manage. Fatigue is significant and completing even simple tasks proves difficult. Sexual activity, financial status, work and home management, hobbies, and recreation are all significantly affected. Family and social life disruption due to severe emotional problems, including depression, often result in suicidal thoughts. General health has deteriorated.

ADLs, activities of daily living.

[a] The specific weights for each of the eight screen questions are added and used to categorize the patient into type A, B, or C. The descriptions described here were developed from the clinical profiles generated from the data.

Modified from Harper et al, 1995.

Low Back Outcome Score

The Low Back Outcome Score (LBOS) was introduced in 1992 (Greenough and Fraser, 1992). This outcome questionnaire was designed take into account the patient's prior abilities and also collect information regarding both small reductions in performance as well as more gross disability. The intended use of this instrument is for tracking treatment outcomes from both conservatively—as well as surgically—treated low back patients. The LBOS includes only subjective data, as tools that include physical measures such as lumbar flexion are subject to variances in patient cooperation and inter-rater technique, and can be influenced by psychological factors. Similarly, straight leg raise ranges vary throughout the day (Porter and Trailescu, 1990) and, hence, may lead to inter- and intraobserver error due to the biological variability. Therefore, the inclusion of physical examination data can reduce the validity and reliability of the instrument since observer bias and intra- and interobserver variation are difficult to control. Rather, several factors that can be used to assess functional outcomes, such as pain via a Visual Analogue Scale; the activity level of employment, such as light, medium, or heavy physical demand characteristics versus unemployment; and sporting levels of activity can be assessed. Even though these factors are also subject to many influences, their utilization will result in a more accurate outcome

gathering approach. Because of the inherent variables, a composite outcome score was devised in an attempt to avoid these influences. It was anticipated in Greenough and Fraser's 1992 study that the comprehensive outcome score would allow measurement of the treatment approach as well as allow for the determination of the causal factors of low back pain.

Greenough and Fraser's 1992 study compared the LBOS to the Oswestry Disability Questionnaire and the Waddell Disability Index in a retrospective study of non-surgically treated low back pain patients. The study results indicated that the LBOS provided a satisfactory spread of data and compared favorably with both the Oswestry and the Waddell Disability Index utilizing several methods of statistical analyses. A prospective study using the LBOS is underway to further test this tool (see Appendix Form C–7).

Clinical Back Pain Questionnaire

The Clinical Back Pain Questionnaire (CBPQ) introduced by Ruta et al (1994), utilizes a stringent reliability and validity process to screen this instrument. These authors established the validity and reliability of the instrument. They also provide a good literature review and include several of the previously mentioned instruments. The authors report findings consistent with previous studies that re-

Table 7–7: Correlation of Pretreatment Variables with Patient Follow-up Ratings

PRETREATMENT VARIABLES	PAIN INTENSITY	RETURN TO ACTIVITIES
Questionnaires		
Activities Discomfort Scale[a]	.48[b]	.28τ
MMPI		
Hypochondriasis	.38[b]	.29[b]
Depression	.27[b]	.16
Psychasthenia	.22τ	.06
Hysteria	.21τ	.13
Physician ratings		
Predicted pain relief[c]	.36[b]	.31[b]
Predicted return to activities[c]	.35[b]	.30[b]
Severity of impairment[a]	.23τ	.21

τ = p < .05.

[a] High scores indicate greater dysfunction.

[b] p < .01.

[c] High scores indicate less likely to improve.

Modified from Turner et al, 1983.

ported a poor correlation between physical impairment and functional disability measures versus measures of pain and physical impairment (Karoly and Jensen, 1987; Turk and Rudy, 1987; Rainville et al, 1992). Ruta et al (1994) compared the CBPQ to the SF-36 in a low back pain population and noted that back pain sufferers were less healthy than the general population as depicted by the SF-36. They also reported a greater responsiveness, or sensitivity to change over time, compared to the SF-36. More specifically, the SF-36 detected only a small degree of change over a 2-week time period compared to the CBPQ. They report the benefits of including both a general health instrument like the SF-36 and the CBPQ in tracking outcomes as the general health questionnaire can shed light on general measures and may detect comorbid factors where the CBPQ is more sensitive in tracking outcomes and discriminating between patients. Finally, they note that they plan to follow-up their sample at 6 months and 1 year to test this theory (see Appendix Form C–8).

Spinal Stenosis Questionnaire

An 18-item spinal stenosis questionnaire made up of a 7-item symptom severity scale, a 5-item physical function scale, and a 6-item satisfaction scale was found to be reproducible, valid, internally consistent, and responsive to clinical change in a geriatric spinal stenosis population pre- and postsurgery (Stucki et al, 1996). This measure is meant to be used in conjunction with other existing generic measures of spinal-related disability and health status instruments. Stucki found the test–retest reliability (range: .82 to .96), internal consistency (.64 to .92), and responsiveness (.96 to 1.07) to be statistically significant. Calculating the unweighted mean of all answered items in the questionnaire completes scoring. If more than two items are missing

from the any of the three scales, the scale score is considered invalid. The possible range of the score is 1 to 5 for the symptom severity scale and a 1 to 4 score for both the 5-item physical functional scale and the 6-item satisfaction scale. Stucki et al (1996) concluded that the questionnaire can be used to complement generic instruments when assessing outcomes in patients with lumbar spinal stenosis. A "Point of View" offered by Timothy S. Carey, MD, MPH is included in this article (p. 803). Carey raises several important points, among them that this instrument does not stand alone, as issues such as the mortality and morbidity rates of the surgical procedure, the necessity for second operations, and the effects of treatment on overall functional status are not gathered by the questionnaire. In addition, overall costs of treatment to satisfy third-party payers as well as modifications of the questionnaire for conservative/nonsurgical treatment are included (see Appendix Form C–9).

Low Back Pain and Other TyPEs

Low Back Pain TyPEs (Technology of Patient Experience specification) is a data collection approach designed to measure and analyze low back pain outcomes and treatment (Deyo, 1990). The instrument is included in the Outcomes Management System (OMS), which is "a technology of patient experience designed to help patients, payers, and providers make more rational medical care-related choices based on better insight into the effect of these choices on the patient's life" (Ellwood, 1988). A key feature of the OMS is a series of questionnaires known as TyPE (Technology of Patient Experience) specifications. The system of TyPEs includes two categories of instruments. The first is a general purpose survey used to capture an individual's personal identifiers, demographic information, health risks, comorbidities, functional status and well-being, and satisfaction with provider services. This tool includes a general health questionnaire derived from the RAND 36-Item Health Status Survey 1.0 called the HSQ-2.0 (see Chap. 5). The second category of instruments is condition-specific and includes a minimum set of information that can be used to describe and compare individual patient's diagnoses, therapies, and clinical outcomes. Each TyPE has a user's manual describing the rationale for included data elements and a recommended approach for collecting data. There are TyPE specifications for 19 diagnoses and conditions as of 1998 (Table 7–8). Other TyPEs not yet ready for publication included the following conditions: blood infections, drug use disorders, gallstones, lung transplant, osteoporosis prophylaxis, panic disorder, peripheral vascular disease, pregnancy, schizophrenia, shoulder disorders, and smoking cessation.

The low back pain TyPEs consists of an initial questionnaire (Form 6.1, 22 items), a "Physicians Examination and Diagnosis—Baseline" (10 items), a "Patient Follow-up Questionnaire" (14 items), a "Physical Examination—Follow-up" (10 items), and a user's manual. The low back pain TyPEs were not designed to result in a single score. Rather, each question is sufficiently important to stand alone and can serve as a baseline for future comparative assessment (Personal correspondence with Deyo: No scoring method intended). This instrument serves as an excellent history and physical examination form specifically designed for low back pain patients and many questions are outcomes-oriented and therefore can be compared to the follow-up questionnaire individually.

An abundance of outcome tools are available from which to choose for tracking outcomes of the lumbar spine. By no means have all of the tools discussed or listed been included in the appendix. Omission of any tool does not represent any bias against that tool. Similarly, the inclusion of any tool in the appendix does not suggest bias for that tool. Some of the "gold standards" were included, but again, not all. Also, there may be some disagreement about which tools represent a "gold standard." The reader should, therefore, remember the caveats rather than becoming overly concerned about which tool to use.

Table 7–8: Various Condition-specific Questionnaires Available from Stratis Health

CONDITION	TYPE DEVELOPER(S)	ORGANIZATION	VERSION DATE
1. Angina	David B. Pryor, MD	Allina Health Systems	10/8/93
2. Asthma	Robert A. Bethel, MD	National Jewish Center	4/20/94
3. Carpal tunnel syndrome	Jeffrey N. Katz, MD, MS, et al	Brigham and Women's Hospital	10/25/93
4. Cataracts	Jonathan C. Javitt, MD, MPH, et al	Georgetown University	3/2/93
5. Chronic obstructive pulmonary disease	Robert A. Bethel, MD	National Jewish Center	10/6/92
6. Chronic sinusitis	Sanford R. Hoffman, MD, et al	Hoffman Healthcare	10/8/93
7. Depression	G. Richard Smith, MD, et al	University of Arkansas	8/15/94
8. Diabetes	Byron J. Hoogwerf, MD	Cleveland Clinic	11/24/92
9. Hip fracture	John F. Fitzgerald, MD	Indiana University	10/12/92
10. Hip replacement	Matthew H. Liang, MD, MPH	Brigham and Women's Hospital	10/1/90
11. Hypertension/Lipid disorders	John M. Flack, MD, MPH Richard H. Grimm, MD, PhD	University of Minnesota University of Minnesota	2/1/92
12. Low back pain	Richard A. Deyo, MD, MPH Daniel C. Cherkin, PhD, et al	Veterans Administration –Washington	10/12/92
13. Osteoarthritis: knee	Robert F. Meenan, MD, MPH Lewis E. Kazis, ScD	Boston University Boston University	5/1/91
14. Prostatism	Floyd J. Fowler, PhD Michael J. Barry, MD	University of Massachusetts Massachusetts Gen. Hosp	1/19/93
15. Rheumatoid arthritis	Robert F. Meenan, MD, MPH Lewis E. Kazis, ScD	Boston University Boston University	10/12/92
16. Stroke	G. Richard Smith, MD	University of Arkansas	10/31/94
17. Substance use: Alcohol	Thomas Baber, PhD	University of Connecticut	4/24/96
18. Panic disorder	Kathryn Rost, PhD	University of Arkansas	4/24/96
19. Osteoporosis risk assessment	Robert Lindasy, MBChB, PhD, FRCP	Helen Hayes Hospital	1/9/98

Reprinted with permission from Stratis Health, 2901 Metro Drive, Suite 400, Bloomington, MN 55425-1525.

CLINICAL TIP 7–2
Guidelines to Using Outcomes Assessment Tools

Three steps that are *essential* to become truly outcomes-based in managing patients are as follows:

1. Choose an outcome tool or tools that best matches your specific patient population.
2. Once you start with a tool, use the same tool at follow-up and at discharge.
3. Review the results of the scored instruments and compare them to the prior scores to help guide the clinical decision-making process.

CERVICAL SPINE ASSESSMENT TOOLS

Although many questionnaires exist regarding the lumbar spine, very little has been published with respect to the cervical spinal region. This section of the chapter discusses the most clinically applicable instrument—the Neck Disability Index—as well as headache, dizziness, and tinnitus questionnaires.

Neck Disability Index

The Neck Disability Index (NDI) is a questionnaire commonly used for spine-related complaints involving the cervical spine (Appendix Form C–10). The NDI was designed by modifying the Oswestry Low Back Pain Disability Questionnaire, producing a similar 10-item scaled instrument. The instrument was utilized on an initial sample of 17 consecutive patients with whiplash injuries with good statistical significance reported (Pearson's r = .89, p ≤ .05) (Vernon and Mior, 1991). The alpha coefficients were calculated from a pool of questionnaires completed by 52 patients, resulting in a total index alpha of .80, with all items having individual alpha scores greater than .75. Concurrent validity was assessed in two different ways with moderately high correlations reported with both methods (.60 and .69 to .70, respectively). The scoring and interpretation of the NDI is analogous to that of the Oswestry Low Back Pain Disability Questionnaire (see Table 7–3). A more complete discussion of alpha coefficients and concurrent validity can be found in Chapter 2.

Headache Disability Inventory

The Headache Disability Inventory (HDI) is a 25-question, condition-specific tool that is often used in conjunction with the NDI for patients suffering from cervicogenic headaches (Jacobson et al, 1994). It is also useful as a standalone instrument for headache sufferers in whom a cervical component is lacking, as in vascular headaches. Several criteria, including internal consistency/reliability, construct validity, and test–retest reliability, must be met. Originally derived from a 40-item version, this 25-question tool includes 12 emotional and 13 functional questions that make up the two subscales, in addition to a total score.

The HDI is applicable in the assessment of the daily living impact and subsequent treatment of headaches. Jacobson et al (1994) reported mean HDI total scores of 32.33 for mild, 33.72 for moderate, and 60.73 for severe when compared to self-perceived headache severity. A minimum of a 29-point total score change based on the 95% confidence interval was described as necessary to conclude positive treatment effects. Over 80% of 67 subjects (mean age, 38 years; SD, 11 years)—of whom 16 were diagnosed with migraine with aura, 35 with migraine without aura, and 16 with tension headache—scored above 29 total points. No difference in the accuracy of the HDI was reported between the various types of headaches. Similarly, no significant gender or age effects were observed (p > .05 for total and subscale scores) (Jacobson et al, 1994). A test–retest comparison to the Headache Scale (HS) (Hunter, 1983) revealed an r = .83 for the HDI in a 60-day test–retest reliability study compared to r = .76 in a 1-week test–retest for the HS.

Jacobson et al (1994) discuss their prediction and observation of increased HDI scores as the patient's self-perceived headache disability increased. However, they did not expect to observe that headache frequency did not significantly affect self-perceived headache disability. They conclude that **treatment should, therefore, be aimed at relieving headache symptoms more so than frequency** (Jacobson et al, 1994). In this respect, as suggested by the International Headache Society (IHS), the use of an index incorporating headache frequency (severity times frequency) would result in an invalid index of self-perceived disability (IHS, 1991). The total score in this 25-item instrument is calculated by assigning point values at a maximum of 4 points for each "yes" response; hence, a score of 100 is the maximum possible total score (if all 25 questions were scored "yes"). A "sometimes" response is assigned a score of 2, while 0 points are assigned for a "no" response. The response to each of the 25 questions determines the total score and the "emotional" (maximum possible 48 points) and "functional" (maximum possible 52 points) scores are calculated as a percent of the patient's total. Table 7–9 demonstrates the scoring method. The questionnaire can be found in the Appendix Form C–11.

Dizziness Handicap Inventory (DHI)

The Dizziness Handicap Inventory (DHI) is a questionnaire developed to evaluate the impact of vestibular system disease, or dizziness, on everyday life. Similar to the set-up of the HDI, the 25 questions contained in the DHI are divided into three, rather than two, content domains. These domains include a functional scale (9 questions/36 points), an emotional scale (9 questions/36 points), and also a physical domain of dizziness and unsteadiness (7 questions/28 points). Scoring is completed by calculating the total score (maximum = 100) with the "yes" column items valued at 4 points, the "sometimes" column items valued at 2 points each, and the "no" items valued at 0 points each. A separate score for each of the three domains can then be calculated and divided by the patient's total score to deter-

Table 7–9: Scoring Method for Headache Disability Index[a]

E = Emotionally based questions (Nos. 1, 3, 5, 6, 8, 9, 10, 11, 12, 14, 20, 22, 23)

    13 questions total

F = Functionally based questions (Nos. 2, 4, 7, 13, 15, 16, 17, 18, 19, 21, 24, 25)

    12 questions total

Score Values

"Yes"	=	4 points
"Sometimes"	=	2 points
"No"	=	0 points

Final Scores

Emotional = total sum of the scores for the "E" questions / patient's total score or,

    Patient's Emotional score (E question total) / Patient's Total score × 100 = % of the patient's total score (represented by emotionally based questions).

Functional = total sum of the scores for the "F" questions / patient's total score or,

    Patient's Functional score (F question total) / Patient's Total score × 100 = % of the patient's total score (represented by functionally based questions).

[a] Scoring can be reported on three scales; a 100-point total score, which is made up of 52 points derived from emotionally based questions, and 48 points from functionally based questions. Hence, since 100 points make up the total score, if the entire questionnaire is completed, the percentage of emotional versus functional components can be easily compared.

mine the percent of the total attributed to each of the domains (functional vs emotional vs physical). In a study of 106 subjects, good internal consistency, reliability, and validity were demonstrated (Jacobson and Newman, 1990). With the exception of the physical subscale, the mean values for the DHI scores increased significantly as dizziness episodes increased in frequency. Test–retest reliability of the instrument was high. This questionnaire was modeled after the Hearing Handicap Inventory for the Elderly (Ventry and Weinstein, 1982). It was also found to correlate with balance function tests that included electronystagmography, rotational testing, and platform posturography (Jacobson et al, 1991) (see Appendix Form C–12).

Tinnitus Handicap Inventory

The Tinnitus Handicap Inventory (THI) was developed to track patients who suffer from tinnitus pre- and post-treatment (Newman et al, 1996) (see Appendix Form C–13). Like the HDI and DHI, the THI was found to be valid (when compared to other measures of tinnitus), reliable (Cronbach's alpha = .93), responsive, and easy to score and interpret. Scoring of the THI is conducted in the same manner as for the HDI and the DHI, with a total score calculated as well as subscales, which in this case include emotional, functional, and catastrophic subscales. The catastrophic subscale was the least internally consistent (alpha) due to its smaller number of items (5 items; alpha = .68) compared to the functional (12 items; alpha = .86) and emotional subscales (8 items; alpha = .87). The catastrophic subscale was retained, however, because of its potential use for identifying the most handicapped individuals who require more aggressive treatment. This subscale identifies patients with psychosocial concerns that may ne-

cessitate referral to other professionals such as psychiatry or psychology. The THI is described as being the companion to the Hearing Handicap Inventory for the Elderly/Adults (Ventry and Weinstein, 1982; Newman et al, 1990) (see Appendix Form C–14). The THI was found to be applicable in a busy clinical setting for quantifying the impact of tinnitus on daily living.

Hearing Handicap Inventory for Adults

This instrument was revised from the Hearing Handicap Inventory for the Elderly (HHIE) for use with younger hearing-impaired adults (<65 years of age) (Newman et al, 1990, 1991). The Hearing Handicap Inventory for Adults (HHIA) is a 25-item self-assessment scale that is comprised of two subscales, addressing emotional and social/situational considerations. The revision was necessary to include items relating to occupational effects of hearing loss. A 67-patient population study demonstrated high internal consistency reliability along with a low standard error of measurement. When correlating audiometric findings with the HHIA, a weak but statistically significant relationship with pure-tone sensitivity and suprathreshold word recognition ability was found. Newman et al (1990) concluded that audiometric measures alone are insufficient to capture a patient's hearing disability, which the HHIA facilitates (see Appendix Form C–14).

Temporomandibular Disorders

Temporomandibular Joint Scale

The Temporomandibular Joint (TMJ) Scale is a 97-item questionnaire that takes approximately 15 minutes to complete and measures the physical and psychosocial aspects of temporomandibular (TM) disorders (Levitt et al, 1987,

1988). The TMJ Scale is administered on a pencil-and-paper symptom inventory, computer scored, and generates scores separated into ten different scales. These scales are categorized into one of three domains: physical (six scales), psychosocial (three scales) and global (one scale). The scales have been found to be reliable, valid, and have predictive power. The following chart shows the scales in each of the domains:

Physical Domain	Psychosocial Domain	Global Domain
Pain report	Psychological	Global
Palpation pain	factors	
Perceived	Stress	
malocclusion	Chronicity	
Joint dysfunction		
Range of motion		
limitation		
Non-TM disorder		

The patient responses to questions in each domain are compared to data derived from large normative reference groups that consist of TM patients, non-TM dental patients, and nonpatient normals segregated by gender. Mean percentile ranks for TMJ disorder patients form the units of analysis, which allows for comparison to two "normal" populations and, therefore, allows for the clinical significance of the score to be assessed. **The Global Domain Scale indicates the overall probability of the presence of TMJ disorder and is the best single predictor of the presence or absence of TMJ disorder (80% to 90% accurate)** (Levitt et al, 1987; Levitt, 1989). History, examination, and radiology report data derived from 20 TMJ disorder patients were reviewed by two clinicians (Brown and Gaudet, 1994a) who then completed clinician rating forms, and compared these to previously completed clinician rating forms (Lundeen, 1988). The kappa coefficients were generated after correlating the two forms completed for each patient by the two clinicians (Table 7–10) (Brown and Gaudet, 1994a). The sensitivity (true-positives) and specificity (true-negatives) of the TMJ Scale were then calculated in a 90-TMJ disorder patient and non-TMJ disorder dental patient population, using history and physical examination. Of the 90 subjects tested, 46 were found to have a TMJ disorder and 44 did not (Table 7–10).

Several researchers have reported that with the passage of time, even in the absence of therapy, TMJ symptoms decrease and become less significant (Pullinger and Seligman, 1987; Randolph et al, 1990; McNeill, 1993). Levitt and McKinney (1994) completed a cross-sectional study of 10,000 cases and reported that different age groups experienced very similar severity levels and prevalence rate for TMJ pain. However, joint dysfunction and range of motion limitation showed the most severe level in the younger patient group, decreasing in severity after 30 years of age. Brown and Gaudet (1994b) found no statistical difference between the second test scale scores of the two groups for chronicity and the perceived malocclusion. They then note that in spite of symptom improvement, patients' condition remains chronic due to the mindset of the individual, as noted by the persistently high chronic scale scores pre- versus post-treatment. However, according to the authors, the perceived malocclusion scale would not be expected to improve due to the high frequency of occurrence of change in the relationship of the maxillary to mandibular skeletal and dental components. A posterior open bite is often observed bilaterally after treatment (Brown and Gaudet, 1994a). Thus, the theory is supported that younger patients with acute TMJ symptoms respond better to therapy than older patients with chronic problems. As a result, early detection in the younger patient may significantly affect long-term prognosis.

The use of the TMJ Scale can help the HCP track outcomes with treatment or nontreatment approaches to TMJ disorders. However, studies using larger sample sizes are recommended before firm conclusions are drawn about the

Table 7–10: Outcome Measurement Using the TMJ Scale[a]

SCALE	SENSITIVITY %	SPECIFICITY %	KAPPA COEFFICIENTS (BETWEEN CLINICAL RATINGS BY TWO CLINICIANS)
Pain report	91.7	97.6	1.00
Palpation pain	82.4	94.9	1.00
Joint dysfunction	95.2	87.5	1.00
Range of motion	86.1	83.3	0.46
Non-TMJ disorders	84.4	93.3	1.00
Global scale	93.5	93.2	1.00

TMJ, temporomandibular joint.
[a] The high levels of sensitivity and specificity of the TMJ scale are noted. Also, the high level of consistency supported by the high kappa coefficients are noted with the exception of the range of motion scale.
Modified with permission from Brown and Gaudet, 1994a.

findings that Joint Dysfunction and Range of Motion Scale scores were worse (not statistically significant) in the untreated patient group (Brown and Gaudet, 1994a).

TMD Disability Index

The TMD (Temporomandibular Disorder) Disability Index is another outcome generating method reported recently in an alpha-version (Steigerwald and Maher, 1997). This instrument utilizes many of the symptoms and disabilities with which TMD can present clinically, and scores these in an approach similar to that of the Oswestry Low Back Pain Disability Questionnaire and the Neck Disability Index. Two visual analogue scales that address symptom intensity and frequency (see Appendix Form C–15b) and a pain drawing to capture pain quality and location are also included in the total instrument. Because this is an alpha-version, the authors are requesting feedback regarding its clinical application. This instrument has not been validated nor tested in any retrospective or prospective study at the time of this writing. However, the tool has "face-validity," as it is based on information previously published in a peer review study involving 43 patients who, after undergoing arthroscopic surgery for arthrogenous TMD, had a significant reduction of neck pain, shoulder pain, headache, and jaw pain within 24 hours following the procedure (Steigerwald et al, 1996). I have applied minor modifications to the questionnaire and numerical rating scales to improve their utility. In addition, a scoring method has been devised based on my experience (see Appendix Form C–15c). These modifications and the scoring method have been met with approval from the originating authors and permission has been granted to include them in this text. Feedback from users is encouraged, and it is hoped that this tool will be used in a large prospective study involving the management of TMD (see Appendix Forms 7–15a, b, and c).

UPPER EXTREMITY ASSESSMENT TOOLS

Wrist

Carpal Tunnel Syndrome Questionnaire

A patient-administered questionnaire called the Carpal Tunnel Syndrome Questionnaire (CTSQ) tracks both symptoms and functional status (Levine et al, 1993). The criteria that are commonly utilized, including reproducibility, internal consistency, validity, and responsiveness to clinical change, were evaluated.

The CTSQ was constructed after interviewing a panel of hand surgeons, rheumatologists, and patients who identified six domains: pain, paresthesia, numbness, weakness, nocturnal symptoms, and overall functional status. The first part of the questionnaire, the Symptom Severity Scale, is made up of 11 questions, while the second part, the Functional Status Scale, is comprised of 8 questions. Each question is scored on a 5-point Likert scale scored from 1 point (mildest) to 5 points (most severe). Scoring is accomplished by calculating the mean of the 11 scores. The Functional Status Scale is made up of ADLs that are commonly performed by a broad range of patients, including younger workers, which include those with occupation-associated carpal tunnel syndrome, as well as the elderly. The same scoring approach is used as previously discussed, or the mean of the 8 items is calculated. Unanswered or not applicable items are not included in the calculation of the total score.

The CTSQ was tested on a 67-patient prospective cohort to determine the instrument's reproducibility, internal consistency, validity, and responsiveness to change. A separate cohort, consisting of previously released surgical patients with carpal tunnel syndrome, was studied to further document responsiveness to change. The study was composed of 39 patients (58%) who were evaluated presurgically, and 28 patients (42%) who were being managed conservatively (without surgery). Seventeen (25%) of the subjects studied were men, while 50 (75%) were women. A total of 9 patients (13%) had applied for workers' compensation, the median age was 57 years (range 19 to 88 years old), and the median duration of symptoms was 18 months (range 3 to 58 months) (Levine et al, 1993).

The reproducibility, or the ability to obtain the same result on repeated administrations assuming no clinical change, revealed Pearson correlation coefficients of $r = .91$ and .93 for severity of symptoms and functional status, respectively. The internal consistency, or the extent to which a scale of questions measures a single concept (in this case, symptom severity and functional status of the hand), revealed a Cronbach alpha of .89 and .91 for severity of symptoms and functional status, respectively (Levine et al, 1993). In comparing inter-rater agreement to objective measures previously reported, Levine et al point out the superior scores gathered by the CTSQ compared to the inter-rater agreement in electrocardiograph interpretation of .7 and between radiologists regarding the presence of osteoarthritis of .35 (Koran, 1975). This discussion was included to dispel the myth that so-called soft (subjective) outcomes such as the CTSQ are less valuable when compared to objective measures when, in fact, **the subjective measures are often more sensitive, specific, and responsive than many objective measures.** In a 38-patient group that was treated surgically and evaluated at a mean of 14 months postoperatively, the mean symptom-severity score improved from 3.4 points preoperatively to 1.9 points postoperatively. The functional status score improved from 3 to 2 points (5 being the worst and 1 point being the best score). Similar improvements were noted in an ongoing study in which 26 patients were studied preoperatively and then 3 months postoperatively (Levine et al, 1993).

The questionnaire was also compared to physical examination (objective) tests to test validity. Levine et al (1993) discuss the difficulty in assessing validity using physical examination methods due to the absence of universally accepted standards for measurement of severity of symptoms or functional status. More specifically, when taken together, both scales had positive, but weak, correlation with two-point discrimination and Semmes-Weinstein monofilament testing (Spearman coefficient, r = .12 to .42). When taken separately, scores for severity of symptoms had moderate correlation with grip and pinch strength and weak correlation with Semmes-Weinstein monofilament testing, two-point discrimination, and median nerve sensory conduction velocity. High correlation was noted when comparing the functional status scores to the severity of symptoms where major functional limitations were strongly correlated with severe symptoms. Moderate correlation with grip and pinch strength and a fair or poor correlation with objective measures of sensory function of the median nerve was also noted. **Levine et al (1993) conclude that the two questionnaire scales and traditional physical examination measures of median nerve function capture different but complementary outcome information. Therefore, symptom severity and functional status cannot be reliably compared to sensibility or nerve conduction testing.**

The strength of the CTSQ lies in its ability to track outcomes based on symptom severity and function, which are two of the primary reasons why patients with carpal tunnel syndrome present to HCPs in the first place. The CTSQ was developed for use in a broad-spectrum group of patients (including both young and old workers). If certain information is missing regarding a specific group of patients, for example, a group of assembly-line workers, items can be added to the Functional Status Scale that are germane to that population. Levine et al (1993) recommend that future outcome studies should include objective measures of impairment, complications, demographic data, and workers' compensation status. Therefore, the symptom severity and functional scales presented here were meant to supplement, not replace the variables usually measured in clinical studies. The CTSQ takes less than 10 minutes to complete (see Appendix Form C–16).

Shoulder

Shoulder Evaluation Form

The Shoulder Evaluation Form (SEF) is an instrument that combines both subjective data and physical examination findings (Rowe, 1987). This instrument was developed by the American Shoulder and Elbow Surgeons and has been utilized in several studies in its entirety or in a modified form (Barrett, 1987; Rowe, 1987; Hawkins and Dunlap, 1995). The first of the five categories of tests included in the SEF is a numerical pain rating using a 6-point (0–5) Likert scale, where 5 equals no pain and 0 equals complete disability. The second category is made up of various functional range of motion tests, including a goniometric evaluation of forward flexion and external rotation both from a neutral position (both sitting and lying supine) and from a 90-degree abducted shoulder starting position (sitting only). Internal rotation is also evaluated by measuring the distance the patient can reach up the back by approximating the thumb to the spinous processes; a score is then given for the level reached. The third category includes strength measurements of the anterior and middle deltoid muscles and the strength in internal and external rotation using a 6-point (0–5) grading scheme, where 5 equals normal and 0 equals paralysis. Stability of the shoulder graded on a 6-point scale, where 5 equals normal and 0 equals fixed dislocation, makes up the fourth category. The fifth and last category of the SEF is the assessment of function using 15 ADLs. The point values are defined as follows: 4 = normal; 3 = mild compromise; 2 = difficulty; 1 = with aid; 0 = unable, and NA = other/cannot say (Barrett, 1987; Rowe, 1987) (see Appendix Forms C–17a and b).

Shoulder Injury Self-Assessment of Function

The Self-Assessment of Function is the same 15-item ADL tool that is included in the American Shoulder and Elbow Surgeons SEF (Barrett, 1987; Rowe, 1987). This portion was used as a standalone tool in a study of nonoperative treatment of rotator cuff tears (Hawkins and Dunlop, 1995). These authors also used an instrument similar to the remaining categories of the SEF called the Constant-Murley Scoring of Shoulder Function (Constant and Murley, 1987) (see Appendix Form C–17b).

Rating Scale of the American Shoulder Elbow Surgeons

The Rating Scale of the American Shoulder Elbow Surgeons is quite similar to the SEF as it includes the same 6-point (0–5) pain scale. However, only 12, as compared to 15, ADLs used in the SEF are utilized, including one additional ADL ("reach behind back, fasten brassiere"), while three of the remaining four items ("perineal care," "throwing," and "do usual work") are omitted. The "do usual sport" item of the SEF is replaced with a 5-point (0–4) "Sports" section that grades the patient's ability to participate in the same or in different sporting events (see Appendix Form C–18).

Simple Shoulder Test Questionnaire

The Simple Shoulder Test Questionnaire (SSTQ) is a 12-item "yes/no" type of questionnaire that, as its name implies, is very simple (Matsen et al, 1995). This tool includes information regarding patient biographical data, dominant hand, and which shoulder is being evaluated (left or right). Also, a section for "office use only" allows for the diagnosis, patient identification number, physician name, point of evaluation (initial, preop, or follow-up at 6 months, 1 year, 18 months, or 2, 3, 4, or 5 years), first date of visit, treatment description, and surgery date (see Appendix Form C–19).

University of California at Los Angeles Shoulder Rating Scale

The University of California at Los Angeles Shoulder Rating Scale includes both subjective information, such as pain, function, and patient satisfaction, as well as range of motion and strength (Ellman et al, 1986). This instrument contains a maximum score of 35 points and appears quite similar to the SEF (see Appendix Form C–20).

LOWER EXTREMITY ASSESSMENT TOOLS

Knee Joint
Functional Index Questionnaire
The Functional Index Questionnaire (FIQ) is a valid and reliable method of tracking outcomes in patients being treated for patellofemoral pain syndrome (PFPS) (Chesworth et al, 1989). One study compared five different tools, including the FIQ, for their ability to measure outcomes pre- and post-treatment (Harrison et al, 1995). The different tools included the FIQ, a VAS for pain, the Patellofemoral Function Scale (PFS) (Reid, 1992), a step test, and a subjective report of functional limitations (Harrison et al, 1995). The goal of the study was to evaluate the ability of the clinical tool to measure the subject's changes prior to and 1 month after treatment, but not the specific treatment regimens utilized. A 56-patient population was used in a randomized clinical trial.

The VAS included three components: pain at worst, pain at least, and average pain. Each of the three VAS questions was analyzed separately rather than formulating one composite score. Functional limitations were measured on a 0–4 scale (with 0 = none and 4 = completely disabling) and the "change in condition" was measured on a 1–4 scale (with 1 = significant improvement noted and 4 = condition worse) (Table 7–11) (Harrison et al, 1995).

Patellofemoral Function Scale
The Patellofemoral Function Scale (PFS) was initially presented by Reid in 1992 for evaluating patients with PFPS. This instrument includes parts of a physical examination, as well as activity intolerance derived from the patient's history which includes pain, activity, functional restrictions, and the use of orthoses. In 1988, Schwarz et al developed a patellofemoral rating scale for postoperative evaluation of patients with osteochondritis dissecans of the knee. The patellofemoral index was developed by Saltzman et al in 1990, based on the Cincinnati Knee Rating system (Noyes, 1990) to evaluate patients over a treatment period. Other methods of measuring treatment effects of PFPS, such as decreased muscle strength and, to some degree, disabilities

such as stair climbing, have also been reported (McConnell, 1986; Doucette and Goble, 1992; O'Neill et al, 1992). However, none of these tools have been evaluated for validity (Harrison et al, 1995). Studies of PFPS have reported poor correlation with the condition's severity. For example, patellofemoral alignment (Fairbank et al, 1984; Reikeras, 1992), electromyographic (EMG) variables, and gait functional changes are poorly correlated (Chesworth et al, 1989). More specifically, a VAS for measuring pain as well as a functional index were found effective to measure pain and function changes, while gait and EMG variables did not change in spite of reported improvement in the patient's condition (Chesworth et al, 1989).

The step test that was described by Reid (1992) was performed with the patient stepping down from a 6-inch step, leading with the least affected or normal leg, then leading with the affected leg back up the step. The test was terminated when subjects indicated that they felt knee pain. Time was recorded in seconds. A tape-recorded musical beat was used to set the step rate but the metronome setting was not given. A 5-minute maximum was used if no knee pain was reported. A second step test was performed in most cases within 2 weeks of the initial evaluation. Refer to the YMCA 3-Minute Bench Step Test in Chapter 18 for specific instructions for assessing cardiovascular function. Note that the step test suggested here is a modification of the YMCA approach, but cardiac risk must not be forgotten simply because the focus is on knee function. Table 7–12 lists the descriptive statistics for the VAS, FIQ, step test, PFS, and self-report of functional limitation.

Modest test–retest reliability for the FIQ, VAS, and step tests were found in Reid's study (1992). High internal consistency for the FIQ and modest internal consistency for the PFS were demonstrated. The FIQ and VAS were found to be good discriminators for measuring changes in clinical status. The step test, on the other hand, while reliable, was poor at detecting clinical change. The PFS demonstrated potential to detect clinical change but had not previously been tested for reliability (see Appendix Form C–21).

Subjective Knee Score Questionnaire
The Subjective Knee Score Questionnaire, adapted from Noyes (1990), was utilized together with two clinical tests, the single-leg hop test and an isokinetic isolated knee concentric muscular test. The purpose of the study was to determine if a correlation existed between these three testing approaches and if the information would be beneficial to clinicians in determining patient progression, treatment modification, and in making return-to-sport decisions. The questionnaire rated symptoms (pain, swelling, giving way) and specific sport function, resulting in an overall knee score assessment. The three one-legged hopping functional tests included (1) hop for distance, (2) timed hop, and (3) cross-over triple hop. The isokinetic tests were performed on a Biodex dynamometer at 180, 300, and 450 degrees per second for knee extension/

Table 7–11: Functional Limitations and Change in Condition Scales Used to Compare and Contrast to the FIQ

FUNCTIONAL LIMITATIONS	CHANGE IN CONDITION
0 None	
1 Annoying	1 Significant improvement noted
2 Limits some activities	2 Some improvement noted
3 Limits most activities	3 No improvement noted
4 Completely disabling	4 Condition worse

Modified from Harrison et al, 1995.

Table 7–12: Descriptive Statistics of Five Tests Measuring Outcomes in Patients with Patellofemoral Pain Syndrome

	MEAN	STANDARD DEVIATION	RANGE	NUMBER
Visual Analogue Scale[a]				
Pre-treatment	2.64	1.66	.11–6.33	50
Post-treatment	1.64	1.58	0–5.33	46
Functional Index Questionnaire[b]				
Pre-treatment	1.27	.39	0–2	51
Post-treatment	1.46	.44	.38–2	46
Step Test[c]				
Pre-treatment	2.46	1.49	1–5	56
Post-treatment	3.34	1.7	1–5	56
Patellofemoral Function Scale[d]				
Pre-treatment	51.73	13.95	24–88	56
Post-treatment	59.73	16.65	28–92	56
Functional Limitation[e]				
Pre-treatment	1.84	.71	0–4	56
Post-treatment	1.5	.93	0–3	56

[a] Worst, least, and usual pain ratings for 3 days.
[b] Eight questions over 3 days, based on a scale of 0 to 2.
[c] Two tests pre-treatment and one test post-treatment, in minutes.
[d] Maximum score of 100, representing normal.
[e] Ordinal scale of 0 to 4 (operational definitions—See Table 7–11).
Modified from Harrison et al, 1995.

flexion. The questionnaire results revealed a mean value of 86 points. Sixty-four percent of the subjects tested exhibited normal limb symmetry (within 85%) on all three single-leg hop tests, and 16% exhibited quadriceps strength at least 90% of the contralateral limb isokinetically. A positive correlation was noted between isokinetic knee extension peak torque (180, 300 degrees per second), subjective knee scores, and the three-hop tests ($p < .001$). A statistical trend was observed between knee extension acceleration and deceleration range at 180 and 300 degrees per second for timed hop test and cross-over triple hop ($r = .48$, $r = .49$, $r = .51$, $r = .49$). There were no positive correlations noted for isokinetic test results for the knee flexors (see Appendix Form C–22). These results suggest that these tests correlated well with the exception of isokinetic tests of the knee flexors. Where used together, return-to-sport decisions can be made utilizing these testing approaches (Noyes, 1990).

Rating Knee Replacement Results

The Rating Knee Replacement Results form includes six categories, which include pain, range of motion, stability, flexion contracture, extension lag, and alignment (Insall et al, 1989). Pain is graded from "none" (50 points) to "severe" (0 points); range of motion is given 1 point per 5 degrees, with a maximum of 25 points (125 degrees); and stability is assessed in the anteroposterior direction (0–10 points) and mediolateral (0–15 points). The maximum number of points possible is 100. Deductions of points are subtracted from the total points calculated from the three items previously listed. The deductions include the following categories: flexion contracture (2–20 points); extension lag (5–15 points); and alignment (0–20 points). A maximum deduction point total is 55 points. The calculation of permanent impairment and categorizing the replacement result as good, fair, or poor, is accomplished by identifying the total points calculated with the proper category in the chart located at the bottom of the form and reprinted in Table 7–13 (see Appendix Form C–23).

Other knee scoring methods that combine history and/or examination elements also exist but are not individually discussed here. They include the following:

- Cincinnati Rating System (Noyes et al, 1984)
- Isometric and Isokinetic Scoring Scale (Kannus et al, 1987)

Table 7–13: Total Knee Replacement Rating System

RESULT	POINTS
1. Good results	85–100
2. Fair results	50–84
3. Poor result	Less than 50

Modified from Insall et al, 1989.

- International Knee Documentation Committee Questionnaire (Miller and Carr, 1993)
- Knee Scoring Scale I (Kettlalkamp and Thompson, 1975)

Of note, a portion of the Knee Society clinical rating system is utilized in the rating of permanent impairment regarding knee replacement (AMA, 1993). In addition, high-tech approaches to the assessment of gait using videotape and computer equipment have been used to evaluate knee hyperextension gait abnormalities in unstable knees (Noyes et al, 1996).

Hip Joint

Rating of Hip Replacement Results

The rating scheme for the hip joint is a modification that was presented in the AMA *Guides to the Evaluation of Permanent Impairment*, 4th edition (1993). The assessment includes both patient-driven information, which includes pain, function, and activity restriction, and physical examination information, which includes fixed deformities and range of motion (Callaghan et al, 1990). More specifically, **pain** is scored from "none" (44 points) to "marked" (10 points). **Function** comprises three subcategories, including "limp" (0–11 points), "supporting device" (0–11 points), and "distance walked" (0–11 points). The **activities** category consists of four subcategories, including "stair climbing" (0–4 points), "putting on shoes and socks" (0–4 points), "sitting" (0–4 points), and "public transportation" (0–1 point). The examination portion includes **deformity** and its five subcategories of fixed adduction (0–1 points), fixed internal rotation, fixed external rotation, flexion contracture, and leg length discrepancy, all using a 0–1 point value. The **range of motion** category comprises five subcategories, including flexion, abduction, adduction, external rotation, and internal rotation, all using a 0–1 point value. The points from each category are added together and compared to a chart (Table 7–14). Note that the higher the score, the lesser the impairment. The total number of possible points is 100. The calculation of permanent impairment and categorizing the replacement re-

Table 7–14: Total Hip Replacement Rating System[a]

RESULT	POINTS
1. Good results	85–100
2. Fair results	50–84
3. Poor result	Less than 50

[a] The total hip replacement includes endoprosthesis and unipolar or bipolar varieties.
Modified from Callaghan et al, 1990.

sult as good, fair, or poor, is accomplished by identifying the total points calculated with the proper category in the chart located at the bottom of the form (see Appendix Form C–24).

PSYCHOMETRIC ASSESSMENT TOOLS

The presence of depression is common when patients have had lingering pain. Unfortunately this result is prevalent in patients dealing with musculoskeletal complaints that become chronic. Clinically significant depression has been reported to be present in more than 50% of chronic pain patients who present to chiropractors (Carroll, 1997).

Two models are used when describing musculoskeletal pain. The **biomedical model** refers to pain associated with a physical injury or disease. This model is applicable to those with pain arising from, for example, a fracture and usually has a straightforward course of resolution without complications. This model is inadequate for the majority of patients with recurring or chronic pain due to the psychological component associated with chronic pain. The **biopsychosocial model** consists of a combination of the physical and associated psychological elements associated with chronicity. This is clearly the better model for explaining, understanding, and managing the psychological component associated with chronic pain. This model also addresses "yellow flags," which include psychosocial issues such as work dissatisfaction, marital discord, financial strain, depression, and others (see Chap. 21 for a discussion of "yellow flags"). In the biopsychosocial model, the responsibility for recovery is a partnership between the HCP and the patient, with the role of the HCP being primarily that of "coach."

Beck Depression Inventory

Depression is a significant feature of chronic pain. At any one time, 9% to 20% of the population in the United States suffers from depression, of which 5% have major depression (Regier et al, 1988). Above this rate of depression, 50% of chronic pain patients are depressed, of which only 10% had depression preceding their chronic illness and 90% developed it because of the chronic condition (Sullivan et al, 1992). Approximately 10% to 15% of those suffering with clinical depression commit suicide.

CLINICAL TIP 7–3
Choosing a Subjective Questionnaire

The strength of a subjective questionnaire lies in its ability to:
- Sensitively discriminate the clinical changes that occur between examinations
- Remain practical in a private clinic setting

Therefore, the FIQ may be the favored knee questionnaire since it is the shortest, easiest to score and interpret, and can validly and reliably discriminate between patient groups and controls.

With these rather startling statistics, it becomes clear that a method of screening for depression is essential. Although many tools have been introduced over the past two to three decades, the Beck Depression Inventory (BDI) has been utilized in many studies and has been found to be a reliable screening approach that can be repeated at regular intervals (Appendix Form C–25). Burns, a pupil of Aaron Beck, Professor of Psychology at the University of Pennsylvania Medical School, helped make the BDI more widely available through his best selling book (1992). Scoring of the BDI allows for assessment of progress, which is recommended at regular intervals suggested at once a week; "compare it to weighing yourself regularly when on a diet" (Burns, 1992). Scoring of the BDI is easy, as there is a 0 to 3 possible score for each of a total of 21 items, yielding a maximum possible total score of 63 points if all items are completed. Simply add up the total points and compare it to the following interpretation scale:

1–10	These ups and downs are considered normal
11–16	Mild mood disturbance
17–20	Borderline clinical depression
21–30	Moderate depression
31–40	Severe depression
Over 40	Extreme depression

A cut-off score of 17 or higher upon repeat assessments may be suggestive of the need for professional treatment.

Caution must be exercised when addressing depression with a patient, especially early on in care, prior to establishing a certain level of trust. The BDI or a similar tool should not be used prior to a careful history, and the BDI should be considered only when depression is suspected. This is not a routine intake questionnaire to be completed by a patient on an initial visit. It contains questions concerning suicide and other very sensitive and personal issues that should not be completed unless the patient has gained an appropriate level of trust and understanding. Further, **it is inappropriate to establish a diagnosis from the administration of the BDI. This is meant to be a screen** to facilitate discussion and stimulate referral to a mental health professional, who can then accurately assess the patient's condition. Carroll (1997) urges HCPs not to fear patient anger or rejection as the contrary often occurs as "most sui-cidal individuals are actually relieved to be able to talk about this problem." If many of the following risk factors of depression are present, further assessment may be wise (Carroll, 1997):

- Age over 45
- Divorced, separated, widowed, or single
- Poor economic status
- Recent losses (loss of a job or a spouse or new disability)
- Previous attempts at suicide
- Recent discharge from hospital

Distress and Risk Assessment Method

The Distress and Risk Assessment Method (DRAM) was designed to identify psychosocial patterns in patients with acute pain in order to select proper management approaches from the beginning of care (Moffroid and Haugh, 1995). **The DRAM is based on the concept that some pain and illness behaviors are due to unresolved pain** (Feuerstein et al, 1987). It combines physical and psychological measures in an attempt to differentiate between patients displaying distress, those at risk of developing major psychological overlay, and those who are clearly depressed. The objective of the instrument was to provide a simple screening tool that has both utility and clincial validity. The authors utilized two previously introduced tools to determine the score of the DRAM: the Modified Somatic Perception Questionnaire (MSPQ), a test of heightened autonomic or somatic awareness ("somatic anxiety"), and the Zung Depression Index to capture depressive features (see Appendix Forms C–26 and C–27). It has been reported that these two instruments were much more highly associated with patients' level of disability when compared to other assessment methods (Main and Waddell, 1989). Based on these two instruments, four cluster groups were reported as normal (type N), at risk (type R), distress/depressive (type DD), and distressed/somatic (type DS) (Table 7–15).

Taken as an aggregate, the four cluster groups were reported to be clearly distinguishable from each other in this study of 567 initial subjects, of which 98 patients successfully completed a 1- to 4-year follow-up (Main et al, 1992). There was clear differentiation between the type N, R, and

Table 7–15: The Distress and Risk Assessment Method

TYPE[a]	MODIFIED ZUNG	MSPQ
N (Normal)	<17	NA
R (At risk)	17–33	<12
DD (Distressed/Depressive)	>33	NA
DS (Distressed/Somatic)	17–33	>12

NA, not available.

[a] The four cluster groups are shown with display of the cutoff scores.

Modified from Modified Zung Depression Index; from Main et al, 1992.

DD or DS groups, although more work is recommended to appraise the significance of the difference between the type DD and DS groups.

Many tools are available for assessing depression, anxiety, coping strategies, fear avoidance, disability prediction, and other biopsychological issues. Further discussion of this important aspect of chronic pain exceeds the scope of this chapter. Refer to Chapters 8, 10, and 21 for different perspectives on assessing these and other "yellow flags."

CLINICAL TIP 7–4
Recommendations for Using the DRAM

Recommendations for assessment and management using the DRAM include the following:

- The DRAM is recommended as a screening tool to aid in the clinical appraisal of the patient.
- Its use is especially recommended in problem back clinics and pain centers.
- Consider the DRAM as a first-step screen, not a complete psychological assessment or a malingering test.
- The management of distress must be addressed in addition to conservative or surgical therapy.

A multidisciplinary management approach is appropriate for nonsurgical distressed patients (Main et al, 1992).

Conclusion

Condition-specific questionnaires are appropriate to include in the battery of outcomes assessment tools for a specific condition due to the superior responsiveness of these tools when compared to noncondition-specific tools. **However, many studies recommend the use of a specific tool with a general health questionnaire such as the SF-36/HSQ-2.0 as the latter captures the impact the specific condition is having on the patient's quality of life and general health.** Thus, combining tools that measure pain (the VAS), activity intolerance (Oswestry, Neck Disability Index), and general health (SF-36, HSQ-2.0, or Dartmouth COOP Health Charts) will capture several different outcome domains, all of which are important treatment goals of the presenting patient.

As noted, many questionnaires are available for the lumbar spine but only one specifically for the cervical region and a handful for conditions sometimes associated with cervical spine complaints such as dizziness, tinnitus, temporomandibular dysfunction, hearing loss, and headache. Many new questionnaires are being presented regarding the lumbar spine which may, in time, take over the reign of "gold standard."

Until that time, the Oswestry and Roland-Morris questionnaires are still utilized in the current studies as benchmarks and, therefore, remain gold standards.

Various outcome tools for the extremities were introduced in this chapter. Just like their spinal OA counterparts, these tools reflect information on pain and activity intolerance, and some even address emotional or affective dimensions of a patient's health. Outcome measures for injuries sustained to the shoulder, upper extremity (in general), wrist, hip, and knee are included. Many other tools could have been included. However, the objective was not to try to include every possible published tool or questionnaire. Rather, offering an assortment of tools from which to choose allows HCPs to decide how they wish to manage their own practices. **The primary requirement of outcomes management is to start and end treatment with the same tool(s), score the tool(s), and most importantly, review the results and make treatment plans or decisions based from the outcome tool results. Only until the latter point is practiced can the HCP realize and appreciate the benefits of practicing in a literature- and outcomes-based manner.**

REFERENCES

AMA. *Guides to the Evaluation of Permanent Impairment.* 4th ed. Chicago, Ill: American Medical Association; 1993:88.

Baker DJ, Pynsent PB, Fairbank JCT. The Oswestry disability index revisited: Its reliability, repeatability and validity, and a comparison with the St. Thomas's disability index. In: Roland M, Jenner JR, eds. *Back Pain: New Approaches to Rehabilitation and Education.* Manchester, England: Manchester University Press; 1989:174–86.

Barrett NWP, Franklin JL, Jackins SE, Wyss CR, Matsen FA. Total shoulder arthroplasty. *J Bone Joint Surg.* 1987;69A:865–872.

Beck AT, Ward CH, Mendelson M, Mock J, Erbaugh J. An inventory for measuring depression. *Arch Gen Psychiat.* 1961;4:561–571.

Bergner M, Bobbit RA, Canter WB, Gilson BS. The sickness index profile: Development and final revision of a health status measure. *Medical Care.* 1981;19:787–809.

Brown DT, Gaudet EL. Outcome measurement for treated and untreated TMD patients using the TMJ scale. *J Craniomandib Pract.* 1994a;12:216–221.

Brown DT, Gaudet EL Jr, Phillips C. Changes in vertical tooth position and face height related to long term anterior repositioning splint therapy. *J Craniomandib Pract.* 1994b;12:19–22.

Burns DD. *Feeling Good: The New Mood Therapy.* New York, NY: Avon Books; 1992.

Callaghan JJ, Dysart SH, Savory CF, Hopkinson WJ. Assessing the results of hip replacement: A comparison of five different rating systems. *J Bone Joint Surg [Br].* 1990;72B:1008–1009.

Carroll L. Psychological problems encountered in chiropractic clinical practice. In: Lawrence DJ, ed. *Advances in Chiropractic.* Vol. 4. Baltimore, Md: Mosby; 1997:155–180.

Chesworth BM, Culham EG, Tata GE, Peat M. Validation of oucome measures in patients with patellofemoral syndrome. *J Orthop Sports Phys Ther.* 1989;11:302–308.

Constant CR, Murley AHG. A clinical method of functional assessment of the shoulder. *Clin Orthop.* 1987;214:160–164.

Daltroy LH, Cats-Baril WL, Katz JN, Fossel AH, Liang MH. The North American Spine Society lumbar spine outcome assessment instrument: reliability and validity tests. *Spine.* 1996;21:741–749.

Deyo RA. Comparative validity of the Sickness Impact Profile. *Spine.* 1986;11:951–954.

Deyo RA. Measuring the functional status of patients with low back pain. *Arch Phys Med Rehabil.* 1988; 69:1044–1053.

Deyo RA, et al. The Low Back TyPE. 1990. Available: Stratis Health, 2901 Metro Drive, Suite 400, Bloomington, MN 55425-1525; (612) 858-9188 (O); (612) 858-9189 (Fax).

Deyo RA, Andersson G, Bombardier C, et al. Outcome measures for studying patients with low back pain. *Spine.* 1994;19:2032S–2036S.

Doucette SA, Goble EM. The effect of exercise on patellar tracking in lateral patellar compression syndrome. *Am J Sports Med.* 1992;20:434–440.

Ellman H, Hanker G, Bayer M. Repair of the rotator cuff: End-result study of factors influencing reconstruction. *J Bone Joint Surg.* 1986;68A:1136–1144.

Ellwood PM. Outcomes management: A technology of patient experience. *N Engl J Med.* 1988;318:1549–1556.

Erhard RE, Delitto A, Cibulka MT. Relative effectiveness of an extension program and a combined program of manipulation and flexion and extension exercises in patients with acute low back syndrome. *Phys Ther.* 1994;74:1093–1100.

Fairbank JCT, Couper C, Davies JB, O'Brien JP. The Oswestry Low Back Pain Disability Questionnaire. *Physiotherapy.* 1980;66(18):271–273.

Fairbank JCT, Pynsent PB, van Poortvliet JA, Phillips H. Mechanical factors in the incidence of knee pain in adolescents and young adults. *J Bone Joint Surg [Br].* 1984;66B:685–693.

Feuerstein M, Carter RL, Papciak AS. A prospective analysis of stress and fatigue in recurrent low back pain. *Pain.* 1987;31:333–344.

Greenough CG, Fraser RD. Assessment of outcome in patients with low back pain. *Spine.* 1992;17:36–41.

Haas M, Jacobs GE, Raphaei R, Petzing K. Low back pain outcome measurement assessment in chiropractic teaching clinics: Responsiveness and applicability of two functional disability questionnaires. *J Manipulative Physiol Ther.* 1995;18:79–87.

Harrison E, Quinney AH, Magee D, Sheppard MS, McQuarrie A. Analysis of outcome measures used in the study of patellofemoral pain syndrome. *Physiother Can.* 1995;47:264–272.

Harper AC, Harper DA, Lambert LJ, et al. Development and validation of the Curtin Back Screening Questionnaire (CBSQ). *Pain.* 1995;6:73–81.

Hawkins RH, Dunlop R. Nonoperative treatment of rotator cuff tears. *Clin Ortho Rel Res.* 1995;321:178–188.

Hsieh C, Phillips R, Adams A, Pope M. Functional outcomes of low back pain: Comparison of four treatment groups in a randomized controlled trial. *J Manipulative Physiol Ther.* 1992;15:4–9.

Hudson-Cook N, Tomes-Nicholson K. *The Revised Oswestry Low Back Pain Disability Questionnaire.* England: Anglo-European College of Chiropractic; 1988. Thesis.

Hunter M. The headache scale: A new approach to the assessment of headache pain based on pain descriptions. *Pain.* 1983;16:361–373.

Insall JN, Dorr LD, Scott RD. Rationale of the Knee Society clinical rating system. *Clin Orthop Relat Res.* 1989;248:14.

International Headache Society Committee on Clinical Trials in Migraine. Guidelines for controlled trials of drugs in migraine. *Cephalgia.* 1991;1:1–12.

Jacobson GP, Newman CW. The development of the dizziness handicap inventory. *Arch Otolarngol Head Neck Surg.* 1990;116:424–427.

Jacobson GP, Newman CW, Hunter L, Balzer GK. Balance function test correlates of the Dizziness Handicap Inventory. *J Am Audiol.* 1991;2:253–260.

Jacobson GP, Ramadan NM, Aggarwal SK, Newman CW. The Henry Ford Hospital headache disability inventory (HDI). *Neurology.* 1994;44:837–842.

Kames LD, Naliboff BD, Heinrich RL, Coscarelli Schag C. The chronic illnesses problem inventory: Problem oriented psychosocial assessment of patients with chronic illness. *Int J Psychiatry Med.* 1984;14:65–75.

Kannus P, Jarvinea M, Latvala K. Kenn strength evaluation. *Scand J Sport Sci.* 1987;9:9.

Karoly P, Jensen MP. *Multimethod Assessment of Chronic Pain.* Oxford, England: Pergamon Press; 1987.

Kettlalkamp DB, Thompson C. Development of a knee scoring scale. *Clin Orthop Relat Res.* 1975;107:96.

Kopec JA, Esdaile JM. Spine update: Functional disability scales for back pain. *Spine.* 1995a;20:1943–1949.

Kopec JA, Esdaile JM, Abrahamowicz M, Abenhaim L, Wood-Dauphinee S, Lamping DL. The Quebec Back Pain Disability Scale: Measurement properties. *Spine.* 1995b;20:341–352.

Koran LM. The reliability of clinical methods, data and judgements (first of two parts). *N Engl J Med.* 1975;293:642–646.

Lawlis GF, Cuencas R, Selby D, McCoy CE. The development of the Dallas pain questionnaire. An assessment of the impact of spinal pain on behavior. *Spine.* 1989;14:510–516.

Leclaire R, Blier F, Fortin L, Proulx R. A cross-sectional study comparing the Oswestry and Roland-Morris functional disability scales in two populations of patients with low back pain of different levels of severity. *Spine.* 1997;22:68–71.

Levine DW, Simmons HP, Koris MJ, et al. A self-administered questionnaire for the assessment of severity of syptoms and functional status in carpal tunnel syndrome. *J Bone Joint Surg.* 1993;75A:1585–1592.

Levitt SR. Clinical research with the TMJ scale. *J Craniomandib Pract.* 1989;7:253.

Levitt SR, Lundeen TF, McKinney MW. *The TMJ Scale Manual.* Durham, NC: Pain Resouce Center; 1987.

Levitt SR, Lundeen TF, McKinney MW. Initial studies of a new assessment method for temporomandibular joint disorders. *J Prosthet Dent.* 1988;59:490–495.

Levitt SR, McKinney MW. Validating the TMJ scale in a national sample of ten thousand patients. *J Orofacial Pain.* 1994;8:25–35.

Luck JV Jr, Florence DW. A brief history and comparative analysis of disability systems and impairment rating guides. *Orthop Clin North Am.* 1988;19:839–844.

Lundeen TF, Levitt SR, McKinney MW. Evaluation of temporomandibular joint disorders by clinician ratings. *J Prosthet Dent.* 1988;59:202–211.

Main CJ, Waddell G. Personality assessment in the management of low back pain. *Clin Rehabil.* 1987;1:139–142.

Main CJ, Wood PLR, Hollis S, et al. The distress and risk assessment method. A simple patient classification to identify distress and evaluate the risk of poor outcome. *Spine.* 1992;17:42–52.

Matsen FA III, Ziegler DW, DeBartolo SE. Patient self-assessment of health status and function in glenohumeral degenerative joint disease. *J Shoulder Elbow Surg.* 1995;4:345–351.

McConnell J. The management of chondromalacia patellae: A long term solution. *Aust J Physiother.* 1986;32:215–223.

McNeill C. Craniomandibular disorders: Guidelines for evaluation, diagnosis and management. Chicago, Ill: Quintessence Publishing; 1993.

Millard RW. The functional assessment screening questionnaire: Application for evaluating pain-related disability. *Arch Phys Med Rehabil.* 1989;70:303–307.

Miller RK, Carr AJ. The knee. In: Pysent PB, ed. *Outcome Measures in Orthopaedics.* Oxford, England: Butterworth-Heinemann; 1993:228–244.

Million R, Hall W, Nilsen KH, Baker RD, Jayson MIV. Assessment of the progress of the back pain patient. *Spine.* 1982;7:204–12.

Moffroid MT, Haugh LD. Classification schema for acute and subacute low back pain. *Ortho Phys Ther Clin North Am.* 1995;4:179–192.

Newman CW, Jacobson GP, Spitzer JB. Development of the Tinnitus Handicap Inventory. *Arch Otolaryngol Head Neck Surg.* 1996;122:143–148.

Newman CW, Weinstein BE, Jacobson GP, Hug GA. The Hearing Handicap Inventory for adults: Psychometric adequacy and audiometric correlates. *Ear Hear.* 1990;11:430–433.

Newman CW, Weinstein BE, Jacobson GP, Hug GA. Test–retest reliability of the Hearing Handicap Inventory for Adults. *Arch Otolarngol Head Neck Surg.* 1991;12:355–357.

Noyes FR. Functional disability in the anterior cruciate insufficient knee syndrome. *Sports Med.* 1984; 1:286–287.

Noyes FR. The Noyes Knee Rating System: An assessment of subjective, objective, ligamentous, and functional parameters. Cincinnati, Ohio: Internal Publication of Sports Medicine Research and Education Foundation; 1990.

Noyes FR, Dunworth LA, Andriacchi TP, Andrews M, Hewett TE. Knee hyperextension gait abnormalities in unstable knees: Recognition and preoperative gait retraining. *Am J Sport Med.* 1996;24:35–45.

O'Neill DB, Micheli LJ, Warner JP. Patellofemoral stress. *Am J Sports Med.* 1992;20:151–156.

Pollard AC. Preliminary validity study of the Pain Disability Index. *Percept Motor Skills.* 1984;54:54–74.

Porter RW, Trailescu IF. Diurnal changes in straight leg raising. *Spine.* 1990;15:103–106.

Pullinger A, Seligman D. TMJ osteoarthrosis: A differentiation of diagnostic subgroups by symptom history and demographic. *J Craniomandib Disord Facial Oral Pain.* 1987;1:251–256.

Rainville J, Ahern DK, Phalen L, Childs LA, Sutherland R. The association of pain with physical activities in chronic low back pain. *Spine.* 1992;17:1060–1064.

Randolph CS, Green CS, Moretti R, Forbes D, Perry HT. Conservative management of temporomandibular disorders: A post treatment comparison between patients from a university clinic and from private practice. *Am J Orthod Dentofac Orthop.* 1990;98:77–82.

Reid DC. *Sports Injury Assessment and Rehabilitation.* New York, NY: Churchill Livingstone; 1992.

Reikeras D. Patellofemoral characteristics in patients with increased femoral anteversion. *Skel Radiol.* 1992;21:311–313.

Regier DA, Boyd JH, et al. One month prevalence of mental disorders in the United States. *Arch Gen Psychiatry.* 1988;41:977–986.

Riley JF, Ahern DK, Follick MJ. Chronic pain and functional impairment: Assessing beliefs about their relationship. *Arch Phys Med Rehabil.* 1988;69:579–582.

Roland M, Morris R. A study of the natural history of back pain: Part I: Development of a reliable and sensitive measure of disability in low-back pain. *Spine.* 1983a;8:141–144.

Roland M, Morris R. A study of the natural history of low back pain, Part II. *Spine.* 1983b;8(2):145–150.

Rowe CR. Evaluation of the shoulder. In: Rowe CR, ed. *The Shoulder.* New York, NY: Churchill Livingstone; 1987:633.

Ruta DA, Garratt AM, Wardlaw D, Russell IT. Developing a valid and reliable measure of health outcome for patients with low back pain. *Spine.* 1994;19:1887–1896.

Saltzman CL, Goulet JA, McMellan RT, Schneider LA, Matthews LS. Results of treatment of displaced patellar fractures by partial patellectomy. *J Bone Joint Surg [Am].* 1990;72A(9):1270–1284.

Schwarz C, Blazina ME, Siston DJ, Hirsch LC. The results of operative treatment of osteochondritis dissecans of the patella. *Am J Sports Med.* 1988;16:522–529.

Seltzer GB, Granger CV, Winebery DE. Functional assessment: Bridge between family and rehabilitation medicine within an ambulatory practice. *Arch Phys Med Rehabil.* 1982;63:453–457.

Slater MA, Hall HF, Atkinson JH, Garfin SR. Pain and impairment beliefs in chronic low back pain: Validation of the pain and impairment relationship scale (PAIRS). *Pain.* 1991;44:51–56.

Steigerwald DP, Maher JH. The Steigerwald/Maher TMD Disability Questionnaire. *Today's Chiro.* 1997; 26:86–91.

Steigerwald DP, Verne SV, Young D. A retrospective evaluation of the impact of temporomandibular joint arthroscopy on the symptoms of headache, neck pain, shoulder pain, dizziness, and tinnitus. *J Craniomandibular Prac.* 1996;14:46–54.

Stratford PW, Binkley JM. Measurement properties of the RM18: A modified version of the Roland-Morris Disability Scale. *Spine.* 1997;22:2416–2421.

Stratford PW, Binkley JM, Riddle DL, Guyatt GH. Sensitivity to change of the Roland-Morris back pain questionnaire: part 1. *Phys Ther.* 1998;78:1186–1196.

Stucki G, Daltroy L, Liang MH, Lipson SJ, Fossel AH, Katz JN. Measurement properties of a self-administered outcome measure in lumbar spinal stenosis. *Spine.* 1996;21:796–803.

Sullivan MJL, Reesor K, et al. The treatment of depression in chronic low back pain: Review and recommendations. *Pain.* 1992;50:5–13.

Turner JA, Robinson J, McCreary CP. Chronic low back pain: Predicting response to nonsurgical treatment. *Arch Phys Med Rehabil.* 1983;64:560–563.

Turk DC, Rudy TE. Towards a comprehensive assessment of chronic pain patients. *Behav Res Ther.* 1987;25:237–49.

Ventry IM, Weinstein B. The hearing handicap inventory for the elderly: A new tool. *Ear Hear.* 1982;3:128–134.

Vernon H, Mior S. The Neck Disability Index: A study of reliability and validity. *J Manipulative Physiol Ther.* 1991;14:409–415.

Von Korff M, Saunders K. The course of back pain in primary care. *Spine.* 1996;21:2833–2839.

Waddell G, Main CJ. Assessment severity in low back disorders. *Spine.* 1984;9:204–208.

Yang Y, Eaton S, Maxwell MW. The relationship between the St. Thomas and Oswestry Disability scores and the severity of low back pain. *J Manipulative Physiol Ther.* 1983;16:14–18.

Yellen AN. California School of Professional Psychology; 1978. Doctoral Dissertation.

CHAPTER 8

Measuring Psychosocial Outcomes in Clinical Practice

DAVID A. WILLIAMS AND MICHAEL FEUERSTEIN

INTRODUCTION

As health care evolves, there is greater need to identify the impact of health care procedures on a variety of outcomes. For example, with the increased focus on functional restoration, health care providers (HCPs) have begun to measure functional status and return to work in addition to pain and symptoms. Additionally, cost-effectiveness and patient satisfaction are being included in the evaluation of treatment efficacy.

The focus of this chapter is on a class of outcome measures often referred to as "psychosocial." Historically, the term "psychosocial" has been used to describe a broad range of concepts and, as such, many nonmental health professionals find psychosocial measures confusing, complex, and their utility in daily practice unclear. **Since the primary presenting symptom of most patients with back complaints is pain, and pain relief is often the major goal of patients, patients and HCPs alike frequently fail to consider the important role psychosocial factors play in influencing the effectiveness of pain treatments.**

As will be described in this chapter, psychosocial factors can influence pain perception, ability to adjust to pain, ability to function with pain, and quality of life. Since psychosocial factors are highly influential when treating pain, it is argued that the strategic inclusion of carefully selected psychosocial measures are critical for providing a comprehensive picture of outcome and for interpreting the patterns of findings in a battery of outcome measures. Thus, this chapter hopes to acquaint nonmental health practitioners who evaluate recurrent and chronic back pain with some of the more commonly used assessment tools that measure psychosocial factors relevant to pain. Through this chapter, the HCP should gain an appreciation for the number and variety of assessment tools that are available. Readers of this chapter will become more informed consumers when selecting psychosocial measures that serve the goals and evaluation process of their specific clinics, as well as being informed about the measures being used by other professional colleagues. Readers, specifically those who treat a large number of patients with recurrent and chronic pain, should gain an appreciation for the need to assess specific psychosocial factors for the purposes of understanding why a particular intervention failed and/or when psychosocial factors are assessed to be prominent, to more appropriately plan the overall course of treatment from the beginning.

The chapter focuses on methods for outcomes assessment in two domains: (1) improvement in comorbid psychiatric/psychological disorders; and (2) improvement in psychosocial factors related to pain and function. The section on comorbid psychiatric/psychological disorders addresses outcome measures that focus on changes in psychopathology, and personality disorders, whereas the section on psychosocial factors related to pain and function focuses on measures of pain-specific beliefs and attributions, coping resources, affective responses, environmental and social factors, and pain behaviors. Each of the two sections includes a brief overview of why the domain is thought to be important to outcomes assessment, the assessment tools that are available and frequently used, and clinical recommendations for effectively using the measurement tools.

COMORBID PSYCHIATRIC/PSYCHOLOGICAL DISORDERS

Psychological and psychiatric disorders strongly influence the transition from acute to chronic pain in patients with back and other forms of pain. Several reports have identified depression, anxiety, and personality disorders to be the most frequently occurring psychiatric conditions associated with persistent pain (Large, 1980; Merskey, 1990; Gatchel & Turk, 1996; Gatchel, 1997). Since pain and these psychiatric conditions become interwoven, and may in fact support the maintenance of each other, treatment and assessment of outcomes should address improvements in both pain and the psychiatric/psychological condition if the effectiveness of the treatment is to be adequately understood.

PREVALENCE IN PAIN CONDITIONS

The Epidemiologic Catchment Area (ECA) study estimated that **depression** has a 1 month prevalence of 1.6% in males and 2.9% in females in community samples (Blazer et al, 1994). A review of studies reporting the rate of depression in pain clinic populations, estimates it to range between 31% and 100% (Romano and Turner, 1985). **While the debate continues as to whether depression develops in response to pain or whether pain follows the onset of depression, there is evidence that in at least 50% of patients, pain and depression develop simultaneously and must be treated concomitantly (Hollander and Wong, 1995).**

Anxiety has been well studied as an emotion that influences the perception of acute pain as **it tends to lower both pain threshold and tolerance** (Dworkin, 1967; Chapman and Turner, 1990; Gil, 1992). The point prevalence of an anxiety disorder in the general population is 7%; however, a recent study examining anxiety with one type of chronic pain (temporomandibular disorder) found anxiety to be a comorbid concern in 47% of acute cases and 12% of chronic cases (Gatchel et al, 1996). Similarly, anxiety disorders such as panic disorder and post-traumatic stress disorder were found to be fairly common in patients with chronic pain (Krishnan et al, 1985; Kuch et al, 1985; Muse, 1985; Eisendrath, 1995). Like depression, both pain and anxiety need to be treated together and any outcome measures should identify changes in the combined symptoms of these overlapping conditions.

Personality disorders are characterized by a **persistent constellation of behaviors and inner experiences that are associated with problematic functioning.** The prevalence of personality disorders in the general adult population is estimated at between 5% and 15% (American Psychiatric Association, 1994). In several studies of chronic low back pain patients, however, personality disorders have been diagnosed with a much higher incidence; for example, 58.4% (Fishbain et al, 1986) and 51% (Polatin et al, 1993). The current *Diagnostic and Statistical Manual of Mental Disorders*, edition 4 *(DSM IV)* (American Psychiatric Association, 1994) identifies ten personality disorders and has grouped them into three clusters: "odd or eccentric" (Cluster A: schizoid, schizotypal, paranoid personality disorders), "dramatic emotional, or erratic" (Cluster B: histrionic, borderline, narcissistic, antisocial personality disorders), and "anxious or fearful" (Cluster C: avoidant, dependent, obsessive-compulsive personality disorders) (see Table 8–1 for a more detailed delineation of personality disorders).

In one study of chronic low back pain patients with personality disorders, 44% had Cluster A disorders, 31% Cluster B disorders, and 25% Cluster C disorders (Polatin

Table 8–1: Brief Description of Personality Disorders[a]

PERSONALITY DISORDER	BRIEF DESCRIPTION
Cluster A (odd or eccentric)	
Schizoid	Such individuals display little desire or need of others socially or sexually, tend to choose solitary activities, lack spontaneity and initiative, and find pleasure in few activities. They tend to be indifferent to either praise or criticism, are emotionally cold and detached, and yet, are deficient in self-reliance.
Schizotypal	Such individuals have a decreased need for close relationships and experience cognitive and perceptual distortions as well as eccentricities of behavior such as odd beliefs and magical thinking, odd speech patterns, bodily illusions, and odd and peculiar appearance.
Paranoid	Such individuals distrust others and assume that others' motives are malevolent. They tend to resist external authority and control, are self-reliant, and respond impulsively, and with anger to perceived threat.
Cluster B (dramatic, emotional, or erratic)	
Histrionic	Such individuals are excessively emotional and hedonistic in their pursuit of social attention. They are motivated to avoid pain and boredom and act in a calculated fashion to solicit attention, praise, reassurance, and approval from others.
Borderline	Such individuals tend to have marked instability of interpersonal relationships, self-image, and affect such that their behavior and moods may seem conflicting, contradictory, impulsive, and paradoxical.
Narcissistic	Such individuals tend to be grandiose, self-important, self-absorbed, expect to be admired and respected, and tend to lack genuine empathy for others.
Antisocial	Such individuals actively seek pleasure which typically results in the disregard and violation of the rights of others.
Cluster C (anxious or fearful)	
Avoidant	Such individuals display social inhibition, feel inadequate, and are highly sensitive to negative evaluation. Although desired, interpersonal contact is assumed to result in humiliation and therefore considerable effort is placed in avoiding social exchanges.
Dependent	Such individuals have a strong need to be taken care of and therefore are submissive, clinging, and fear separation from social support.
Obsessive-compulsive	Such individuals are preoccupied with orderliness, perfection, mental control, and interpersonal control at the expense of flexibility, openness, and efficiency.

[a] These ten personality disorders are derived from the current *Diagnostic and Statistical Manual of Mental Disorders*, edition 4 (*DSM IV*). See also Comer (1995).
Modified from American Psychiatric Association, 1994.

et al, 1993). The presence of a personality disorder has been found to be an important predictor of which patients will transition from acute to chronic pain (Gatchel et al, 1995). While no single category of personality disorder appears to be uniquely predictive of chronicity, the personality disorders share traits and behavioral features that appear to influence pain and pain treatment when present even at subdiagnostic levels (Gatchel, 1997).

Outcome assessment tools for comorbid psychiatric conditions can be grossly categorized into three groups: (1) psychological/psychiatric diagnostic assessment, (2) general assessment of psychological/psychiatric status and personality, and (3) measures of specific psychological/psychiatric symptoms. Some of these tools are widely available and are in the public domain, whereas others must be purchased from a distributor along with verification that the

---

CLINICAL TIP 8–1
Personality Disorders and the Long-term Management of Persistent Pain

The establishment of a mutually satisfying interpersonal relationship is problematic for any of the personality disorders. Personality disorders can greatly tax the HCP–patient relationship where trust and cooperation is essential for long-term management of persistent pain. Quick identification of the disorder is essential so that treatment plans can be changed appropriately early in the HCP–patient relationship.

tool will be used by a credentialed mental health professional. Although the listing in this chapter is not exhaustive, it does provide a useful overview of many of the psychometric assessment tools currently in use in clinical pain practices.

PSYCHOLOGICAL/PSYCHIATRIC DIAGNOSTIC ASSESSMENT

If the goal of outcomes assessment is to classify a patient into a diagnostic category reflective of the *Diagnostic and Statistical Manual (DSM-III)*, the gold standard for research is the Structured Clinical Interview for DSM-III-R **(SCID)** (Spitzer et al, 1990). The SCID is widely used to identify current and lifetime psychiatric disorders and produces a valid, objective psychiatric diagnosis at the conclusion of the structured interview. The SCID must be administered by a trained mental health professional or someone under the supervision of the mental health provider. Training is also required in the administration of the interview since adequate standardization is essential for this instrument to be useful. Typical of many well-validated instruments, the SCID is lengthy and might not be practically administered outside of research settings since administration time is approximately 1.5 hours for clinical disorders and an additional 45 minutes for the personality disorders. A potential disadvantage of the SCID is that its product (ie, a clinical diagnosis) is simply a label rather than a numerical value of psychopathology. Thus, patients cannot be identified as having greater or lesser amounts of a disorder. When compared to numerical measures of psychiatric status, labels are more limited in how they can be used statistically, information is often lost when patients fall near the cut-off boundaries of a category, and difficulties in dealing with the heterogeneity that accompanies many diagnostic categories detracts from the utility of this measure (Gatchel, 1997). From the perspective of being an outcomes measure, the SCID can assist in verifying whether a given intervention was helpful in reducing the symptoms that qualified the individual as having a given psychiatric diagnosis. For example, a specific intervention might relieve both the perception of pain and the comorbid depression that maintains the pain. The SCID could verify that the constellation of symptoms needed for an established and widely accepted clinical diagnosis of depression indeed resolves following treatment.

GENERAL ASSESSMENT OF PSYCHIATRIC STATUS AND PERSONALITY

The Minnesota Multiphasic Personality Inventory **(MMPI)** (Hathaway and McKinley, 1967) is one of the most widely used assessment tools of general psychiatric status in both psychiatric and traditional medical arenas. It does not provide a psychiatric/psychological diagnosis; however, it does provide quantitative information on multiple dimensions of psychological functioning. A high score on any one of the ten clinical scales is not necessarily in-

dicative of psychopathology; however specific patterns of elevations across various scales have been empirically associated with different forms of psychiatric disturbance (Greene, 1980). Thus, the profile of a given patient can be compared to the standardized profile of a sample of individuals with known disorders or behavioral problems. The MMPI has been widely used in assessments of chronic pain patients for both clinical care and forensic use. Numerous researchers have developed special interpretations of MMPI scale profiles specifically for patients with pain (Hanvik, 1951; Sternbach, 1974; Fordyce, 1979; Armentrout, 1982; Bradley and Vander Heide, 1984; Moore et al, 1986; Costello et al, 1987; Riley et al, 1993).

Patients frequently complain about the length and wording of questions for this paper-and-pencil self-report measure (566 true/false items) which can take up to 1 to 2 hours to complete. Since so many pain clinics continue to use the MMPI as both an assessment tool and an outcome measure, patients who are seen by multiple pain centers soon grow tired of taking this test. Additionally, taking the MMPI over many administrations can have unknown effects on its validity. There are currently briefer versions of the MMPI (eg, 168 items), with good validity compared to the full version for low back pain patients (Harasymiw et al, 1983) and some versions are available for computer administration. The full MMPI has also been updated into the **MMPI-2** (Butcher et al, 1989), which retains its length of 566 items.

While not particularly good as a predictor of outcome (Keller and Butcher, 1991), the MMPI or MMPI-2 has served as a measure of psychological change pre- to post-treatment and therefore can have utility as an outcome measure (Naliboff et al, 1998; Barnes et al, 1990). At present, there is no clear evidence to favor the MMPI or the MMPI-2 as being the better outcomes measure (Helms, 1994). Like the SCID, however, interpretation of the MMPI should be done by someone well trained in a mental health discipline with specific training in the MMPI. Because interpretation can appear to be easy by the naive, untrained HCP, misinterpretation of this instrument is common in clinical practice. Under these circumstances the use of this assessment tool can be a great disservice to patients. For example, based simply on the computer generated MMPI report, or by simply looking at an MMPI profile, nonmental health professionals frequently and inappropriately label patients as "malingerers," "alcoholics," "symptom magnifiers," or as "depressed." A valid interpretation can only be made by integrating the values across many scales (high and low) and comparing the patient profile to that of a profile from a group of individuals with a known condition. Even then, it should only be used to support the clinical impression of the mental health professional and does not indicate that a given patient has a specific condition. The labeling of anyone based solely on the MMPI is an inappropriate use of the measure.

The Personality Assessment Inventory **(PAI)** (Morey, 1991) is a 344-item self-report inventory of adult personality and takes approximately 50 minutes to complete. It has 22 nonoverlapping scales, including 4 validity scales, 11 clinical scales, 5 treatment-relevant scales, and 2 interpersonal scales. This inventory has advantages over traditional diagnostic methods of assessing personality disorders in that it is sensitive to normal personality features that may serve as both strengths or weaknesses in an individual's attempt to adapt to a chronic pain condition. Although more recently developed than the MMPI and less studied than the MMPI, the PAI is being used more and more frequently with medical populations and allows for greater differentiation of some psychological conditions; for instance, anxiety is broken down into physiological, emotional, and cognitive elements (Helms, 1994). These breakdowns are useful for maximizing an integrated approach to clinical treatment. For example, biofeedback might be helpful for addressing the physiological aspects of anxiety, whereas cognitive-behavioral therapy might be useful for the cognitive and affective aspects. Like the MMPI, the PAI can be computer scored, and computer-generated interpretations are available; however, it is recommended that a trained mental health professional use the computer generated interpretations to support rather than replace a thorough clinical interview. Evidence of mental health credentialing is required to obtain this instrument.

The NEO Personality Inventory–Revised (NEO-PI-R) (Costa et al, 1991), is based on the five-factor theoretical model of personality. According to this theory, there are five elements of personality: neuroticism, extroversion, openness, agreeableness, and conscientiousness (Costa and McCrae, 1990). For some of the factors, additional breakdown of the facets making up the factors comprise separate scales. The inventory is specifically designed to assess normal personality as opposed to disordered personalities and was not developed to be used as a diagnostic tool for psychopathology; therefore, it may be more useful for less chronic pain cases. Like the other personality inventories previously described, the NEO-PI-R is a paper-and-pencil self-report instrument but is relatively brief when compared to the measures discussed so far (ie, 180 items) and also comes in a briefer 60-item version that does not permit the more fine grade analysis of the factors.

MEASUREMENT OF SPECIFIC PSYCHOLOGICAL/PSYCHIATRIC SYMPTOMS

At times, the HCP may be more interested in the effect of treatment on specific psychological symptoms rather than on the global psychological status or diagnostic status of a patient. Quantitative assessment of specific symptoms has the advantage of being less time consuming, less difficult to interpret, easier to accomplish over repeated follow-up administrations, and for some symptoms, easier to accomplish over the phone or via mail. The disadvantages of greater efficiency are the loss of information, the loss of "the bigger

mental health picture," the loss of interacting facets of psychopathology, and depending on the instrument, the trade off of brevity for reliability and validity. The following discussion presents several of the most commonly used instruments for symptoms of depression and anxiety.

The Beck Depression Inventory (BDI) (Beck et al, 1979) **is perhaps the most frequently used depression screen and outcomes measure used in clinical pain practices.** It is a 21-item, paper-and-pencil, self-report inventory that takes 10 minutes to complete and 2 minutes to score. It has standardized cut-offs for normal, mild, moderate, and severe levels of depressive symptomatology. As is true of all symptom measures discussed in this section, scoring highly on this measure does not mean that the patient can be diagnosed as being depressed (as could be done using the SCID described earlier); rather it can simply be interpreted as the patient endorsing a large number of items that have been associated with individuals who are depressed. More specific to patients with pain, scores on the BDI have been correlated with a diagnosis of major depression in chronic pain patients (Turner and Romano, 1984). The BDI has been broken down by several researchers into separate scales that separate the more physiological items from the more cognitive and affective items (Wesley et al, 1991; Williams and Richardson, 1993). It has been argued that some of the somatic signs of depression overlap with the reduced functioning expected by anyone with low back pain. Thus, the purely cognitive items found on the cognitive-depression scale are thought to be a cleaner measure of depressive processes in patients with low back pain. Regardless of the approach, this instrument appears to be an excellent choice for sampling depressive symptomatology in patients with pain (Novy et al, 1995).

The Hamilton Psychiatric Rating Scale for Depression (HAM-D) (Hamilton, 1960) is another measure of depressive symptoms that is an HCP- or provider-administered instrument composed of 17 items. It has the advantage of being brief but the disadvantage of requiring provider time and is less objective in that it requires an HCP's subjective impression of the patient. The Zung Self-Rating Depression Scale (The Zung) (Zung, 1965) is another brief patient self-report measure of depression composed of 20 items. **Although the Zung is about the same length as the BDI, it performed less well than the BDI when correlated with diagnosed depression in chronic pain patients** (Turner and Romano, 1984). An additional scale with good psychometric properties is the Center for Epidemiologic Studies–Depression Scale (CES-D) (Radloff, 1977). This 20-item scale was developed to measure depressive symptoms in the general population.

The State–Trait Anxiety Inventory (STAI) (Spielberger et al, 1979) **is perhaps the most commonly used measure of anxiety symptoms in the pain literature.** The STAI is composed of 20 items assessing state anxiety (ie, as you feel right now), and 20 items assessing trait anxiety (ie, the tendency toward being a generally anxious person). A related instrument by the same author is the State–Trait

Anger Expression Inventory **(STAXI)** (Spielberger, 1991). This is a 20-item inventory with 10 items each assessing the state and trait aspects of anger. This instrument is gaining popularity as the role of anger in the maintenance and exacerbation of pain is being increasingly studied (Ham et al, 1994; Kerns et al, 1994; Fernandez and Turk, 1995; Burns et al, 1996).

Similar to the BDI, the Beck Anxiety Inventory **(BAI)** (Beck and Steer, 1990) has 21 items and is frequently used as both a screening tool and an outcomes measure of anxiety symptoms in chronic pain patients. The instrument is well developed and serves as an excellent companion to the BDI. Like the BDI, the BAI only takes 10 minutes to complete. Table 8–2 offers a summary of the tools belonging to the category of comorbid psychiatric factors.

OUTCOMES ASSESSMENT FOR COMORBID PSYCHOLOGICAL/ PSYCHIATRIC FACTORS: A CRITIQUE

The dichotomous view of (1) pain—being a medical problem, and (2) the response to pain—being a mental health problem, has contributed to many patients having only half of their pain condition treated. Failure to treat the whole problem reduces the effectiveness of any single modality, as the literature on spinal cord stimulation for pain control has highlighted (Long et al, 1981). **The HCP, patient, and third-party reimbursors must value both sides of this artificial division if adequate *relief* from pain is going to occur.** Equally important, adequate *assessment* of both sides of the division must be made if a fair evaluation of treatment and patient improvement is to be made.

When selecting a set of outcome measures for psychiatric/psychological improvement, it is important to do so with a working model of pain and disability in mind so that the measures chosen support the goals of the clinic. For example, if the clinic understands that both depression, and elevated pain intensity interfere with return to work, and the goal of the clinic is to demonstrate that a specific intervention helps patients to return to work, then assessment of depression would be essential in evaluating the efficacy of the intervention. Similarly, if the goal of the clinic is to treat all aspects of pain, then it would be important to demonstrate that the clinic's interventions reduced both the nociceptive complaint of pain and the psychiatric/psychological factors known to exacerbate chronic pain (eg, personality disorders, depression, anxiety/fear of reinjury, anger). If the goal of the clinic is to improve the quality of life of patients, then it would be important to demonstrate that the clinic's interventions removed interwoven pain and psychiatric distress and were able to enhance certain functional outcomes that the patient identified as important to quality of life. Since different clinics have different goals, there is no gold standard that will support the goals and associated working hypotheses of every clinic. There-

Table 8–2: Outcome Assessment Tools for Comorbid Psychiatric Factors

MEASUREMENT DEVICE[a]	DESCRIPTION
Psychological/Psychiatric Diagnosis	
SCID	Based on *DSM-III-R* diagnostic criteria; produces a valid psychiatric diagnosis
Psychiatric Status and Personality	
MMPI	Self-report; empirically keyed profiles of psychiatric status
PAI	Self-report; empirically keyed profiles of psychiatric status and personality
NEOPI-R	Self-report profiles of normal personality based on five-factor theory of personality
Specific Psychiatric Symptoms	
BDI	Self-report measure of depressive symptoms
BAI	Self-report measure of anxiety symptoms
Hamilton Rating Scale	HCP-rated measure of depressive symptoms
Zung	Self-report measure of depressive symptoms
CES-D	Self-report measure of depressive symptoms
STAI	Self-report measure of state and trait anxiety
STAXI	Self-report measure of state and trait anger

BAI, Beck Anxiety Inventory; BDI, Beck Depression Inventory; CES-D, Center for Epidemiologic Studies–Depression Scale; MMPI, Minnesota Multiphasic Personality Inventory; NEOPI-R, NEO Personality Inventory–Revised; PAI, Personality Assessment Inventory; SCID, Structured Clinical Interview for DSM-III-R; STAI, State–Trait Anxiety Inventory; STAXI, State–Trait Anxiety Inventory.

[a] Due to the complexity and length of many of the measurement devices listed, their use is restricted to licensed mental health practitioners.

fore, a clearer specification of the treatment goals along with knowledge of what tools are available for measuring those target treatment goals is important in selecting the tools that will best serve the needs of any given practitioner/clinic.

One overriding rule for choosing an assessment tool is to select an outcome measure that is psychometrically sound—that is, one that is both reliable and valid. A *reliable* test is stable (ie, it performs the same way every time it is given). If a depressed patient is given a reliable depression measure at two points in time, and the patient's depression remains unchanged, then the scores on the depression measure should also remain unchanged. An unreliable measure might produce two different scores under these circumstances; but the change would be due to instability in the test itself rather than any change in the patient. A *valid* test measures what it purports to measure. For example, if a test claims to measure depression, then it should truly measure depression rather than other characteristics such as anger or hostility. It is important to note that a test can be *reliable* without being *valid*; that is, it can be highly consistent at measuring the wrong thing. The tests mentioned in this chapter are both *reliable and valid* for use with pain patients and have been used with many individuals before being marketed to HCPs. Each of the instruments reviewed in this chapter has followed careful methodology in its development, which is why some of the questionnaires may seem to be more lengthy than is necessary; in fact, they would probably be less psychometrically sound if they were shorter. In an age when almost anything can be mass produced quickly for a buck, or when anyone can post a self-developed outcome measure on the Internet, the HCP is warned to carefully discern whether the measure proposed to be used is *reliable* and *valid*.

PAIN-SPECIFIC PSYCHOSOCIAL OUTCOMES

Comorbid psychiatric disturbances are not the only psychological factors that can influence the course of pain treatment. **Because pain, particularly persistent pain, is not often directly tied to specific pathophysiology, but rather is linked to integrated perceptions arising from neurochemical input, cognition, and emotion, the mind greatly influences the intensity of the pain** (Melzack and Wall, 1982). Similarly, past experiences with pain and coping with adversity influence the impact of pain on functioning. In a sample of mixed pain patients with pain duration of greater than 2 years, 80% had fair to poor psychosocial adjustment to their condition. Annual medical costs of fair to poorly adjusted patients are 2.5 to 3 times greater than in well-adjusted patients (Weir et al, 1992). This section highlights several areas that have recently gained support as being critically important to the progression of and adjustment to pain in its treatment and rehabilitation. These areas include pain-specific **beliefs and**

attitudes, coping ability for pain, **affective responses** to pain, **environmental and social factors,** and **pain behaviors.**

BELIEFS AND ATTITUDES

Beliefs and attitudes about the nature of pain, and its treatment influence patients' compliance with chronic pain treatment (Williams and Thorn, 1989; Williams and Keefe, 1991; Williams et al, 1994; Jensen and Karoly, 1991). Similarly, beliefs regarding the efficacy of treatments and personal efficacy to control pain, influence outcomes (Keefe et al, 1989; Shutty et al, 1990; Jensen et al, 1991). **Although some beliefs may be alterable through simple education, others represent substantial barriers to treatment and may need to be addressed before treatment can continue** (Turner and Jensen, 1993). Such beliefs might include strong conviction that pain and illness encompass all aspects of life (Waddell et al, 1989), that pain is mysterious and will be enduring regardless of treatment (Williams and Keefe, 1991), and that a cause and cure must be found for the pain before attempts at functioning are worthwhile (Jensen et al, 1994).

Assessment measures for beliefs and attitudes may be broken down into the following domains: (1) locus of control beliefs, (2) catastrophic beliefs regarding pain, (3) self-efficacy and expectancies, and (4) beliefs regarding the nature and impact of pain. Locus of control measures are usually concerned with whether patients attribute control over pain to themselves (internal locus), to others (external locus), or to chance. Catastrophic beliefs regarding pain may or may not reflect the reality of the pain condition; however, the presence of catastrophic beliefs (eg, believing the pain will never get any better, or that life is not worth living with pain) has been associated with increased pain, greater activity interference, and greater psychological distress (Sullivan and D'Eon, 1990; Keefe et al, 1991; Geisser et al, 1994; Lester et al, 1996). Self-efficacy and expectancy beliefs refers to personal beliefs regarding one's ability to control pain, to perform the needed tasks to control pain or to function with pain. A belief in personal efficacy to function with pain has been associated with both coping strategy use and adjustment to chronic pain, since functioning with pain appears to be closely tied to what people believe they are capable of doing (Jensen and Keefe, 1991; Lackner et al, 1996). Finally, beliefs regarding the nature and impact of pain have been associated with treatment compliance and maintenance of pain (Williams et al, 1989; Jensen et al, 1994). A number of instruments have been developed to assess beliefs and attitudes about pain. Several of these measures are described next.

Form C of the The Multidimensional Health Locus of Control Scale **(MHLC)** (Wallston et al, 1978, 1994) is an 18-item inventory that can be tailored to specific medical symptoms and provides four scores: internality, chance, HCPs, and other powerful people. Studies of health locus of control have found that people with an internal locus of control are better able to make good use of cognitive coping strategies for pain (Crisson and Keefe, 1988; Buckelew et al, 1990) and are generally less depressed (Skevington, 1983). The belief that pain control was in the hands of "powerful others" such as HCPs has been associated with greater depression (Affleck et al, 1987), and the belief that pain control was a chance event was associated with greater distress and helplessness (Crisson and Keefe, 1988). **In general, the belief in greater personal control over pain was associated with lowered reporting that pain interfered with daily functioning** (Strong et al, 1990). The Beliefs about Controlling Pain Questionnaire **(BCPQ)** (Skevington, 1990) also assesses the locus of control construct specifically for pain. This 15-item self-report scale taps into internal locus of control for pain, beliefs about powerful others (HCPs) controlling pain, and beliefs about pain being controlled by chance events.

The Coping Strategies Questionnaire **(CSQ)** (Rosenstiel and Keefe, 1983) contains a scale that assesses **catastrophic beliefs** about pain. This 6-item scale is highly predictive of pain and poor outcomes in a variety of populations, including arthritic and low back pain populations (Rosenstiel and Keefe, 1983; Keefe et al, 1989, 1990a, 1990b, 1990d, 1991). A second measure of catastrophizing is the Inventory of Negative Thoughts in Response to Pain **(INTRP)** (Gil et al, 1990). The INTRP is a 21-item self-report measure with three factor-derived scales: negative self-statements, negative social cognitions, and self-blame. This instrument actually evolved out of the catastrophizing concept in an attempt to further refine specific components of catastrophizing that influence exacerbation of pain symptoms. The INTRP has been found useful in outcomes assessment of multidisciplinary pain treatment (Tota-Faucette et al, 1993). A third, more general measure of negative thinking is the Automatic Thoughts Questionnaire **(ATQ)** (Hollon and Kendall, 1980) shown to be sensitive to cognitive changes following treatment using cognitive behavioral therapy.

There are many brief and task specific measures that attempt to assess **personal efficacy** to: (1) control pain, (2) perform health behaviors such as exercise to manage pain, and (3) manage pain in the future. **Such instruments are useful in determining how much effort will be needed to assist the patient in overcoming attitudinal barriers to achieve a positive treatment outcome.** The **Arthritis Self-Efficacy Scale** (Lorig et al, 1989) is one instrument that assesses patients' beliefs about their ability to perform nine basic functional tasks (eg, walking, managing frustration, dressing, etc). Greater belief in one's ability to perform these tasks was associated with decreased pain level, decreased depressive symptoms, and decreased disability (O'Leary et al, 1988; Lorig et al, 1989). Other briefer and more specific measures have been published that assess **self-efficacy** to engage in exercise for pain management (Dolce et al, 1986; Dolce, 1987), ability to cope with pain (Jensen et al, 1991a, 1991b), ability to control and decrease pain using cognitive and behavioral coping skills (Rosenstiel and Keefe, 1983), and ability to return to work (Papciak and Feuerstein, 1991).

Several measures tap into general beliefs about the **nature and impact of pain.** The Survey of Pain Attitudes **(SOPA)** (Jensen et al, 1994) is one such measure. The SOPA is a 57-item measure that can be scored to produce seven scales tapping beliefs about pain: control, disability, harm, emotion, medication, solicitude, and medical cure. Treatment compliance and outcome have been associated with the beliefs assessed by this instrument. A second, brief measure, is the 16-item Pain Beliefs and Perceptions Inventory **(PBPI)** (Williams and Thorn, 1989; Williams et al, 1994). The PBPI was developed empirically by asking injured workers to identify beliefs about their pain condition. The resulting measure is a condensation of their responses and is scored to produce four scales: the belief that pain is mysterious, the belief that pain is constant, the belief that pain is permanent, and blaming oneself for causing the pain. High scores on beliefs such as mystery and permanence are strongly associated with distress, and poorer treatment compliance, whereas constancy is associated with greater perception of pain intensity and decreased tolerance. Self-blame is associated with depressive symptoms. **Assessment of these beliefs gives the HCP an idea about how the patient thinks about his or her pain, which may differ significantly from how the HCP understands the problem.** Since some beliefs are associated with pain intensity, depression, and compliance, the HCP may want to alter beliefs and track those changes. Recently, the PBPI has been used as an outcome measure in several treatment intervention studies. In the first study, a 4-week multidisciplinary pain program reported pre- to post-treatment declines in the strength by which patients endorsed beliefs in pain permanence and mystery, which in turn was associated with positive outcome in pain (Cole et al, 1993). A second study demonstrated significant decreases in the belief that pain was mysterious following a 3- to 4-week inpatient pain management program consisting of biofeedback; assertiveness training; individual, group, and family psychotherapy; stress management; physical therapy; behavioral modification; physical exercise; occupational therapy; detoxification from narcotics; and medication management (Lipchik et al, 1993).

COPING ABILITY FOR PAIN

Coping effectively with pain is a skill that is attracting great attention from treatment outcomes researchers. **Currently, there is a very poor association between objective measures of physical pathology and the amount of pain and disability a patient with pain will express** (Haldeman, 1990; Feuerstein and Beattie, 1995). A more effective predictor of pain and disability is the patient's ability to adjust and adapt to a prolonged physical problem (Browne et al, 1990). An inability to adjust appears to be a problem facing greater than 50% of patients with pain (Weir et al,

1992). Coping skills, an integral part of cognitive-behavioral therapy for pain (CBT), has become an important predictor of treatment outcome, improvement in treatment, and subsequent health resources utilization (Aronoff et al, 1983; Jacobs, 1987; Linton and Bradley, 1996).

The most widely used assessment tool for the assessment of coping is the Coping Strategies Questionnaire (CSQ) (Rosenstiel and Keefe, 1983). This 48-item self-report measure produces nine scales: diverting attention, reinterpreting pain sensation, calming self-statements, ignoring pain, praying and hoping, catastrophizing, increasing behavioral activity, and pain behavior. The ninth scale is driven by two single-item questions that assess the patient's ability to use the assessed coping skills to control and to decrease pain. While initially there were no qualitative assumptions about the various coping strategies, this initial study did find some coping responses to be associated with poorer outcomes (eg, catastrophizing, praying and hoping). Other instruments have set out to make clearer distinctions about the quality of various coping strategies. The Vanderbilt Pain Management Inventory (VPMI) (Brown and Nicassio, 1987) is an 18-item inventory that assesses the tendency of patients to use active (thought to be more adaptive) versus passive approaches to pain management. Examples of active strategies include exercise, use of cognitive coping abilities, and activity; whereas passive strategies include rest and passive medication use. A third instrument is the Ways of Coping Checklist (WCCL) (Folkman and Lazarus, 1980), which is a theoretically driven instrument based on the transactional model of stress that suggests that coping responses to aversive situations are determined first by one's appraisal of the situation (Lazarus and Folkman, 1984). For example, the appraisal that pain is a life-threatening symptom is likely to lead to a different set of coping responses than the appraisal that pain is a challenge through which the individual will become a better person. Although not specific to pain, this instrument has been used widely to assess coping for both medical and nonmedical concerns. It is a 42-item inventory that measures five coping categories: problem-focused coping, self-blame, avoidance, wishful thinking, and seeking of social support (Vitaliano et al, 1985) and has been used with low back pain populations (Turner et al, 1987), and arthritis patients (Parker et al, 1988; Manne and Zautra, 1990) to evaluate the ways these pain patients were naturally dealing with and evaluating their pain condition.

AFFECTIVE RESPONSES

Affective responses to pain need not be diagnosable as clinical depression, abnormal personality, or otherwise considered "psychopathology" or "illness" in order to influence the course of pain treatment. **Subclinical levels of these emotions can influence pain perception and functioning in both acute and chronic forms of pain** (Melzack and Wall, 1982; Turk et al, 1983; Gatchel et al, 1996). **Stress** also influences how pain is perceived and handled. Stress can disrupt numerous systems in the body (Huether, 1996). This disruption, which includes both hyperarousal of the autonomic nervous system and hyporesponsivity of the central nervous system, has been hypothesized to be associated with numerous types of chronic pain syndromes. Examples include migraine headache, fibromyalgia, irritable bowel pain (Chrousos and Gold, 1992; Yunus, 1992; Clauw, 1995), which can play both a causal and maintaining role in pain and suffering. **Physiological, emotional, and cognitive changes associated with prolonged stressors are important measures of treatment outcome and predictors of future function** (Kerns and Jacob, 1995; Main and Watson, 1995). A related emotional concern that has an impact on pain maintenance and physical functioning, particularly in low back pain, is the fear of reinjury and increased pain. The fear of increased pain can lead to the active avoidance of activities that the patient believes could exacerbate pain. As the theory suggests, once activity is reduced, so is the fear of reinjury—at least temporarily. However, with deconditioning, pain can increase even at low levels of activity, which can lead the patient to avoid a broader range of activities which further diminishes physical functioning (McCracken et al, 1992, 1993). Anxiety sensitivity is a closely related psychological characteristic that is based on the belief that the anxiety-related bodily sensations themselves will have harmful somatic, social, or psychological consequences. Anxiety sensitivity has recently been associated with negative affect and decreased function even after controlling for severity of pain (Asmundson and Norton, 1995; Asmundson and Taylor, 1996).

There are many assessment tools for affect. The choice of the tool depends on the goal of assessment. If the goal of assessment is to assess disordered emotions, then the assessment tools mentioned earlier under specific psychiatric symptoms are recommended. If, however, very brief assessment of **general mood state** is desired, then a tool such as the POMS-LASA can be useful. The Profile of Moods States (POMS) (McNair et al, 1971) is a relatively lengthy emotions assessment tool; however, the briefer **POMS-LASA** provides a quick screen for self-reported anxiety, depression and anger (Sutherland et al, 1989). These three visual analogue scales (VASs) simply ask the patient to indicate their mood along a line with descriptors of the mood (eg, none, extremely) anchoring each end of the line. This assessment can be completed in under 1 minute and these scales have shown good validity for assessing mood when compared with the full POMS and with the Symptom Checklist 90–Revised (to be discussed later in this section).

The Illness Behavior Questionnaire (IBQ) (Pilowski, 1978) is a well-established assessment tool that taps into **anxiety-related concerns** about health such as disease phobia, disease conviction, somatic versus psychological perceptions of illness, inhibition of affect, affective disturbance, denial, dysphoria, hypochondria, and irritability. This 62-item questionnaire has been shown to be significantly related to affective disturbance and psychological distress in low back pain patients (Waddell et al, 1989), health care utilization of low back pain patients (Miller and Haffner, 1991), and depression in fibromyalgia patients (Ercolani et al, 1994).

The Symptom Checklist 90–Revised (**SCL-90-R**) (Derogatis, 1983) also assesses **emotional distress** that is associated with or affects physical health. It is of average length (eg, 90 items) and requires 15 to 30 minutes to complete. One drawback of the SCL-90-R is that many of the scales are highly interrelated and, therefore, may tap into a single general distress factor. If this is the case, then the SCL-90-R might be a very good measure of general distress but less good at teasing out the specific aspects of distress (anxiety, somatic concerns, etc) that have an impact on pain and function. Regardless, the SCL-90-R has been used in numerous pain studies as an indicator of the role distress plays on pain and functioning (Cassissi et al, 1993; Ham et al, 1994; Robbins et al, 1996; ter Kuile et al, 1996). Also, it has been used to identify groupings of patients with similar symptom profiles so as to better predict outcome and/or tailor psychosocial interventions (Shutty et al, 1986; Shutty and DeGood, 1987; Jamison et al, 1988; Williams et al, 1995). A similar but briefer instrument by the same author is the Brief Symptom Inventory (**BSI**) (Derogatis and Spenser, 1983). This inventory produces scores on constructs that are similar to the SCL-90-R (eg, anxiety and depression) but is only 53 items in length and, therefore, may be better suited for outcomes assessment where efficiency is a priority.

The Anxiety Sensitivity Index (**ASI**) (Reiss et al, 1986) is a 16-item self-report measure assessing the potential of an individual to develop conditioned **fear/anxiety** to unpleasant bodily sensations such as pain (discussed earlier). Such fear could result in decreased activity and function (Asmundson and Norton, 1995). **Fear of pain** can also be assessed with the Pain Anxiety Symptoms Scale (**PASS**) (McCracken et al, 1992). This is a 53-item self-report inventory that produces four scales: somatic anxiety, cognitive anxiety, fear, and escape-avoidance. In the prediction of disability, fear of pain stands on its own and does not overlap with trait anxiety, depression, and pain sensation (McCracken et al, 1992). In addition, fear of pain is associated with overestimates of reported pain, and restricted range of motion during passive movement (McCracken et al, 1993). The Fear-Avoidance Beliefs Questionnaire (**FABQ**) (Waddell et al, 1993) captures patients' fears about pain and work, and about pain and physical activity. These authors found these fears to be strong and specific predictors of work loss due to low back pain.

ENVIRONMENTAL AND SOCIAL FACTORS

Environmental and social factors play a more influential role than most patients and HCPs initially expect. From a clinical perspective it is well recognized that persistent pain can affect a patient's ability to optimally fulfill his or her family and occupational roles. Similarly, family and work related stressors can influence both pain (Feuerstein et al, 1985a) and disability (Feuerstein and Beattie, 1995). Therefore, brief assessment of the impact of an intervention on the family and work environments represent an important dimension of clinical outcome assessment. **Such an assessment can inform the HCP as to whether the chosen intervention has influenced the impact that pain and disability may be exerting on dimensions of the quality of family and work life.**

Although many scales measure family distress and job stress, the Work Environment and Family Environment Scales (**WES** and **FES**) are the two that we would recommend when considering simple scales that measure multiple dimensions of these environments in efficient and easy to understand formats (Moos, 1981; Moos and Moos, 1981). Some of the dimensions the FES measures include cohesion, expressiveness, and conflict. Examples of scales the WES measures include coworker support, supervisor support, and work pressure. These 90-item scales are easy to administer and score and provide understandable profiles of the sources of stress within the family and work environment, highlighting how the patient perceives these important environments. The scales have been related to increased levels of pain (Feuerstein et al, 1985a) and have acceptable reliability and validity. The scales could also be reduced to measure a few of the key dimensions (eg, those listed above) that the HCP thought were the critical factors of work and family environments that should be affected by the intervention under question.

PAIN BEHAVIOR ASSESSMENT METHODS

Assessment of **pain behaviors** has long been an important treatment outcome measure in both research and clinical practice. There is often great discrepancy between what people say about their pain and how they behave (Fordyce, 1976, 1995). **Because pain cannot be objectively measured by lab test or probe, a useful collateral measure of pain is the direct observation of pain behavior** (Kremer et al, 1981). Numerous outcome assessment tools utilize systematic behavioral measures of pain since the presence or absence of such behaviors are objectively quantified and can be standardized. One caveat in the use of behavioral assessment is that one cannot assume that the patient is pain-free if no behavioral manifestations of pain are present. Similarly pain is not necessarily more severe if greater amounts of pain behavior are present. Behavioral measures of pain are simply collateral measures that help the HCP obtain a more comprehensive picture of the total pain experience of the patient.

Keefe and Block (1982) developed one of the most widely used direct methods of **pain behavior observation.** This method uses a highly standardized protocol for having patients engage in common physical activities, video recording the activities and responses, and coding of the various pain behaviors that are observed. The **back pain** observation protocol codes for guarding, bracing, rubbing, grimacing, and sighing which can be reliably replicated across patients and between coders (Keefe and Bradley, 1984; Keefe et al, 1990a). Other protocols based on the same methods search for slightly different behaviors and have been developed for **arthritis,** (McDaniel et al, 1986; Anderson et al, 1987a, 1987b, 1992), and **fibromyalgia** (Baumstark et al, 1993). **Pain behaviors have shown good association with pain intensity, and predict functional status even after controlling for traditional medical status variables** (Keefe and Bradley, 1984). One drawback of many of these protocols is that they are time and labor intensive (eg, requiring 10 minutes of videotaping and rigorous training of coders who must view the 10 minute video at a later date) and are probably best used in outcomes research rather than in daily clinical practice. This is, however, the method of choice if scientific rigor and clean methodology in assessing pain behavior is desired.

The Waddell Non-organic Low Back Pain (LBP) Signs are used to identify abnormal illness behavior, which may manifest itself as an observed pain behavior (Waddell, 1980). Refer to Chapter 16 for a more detailed description of these measures.

Other direct observation methods include one developed by Follick, Ahern, and Aberger, (1985) that had patients engage in a wider array of tasks (such as climbing stairs or performing other daily tasks) and also included verbal behavior. This measure has been found to be useful in predicting outcomes from a multidisciplinary pain clinic (Kleinke and Spangler, 1988). While usually less reliable than the methods that utilize standardized tasks and videotaped records for coders, several methods have been developed that are designed to be used by nurses in inpatient settings (Cinciripini and Floreen, 1983) or by HCPs on their daily rounds or during examinations (Richards et al, 1982). A brief measure called the Pain Behavior Scale **(PBS)** (Richards et al, 1982) is a 10-item scale that is completed by the HCP and has high inter-rater agreement. A modified version with equally good psychometric properties was developed by Feuerstein **(PBS-revised)** for outpatient settings (Feuerstein et al, 1985b).

MULTIDIMENSIONAL MEASURES OF PAIN AND FUNCTIONING

Some measures assess multiple dimensions that are important to the assessment of psychosocial considerations. One such instrument is the Short Form-36 **(SF-36)** (Ware and Sherbourne, 1992). This self-report measure was developed as part of the RAND Medical Outcomes Study and has good psychometric qualities based on a large medical sample (n = 2471) and has been used extensively in treatment outcome research (Hays et al, 1993). The survey can be scored to produce the following subscales: physical functioning, physical role functioning, emotional role functioning, mental health, pain, social functioning, energy, and general health. A new version of the SF-36, the 12-item **SF-12** (Ware et al, 1995) utilizes a subsample of the SF-36 items to produce a Physical Health and a Mental Health scale. This is a good example of an instrument that has been made useful and brief but at the same time has not sacrificed any of the steps needed to assure methodological rigor in its refinement. While useful for the assessment of a broad range of medical and psychiatric outcomes, this instrument was not designed specifically for pain. Refer to Chapter 5 for additional information regarding the SF-36 and SF-12.

The West Haven–Yale Multidimensional Pain Inventory **(WHYMPI)** (Kerns et al, 1985) attempts to assess multiple factors that are specifically relevant to pain treatment in one psychometrically sound instrument. This 52-item inventory assesses general pain and suffering, interference with family and work functioning, social support, the patients' perceptions about how others respond to displays of pain and suffering, and frequency of being able to engage in daily activities. The WHYMPI (also referenced as the MPI) has been used to successfully document change along numerous dimensions of treatment in multidisciplinary pain programs (Flavell et al, 1996). Although not every scale will be of use to every HCP, individual scales can be selected that address specific hypotheses of the practitioner.

A third multidimensional measure is the Biobehavioral Pain Profile **(BPP)** (Dalton et al, 1994). The BPP is a 41-item self-report scale that assesses six factors associated with the progression of pain problems: environmental influences, loss of control, health care avoidance, past and current experiences, physiological responsivity, and thoughts of disease progression. The scale has strong psychometric properties and is easily administered and scored. Table 8–3 offers a summary of tools that are practical regarding the assessment of pain-specific psychosocial factors.

OUTCOMES ASSESSMENT OF PSYCHOSOCIAL FACTORS: HOW TO SELECT A MEASURE

It is recognized that the busy HCP has neither the time nor the resources to conduct lengthy outcome assessments. Also, many patients may choose to go elsewhere if they are confronted with a huge set of scales to complete. The purpose of this chapter was to alert the HCP to the range of outcome measures that assess different aspects of what is generally referred to as psychosocial outcomes.

The selection of any one of these options relates to the purpose of the evaluation. If, for example, a third-party payer is interested in the impact of treatment intervention on return to work (RTW) and future health care use, several approaches can be taken. One would be to measure only return to work and related health care costs. This approach is very practical and perhaps less costly than a more comprehensive assessment strategy. The problem with this approach, however, rests in its inability to explain the

Table 8–3: Outcome Assessment Tools for Pain-Specific Psychosocial Factors

MEASUREMENT DEVICE	DESCRIPTION
Beliefs	
MHLC Form C	Self-report locus of control measure for general medical illnesses; can be tailored for pain
BCPQ	Self-report locus of control measure for pain
CSQ-CAT	Subscale of the CSQ; self-report measure of catastrophizing beliefs about pain
INTRP	Self-report measure that defines components of catastrophizing the influence of pain flare-ups
ATQ	Process measure that assesses cognitive change; usually used in CBT
ASES	Self-report measure of self-efficacy to perform basic functional tasks; developed for arthritis
Brief Self-Efficacy Scales	
Dolce et al (1986)	Ability to engage in exercise
Jensen et al (1994)	Ability to cope with pain
Rosensteil and Keefe (1983)	Ability to control and decrease pain
Papciak and Feuerstein (1991)	Ability to return to work
SOPA	Self-report measure of seven different pain beliefs influencing treatment outcome and compliance
PBPI	Brief self-report measure of four pain beliefs influencing treatment outcome and compliance
Coping	
CSQ	Self-report measure of nine different coping strategies for pain and two scales assessing self-efficacy to use coping strategies to control and decrease pain
VPMI	Self-report measure of active and passive coping strategies
WCCL	Self-report theoretically derived measure of coping skills based on the transactional model of stress
Affective Responses	
POMS-LASA	Self-rated VAS for three mood states
IBQ	Self-report measure of anxiety-related health concerns
SCL-90-R	Self-report empirically keyed profiles of global symptoms of distress
BSI	Self-report of general psychiatric symptoms and distress
ASI	Self-report measure of anxiety sensitivity to conditioned fear responses
PASS	Self-report measure of fear associated with pain and functioning with pain
FABQ	Measure of patient's fear about pain, work, and physical activity
Environmental and Social Factors	
FES	Self-report measure of patient's family functioning in eight domains important to pain and disability
WES	Self-report measure of patient's work functioning in eight domains important to pain and disability
Pain Behavior	
Keefe and Block (1982)	Direct pain behavior observation method
Follick et al (1985)	Direct pain behavior observation method
Brief Methods of Direct Observation	
Cinciripini and Floreen (1983)	Observer rated for inpatient use
Richards et al (1982)	Observer rated for inpatient use on rounds
Shutty et al (1990)	Observer rated for outpatient use
PBS	Observer rated for inpatient use
PBS-R	Observer rated for outpatient use

Table 8–3: (cont.)

MEASUREMENT DEVICE	DESCRIPTION
Multidimensional Measures	
SF-36 and SF-12	Self-report measure of general physical and mental health functioning
WHYMPI	Self-report measure of psychosocial and functional status along multiple dimensions
BPP	Self-report measure of psychosocial and functional status along multiple dimensions

ASES, The Arthritis Self-Efficacy Scale (Long et al, 1989); ASI, Anxiety Sensitivity Index; ATQ, Automatic Thoughts Questionnaire; BCPQ, Beliefs about Controlling Pain Questionnaire; BPP, Biobehavioral Pain Profile; BSI, Brief Symptom Inventory; CSQ, Coping Strategies Questionnaire; FABQ, Fear-Avoidance Beliefs Questionnaire; FES, Family Environment Scale; IBQ, Illness Behavior Questionnaire; INTRP, Inventory of Negative Thoughts in Response to Pain; MHLC, Multidimensional Health Locus of Control; PASS, Pain Anxiety Symptom Scale; PBPI, Pain Beliefs and Perception Inventory; PBS, Pain Behavior Scale; POMS, Profile of Mood States; SCL-90-R, Symptom Checklist 90–Revised; SF, Short Form; SOPA, Survey of Pain Attitudes; VPMI, Vanderbilt Pain Management Inventory; WCCL, Ways of Coping Checklist; WES, Work Environment Scale; WHYMPI, West Haven–Yale Multidimensional Pain Inventory.

treatment failures, the failure to meet specified goals of treatment, or greater than usual utilization of health care resources. For example, suppose your data on RTW and health care indicated that a subgroup of patients returned to work and used less care while another subgroup had very limited improvement on these same measures. If all had the same intervention, why was this observed? Such a question could not begin to be answered if your assessment battery lacked measures that assessed factors that contribute to delayed functional recovery and increased health care use (eg, various psychosocial measures). **This example illustrates the importance of clearly defining the clinical outcome question(s) up front and delineating what you think might occur in very specific terms (ie, state your clinical hypotheses).** This "hard thinking" up front can potentially save you time and money in the long run. While the use of outcome methodologies in daily practice

is not identical to running large clinical trials, the thinking processes are very similar. Indeed, even well-funded clinical trials are concerned with the costs and practical aspects of conducting such evaluations.

When deciding on whether or not to include a psychosocial measure in your outcomes assessment battery, you might want to ask yourself the following questions. What is the nature of my practice? Am I seeing primarily recurrent and chronic cases of back pain? Are many of my patients exhibiting high levels of psychological distress? Is it the case that despite my best efforts at facilitating compliance with exercise and other health behaviors and encouraging self-management approaches, a large percentage of patients are not complying? Does pain persist at pre-treatment levels despite improvements in function? Do I have an integrated rehabilitation approach that involves mental health professionals in the community for selected cases? **Affirmative answers to any of these questions suggests that psychosocial factors may be affecting outcomes and that measurement of such factors could assist in understanding outcomes and in making adjustments to your clinical approach so as to reduce the impact of such factors on your outcomes.**

Once it has been decided that certain psychosocial measures should be included in an outcome assessment, which ones should be selected? Again, this is based in part on what one expects or what working hypotheses are being considered. Clearly, if the intent is to determine whether there is a change in the percentage of cases that demonstrate patterns of classic psychological disorders, the screening procedures for assessing such conditions should be considered (eg, SCID). If the intent is to assess whether significant reductions in certain dimensions of psychopathology have occurred (hypochondriasis, somatization, depression, anxiety) the standard self-administered scales that assess these clinical features would be useful. When the interest is in briefly assessing the impact of your treatment on mood or distress, the brief mood scales or standardized scales for measuring depression and anxiety should prove useful. In terms of measuring factors that may directly modulate pain such as beliefs,

---

CLINICAL TIP 8–2
Obtaining Copies of Specific Scales

We could not provide specific scales due to ethical restrictions as per the American Psychological Association. However, many scales are available in the references cited or can be made available by the distributor of the test. For those interested in obtaining copies of scales, it is recommended that you follow the procedure below:

1. Search the article referenced for the scale. If not present, request a copy from the author of the scale.
2. For those scales or screening protocols for which the reference indicates a distributor (eg, Educational Testing Service, Consulting Psychologists Press, Psychological Assessment Resources, etc), obtain the necessary clearance from the distributor. This may require working in collaboration with a licensed mental health professional.

attitudes, and coping strategies, first be clear on what factor(s) is of interest and select the measure(s) that best taps the multiple constructs of interest. It is important to choose measures that are not highly correlated with one another, because this indicates that the measures may be assessing the same construct and in the interest of time and cost, a single, all-encompassing measure (eg, self-efficacy) may be the optimal choice. When the interest is in evaluating the effects of an intervention on work and family, selected subscales of the WES and FES are suggested. Lastly, for pain behavior a brief pain behavior scale may provide a useful, easy to use measure of pain behavior.

Conclusion

Psychosocial indices provide a unique and valuable source of outcome measures. The present chapter provides the HCP interested in broadening the scope of outcomes to include psychosocial factors with an overview of the various options. There is no cookbook solution to the selection and use of psychosocial outcomes in clinical practice. The challenge to the reader is to develop a strategy that best fits his or her individual practice. **It is hoped that when these measures are used, the HCP and other members of a "multidisciplinary treatment team" will be better able to determine the effects of their treatment on the multiple dimensions of pain and disability as well as identify factors that have an impact on treatment outcomes.** Through the use of such a comprehensive measurement strategy, the HCP will be more skilled at measuring and understanding complex clinical outcomes in individual cases and groups of patients.

The systematic use of the various measures discussed in this chapter should also help **facilitate communication** among the many participants involved in the care of these patients (eg, chiropractor, orthopedic surgeon, internist, physical therapist, psychologist, nurse case manager, claims adjuster, employer). Using multiple sources of systematically collected information, HCPs can redesign individual treatment plans as well as fine-tune general approaches to certain groups of patients to further enhance outcomes. Such a process is in the best interests of patients, providers, and third-party payers.

(The opinions or assertions contained herein are the private ones of the authors and are not to be construed as official views of the Department of Defense or the Uniformed Services University of the Health Sciences.)

REFERENCES

Affleck G, Tennen H, Pfeiffer C, Fifield J. Appraisals of control and predictability in adapting to a chronic disease. *J Pers Soc Psychol.* 1987;53(2):273–279.

American Psychiatric Association. *Diagnostic and Statistical Manual of Mental Disorders* 4th ed. Washington, DC: American Psychiatric Press; 1994.

Anderson KO, Bradley LA, McDaniel LK, et al. The assessment of pain in rheumatoid arthritis: Disease differentiation and temporal stability of a behavioral observation method. *J Rheumatol.* 1987a;14(4):700–704.

Anderson KO, Bradley LA, McDaniel LK, et al. The assessment of pain in rheumatoid arthritis. Validity of a behavioral observation method. *Arthritis Rheum.* 1987b;30(1):36–43.

Anderson KO, Bradley LA, Turner RA, et al. Observation of pain behavior in rheumatoid arthritis patients during physical examination. Relationship to disease activity and psychological variables. *Arthritis Care Res.* 1992;5(1):49–56.

Armentrout DP. Pain-patient MMPI subgroups: The psychological dimensions of pain. *J Behav Med.* 1982; 5(2):201–211.

Aronoff GM, Evans WO, Enders PL. A review of follow-up studies of multidisciplinary pain units. *Pain.* 1983;16(1):1–11.

Asmundson GJ, Norton GR. Anxiety sensitivity in patients with physically unexplained chronic back pain: A preliminary report. *Behav Res Ther.* 1995;33(7):771–777.

Asmundson GJ, Taylor S. Role of anxiety sensitivity in pain-related fear and avoidance. *J Behav Med.* 1996;19(6): 577–586.

Barnes D, Gatchel RJ, Mayer TG, Barnett J. Changes in MMPI profile levels of chronic low back pain patients following successful treatment. *J Spinal Disord.* 1990;3(4):353–355.

Baumstark KE, Buckelew SP, Sher KJ, et al. Pain behavior predictors among fibromyalgia patients. *Pain.* 1993;55(3):339–346.

Beck AT, Rush AJ, Shaw BF, Emery G. *Cognitive Therapy and Depression*. New York, NY: Guilford Press; 1979.

Beck AT, Steer RA. *Beck Anxiety Inventory: Manual*. 2nd ed. New York, NY: Psychological Corporation/Harcourt Brace Jovanovich, 1990.

Blazer DG, Kessler RC, McGonagle KA, Swartz MS. The prevalence and distribution of major depression in a national community sample: The national comorbidity survey. *Am J Psychiatry*. 1994;151(7):979–986.

Bradley LA, Van der Heide LH. Pain-related correlates of MMPI profile subgroups among back pain patients. *Health Psychology*. 1984;3:157–174.

Brown GK, Nicassio PM. The development of a questionnaire for the assessment of active and passive coping strategies in chronic pain patients. *Pain*. 1987;31:53–65.

Browne GB, Arpin K, Corey P, Fitch M, Gafni A. Individual correlates of health services utilization and the cost of poor adjustment to chronic illness. *Medical Care*. 1990;28:43–58.

Buckelew SP, Shutty MS Jr, Hewett J, Landon T, Morrow K, Frank RG. Health locus of control, gender differences and adjustment to persistent pain. *Pain*. 1990;42(3):287–294.

Burns JW, Johnson BJ, Mahoney N, Devine J, Pawl R. Anger management style, hostility and spouse responses: gender differences in predictors of adjustment among chronic pain patients. *Pain*. 1996;64(3):445–453.

Butcher JN, Dahlstrom WG, Graham JR, Tellegen A, Kaemmer B. *Manual for Administration and Scoring MMPI-2: Minnesota Multiphasic Personality Inventory-2*. Minneapolis, Minn: University of Minnesota Press; 1989.

Cassisi JE, Sypert GW, Lagana L, Friedman EM, Robinson ME. Pain, disability, and psychological functioning in chronic low back pain subgroups: Myofascial versus herniated disc syndrome. *Neurosurgery*. 1993; 33(3):379–85; discussion 385–386.

Chapman CR, Turner JA. Psychologic and psychosocial aspects of acute pain. In: Bonica JJ, ed. *The Management of Pain*. Philadelphia, Pa: Lea & Febiger; 1990:122–132.

Chrousos GP, Gold PW. The concepts of stress and stress system disorders: overview of physical and behavioral homeostasis. *J Am Med Assoc*. 1992;267(9):1244–1252.

Cinciripini PM, Floreen A. An assessment of chronic pain behavior in a structured interview. *J Psychosom Res*. 1983;27(2):117–123.

Clauw DJ. The pathogenesis of chronic pain and fatigue syndromes, with special reference to fibromyalgia. *Medical Hypotheses*. 1995;44:369–378.

Cole BC, Fishbain DA, Rosomoff HL, Steele-Rosomoff R. Patient's pain beliefs and treatment response at admission, discharge, and follow-up from a multidisciplinary pain center. [Abstract]. *Proceedings of the 12th Annual Scientific Meeting of the American Pain Society*. 1993:A97.

Comer RJ. *Abnormal Psychology*. 2nd ed. New York, NY: W.H. Freeman; 1995.

Costa PT, McCrae RR. Personality disorders and the five-factor model of personality. *J Personal Disord*. 1990;4(4):362–371.

Costa PT, McCrae RR, Dye DA. Facet scales for agreeableness and conscientiousness: a revision of the Neo-Personality Inventory. *Personal Individ Differences*. 1991;12:887–898.

Costello RM, Hulsey TL, Schoenfeld LS, Ramamurthy S. P-a-i-n: A four-cluster MMPI typology for chronic pain. *Pain*. 1987;30(2):199–209.

Crisson JE, Keefe FJ. The relationship of locus of control to pain coping strategies and psychological distress in chronic pain patients. *Pain*. 1988;35(2):147–154.

Dalton JA, Feuerstein M, Carlson J, Roghman K. Biobehavioral pain profile: Development and psychometric properties. *Pain*. 1994;57(1):95–107.

Derogatis LR. *SCL-90-R Administration, Scoring and Procedures Manual-II*. 2nd ed. Towson, Md: Clinical Psychometric Research; 1983.

Derogatis LR, Spencer PM. *The Brief Symptom Inventory: Administration, Scoring, and Procedures Manual-I*. Baltimore, Md: Clinical Psychometric Research; 1983.

Dolce JJ. Self-efficacy and disability beliefs in behavioral treatment of pain. *Behav Res Ther*. 1987; 25(4):289–299.

Dolce JJ, Crocker MF, Moletteire C, Doleys DM. Exercise quotas, anticipatory concern and self-efficacy expectancies in chronic pain: A preliminary report. *Pain*. 1986;24(3):365–372.

Dworkin SF. Anxiety and performance in the dental environment: An experimental investigation. *J Am Soc Psychosom Dent Med*. 1967;14:88–102.

Eisendrath SJ. Psychiatric aspects of chronic pain. *Neurology*. 1995;45(Suppl 9):s26–s36.

Ercolani M, Trombini G, Chattat R, et al. Fibromyalgic syndrome: Depression and abnormal illness behavior. Multicenter investigation. *Psychother Psychosom*. 1994;61(3–4):178–186.

Fernandez E, Turk DC. The scope and significance of anger in the experience of chronic pain. *Pain*. 1995;61(2):165–175.

Feuerstein M, Beattie P. Biobehavioral factors affecting pain and disability in low back pain: Mechanisms and assessment. *Phys Ther.* 1995;75(4):267–280.

Feuerstein M, Greenwald M, Gamache MP. The pain behavior scale: Modification and validation for outpatient use. *J Psychopathol Behav Assess.* 1985b;7:301–315.

Feuerstein M, Sult S, Houle M. Environmental stressors and chronic low back pain: Life events, family, and work environment. *Pain.* 1985a;22:295–307.

Fishbain D, Goldberg D, Meagher R, Steele R, Rosomoff H. Male and female chronic pain patients categorized by DSM-III psychiatric diagnostic criteria. *Pain.* 1986;26:181–197.

Flavell HA, Carrafa GP, Thomas CH, Disler PB. Managing chronic back pain: Impact of an interdisciplinary team approach. *Med J Aust.* 1996;165(5):253–255.

Folkman S, Lazarus RS. An analysis of coping in a middle-aged community sample. *J Health Social Behav.* 1980;21:219–239.

Follick MJ, Ahern DK, Aberger EW. Development of an audiovisual taxonomy of pain behavior: Reliability and discriminant validity. *Health Psychol.* 1985;4(6):555–568.

Fordyce WE. *Behavioral Methods of Chronic Pain and Illness.* St. Louis, Mo: CV Mosby; 1976.

Fordyce WE. Use of the MMPI in the assessment of chronic pain. In: Butcher JJ, Dahlstrom G, Gynther M, Schofield W, eds. *Clinical Notes on the MMPI.* Roche Psychiatric Service Institute; 1979:2–13.

Fordyce WE. *Back Pain in the Workplace: Management of Disability in Nonspecific Conditions.* Seattle, Wash: International Association for the Study of Pain Press; 1995.

Gatchel RJ. The significance of personality disorders in the chronic pain population. *Pain Forum.* 1997;6(1):12–15.

Gatchel RJ, Garofalo BA, Ellis E, Holt C. Major psychological disorders in acute and chronic TMD: An initial examination. *J Am Dental Assoc.* 1996;127:1365–1374.

Gatchel RJ, Polatin PB, Kinney RK. Predicting outcome of chronic back pain using clinical predictors of psychopathology: A prospective analysis. *Health Psychology.* 1995;14(5):415–420.

Gatchel RJ, Turk DC. *Psychological Approaches to Pain: A Practitioner's Handbook.* New York, NY: Guilford Press; 1996.

Geisser ME, Robinson ME, Keefe FJ, Weiner ML. Catastrophizing, depression and the sensory, affective and evaluative aspects of chronic pain [see comments]. *Pain.* 1996;59(1):79–83.

Gil KM. Psychological aspects of acute pain. In: Sinatra RS, Hord AH, Ginsberg B, Preble LM, eds. *Acute Pain: Mechanisms and Management.* St. Louis, Mo: Mosby-Year Book; 1992.

Gil KM, Williams DA, Keefe FJ, Beckham JC. The relationship of negative thoughts to pain and psychological distress. *Behavior Ther.* 1990;21:349–362.

Greene RL. *The MMPI: An Interpretive Manual.* New York, NY: Grune & Stratton; 1980.

Haldeman S. North American Spine Society: Failure of the pathology model to predict back pain. *Spine.* 1990;15(7):718–724.

Ham LP, Andrasik F, Packard RC, Bundrick CM. Psychopathology in individuals with post-traumatic headaches and other pain types. *Cephalalgia.* 1994;14(2):118–126; discussion 78.

Hamilton M. A rating scale for depression. *J Neurol Neurosurg Psychiatry.* 1960;23:56–62.

Hanvik LJ. MMPI profiles in patients with low back pain. *J Consult Psychology.* 1951;15:350–353.

Harasymiw SJ, McKian PM, Herz GI. Comparative analysis of MMPI Form R and MMPI-168 profiles in low back pain patients. *Scand J Rehabil Med.* 1983;15:147–153.

Hathaway SR, McKinley JC. *MMPI Manual.* Rev. ed. Psychological Corporation; 1967.

Hays RD, Sherbourne CD, Mazel RM. The RAND 36-item health survey 1.0 [see comments]. *Health Econ.* 1993;2(3):217–227.

Helms E. What types of useful information do the MMPI and MMPI-2 provide on patients with chronic pain? *APS Bulletin.* 1994;4(1):1–5.

Hollander E, Wong CM. Obsessive-compulsive spectrum disorders. *J Clin Psychiatry.* 1995;56(Suppl 4):3–6; discussion 53-55.

Hollon SD, Kendall PC. Cognitive self-statements in depression: Development of an automatic thoughts questionnaire. *Cognitive Ther Res.* 1980;4:383–395.

Huether G. The central adaptation syndrome: Psychosocial stress as a trigger for adaptive modifications of brain structure and brain function. *Prog Neurobiol.* 1996;48:569–612.

Jacobs DF. Cost-effectiveness of specialized psychological programs for reducing hospital stays and outpatient visits. *J Clin Psychol.* 1987;43(6):729–735.

Jamison RN, Rock DL, Parris WC. Empirically derived symptom checklist 90 subgroups of chronic pain patients: A cluster analysis. *J Behav Med.* 1988;11(2):147–158.

Jensen MP, Karoly P. Control beliefs, coping efforts, and adjustment to chronic pain. *J Consult Clin Psychol.* 1991;59(3):431–438.

Jensen MP, Turner JA, Romano JM. Self-efficacy and outcome expectancies: Relationship to chronic pain coping strategies and adjustment. *Pain.* 1991a;44(3):263–269.

Jensen MP, Turner JA, Romano JM, Karoly P. Coping with chronic pain: A critical review of the literature. *Pain.* 1991b;47(3):249–283.

Jensen MP, Turner JA, Romano JM, Lawler BK. Relationship of pain-specific beliefs to chronic pain adjustment. *Pain.* 1994;57(3):301–309.

Keefe FJ, Block AR. Development of an observation method for assessing pain behavior in low back pain patients. *Behav Ther.* 1982;13:363–375.

Keefe FJ, Bradley LA. Behavioral and psychological approaches to the assessment and treatment of chronic pain. *Gen Hosp Psychiatry.* 1984;6(1):49–54.

Keefe FJ, Bradley LA, Crisson JE. Behavioral assessment of low back pain: Identification of pain behavior subgroups. *Pain.* 1990a;40(2):153–160.

Keefe FJ, Brown GK, Wallston KA, Caldwell DS. Coping with rheumatoid arthritis pain: catastrophizing as a maladaptive strategy. *Pain.* 1989;37(1):51–56.

Keefe FJ, Caldwell DS, Martinez S, Nunley J, Beckham J, Williams DA. Analyzing pain in rheumatoid arthritis patients: Pain coping strategies in patients who have had knee replacement surgery. *Pain.* 1991; 46(2):153–160.

Keefe FJ, Caldwell DS, Williams DA, et al. Pain coping skills training in the management of osteoarthritic knee pain-II: Follow-up results. *Behav Ther.* 1990b;21:435–447.

Keefe FJ, Caldwell DS, Williams DA, et al. Pain coping skills training in the management of osteoarthritic knee pain: A comparative study. *Behav Ther.* 1990c;21:49–62.

Keefe FJ, Crisson J, Urban BJ, Williams DA. Analyzing chronic low back pain: The relative contribution of pain coping strategies. *Pain.* 1990d;40(3):293–301.

Keller LS, Butcher JN. *Assessment of Chronic Pain Patients with the MMPI-2.* Minneapolis, Minn: University of Minnesota Press; 1991.

Kerns RD, Jacob MC. Toward an integrated diathesis-stress model of chronic pain. In: Goreczny AJ, ed. *Handbook of Health and Rehabilitation Psychology.* New York, NY: Plenum Press; 1995:325–340.

Kerns RD, Rosenberg R, Jacob MC. Anger expression and chronic pain. *J Behav Med.* 1994;17(1):57–67.

Kerns RD, Turk DC, Rudy TE. The West Haven-Yale Multidimensional Pain Inventory (WHYMPI). *Pain.* 1985;23(4):345–356.

Kleinke CL, Spangler AS Jr. Predicting treatment outcome of chronic back pain patients in a multidisciplinary pain clinic: Methodological issues and treatment implications. *Pain.* 1988;33(1):41–48.

Kremer EF, Block A, Gaylor MS. Behavioral approaches to treatment of chronic pain: The inaccuracy of patient self-report measures. *Arch Phys Med Rehabil.* 1981;62(4):188–191.

Krishnan KRR, France RD, Pelton S, McCann UD, Davidson J, Urban B. Chronic pain and depression. II. Symptoms of anxiety in chronic low back pain patients and their relationship to subtypes of depression. *Pain.* 1985;22:289–294.

Kuch K, Swinson RP, Kirby N. Post-traumatic stress disorder after car accidents. *Can J Psychiatry.* 1985; 30(6):426–427.

Lackner JM, Carosella AM, Feuerstein M. Pain expectancies, pain, and functional self-efficacy expectancies as determinants of disability in patients with chronic low back disorders. *J Consult Clin Psychol.* 1996;64(1):212–220.

Large RG. The psychiatrist and the chronic pain patient. *Pain.* 1980;9:253–263.

Lazarus RR, Folkman S. *Stress, Appraisal, and Coping.* New York, NY: Springer; 1984.

Lester N, Lefebvre JC, Keefe FJ. Pain in young adults—III: Relationships of three pain-coping measures to pain and activity interference. *Clin J Pain.* 1996;12(4):291–300.

Linton SJ, Bradley LA. Strategies for the prevention of chronic pain. In: Gatchel RJ, Turk DC, eds. *Psychological Approaches to Pain Management.* New York, NY: Guilford Press; 1996:438–457.

Lipchik GL, Milles K, Covington EC. The effects of multidisciplinary pain management treatment on locus of control and pain beliefs in chronic non-terminal pain. *Clin J Pain.* 1993;9(1):49–57.

Long DM, Erickson D, Campbell J, North RB. Electrical stimulation of the spinal cord and peripheral nerves for pain control: A 10 year experience. *Appl Neurophysiol.* 1981;44:207–217.

Lorig K, Chastain RL, Ung E, Shoor S, Holman HR. Development and evaluation of a scale to measure perceived self-efficacy in people with arthritis. *Arthritis Rheum.* 1989;32(1):37–44.

Main CJ, Watson PJ. Screening for patients at risk of developing chronic incapacity. *J Occup Rehabil.* 1995;5(4):207–217.

Manne SL, Zautra AJ. Couples coping with chronic illness: Women with rheumatoid arthritis and their healthy husbands. *J Behav Med*. 1990;13:327–342.

McCracken LM, Gross RT, Sorg PJ, Edmands TA. Prediction of pain in patients with chronic low back pain: Effects of inaccurate prediction and pain-related anxiety. *Behav Res Ther*. 1993;31(7):647–652.

McCracken LM, Zayfert C, Gross RT. The pain anxiety symptoms scale: Development and validation of a scale to measure fear of pain. *Pain*. 1992;50(1):67–73.

McDaniel LK, Anderson KO, Bradley LA, et al. Development of an observation method for assessing pain behavior in rheumatoid arthritis patients. *Pain*. 1986;24(2):165–184.

McNair D, Lorr M, Droppleman L. *Manual for the Profile of Mood States*. San Diego, Calif: Educational Testing Service; 1971.

Melzack R, Wall PD. *The Challenge of Pain*. New York, NY: Basic Books; 1982.

Merskey H. Chronic pain and psychiatric illness. In: Bonica JJ, ed. *The Management of Pain*. Philadelphia, Pa: Lea & Febiger; 1990:320–327.

Miller RJ, Hafner RJ. Medical visits and psychological disturbance in chronic low back pain. A study of a back education class. *Psychosomatics*. 1991;32(3):309–316.

Moore JE, Armentrout DP, Parker JC, Kivlahan DR. Empirically derived pain-patient MMPI subgroups: Prediction of treatment outcome. *J Behav Med*. 1986;9:51–63.

Moos RH. *Work Environment Scale: Manual*. Palo Alto, Calif: Consulting Psychologist Press; 1981.

Moos RH, Moos BS. *Family Environment Scale: Manual*. Palo Alto, Calif: Consulting Psychologist Press; 1991.

Morey LC. *The Personality Assessment Inventory (manual)*. Odessa, Fl: Psychological Assessment Resources; 1991.

Muse M. Stress-related post-traumatic chronic pain syndrome: Criteria for diagnosis and preliminary report on prevalence. *Pain*. 1985;23:295–300.

Naliboff BD, McCreary CP, McArthur DL, Cohen MJ, Gottlieb HJ. MMPI changes following behavioral treatment of chronic low back pain. *Pain*. 1988;35(3):271–277.

Novy DM, Nelson DV, Berry LA, Averill PM. What does the Beck Depression Inventory measure in chronic pain?: A reappraisal. *Pain*. 1995;61(2):261–270.

O'Leary A, Shoor S, Lorig K, Holman HR. A cognitive-behavioral treatment for rheumatoid arthritis. *Health Psychol*. 1988;7(6):527–544.

Papciak AS, Feuerstein M. *Fear of Pain in Work Rehabilitation*. Presented at the 25th Annual Meeting of the Advancement of Behavioral Therapy: New York, NY; 1991.

Parker J, McRae C, Smarr K, et al. Coping strategies in rheumatoid arthritis. *J Rheumatol*. 1988;15:1376–1383.

Pilowski I. A general classification of abnormal illness behavior. *Br J Med Psychol*. 1978;51:131–137.

Polatin PB, Kinney RK, Gatchel RJ, Lillo E, Mayer TG. Psychiatric illness and chronic low back pain: The mind and the spine—which goes first? *Spine*. 1993;18(1):66–71.

Radloff LS. The CES-D Scale: A self-report depression scale for research in the general population. *Appl Psychol Measurement*. 1977;1(3):385–401.

Reiss S, Peterson RA, Gursky DM, McNally RJ. Anxiety sensitivity, anxiety frequency, and the prediction of fearfullness. *Behav Rese Ther*. 1986;24:1–8.

Richards R, Nepomuceno C, Riles M, Suer A. Assessing pain behavior: The UAB Pain Behavior Scale. *Pain*. 1982;14:393–398.

Riley JL, Robinson ME, Geisser ME, Wittmer VT. Multivariate cluster analysis of the MMPI-2 in chronic low-back pain patients. *Clin J Pain*. 1993;9(4):248–252.

Robbins RA, Moody DS, Hahn MB, Weaver MA. Psychological testing variables as predictors of return to work by chronic pain patients. *Percept Mot Skills*. 1996;83(3 Pt 2):1317–1318.

Romano JM, Turner JA. Chronic pain and depression: Does the evidence support a relationship? *Psychol Bull*. 1985;97(1):18–34.

Rosenstiel AK, Keefe FJ. The use of coping strategies in chronic low back pain patients: Relationship to patient characteristics and current adjustment. *Pain*. 1983;17(1):33–44.

Shutty MS, DeGood DE. Cluster analyses of responses of low back pain patients to the SCL–90: Comparison of empirical versus rationally derived subscales. *Rehabil Psychol*. 1987;32:133–143.

Shutty MS, DeGood DE, Schwartz DP. Psychological dimensions of distress in chronic pain patients: A factor analytic study of Symptom Checklist-90 responses. *J Consult Clin Psychol*. 1986;54(6):836–842.

Shutty MS, DeGood DE, Tuttle DH. Chronic pain patients' beliefs about their pain and treatment outcomes. *Arch Phys Med Rehabil*. 1990;71(2):128–132.

Skevington SM. Chronic pain and depression: Universal or personal helplessness? *Pain*. 1983;15(3):309–317.

Skevington SM. A standardized scale to measure beliefs about controlling pain (B.P.C.Q.): A preliminary study. *Psychol Health*. 1990;4:221–232.

Spielberger CD. *State–Trait Anger Expression Inventory: Professional Manual*. Odessa, Fl: Psychological Assessment Resources; 1991.

Spielberger CD, Gorsuch RL, Lushene R. *Manual for the State–Trait Anxiety Inventory: (STAI) "(Self-Evaluation Questionnaire)."* Palo Alto, Calif: Consulting Psychologists Press; 1979.

Spitzer RL, Williams JBW, Gibbon M, First MB. *Structured Clinical Interview for DSM-IIIR*. Washington, DC: American Psychiatric Press; 1990.

Sternbach RA. *Pain Patients: Traits and Treatments*. New York, NY: Academic Press; 1974.

Strong J, Ashton R, Cramond T, Chant D. Pain intensity, attitude, and function in back pain patients. *Aust Occup Ther J*. 1990;37:179–183.

Sullivan MJ, D'Eon JL. Relation between catastrophizing and depression in chronic pain patients. *J Abnorm Psychol*. 1990;99(3):260–263.

Sutherland HJ, Lockwood GA, Cunningham AJ. A simple, rapid method for assessing psychological distress in cancer patients: Evidence for linear analog scales. *J Psychosocial Oncol*. 1989;7:31–43.

ter Kuile MM, Spinhoven P, Linssen AC, van Houwelingen HC. Cognitive coping and appraisal processes in the treatment of chronic headaches. *Pain*. 1996;64(2):257–264.

Tota-Faucette ME, Gil KM, Williams DA, Keefe FJ, Goli V. Predictors of response to pain management treatment. The role of family environment and changes in cognitive processes. *Clin J Pain*. 1993;9(2):115–123.

Turk DC, Meichenbaum D, Genest M. *Pain and Behavioral Medicine: A Cognitive–Behavioral Perspective*. New York, NY: Guilford Press; 1983.

Turner JA, Clancy S, Vitaliano PP. Relationships of stress, appraisal and coping to chronic low back pain. *Behav Res Ther*. 1987;25:281–288.

Turner JA, Jensen MP. Efficacy of cognitive therapy for chronic low back pain. *Pain*. 1993;52(2):169–177.

Turner JA, Romano JM. Self-report screening measures for depression in chronic pain patients. *J Clin Psychol*. 1984;40(4):909–913.

Vitaliano PP, Russo J, Carr JE, Maiuro RD, Becker J. The Ways of Coping Checklist: Revision and psychometric properties. *Multivar Behav Res*. 1985;20:3–26.

Waddell G, McCulloch JA, Kummel E, Venner RM. Nonorganic physical signs in low-back pain. *Spine*. 1980;5:117–125.

Waddell G, Newton M, Henderson I, Somerville D, Main CJ. A fear-avoidance beliefs questionnaire (FABQ) and the role of fear-avoidance beliefs in chronic low back pain and disability. *Pain*. 1993;52(2):157–168.

Waddell G, Pilowsky I, Bonds MR. Clinical assessment and interpretation of abnormal illness behavior in low back pain. *Pain*. 1989;39:41–53.

Wallston KA, Stein MJ, Smith CA. Form C of the MHLC scales: A condition-specific measure of locus of control. *J Personality Assess*. 1994;63(3):534–553.

Wallston KA, Wallston BS, DeVellis R. Development of the Multidimensional Health Locus of Control (MHLC) scales. *Health Education Monographs*. 1978;6:160–170.

Ware JE, Kosinski M, Keller SD. *SF-12: How to Score the SF-12 Physical and Mental Health Summary Scales*. 2nd ed. Boston, Ma: The Health Institute, New England Medical Center; 1995.

Ware JE Jr, Sherbourne CD. The Mos 36-item Short-form Health Survey (SF-36). Conceptual framework and item selection. *Med Care*. 1992;30(6):473–483.

Weir R, Browne GB, Tunks E, Gafni A, Roberts J. A profile of users of speciality pain clinic services: Predictors of use and cost estimate. *J Clin Epidemiol*. 1992;45:1339–1415.

Wesley AL, Gatchel RJ, Polatin PB, Kinney RK, Mayer TG. Differentiation between somatic and cognitive/affective components in commonly used measures of depression in patients with chronic low-back pain. *Spine*. 1991;16(suppl 6):s213–s215.

Williams AC, Richardson PH. What does the BDI measure in chronic pain? *Pain*. 1993;55(2):259–266.

Williams DA, Keefe FJ. Pain beliefs and the use of cognitive-behavioral coping strategies. *Pain*. 1991;46:185–190.

Williams DA, Robinson ME, Geisser ME. Pain beliefs: Assessment and utility. *Pain*. 1994;59:71–78.

Williams DA, Thorn BE. An empirical assessment of pain beliefs. *Pain*. 1989;36:351–358.

Williams DA, Urban B, Keefe FJ, Shutty MS, France R. Cluster analyses of pain patients' responses to the SCL-90R. *Pain*. 1995;61(1):81–91.

Yunus MB. Towards a model of pathophysiology of fibromyalgia: Aberrant central pain mechanisms with peripheral modulation. *J Rheumatol*. 1992;19(6):846–850.

Zung WWK. A self-rating depression scale. *Arch Gen Psychiatry*. 1965;12:63–70.

CHAPTER 9

Patient Satisfaction
and Experience

THOMAS R. ZASTOWNY

INTRODUCTION

Many factors have prompted renewed interest in the relationship between patient satisfaction, health care quality, and outcome, including: (1) a re-emergence of interest in the basic subject of quality, (2) an increase in the attention to outcome assessment more broadly and use of "clinical indicators," (3) implementation of the concepts of total quality management (TQM) and continuous quality improvement (CQI) in health care, and (4) greater recognition that patient satisfaction is an important measure of health care "system" performance and outcome. Within managed care settings, these factors have also translated directly into market share, health care plan and provider (HCP) selection, and creation of significant "cost–offset" opportunities.

The assessment of satisfaction and patient experience as an indicator of quality and outcome of care is important. The current literature is rich with excellent ideas about how satisfaction, quality of care, and outcome can be joined. This chapter discusses the use of patient satisfaction and personal health care experiences as a measure of health care quality and outcome. It traces the development of satisfaction from a theoretical and methodological perspective using a variety of research publications and literature reviews. It also presents a field-proven patient experience and satisfaction assessment methodology known as the Patient Experience Survey (PES) that has been employed throughout the country for the past decade. Contemporary models of satisfaction assessment are also highlighted which identify factors that can serve as "drivers" of continuous quality improvement. Finally, it offers recommendations and comments on the use of patient satisfaction data in quality assessment and improvement building on the concept of "patient-based" quality systems.

(TQM) in which various "work and clinical processes" are defined, developed and improved. It is now routine to see patient satisfaction measures included as part of quality improvement efforts in the United States and in many countries across the world (eg, Cardosa and Rudkin, 1994; Holm and Henriksen, 1994; Raspe et al, 1996).

MEASUREMENT ISSUES

A second general set of issues concerning satisfaction measures as quality and outcome indicators includes the problem of highly positive ratings of satisfaction and the limited availability of comparative standards in the field (Lehman and Zastowny, 1983). It is common for a majority of patients to express strong positive attitudes about their health care despite negative experiences. For example, **only rarely is it that fewer than 70% of clients surveyed report anything less than "being satisfied" with care and fewer than 10% of patients can be expected to report any specific dissatisfaction** (Lebow, 1983a; Lehman and Zastowny, 1983.) This situation makes clear the need for meaningful guidelines to assist HCPs and program evaluators in interpreting the typically high levels of satisfaction expressed by their patients. It also suggests the need for refinements in the measurement approach to, and analysis of, satisfaction data. The more recent satisfaction measurement tools developed and used in the last several years have greatly reduced this problem. Additionally, the conceptualization of satisfaction has also been significantly broadened to include patient experience and personal preferences. For example, asking patients specifically about problems encountered and personal experience in their health care encounters has permitted a much more comprehensive view of their opinions and generated satisfaction distributions with much greater variability (ie, greater satisfaction and dissatisfaction ratings). This is especially true if the assessment questionnaires are "problem" sensitive (see the section entitled "A Measurement Approach and Some Available Measures" later in this chapter).

Finally, the use of satisfaction as an "outcome" measure and a quality of care indicator has some special methodological difficulties (Scheirer, 1978; LeVois et al, 1981; Nguyen et al, 1983). One important area is the limited availability of standardized instruments in the field and the number of potential dimensions underlying these measures (Pascoe, 1983; Ware et al, 1983). One conservative approach to handle this difficulty is to use those aspects of care most frequently measured in the literature (refer to Table 9–3) including: (1) personal aspects of care, (2) technical quality of care, (3) accessibility and availability of care, (4) continuity of care, (5) patient convenience, (6) physical setting, (7) financial considerations, and (8) efficacy of treatment (Ware and Snyder 1975; Ware et al, 1976a, 1976b, 1978, 1983).

To complicate matters further, both global and highly specific measures and dimensions of satisfaction have also been used. As a help in this area, it has been suggested that more global measures and dimensions of satisfaction may

---

CLINICAL TIP 9–5
Think Like a Patient

Pay attention to the methodological issues noted in this chapter but remember that most of our breakthroughs in this area will come from "thinking and experiencing" like a patient. Walk through your program, experience a visit, sit in the waiting room. What do you see? Is it good? Talk to patients, conduct focus groups, talk to family members. Listen and you will discover.

---

yield more general impressions of the care received and, hence, may not accurately reflect those aspects of care most closely and specifically related to actual quality of care and outcome (Cleary and McNeil, 1988). This may be particularly true if the measures used are focused on the delivery of care at a microanalytic level (eg, specific ratings of HCP–patient interactions). Other problems related to the measurement aspects of satisfaction may include social desirability factors, the "Hawthorne" effect, reward and reinforcement effects, cognitive dissonance/incongruity pressures, questionnaire set "response," multicollinearity (Stratmann, 1994) and experimental and design bias (Scheirer, 1978; LeVois et al, 1981; Pascoe, 1983). These topics are very important to consider when selecting a satisfaction questionnaire and designing an overall assessment approach.

A CONCEPTUAL AND MEASUREMENT MODEL

Prior to a limited review of some available instruments and satisfaction measures, it is helpful to return to some abstract thinking. Figure 9–1 presents an overall conceptual model for factors affecting patient satisfaction and experience. This model was developed from the earlier efforts of myself and colleagues predicting satisfaction and utilization in several clinic populations (Zastowny et al, 1983, 1988) and later work in a variety of health care settings (Zastowny et al, 1995; Zastowney, 1997) (Fig. 9–1). The model includes (1) health care framework components, (2) health care delivery characteristics and illness factors, (3) patient–HCP interactions, and (4) personal factors.

Some of the key assumptions of the model shown in Figure 9–1 include:

- Recognition of a *dynamic interplay* between health care framework components, health care delivery and illness factors, contributions from patient–HCP interactions, and personal factors of the patient.
- Expectations of a *bi-directional relationship* between health care utilization and satisfaction. For example, sometimes satisfaction is an "outcome" of care

Man
tionnaire
approach

- L
  C
  A
  tk
- N
  m
- R
  wi

USE OI
IN REH

Some ad
used in re
pages, wit
studies. V
these stud
Relati
faction wi
specifically
other rest
earliest st
with medi
This study
tion amon
each of th
back pain
form of m
the patient
weeks' dur
frequent f
with failu

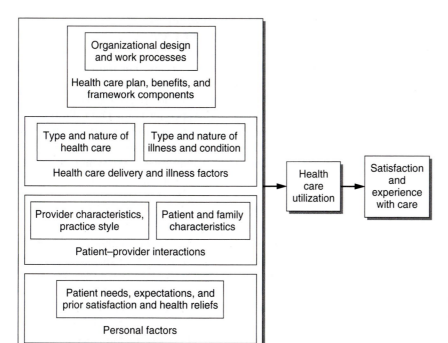

Figure 9–1. Factors affecting patient satisfaction and experience.

From Zastowny, 1997. Reprinted with permission.

and at other times satisfaction is an "input" to future care.

- Awareness that at any one point in time, one particular factor may overshadow the others, especially if there is a *particularly "good" or "bad" health care experience.*
- Recognition of a *complex relationship* between health care utilization, satisfaction, and experience with care, and eventual health care outcome and quality.

The model provides a conceptualization of the contributors to satisfaction and highlights potential content areas for measurement (eg, health care delivery and illness factors). Lastly, it is suggested that part of the overall impression of satisfaction with care is developed out of the day-to-day events associated with health care utilization, including many components that are typically considered dimensions of health care performance (such as appropriateness of care, availability, timeliness, effectiveness, continuity, and efficiency). These dimensions also provide a natural crosswalk to standards of health care accreditation organizations such as the Joint Commission on Accreditation of Health Care Organizations (JCAHO) and the Commission on Accreditation of Rehabilitative Facilities (CARF).

UNDERSTANDING PATIENT SATISFACTION

As we continue to approach more detailed measurement issues in the area of patient satisfaction some key steps to understanding patient satisfaction (Zastowny, 1996) are listed below:

- Patient satisfaction is not the same as customer needs, patient expectations, experience, or quality—although it is often said that there cannot be quality without patient satisfaction (Vuori, 1987).
- Measuring satisfaction can be complex because it often includes different dimensions of care with different attributes.
- The specifics of measuring satisfaction are very different depending on the nature of care. (For example, consider what is important from the patients' perspective in a pediatric continuity clinic, emergency department, or physical therapy practice.)
- It is insufficient (besides being poor business practice) to measure patient satisfaction once a year, report those findings, and not respond to them.
- The tools and methods for measuring patient satisfaction have made quantum leaps in the last several years.

Table 9–4:

Were you sa
Did you hav
Do you feel
Do you feel
Do you feel
Did the doct
Would you li
Was your me
  to a docto
Did you seek

[a] All subjects r
From Deyo and

CLINICAL TIP 9–6
Health Care Accreditation

Even if your organization is not in the accreditation ballgame (eg, JCAHO), it is useful to become knowledgeable about existing health care standards in your area. This can be very important for joint-venture opportunities, many of which will be with larger hospitals and health systems that may require health care standards compliance. Additionally, at this point in time, many of the national standards systems require assessment of patient satisfaction.

Cu

Find, custo
able to yo
existing to
some of yo
tions, do s
format of tl

• Patiel
forma
• Finall
has al
ment
care c

**A MEASU
AND SON**

Following so
ful measuren
some availab
methodologie
satisfaction d
tion, in 1982
tient Experie
a broad pers
patient's pers
and evaluatio
measure hosp
customer sati
tion in the 1
successfully i
was adapted
later to heal
mented in m

*Exploring |
Use of Foc*
From the ex
emerged tha
for measurin
the beginnir
specifically, i
tion instrum
tients to ider
to patients w
also provide
ment measur
and to the ur
periences. T
important "a
manner, pati
for ongoing a

plained by analysis of HCPs' characteristics (eg, years in practice, length of visit) or patient characteristics (eg, sociodemographic features, severity or duration of back pain). **The authors suggest that HCPs who have more confidence in their ability to effectively manage low back pain may, in fact, be more effective patient educators.**

In an earlier study, Cherkin and MacCornack (1989) compared HMO enrollees' evaluation of care received from family physicians and chiropractors for care of low back pain. The study demonstrated that patients of chiropractors were three times as likely (66% vs 22%) as patients of family physicians to report they were satisfied with (1) amount of information given, (2) sense of HCP's concern, and (3) confidence and professional comfort with management of their condition. The authors indicate that the more positive evaluation of chiropractors might be attributable to differences in the case-mix of the provider groups or to the actual benefits of spinal manipulation. However, in addition they suggest an equally, if not more powerful variable (ie, the therapeutic relationship and interaction of the patient and HCP) may be the factor explaining the differences. This finding is clearly reinforced and supported by the specific set of research findings on patient–provider interactions in the broader medical care context (Caterinicchio, 1979; Hall, 1987; Roter et al, 1987).

The Rehabilitative Services Department of British Columbia reported a study in 1989 in the *Quarterly Review Bulletin* (Davis and Hobbs, 1989) measuring outpatient satisfaction with rehabilitative services. Working with an interdisciplinary committee, they developed an operational definition of satisfaction including the following dimensions: (1) access to care, (2) physical environment, and (3) care with three components—human aspect, clinical, and outcome. Out of this conceptualization, they developed and used a satisfaction measure with their rehabilitative outpatients. The survey findings indicated overall satisfaction with specific areas highlighted for improvement, including access, physical comment, need for additional information, and the nature of problems.

A similar study was published in 1994 in *Spine* (Hazard et al, 1994). This study examined the relationship between patient satisfaction and pain, impairment, and disability outcomes among chronic low back pain patients. This study followed 90 chronic low back pain patients who underwent initial pain, impairment, and disability evaluations. A unique aspect of the study was the availability of correlations between initial pain, disability, and impairment ratings, and similar assessments conducted at a 5-year follow-up. Correlation coefficients between self-assessments of pain, disability, and impairment (similar to results seen previously in the literature) were modest but positive. Satisfaction at year 5 correlated poorly with current pain and disability; however, satisfaction levels were much higher among patients who returned to work after 1 year regardless of the specific treatment. One conclusion of the study was that it was not possible to define outcome preferences for all chronic low back pain patients. However, the

---

> **CLINICAL TIP 9–9**
> Musculoskeletal Pain and Disability
>
> Key satisfaction issues for patients with musculoskeletal pain and disability include pain experience, health beliefs, waiting time, interface with primary HCPs, cost of care, HCP understanding, and chronic illness management.

study did suggest an important strategy for improving care. The recommendation indicated that patient satisfaction depends to some extent on meeting patient's pretreatment expectations, and that chronic low back pain patients and their HCPs may improve their therapeutic alliance by mutually setting pain, impairment, and disability treatment goals and judging the "downstream" outcomes accordingly.

Another recent study (Coulter et al, 1994) designed a 14 item measure of satisfaction with chiropractic care entitled *The Chiropractic Satisfaction Questionnaire (CSQ)*. The content of the CSQ includes items on interpersonal quality, technical quality, time spent with the chiropractor, cost of care, and provides an overall satisfaction rating with care. This assessment is shown in Appendix Form D-2. This study was conducted using a sample of 486 patients receiving care from 44 chiropractors within California primarily to provide initial reliability and validity for the CSQ. Using this data, the internal consistency and reliability of the 14 CSQ items was estimated at 0.95. Additionally, to assess construct validity, the CSQ was correlated with patient rating of "confidence of treatment received" and patient perceived efficacy of care. Both correlations (CSQ with confidence and perceived efficacy) were positive and significant. In the discussion of the outcomes of this article, some useful considerations regarding critical dimensions of care and assessment of chiropractic health care emerge. These include the importance of assessing patients' understanding about health and illness, the HCPs' personal set of beliefs and philosophies concerning health and health care delivery, and patients' expectations for care.

METHODOLOGICAL RECOMMENDATIONS

A complete review of methodological issues concerning satisfaction assessment is well beyond the scope of this chapter. However some basic points are important to note and are provided in the following discussion.

Recommendations for Patient Satisfaction Questionnaire Design and Use

• Use focus groups to identify and define aspects of care for measurement.
• Use several items to measure each aspect of care.
• Carefully balance the need for information with demand on patients' time (eg, try to keep questionnaires to a single page).

- Try to assess at least 50 to 100 patients in a given area.
- Design your sampling strategy along the continuum of care for your health care services (eg, admission, continued stay, discharge).
- Use graphic design resources to make the questionnaire appealing and user-friendly.
- Field test your questionnaire with a selected group of patients before conducting the full survey.
- Review the questionnaire with a proofreader for language level and readability.
- Design the questionnaire to facilitate coding and for quick linkage to database for analysis.
- Consider mixed sampling strategies (eg, some telephone surveys, some mail, some in person interviews).

Administering Satisfaction Questionnaires

A related set of issues are associated with the administration of satisfaction questionnaires. **One preferred method is for the assessment to be administered and collected by an independent agency.** This strategy minimizes the bias potential associated with the same individuals being involved in treatment and evaluation activities, and the common "halo" effect of patients perceiving their HCPs in a positive fashion. However this approach can become cost prohibitive especially in smaller clinics. If questionnaires are administered by the treatment facility in which clients are seen, the following points should be considered: (1) use clinic support staff to administer the questionnaires rather than HCPs or administrative staff; (2) use identification numbers rather than patient names whenever possible; (3) provide a "drop-box" in which clients can place completed questionnaires; (4) encourage a patient suggestion system so that assessment of satisfaction is not seen as the only method of change, but rather as a partnership for improvement; (5) as noted previously, use mixed sampling approaches (eg, mail, phone, interview) to avoid method bias; and (6) use event-oriented questions (see "A Measurement Approach" earlier in this chapter) to facilitate specific identification of problem areas.

PRACTICAL APPLICATIONS: BLUEPRINTS FOR ACTION

One goal of measuring patient satisfaction and experience is to improve quality of care and outcomes. These goals can be linked to three key questions tied to the service evaluation process:

1. Is patient satisfaction improving?
2. What are the main drivers of patient satisfaction?
3. What specific things should be done or not be done to improve satisfaction?

Any satisfaction measure should help with regard to answering these questions.

Careful assessment of patients and families is an important first step. What happens after a survey is completed and the data are collected? A useful approach to patient satisfaction and experience data is to organize and analyze the information to create a guide for change and continuous improvement. There are numerous methods available to help accomplish this outcome, including perspective maps, customer windows, and matrix charts.

The idea behind these techniques is a simple one. The task is to score the data and plot it so it guides improvement. Figure 9–2 provides an example of such a map (Perspective Map of Patient and Provider Ratings). In this example both patients' and HCPs' responses are combined. This figure compares staff ratings of importance and patient satisfaction perspectives for a variety of existing services and aspects of care.

In this example, key areas for improvement include Occupational Health Services (A) and Access to Providers (C). Another aspect of this technique is that the dimensions of the map can be defined in whatever way the health care organization chooses. For example, one might select:

- Patients' compared to families' perspective
- HCPs' compared to family
- Perceived importance of a health care activity with satisfaction for patients, or family members

The logistics for completing and using the map are straightforward and as follows:

- Select an assessment scale for satisfaction and performance or any aspect of care to be rated.
- Assess the customers and HCPs with the scales.
- Plot the scores on the map or average the scores to provide a numerical value for the matrix column or row.
- Review the plot and rankings and use as a guide for priority setting.

This method also has direct applicability for emerging care management tools such as "care maps" and "clinical pathways" (Zastowny, 1997).

CLINICAL TIP 9–10
Blueprint for Improvement

Out of any patient satisfaction effort, an actual blueprint for improvement can be developed. Some organizations have enough experience with their measurement systems and costs to also define the relative cost for each increment in expected patient satisfaction associated with planned changes. Every satisfaction report should end with exploration of questions such as: "What can be done better?" "How can we improve?"

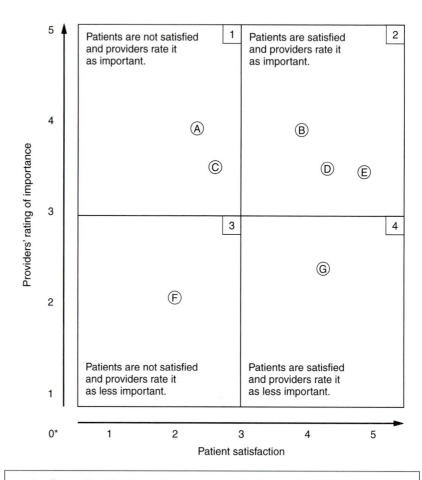

Figure 9–2. Perspective map of patient and HCP ratings.

From Zastowny, 1996. Reprinted with permission. © 1997 Aspen Publishers, Inc.

A = Occupational health services
B = Nursing care
C = Access to providers
D = General medical care

E = Drug and alcohol treatment
F = Parking and office access
G = Therapeutic environment

*Footnote Scale: 1 is lowest, 5 is highest

Conclusion

The evolution of measurement and use of patient satisfaction and experience data in health care will continue. Nelson and Batalden (1993) provide an excellent glimpse of the future for what they term "patient-based" quality systems. They define *patient-based* quality measurement systems as having the following characteristics: (1) patient based (referring to information that is provided by individuals who receive health care), (2) *quality,* as the goodness of the match between patient need and set of services delivered, and (3) *system of measurement* integrating numerous components (eg, sampling, data collecting and analysis, feedback, and distribution of information). Also, the overall quality or "goodness" of health care is determined from the patient's perspective using the above characteristics as well as additional outcome data. The features of such a system, with comparison to approaches, are listed in Table 9–5. The features

listed are important ones and closely parallel many of the issues discussed in this chapter.

On the whole, there is increasing agreement that our understanding of the relationship between patient satisfaction, quality of care, and outcome will advance as we explore more specific hypotheses with carefully constructed evaluation designs, rigorous methodology, and consistent measurement approaches. There is also substantial agreement that soon, assessment of patient satisfaction and experience will become part of routine patient care. Evaluation approaches will also increasingly move toward comprehensive, longitudinal assessments of health care outcomes using valid, reliable measures. Furthermore, these data will directly inform and shape quality improvement efforts in a "real-time" fashion. Table 9–6 offers additional patient satisfaction studies that have been conducted since the early 1960s through the late 1970s.

CASE STUDY 9-1
LOW BACK PAIN

Given the prevalence of low back pain in the general population, this condition serves as an excellent example to further illustrate measurement of patient satisfaction. To begin, a number of general aspects of care might be defined, including assessment, diagnostics and treatment, teaching and counseling, medications, consultations and referrals, psychological outcomes, educational outcomes, psychosocial outcomes, and specific satisfaction with the health care visit. Using these elements as the basic building blocks and anticipating the activities of a series of sequential visits, more specific satisfaction questions can be developed. For example, assume that the patient is in the second or third visit and the goals of the sessions are listed below:

TREATMENT GOALS

- Patient able to correlate activity with pain level
- Patient verbalizes understanding of exercise regimen
- Patient to develop understanding of lifestyle change
- Patient engaging in appropriate exercise with proper body mechanics

Following the goals and approach of the treatment noted above, specific satisfaction questions might include:

SPECIFIC SATISFACTION QUESTIONS

- Treatment room temperature was comfortable.
- Professional staff identified themselves and their roles.
- Once in the treatment room, length of wait to see the HCP was reasonable.

- Sufficient privacy was provided during treatment.
- The HCP gave education on body mechanics.
- The HCP prepared me for the amount of pain I experienced during treatment.
- The HCP explained treatment choices in a way that I could understand.
- Following my visit, I understand more about a healthy lifestyle.
- Following my visit, I understand more about pain control.
- I was given a thorough and careful physical examination.
- Sufficient time was spent on my care.
- I had the opportunity to ask questions about my care.

These specific questions might also be used in combination with an overall rating of the visit, for example, "Overall, how would you rate your treatment today? A (Excellent); A−, B+, B (Good); B−, C+, C (Fair); C−, D+, D (Poor); or F (Unacceptable). If, upon assessment of a number of patients, any of the above questions were checked as problematic, the specific items would serve as targets for improvement. The specific performance can also be compared to existing baseline data within a clinic or compared to local and national benchmarks. Clinical experience in this area reinforces existing research suggesting that for low back pain patients, the psychosocial and personal aspects of service delivery are very important to level of satisfaction and also perceived efficacy of the treatment.

Table 9-5: Features of Patient-Based Quality Measurement Systems

FEATURE	CURRENT	FUTURE
Content	Satisfaction ———————————	Care evaluations, health outcomes
Validation	Rare ———————————	Common
Frequency	Annually or all patients ———————	Continually or representative samples
Sampling	Not rigorous ———————————	Careful specification of sampling frame
Response rates	Low (< 40%) ———————————	High (> 60%)
Comparative data	Rare ———————————	Common
Users and uses	Few and limited ———————————	Many and diverse and educated
Direct link to action	Infrequent ———————————	Common
Feedback	Cross-sectional, tabular ———————	Trends, graphic, layered measures

From Nelson and Batalden, 1993. Reprinted with permission.

Table 9–6: Additional Patient Satisfaction Studies

INVESTIGATOR(S)	SATISFACTION DOMAINS	ASPECT
Freidson E. *Patients' Views of Medical Practice.* New York, NY: Russell Sage Foundation; 1961.	Interest, competence, time spent	Cumulative impressions of one or more physicians in health care organization
Cahal MF. What the public thinks of the family doctor—Folklore and facts. *Gen Practitioner.* 1962;25:146–157.	Finances, interest, humaneness, explanations, quality of care, efficacy of use, competence	Cumulative attitudes toward physicians and health care services
King SH. *Perceptions of Illness and Medical Practice.* New York, NY: Russell Sage Foundation; 1962.	Personal interest, explanations	Cumulative attitudes toward physicians and health care services
Cartwright A. *Human Relations and Hospital Care.* London, England: Routledge & Kegan Paul; 1964.	Physician's authority, information	Cumulative experience with physicians and recent stay in hospital
Deisher RW, Engel WC, Spieholz R, Standafact SJ. Mothers' opinions of their pediatric care. *Pediatrics.* 1965;35:82–90.	Wait time, accessibility, physician's personality, explanations, examinations, fees	Cumulative experience with regular source of care
Apostle D, Oder F. Factors that influence the public's view of medical care. *JAMA.* 1967; 202:140–146.	Accessibility, listening, explanations, thoroughness	Cumulative attitudes toward physicians and health care services
Franklin BJ, McLemore SD. A scale for measuring attitudes toward student health services. *J Psychol.* 1967;66:143–147.	Physician–patient relationship, physician competence, clinic procedures, quality of care	Cumulative experience with staff and physicians and services in clinic
Alpert JJ, Kosa J, Haggerty LJ, Robertson LS, Heagarty MC. Attitudes and satisfaction of low income families receiving comprehensive pediatric care. *Am J Public Health.* 1970;60:499–506.	Wait time, communication, explanations	Cumulative experience with clinic
DeCastro F, Amin H. An ambulatory pediatric unit: Consumers' satisfaction. *Clin Pediatr.* 1970;9:445–448.	Physicians and nurses "handling," explanations	Immediate perceptions of clinic experience
Houston CS, Pasanen WE. Patients perception of hospital care. *Hospitals.* 1972;46:70–74.	Information, admitting procedures, symptom improvement, continuity of care, finances, attention	Recent stay in hospital
Bobilya LJ. Students' view of the Indiana University health service. *J Am Coll Health.* 1974;23:19–21.	Physician–patient relationship, staff courtesy, general satisfaction	Cumulative perceptions of staff and physicians in clinic
Noyes RW, Levy MI, Chase CL, Udry JR. Expectation fulfillment as a measure of patient satisfaction. *Am J Obstet Gynecol,* 1974;118:809–814.	Office practice, fees, wait time, physician–patient relationships, expectation fulfillment	Compared cumulative perceptions of specific clinic with cumulative past experiences in other similar clinics
Kincey J, Bradshaw P, Ley P. Patients' satisfaction and reported acceptance of advice in general practice. *J R Coll Gen Practitioners.* 1975;25:558.	Office practices, information, compliance	Recent visit with private physician
Lebow JL. Evaluation of an outpatient pediatric practice through the use of consumer questionnaires. *Med Care.* 1975;13:250–255.	Physician's interest, wait time, information, symptom relief, compliance, quality of care, clinic procedures	Immediate and follow-up reactions to behavior of nurses and physicians
Linn LS. Factors associated with patient evaluation of health care. *Milbank Q Health Soc.* 1975;53:531–553.	General satisfaction, physician–patient relationship, understanding	Immediate perceptions of specific physician on initial and return visits

Table 9–6: (cont.)

INVESTIGATOR(S)	SATISFACTION DOMAINS	ASPECT
Wrigglesworth JM, Williams JT. The construction of an objective test to measure patient satisfaction. *Int J Nurs Stud.* 1975;12:123–132.	Staff relations, nurse care, confidence in physician, communication, information	Recent stay in hospital
Light HK, Solheim JS, Hunter GW. Satisfaction with medical care during pregnancy and delivery. *Am J Obstet Gynecol.* 1976;125:827–831.	Quality of prenatal and obstetric care in hospital and on follow-up	Cumulative experience with care during hospital and outpatient visits
Bertakis KD. The communication of information from physician to patient: A method for increasing patient retention and satisfaction. *J Fam Pract.* 1977;5:217–222.	Information, concern, time spent, communication, confidence in physician, treatment outcome	Immediate and delayed perceptions of care
Mangelsdorf AD. Patient satisfaction questionnaire. *Med Care.* 1979;17:86–90.	Interaction with physicians and staff, satisfaction with ancillary services (lab and x-rays)	Immediate perceptions of physician and clinic
McDaniel PA. The effects of student satisfaction and attitudes on staffing and policy decisions: A case study and empirical support. *J Am Coll Health.* 1979;27:214–217.	Physician personal interest and competence, communication, wait time, access to care, exam thoroughness, compliance intent	Cumulative experience with specific physician and clinic
Roghmann KJ, Hengst A, Zastowny TR. Satisfaction with medical care: Its measurement and relation to utilization. *Med Care.* 1979;17:461–479.	General satisfaction with medical care	Cumulative experience with specific clinic

REFERENCES

Attkisson CC, Pascoe GC, eds. Patient satisfaction in health and mental health services. *Eval Prog Plan.* 1983;6(Suppl 3, 4):185–418.

Bowers MR, et al. What attributes determine quality and satisfaction with health care delivery? *Health Care Man Rev.* 1994;19(4):49–55.

Brook RH, et al. Assuring the quality of medical care using outcome measures: An overview of the method. *Med Care.* 1977;Sept(Suppl):1–165.

Bush T, Cherkin D, Barlow W. The impact of physician attitudes on patient satisfaction with care for low back pain. *Arch Fam Med.* 1993;2(3):301–305.

Cardosa M, Rudkin GA. Outcome from day-case knee arthroscopy in a major teaching hospital. *Arthroscopy.* 1994;10(6):624–629.

Caterinicchio RP. Testing plausible path models on interpersonal trust in patient–physician treatment relationships. *Soc Sci Med.* 1979;13(A):81–99.

Cherkin DC, MacCornack FA. Patient evaluations of low back pain care from family physicians and chiropractors. *Western J Med.* 1989;150(3):351–355.

Cleary PD, McNeil BJ. Patient satisfaction as an indicator of quality care. *Inquiry.* 1988;25:25–36.

Conquest—A database of clinical performance measures. *Int J Qual Health Care.* 1996;8(4):417–418.

Consumer Reports. How is your doctor treating you? *Consumer Reports.* 1995;Feb:81–88.

Coulter ID, Hays RD, Danielson CD. The chiropractic satisfaction questionnaire. *Top Clin Chiro.* 1994;1(4):40–43.

Davies AR, Doyle MAT, Lansky D, et al. Outcomes assessment in clinical settings: A consensus statement on principles and best practices in project management. *Jt Comm J Qual Improve.* 1994;20:6–16.

Davis D, Hobbs G. Measuring outpatient satisfaction with rehabilitation services. *Q Rev Bull.* 1989;15(6):192–197.

Deming WE. *Out of the Crisis*. Cambridge, Mass: Massachusetts Institute of Technology; 1982.

Deyo RA, Diehl AK. Patient satisfaction with medical care for low-back pain. *Spine*. 1986;11(1):28–30.

Donabedian A. Twenty years of research on quality of medical care, 1965–1984. *Eval Health Professions*. 1985;8:243–265.

Donabedian A. The role of outcomes in quality assessment and assurance. *Q Rev Bull*. 1992;18(11):359.

Elbeck M. Patient contribution to the design and meaning of patient satisfaction for quality assurance purposes: The psychiatric case. *Health Care Man Rev*. 1992;17(1):91–95.

Ellwood PM. Outcomes management: A technology of patient experience. *N Engl J Med*. 1988;318(23):1549–1556.

Epstein AM. The outcomes movement—will it get us where we want to go? *N Engl J Med*. 1990;323:266–270.

Gold M, Wooldridge J. Surveying consumer satisfaction to assess managed-care quality: Current practices. *Health Care Finan Rev*. 1995;16(4):155–173.

Greenfield TK, Attkisson CC. Progress toward a multifactorial Service Satisfaction Scale for evaluating primary care and mental health services. *Eval Prog Plan*. 1989;12:271–276.

Hall JA, et al. Task versus socioemotional behaviors in physicians. *Med Care*. 1987;25(5):399–412.

Hall JA, Dornan MC. What patients like about their medical care and how often they are asked: A meta-analysis of the satisfaction literature. *Soc Sci Med*. 1988;27(9):939.

Hall JA. Meta-analysis of correlates of provider behavior in medical encounters. *Med Care*. 1988;26(7):657–672.

Hall JA. A causal model of health status and satisfaction with medical care. *Med Care*. 1993;31(1):84–94.

Hazard RG, Haugh LD, Green PA, Jones PL. Chronic low back pain: The relationship between patient satisfaction and pain, impairment, and disability outcomes. *Spine*. 1994;19(8):881–887.

Heitoff KA, Lohr KN, eds. *Effectiveness and Outcomes in Health Care: Proceedings of an Invitational Conference by the Institute of Medicine Division of Health Care Services*. Washington, DC: National Academy Press; 1990.

Holm AR, Henriksen CW. Orthopedic ambulatory surgery: A study of patient satisfaction. [Danish]. *Ugeskrift Laeger*. 1994;156(41):6018–6021.

Koehler WF, et al. Physician-patient satisfaction: Equity in the health services encounter. *Med Care Rev*. 1992;49(4):455–484.

Larson CO, Nelson EC, Gustafson D, Batalden PB. The relationship between meeting patients' information needs and their satisfaction with hospital care and general health status outcomes. *Int J Qual Health Care*. 1996;8(5):447–456.

Larson DL, Attkisson CC, Hargreaves WA, et al. Assessment of client/patient satisfaction: Development of a general scale. *Eval Prog Plan*. 1979;2:197–207.

Lebow J. Research assessing consumer satisfaction with mental health treatment: A review of findings. *Eval Prog Plan*. 1983a;6:211–236.

Lebow J. Similarities and differences between mental health and health care evaluation studies assessing consumer satisfaction. *Eval Prog Plan*. 1983b;6:237–245.

Lehman AF, Zastowny TR. Patient satisfaction with mental health services: A meta-analysis to establish norms. *Eval Prog Plan*. 1983;6:265–274.

LeVois M, Nguyen T, Attkisson C. Artifact in client satisfaction assessment: Experience in community mental health settings. *Eval Prog Plan*. 1981;4:139–150.

Linder-Pelz S. Toward a theory of patient satisfaction. *Soc Sci Med*. 1982;16:577–582.

Lohr KN. *Breast Cancer: Setting Priorities for Effectiveness Research. Report of a Study by a Committee of the Institute of Medicine, Division of Health Care Services*. Washington, DC: National Academy Press; 1990.

Mirin SM, Namorow MJ. Why study treatment outcomes? *J Hosp Comm Psychiatry*. 1991;42(10):1007–1013.

Neison EC, et al. Gaining customer knowledge: Obtaining and using customer judgments for hospitalwide quality improvement. *Top Health Record Man*. 1991;11:13–26.

Nelson EC, Batalden PB. Patient-based quality measurement systems. *Q Man Health Care*. 1993;2(1):18–30.

Nelson EC, Hays RD, Larson C, Batalden PB. The patient judgment system: Reliability and validity. *Q Rev Bull*. 1989;15(6):185–191.

Nguyen TD, Attkisson CC, Stegner BL. Assessment of patient satisfaction: Development and refinement of a service evaluation questionnaire. *Eval Prog Plan*. 1983;6:299–314.

Norton PG, et al. Satisfaction of residents and families in long-term care: 1. Construction and application of an instrument. *Q Man Health Care*. 1996;4(3):38–46.

ORYX, Outcomes—The Next Evolution in Accreditation. Oakbrook Terrace, Ill: Joint Commission on Accreditation of Healthcare Organizations; 1997.

Pascoe GC. Patient satisfaction in primary health care: A literature review and analysis. *Eval Prog Plan*. 1983;6:185–210.

Raspe H, et al. Patient "satisfaction" in medical rehabilitation: A useful outcome indicator? [German]. *Gesundheitswesen*. 1996;58(7):372–378.

Relman AS. Assessment and accountability: The third revolution in medical care. *N Engl J Med*. 1988;319(18):1220–1222.

Roghmann KJ, Hengst A, Zastowny TR. Satisfaction with medical care: Its measurement and relation to utilization. *Med Care*. 1979;17(5):461–479.

Ross CK, et al. The importance of patient preferences in the measurement of health care satisfaction. *Med Care*. 1993;31(12):1138–1149.

Ross CK, et al. A comparative study of seven measures of patient satisfaction. *Med Care*. 1995;33(4):393–406.

Roter DL, et al. Relations between physicians' behaviors and analogue patients' satisfaction, recall, and impressions. *Med Care*. 1987;25(5):437–451.

Sato T, Takeichi M, Fukui T, Gude JK. Doctor-shopping patients and users of alternative medicine among Japanese primary care patients. *Gen Hosp Psychiatry*. 1995;17(2):115–125.

Scheirer M. Program participants' positive perceptions: Psychological conflict of interest in social program evaluation. *Eval Quarterly*. 1978;2:53–70.

Strasser S, et al. The patient satisfaction process: Moving toward a comprehensive model. *Med Care Rev*. 1993;50(2):219–248.

Stratmann W, Zastowny TR, Bayer LR, Adams EH, Black GS, Fry PA. Patient satisfaction surveys and multicollinearity. *Qual Man Health Care*. 1994;2:1–12.

Vuori H. Patient satisfaction—An attribute or indicator of quality of care? *Qual Rev Bull*. 1987;March:106–108.

Ware JE Jr, Davies-Avery A, Stewart AL. The measurement and meaning of patient satisfaction: A review of the recent literature. *Health Mental Care Serv Rev*. 1978;1:1–15.

Ware JE, Phillips J, Yody BB, Adamczyk J. Assessment tools: Functional health status and patient satisfaction. *Am J Med Qual*. 1996;11(1):850–853.

Ware JE, Snyder MK. Dimensions of patient attitudes regarding doctors and medical care services. *Med Care*. 1975;13:669–682.

Ware JE, Snyder MK, Wright WR. Development and validation of scales to measure patient satisfaction with health care services: Volume 1 of a final report. Part A: Review of literature, overview of methods, and results regarding construction of scales. Report prepared for the National Center for Health Services Research by School of Medicine, Southern Illinois University, Carbondale, Ill; 1976a.

Ware JE, Snyder MK, Wright WR. Development and validation of scales to measure patient satisfaction with health care services: Volume 1 of a final report. Part B: Results regarding scales constructed from the Patient Satisfaction Questionnaire and measures of other health care perceptions. Report prepared for the National Center for Health Services Research by School of Medicine, Southern Illinois University, Carbondale, Ill; 1976b.

Ware JE, Snyder MK, Wright WR, Davies AR. Defining and measuring patient satisfaction with medical care. *Eval Prog Plan*. 1983;6:247–264.

Weingarten SR, et al. A study of patient satisfaction and adherence to preventive care practice guidelines. *Am J Med*. 1995;99:590–596.

Zastowny TR. Patient satisfaction, family burden, and outcome. *Case Man*. 1996;3(8):1–4. Special Insert.

Zastowny TR. Assessment of satisfaction and patient experience with clinical pathways: A conceptual model. In: Howe RS, ed. *Clinical Pathways for Ambulatory Care Case Management*. Suppl 1. Gaithersburg, Md: Aspen Publishers; July 1997:1–13.

Zastowny TR, Roghmann KJ, Henqst A. Satisfaction with medical care: Replications and theoretical re-evaluation. *Med Care*. 1983;21:294–322.

Zastowny TR, Roghmann KJ. Utilization of services and satisfaction with care: The relevance of health beliefs in a Medicaid population. Unpublished manuscript; 1988.

Zastowny TR, Roghmann KJ, Cafferota GL. Patient satisfaction and the use of health services: Explorations in causality. *Med Care*. 1989;27:705–723.

Zastowny TR, Stratmann WC, Adams EH, Fox ML. Patient satisfaction and experience with health services and quality of care. *Qual Man Health Care*. 1995;3(3):50–61.

CHAPTER 10

Predicting Outcome in Low Back Pain

Jeffery E. Fitzthum

INTRODUCTION

There are many options for assessing the outcomes of treatment for back pain but few for **predicting** outcome. Because up to two thirds of work injury costs derive from lost time wages (Shvartzman et al, 1992) having the ability to determine in advance probable response to treatment would seem vitally important. Those individuals who ultimately do not respond well to standard treatment approaches could be identified early. **If placed in a treatment program tailored to their needs, there is potential for reduction in time lost and consequent reduction in cost.**

Few instruments dedicated to predicting treatment response have been developed and those available have yet to be well validated. Over the past two decades, many studies have addressed the issue of prediction, but the results have been varied and often contradictory. Such lack of robustness in these studies probably derives from having been performed in a wide variety of settings, industrial or clerical, employed or unemployed, with and without workers' compensation; from surveillance of different injuries, including acute, mixed acute and chronic, low back pain only, or back and leg pain; and from assessment of multiple outcomes, including persisting pain, physical capacity, and return to work. Nevertheless, there is a general impression that self-reported pain and disability ratings, demographic, psychosocial, and occupational factors are good predictors of outcome; counterintuitively, the results of imaging studies and physical examination findings seem to be less useful as predictors.

To a first approximation, predicting outcome can be accomplished utilizing one predictive factor alone, but accuracy suffers. For example, the presence of depression has often been found to be related to poor outcome, but many individuals without depression respond poorly to treatment and many with depression respond well. Just as the experience of pain and consequent disability is understood to be multifactorial, the response to treatment undoubtedly depends on multiple issues. Therefore, to improve accuracy of prediction, research efforts in recent years have been directed more toward defining groups of predictive factors. Typically, in such a study, individuals with back pain are examined against a wide variety of potential predictors. Then, at a suitable later date when outcome is known, statistical modeling is used to determine which factors when grouped together are most closely related to outcome. The discussion in this chapter covers single and grouped factors. The single factors are listed first so as to familiarize the health care provider (HCP) with the many potential determinants of outcome.

SINGLE PREDICTIVE FACTORS

For the convenience of the HCP single predictors are presented separately for the clinical interview and the clinical examination.

PREDICTORS FOUND IN THE CLINICAL INTERVIEW

Because patients present at different stages of development in their back pain and because different predictors seem to be important at different stages, an attempt has been made further to categorize single factors into predictor types: primary, secondary, and tertiary (Gatchel et al, 1995a). **Primary indicators predict which uninjured individuals may eventually suffer injury; secondary indicators identify individuals with acute back pain who eventually develop chronic back pain; and tertiary indicators predict those individuals with chronic pain who fail with treatment.**

Primary Predictors

Primary predictors of outcome (Table 10–1) have not been an area of major research interest and may be of limited value for HCPs. Various factors have been identified as raising the risk that a healthy individual will suffer back injury, including smoking, shorter time on the job, lower satisfaction with work, post-traumatic stress disorder, major

depression, personality disorder, substance abuse, and elevations on scale 3 of the Minnesota Multiphasic Personality Inventory (MMPI).

Secondary Predictors

Of greater interest to the HCP are those aspects of the clinical interview that indicate a risk for an acute injury becoming chronic (Table 10–2). A multitude of demographic, occupational, psychosocial, and pain characteristics are statistically associated with poor outcome. **Demographic factors** include older age, minority status, immigrant status, limited proficiency in speaking English, smoking, and lower educational level. Dionne et al (1995) further demonstrated that the relationship between lower education level and poor outcome could largely be explained by strength requirements of the job, materials handling requirements of the job, smoking, body mass index, marital status, financial compensation, Symptom Checklist 90–Revised (SCL-90-R) depression scores, and SCL-90-R somatization scores. Of these, marital status, smoking and somatization were, perhaps, the more important. Cherkin et al (1996), on the other hand, did not find educational level to be important in a highly educated, largely white study population.

Shorter time on the job prior to injury behaves not only as a primary indicator but as a secondary predictor. Similarly, lower satisfaction with work is thought by some to be a primary and a secondary predictor. Lancourt and

Table 10–1: Primary Predictors of Poor Outcome[a]

Demographic Factors	
Smoking	Frymoyer and Cats-Baril (1987)
Occupational Factors	
Shorter time on the job	Bigos et al (1986), Kelsey and Golden (1988), Lancourt and Kettelhut (1992)
Lower satisfaction with work	Bigos et al (1991), Magora (1985), Niemcryck et al (1987), Westin et al (1972)
Psychosocial Factors	
History of post-traumatic stress disorder, major depression, personality disorder, substance abuse	Polatin et al (1993), Bigos et al (1991)

[a] Primary predictors suggest a higher likelihood for an uninjured person to report injury.

Table 10–2: Secondary Predictors of Poor Outcome[a]

Demographic Factors

Older age	Biering-Sorensen (1983), Milhous et al (1989)
Minority status	Gatchel et al (1995a)
Immigrant status	Lee et al (1989)
Limited proficiency in speaking English	LaCroix et al (1990)
Smoking	Lancourt and Kettelhut (1992)
Lower educational level	Cats-Baril and Frymoyer (1987), Dionne et al (1995)

Occupational Factors

Lower wage level	Deyo and Tsio-Wu (1987)
Shorter time on the job	Astrand (1987), Kelsey and Golden (1988)
More than 2 weeks off work, injured	Lehmann et al (1993)
Availability of light work; being fired or terminated; physically difficult work	Lancourt and Kettelhut (1992)
Workers' compensation	Hadler et al (1995)

Pain Profile

Previous back pain	Coste et al (1994), Burton et al (1995)
Gradual rather than sudden onset	Roland and Morris (1983)
Higher self-reported pain/disability	Biering-Sorensen (1983), Mooney et al (1976), Gallon (1989), Murphy and Cornish (1984)
Sciatica	van den Hoogen et al (1997)
Graphically illustrated pain drawing	Cairns et al (1984)

Psychosocial Factors

Child abuse	Schofferman et al (1992), McMahon et al (1997)
Relocation required by injury	Lancourt and Kettelhut (1992)
Poor coping skills	Martin et al (1996)
Financial difficulties	Lancourt and Kettelhut (1992)

[a] The presence of these factors in an acutely injured individual appear to be associated with delayed return to work and other poor outcomes.

Kettelhut (1992), on the other hand, did not find satisfaction with work to affect outcome.

Taking more than 2 weeks off work following injury reflects poorly on the probability of returning to work; conversely, remaining on the job is a favorable sign (Lehmann et al, 1993). Other **occupational factors** that suggest poor outcome include lack of light duty, being fired or terminated, physically difficult work (Lancourt and Kettelhut, 1992), jobs with high psychological stress, lower wage level, and lack of job autonomy. Gatchel et al (1995a) found the physical demands of the job not to make a difference for return to work but surveyed a population of workers whose injuries were less than 6 weeks old; Lancourt evaluated acute and chronic back pain patients who were receiving workers' compensation benefits.

Frequently controversial, the impact of workers' compensation payments on return to work has repeatedly been investigated with mixed results (Ambrosius et al, 1995; Gallagher 1995; Taylor et al, 1996; Mayer et al, 1998). Of interest, Hadler et al (1995) found that workers whose injuries were covered by workers' compensation took more

time from work overall but returned to work in the same time frame as individuals whose injuries were not covered. Even though return to work was not delayed, the covered workers reported a delay in the recovery of sense of wellness compared to the noncovered workers.

Specific aspects of the patient's **pain history** and attributes of the pain complaint also indicate risk of delayed recovery. Such factors include a history of previous back pain, a history of significant pain of any type, a gradual rather than sudden onset, sciatica, and abnormal or more graphically illustrated pain drawings. The most commonly reported aspect of pain that is associated with diminished outcome is higher self-reported pain intensity and related disability. A number of instruments are frequently used to measure self-reported pain and disability such as the Oswestry Low Back Pain Disability Questionnaire, the Roland-Morris Low Back Pain and Disability Questionnaire, and the Visual Analogue Scale. Recently, the Roland-Morris Questionnaire has been validated as an 18-item inventory, the RM-18 (Strathford and Brinkley, 1997).

A history of child abuse is correlated with unsuccessful lumbar spine surgery and with failure of conservative treatment approaches (McMahon et al, 1997). Other **psychosocial factors** include relocation required by injury, financial difficulties, and poor coping skills.

Tertiary Predictors

For individuals already afflicted by chronic back pain, **occupational factors** such as greater duration of employment prior to injury and job availability upon recovery improved the likelihood of return to work (Table 10–3). Milhous et al (1989) found shorter length of unemployment to correlate significantly with return to work, as did fewer weeks of compensation. Greater current activity levels predict a better 6-month return to work in unemployed individuals with chronic low back pain.

Chronicity of pain appears to be predictive of further chronicity. In a study of patients with acute and chronic low back pain, van den Hoogen et al (1997) found that the duration of back pain prior to an initial visit with an HCP indicated a longer time to recovery (also noted by Roland and Morris, 1983). For every week of pain prior to the initial visit, there was a 2% lower likelihood of recovery in the following week (van den Hoogen et al, 1997).

Not surprisingly, self-reported pain intensity and disability also predict poorer responses to treatment in those already afflicted with chronic pain. Waddell (1984) has reported that allodynia, or perception of pain with a non-painful stimulus, reliably indicates poorer outcome. Lack of leg pain in unemployed individuals with chronic low back pain predicts a greater likelihood of return to work (Milhous et al, 1989). A history of spinal surgery also reduces the likelihood of a favorable outcome.

In the chronic pain population, psychosocial factors play a strong role. Personality disorder bodes poorly. Depression as indicated by the Beck Depression Inventory and premorbid pessimism scale of the Millon Behavior Health Index are associated with unfavorable outcome. Milhous et al (1989) noted that lower scores for the MMPI scales of hypochondriasis and hysteria indicated a greater likelihood of return to work at 6 months following injury, as did better scores in a semistructured psychiatric interview looking at psychosocial discomfort, adequacy of coping mechanisms, global psychiatric disability, treatability of psychiatric disorder, and patients' motivation for vocational rehabilitation. Posttraumatic stress disorder may be more prevalent in those with refractory pain that derives from an accident (Geisser et al, 1996).

PREDICTORS FOUND IN THE CLINICAL EXAMINATION

In general there is less convincing evidence that physical measures, diagnostic studies as well as examination findings, are predictive for outcome than the clinical interview.

Table 10–3: Tertiary Predictors of Poor Outcome[a]

Occupational Factors	
Shorter duration of employment prior to injury	Polatin et al (1989)
Job availability upon recovery	Polatin et al (1989)
Shorter duration off work injured; fewer weeks of compensation	Milhous et al (1989)
Pain Profile	
Greater duration of back pain prior to treatment	van den Hoogan et al (1997), Roland and Morris (1983)
History of spinal surgery	Polatin et al (1989), Lancourt and Kettelhut (1992)
Diminished and current activity levels	Milhous et al (1989)
Higher self-reported pain and disability	Polatin et al (1989)
Allodynia	Waddell (1984)
Leg pain	Milhous et al (1989)
Psychosocial Factors	
Personality disorder	Gatchel et al (1995a), Polatin et al (1993)
Depression	Polatin et al (1989)
Post-traumatic stress disorder	Geisser et al (1996)
Psychological discomfort, adequacy of coping, psychiatric disability, treatability	Milhous et al (1989)

[a] When an individual already has chronic back pain the presence of these factors indicates poorer likelihood of responding to treatment.

Of the relatively few studies that included examination findings such as strength, range of motion, posture, reflexes, and sensation, there has been little common agreement as to the findings that were reliable.

Diagnostic studies, including magnetic resonance imaging (MRI), electromyogram (EMG), myelogram, and computed tomography (CT) do not have primary or secondary predictive value for return to work (Lancourt and Kettelhut, 1992; Mayer et al, 1987). Quite likely, there is no tertiary predictive value as well.

Primary Predictors

Recent evidence indicates that at least one aspect of physical performance is predictive of new onset low back pain. Specifically, Luoto et al (1995) found in a population of 126 pain free individuals that endurance for performing static back extension or Sorenson's test (Biering-Sorenson, 1984) strongly correlated with those who would experience their first episode of back pain within the following year. Less than 58 seconds' endurance indicated a 3.4 times greater likelihood of developing low back pain (odds ratio 3.4, confidence interval 1.2–10.0). Refer to Chapter 16 for more information regarding physical performance testing.

Secondary Predictors

Lancourt and Kettelhut (1992) found certain "nonorganic" signs to be predictive for persisting low back pain and disability, including some of the Waddell signs (pain with axial loading, pain with simulated rotation, and inconsistency between supine and sitting straight leg raising), positive response to sham sciatic tension testing (straight leg raise with the foot plantarflexed), pain with simultaneous hip/knee flexion and hip rotation, pain with the Burns test (kneeling, curled in a ball), nonanatomical sensory changes to pinprick, and verbal magnification of symptoms. "Organic/nonorganic" signs that predicted less likelihood of returning to work included slow or limping gait, difficulty with heel walking and with toe walking, abnormal thoracolumbar flexion, slow flexion, reduced extension, decreased lateral bending, tenderness to deep palpation, and performing straight leg raising less than 100 degrees. The only truly organic sign that predicted poorer outcome was muscle atrophy with greater than or equal to $1/4$ inch loss. Reduced trunk strength and endurance have also been noted in those who progress to chronic pain and disability (Alaranta et al, 1994; Beiring-Sorensen, 1984; Luoto, 1995).

Tertiary Predictors

Limitations in true thoracolumbar flexion and hip flexion have been noted to predict persistence of pain and disability for chronic back pain sufferers (Polatin et al, 1989). Milhous et al (1989) failed to find that spinal range of motion, isometric trunk strength, or lifting ability predicted return to work in a population of chronic back pain patients who were unemployed at the time of their study.

GROUPED FACTORS

As the foregoing discussion demonstrates, a wide variety of factors potentially contribute to or are associated with poor outcome. There is only modest agreement across studies, which indicates that no single variable is likely to be useful in all patients or in all situations. By assaying patients across multiple variables, sensitivity and specificity of prediction can be improved. For example, as noted earlier, the presence of depression in a patient, although important, is not an absolute marker of poor response to treatment. On the other hand, an individual over the age of 50 who reports not only depression, but also previous back surgery, longstanding pain complaints, high pain levels, and no availability of modified work, is not likely to do well. The following discussion outlines several studies that have attempted to delineate the most accurate groupings of predictive factors. The HCP is strongly encouraged to compare the populations under study for similarity and, presumably, applicability of findings to his or her own patient population. Only two of these studies have used their results to generate an efficient clinical tool; these instruments are described at the end of this section.

UTILITY OF GROUPING PREDICTIVE FACTORS

Although not the first to make use of multivariate statistics for grouping predictive factors, Burton and Tillotson (1991) specifically examined the accuracy or utility of doing so. In 109 sequential patients with low back and/or leg pain, a wide variety of clinical, occupational, and demographic factors were evaluated but few psychosocial variables. Treatment was at the discretion of the HCPs and included medication, manipulation, injections, advice, exercise, and in four patients, surgery. Two outcomes were assessed—symptom free or not symptom free, and improving or not improving—at 1 month, 3 months, and 1 year. Interestingly, the use of a multivariate statistical approach was felt to be vindicated. That is, groups performed better than any single variable, but for each of the six outcome categories, different groupings of predictors were found to be the most significant. Greatest accuracy was found for predicting two of the outcome categories: those who were improving and those who would not be symptom free at any time point. **The two most common variables included in all but one of the six groupings were length of the current episode of back pain and presence of a trunk list.**

IMPORTANCE OF PSYCHOLOGICAL FACTORS

By following a cross-section of 252 back pain patients in an osteopathic general practice for a year, Burton et al (1995) demonstrated that whether an individual patient recovered or not at 1 year **could be predicted with at least**

VERMONT DISABILITY PREDICTION QUESTIONNAIRE

Utilizing 28 questions from a 1987 predictive model developed by Frymoyer and Cats-Baril, plus 5 more devised through a modified delphi process, Hazard et al (1996) studied 166 people within 15 days of a work-related back injury. Through kappa analysis and logistic regression, 11 of the questions were found in combination to be significantly associated with return to work by the third month following injury. Based on their regression coefficients, differential weighting was applied to the questions. For example, for the question asking how many times a medical doctor had been visited in the past for back problems, a score of 0 was assigned to the responses "never" and "1 to 5 times," but a score of 4 was assigned to the distractors "6 to 10 times," "11 to 20 times," and "more than 20 times." For other questions such as "How many times have you been married?" only the scores of 0 or 1 were assigned. The authors provide a scoring system and list a variety of cutoff scores yielding different specificity and sensitivity results that can then be used for different purposes (see Appendix Form H–9). Although 4 of the questions emphasize past back problems, the remainder touch on occupational, psychosocial factors and the individual's perceptions of pain and disability. Unfortunately, the final form of the questionnaire may reflect a selection bias in that 699 subjects were eligible but only 166 returned questionnaires in the allotted time. A prospective follow-up study (Hazard et al, 1997) found diminished specificity and sensitivity with this instrument but still demonstrated reasonable utility in a population of acute back injuries.

DISABILITY PREDICTION REGARDING NONSPINAL DISORDERS

Although this chapter has been devoted to back pain, researchers have also looked at the factors that bear on chronicity of whiplash injuries and cumulative trauma disorder. In a review of 47 articles discussing whiplash injury, Bannister and Gargan (1993) concluded that several factors were unfavorable prognostically, including duration and severity of symptoms, age greater than 50 at the time of injury, upper extremity pain, and the presence of thoracic or low back pain. Investigations into cumulative trauma disorder have found predictors similar to back pain, including "psychosocial classification" (Bonzani et al, 1997); perceived stress (Hess 1997); age, gender, lack of social support, and low decision latitude (Buckle, 1997); and higher pain levels, greater psychological reactivity to pain, anger toward employers, less time on the job, and greater frequency of previous acute injury (Himmelstein et al, 1995). Quite possibly, factors important for predicting chronic disability will be very similar across all musculoskeletal injuries.

Conclusion

The science of predicting disability is evolving. Because the determinants of response to treatment of back pain are multiple, current research efforts are aimed at developing efficient prediction tools through the use of statistical models. Generally, self-reported pain and disability ratings, and demographic, psychosocial, and occupational factors have been found to be among the most important variables; seemingly of less importance are physical examination findings; and of no demonstrable importance are the results of imaging studies. Different specific factors and different groups of factors may, however, be important at different times in the evolution of an individual's pain and disability (Burton and Tillotson, 1991; Burton et al, 1995; Gatchel et al, 1995b). Being aware of the many potential determinants of outcome should be helpful to HCPs in identifying patients at risk for poor outcome. Additionally, the two clinical instruments discussed previously can be useful in the average clinical practice, although they have shortcomings and may be applicable only to specific back pain populations.

No matter how the HCP screens for those individuals destined to respond poorly to treatment, the purpose for doing so is worthwhile only to the extent that appropriate intervention can make a difference. Because the determinants of poor outcome appear to be multifactorial, a successful treatment approach would logically attempt to address all related factors; hence, a multidisciplinary approach would seem best.

REFERENCES

Alaranta H, Hurri H, Heliovaara M, Soukka A, Harju R. Non-dynamometric trunk performance tests: Reliability and normative data. *Scan J Rehab Med.* 1994;26:211–215.

Ambrosius FM, Kremer AM, Herkner PB, DeKraker M, Hartz S. Outcome comparison of workers' compensation and noncompensation low back pain in a highly structured functional restoration program. *J Orthop Sports Phys Ther.* 1995;21:7–12.

Astrand N. Medical, psychological and social factors associated with back abnormalities and self-reported back pain. *Br J Med.* 1987;44:327–336.

Bannister G, Gargan M. Prognosis of whiplash injuries: A review of the literature. In: White LA. *Cervical Flexion-Extension/Whiplash Injuries. Spine: State of the Art Reviews.* Philadelphia, Pa: Hanley & Belfus; 1993:7:557–569.

Biering-Sorensen F. A prospective study of LBP in a general population, II: Location, character, aggravating and relieving factors. *Scand J Rehab Med.* 1983;15:15–81.

Biering-Sorensen F. Physical measurements as risk indicators for low-back trouble over a one-year period. *Spine.* 1984;9:106–119.

Bigos S, Battie MC, Spengler DM, et al. A prospective study of work perceptions and psychosocial factors affecting the report of back injury. *Spine.* 1991;16:1–6.

Bigos S, Spengler D, Martin N, et al. Back injuries in industry: A retrospective study. II injury factors and III employee factors. *Spine.* 1986;11:252–256.

Bonzani PJ, Millender L, Keelan B, Mangieri MG. Factors prolonging disability in work-related cumulative trauma disorders. *J Hand Surg [Am].* 1997;22:30–4.

Buckle P. Upper limb disorders and work: the importance of physical and psychosocial factors. *J Psychosom Res.* 1997;43:17–25.

Burton AK, Tillotson KM. Prediction of the clinical course of low back trouble using multivariable models. *Spine.* 1991;16:7–14.

Burton AK, Tillotson KM, Main CJ, Hollis S. Psychosocial predictors of outcome in acute and subchronic low back trouble. *Spine.* 1995;20:722–728.

Cairns D, Mooney V, Crane P. Spinal pain rehabilitation: Inpatient and outpatient treatment results and development of predictors of outcome. *Spine.* 1984;9:91–94.

Cats-Baril WL, Frymoyer JW. Identifying patients at risk of becoming disabled because of low-back pain: The Vermont Rehabilitation Engineering Center predictive model. *Spine.* 1991;16:605–607.

Cherkin DC, Deyo RA, Street JH, Barlow W. Predicting poor outcomes for back pain seen in primary care using patients' own criteria. *Spine.* 1996;24:2900–2907.

Coste J, Delecoeuillerie G, Cohen de Lara A, Le Pare JM, Paolaggi JB. Clinical course and prognostic factors in acute low back pain: An inception cohort study in primary care practice. *BMJ.* 1994;308:577–80.

Deyo R. Practice variations, treatment fads, rising disability: Do we need a new clinical research paradigm? *Spine.* 1993;18:2153–62.

Deyo RA, Diehl AK. Psychosocial predictors of disability in patients with low back pain. *J Rheumatol.* 1988;15:1557–1564.

Deyo R, Tsio-Wu W. Functional disability due to back pain: A population based study indicating the importance of socioeconomic factors. *Arthr Rheumatol.* 1987;30:1247–1253.

Dionne C, Koepsell TD, Von Korff M, Deyo RA, Barlow WE, Checkoway H. Formal education and back-related disability: In search of an explanation. *Spine.* 1995;20:2721–2730.

Frymoyer JW, Cats-Baril W. Predictors of low back disability. *Clin Orthop.* 1987;221:89–98.

Gallagher RM, Williams RA, Skelly J, Haugh LD, Milhous R, Frymoyer J. Workers' compensation and return-to-work in low back pain. *Pain.* 1995;61:299–307.

Gallon R. Perception of disability in chronic back pain patients: A long-term follow-up. *Pain.* 1989;37:67–75.

Gatchel R, Polatin R, Kinney R. Predicting outcome of chronic back pain using clinical predictors of psychopathology: a prospective analysis. *Health Psychology.* 1995a;14:415–420.

Gatchel RJ, Polatin PB, Mayer TG. The dominant role of psychosocial risk factors in the development of chronic low back pain disability. *Spine.* 1995b;20:2702–2709.

Geisser ME, Roth RS, Bachman JE, Eckert TA. The relationship between symptoms of post-traumatic stress disorder and pain, affective disturbance and disability among patients with accident and non-accident related pain. *Pain.* 1996;66:207–214.

Hadler NM, Carey TS, Garreet J. The influence of indemnification by workers' compensation insurance on recovery from acute backache. *Spine*. 1995;20:2710–2715.

Hansen FR, Biering-Sorensen F, Schroll M. Minnesota Multiphasic Personality Inventory profiles in persons with or without low-back pain: A 20 year follow-up study. *Spine*. 1995;20:2716–20.

Hasenbring M, Marienfeld G, Kuhlendahl D, Soyka D. Risk factors of chronicity in lumbar disc patients. *Spine*. 1994;19:2759–2765.

Hazard RG, Gaugh LD, Reid S, Preble JB, MacDonald L. Early prediction of chronic disability after occupational low back injury. *Spine*. 1996;21:945–951.

Hazard RG, Haugh LD, Reid S, McFarlane G, MacDonald L. Early physician notification of patient disability risk and clinical guidelines after low back injury: A randomized, controlled trial. *Spine*. 1997;12(24):2951–2958.

Hess D. Employee perceived stress. Relationship to the development of repetitive strain injury symptoms. *AAOHN J*. 1997;45:115–123.

Himmelstein JS, Feuerstein M, Stanek EJ, et al. Work-related upper-extremity disorders and work disability: clinical and psychosocial presentation. *J Occup Environ Med*. 1995;37:1278–1286.

Junge A, Frohlich M, Ahrens S, et al. Predictors of bad and good outcome of lumbar spine surgery. *Spine*. 1996;21:1056–1065.

Kelsey J, Golden A. Occupational and workplace factors associated with low back pain. *J Occup Med*. 1988;3:7–15.

Klenerman L, Slade PD, Stanley M, et al. The prediction of chronicity in patients with an acute attack of low back pain in a general practice setting. *Spine*. 1995;20:478–484.

LaCroix J, Powell J, Lloyd G, Doxey N, Mitson G, Aldam C. Low back pain: factors of value in predicting outcome. *Spine*. 1990;15:495–499.

Lancourt J, Kettelhut M. Predicting return to work for lower back pain patients receiving worker's compensation. *Spine*. 1992;17:629–640.

Lee P, Chow S, Lieh-Mak F, Chan K, Wong S. Psychosocial factors influencing outcome in patients with low back pain. *Spine*. 1989;14:838–842.

Lehmann TR, Spratt KF, Lehmann KK. Predicting long-term disability in low back injured workers presenting to a spine consultant. *Spine*. 1993;18:1103–1112.

Luoto S, Heliovaara M, Hurri H, Alaranta H. Static back endurance and the risk of low-back pain. *Clin Biomech*. 1995;10:323–324.

Magora A. Investigation of the relationship between low back pain and occupation. *Scand J Rehabil Med*. 1985;17:1–4.

Main CJ. The Modified Somatic Perception Questionnaire (MSPQ). *J Psychosom Res*. 1983;27:503–514.

Main CJ, Waddell G. A comparison of cognitive measures in low back pain: Statistical structure and clinical validity at initial assessment. *Pain*. 1991;46:287–298.

Martin MY, Bradley LA, Alexander RW, et al. Coping strategies predict disability in patients with primary fibromyalgia. *Pain*. 1996;68:45–53.

Mayer TG, Gatchel RJ, Mayer H, Kishino ND, Keeley J, Mooney V. A prospective two year study of functional restoration in industrial low back injury. *JAMA*. 1987;258:1763–1767.

Mayer T, McMahon MJ, Gatchel RJ, Sparks B, Wright A, Pegues P. Socioeconomic outcomes of combined spine surgery and functional restoration in workers' compensation spinal disorders with matched controls. *Spine*. 1998;23:598–605.

McMahon, MJ, Gatchel RJ, Polatin PB, Mayer TG. Early childhood abuse in chronic spinal disorder patients: A major barrier to treatment success. *Spine*. 1997;22:2408–2415.

Milhous RL, Haugh LD, Frymoyer JW, et al. Determinants of vocational disability in patients with low back pain. *Arch Phys Med Rehabil*. 1989;70:589–593.

Mooney V, Cairns D, Robertson J. A system for evaluating and treating chronic back disability. *Western J Med*. 1976;124:370–376.

Murphy KA, Cornish RD. Prediction of chronicity in acute low back pain. *Arch Phys Med Rehabil*. 1984;65:334–337.

Niemcryck SJ, Jenkins CD, Rose RM, Hurst MW. The prospective impact of psychosocial variables on rates of illness and injury in professional employees. *J Occup Med*. 1987;29:645–652.

Oland G, Tveiten G. A trial of modern rehabilitation for chronic low-back pain and disability: vocational outcome and effect of pain modulation. *Spine*. 1991;16:457–459.

Pederson PA. Prognostic indicators in low back pain. *J R Coll Gen Practitioners*. 1983;31:209–216.

Polatin PB, Gatchel RJ, Barnes D, Mayer H, Ahrens C, Mayer TG. A psychosociomedical prediction model of response to treatment by chronically disabled workers with low back pain. *Spine*. 1989;14:956–961.

Polatin PB, Gatchel RJ, Cox B, Mayer T. Waddell signs in chronic low back patients: When they may not be predictive. North American Spine Society homepage; Oct 1996.

Polatin P, Kinney RK, Gatchel RJ, Lillo E, Mayer TG. Psychiatric illness and chronic low back pain: The mind and the spine: Which goes first? *Spine*. 1993;18:66–71.

Roland M, Morris R. A study of the natural history of low-back pain. Part II: Development of guidelines for trials of treatment in primary care. *Spine*. 1983;8:145–150.

Sanders SH. Risk factors for the occurrence of low back pain and chronic disability. *Am Pain Soc Bull*. 1995;5:1–6.

Schofferman J, Anderson D, Hines R, Smith G, White A. Childhood psychological trauma correlates with unsuccessful lumbar spine surgery. *Spine*. 1992;17:5138–5144.

Shvartzman L, Weingarten E, Sherry H, Levin S, Persaud A. Cost effectiveness analysis of extended conservative therapy versus surgical intervention in the management of herniated intervertebral disc. *Spine*. 1992;17:176–182.

Slade PD, Troup JDG, Lethem J. The fear-avoidance model of exaggerated pain perception—2. Preliminary studies of coping strategies for pain. *Behav Res Ther*. 1983;21:409–416.

Sobel J, Rainville J, Hartigan C. Does abnormal illness behavior affect the outcome from functionally oriented rehabilitation in chronic low back pain? North American Spine Society homepage; Oct 1996.

Spengler D, Bigos S, Martin N, et al. Back injuries in industry: I. A retrospective study. *Spine*. 1986;11:241–245.

Strathford PW, Binkley JM. Measurement properties of the RM-18: A modified version of the Roland-Morris Disability Scale. *Spine*. 1997;22:2416–21.

Symonds TL, Burton AK, Tillotson KM, Main CJ. Absence resulting from low back trouble can be reduced by psychosocial intervention at the work place. *Spine*. 1995;20:2738–2745.

Symonds TL, Burton AK, Tillotson KM, Main CJ. Do attitudes and beliefs influence work loss due to low back trouble? *Occup Med*. 1996;46:25–32.

Taylor VM, Deyo RA, Ciol M, Kreuter W. Surgical treatment of patients with back problems covered by workers' compensation versus those with other sources of payment. *Spine*. 1996;21:2255–2259.

Tyre TE, Walworth DE, Tyre EM. The outcome status of chronic pain patients 4 years after multidisciplinary care. *Wisconsin Med J*. 1994;Jan:9–12.

van den Hoogen HJM, Koes BW, Deville W, van Eijk JTM, Bouter LM. The prognosis of low back pain in general practice. *Spine*. 1997;22:1515–1521.

Waddell G, Main CJ. Assessment of severity in low-back disorders. *Spine*. 1984;9:204–208.

Werneke MW, Harris DE, Lichter RL. Clinical effectiveness of behavioral signs for screening chronic low-back pain patients in a work-oriented physical rehabilitation program. *Spine*. 1993;18:2142–2418.

Westin C, Hirsch C, Lindegard B. The personality of the back patient. *Clin Orthop*. 1972;87:209–216.

SECTION

III

Objective Outcome Assessment Tools

As the term "objective" implies, this section describes "health care provider (HCP)–driven" tests that, when utilized, can help support the "medical necessity" of a treatment approach. The prescriptive power of these tests also provides information that the HCP can utilize when forming patient treatment plans, which is particularly useful in a rehabilitation setting. The first chapter in this section (Chap. 11) addresses low-tech assessment approaches and compares these to various available high-tech methods. Strength and endurance testing of the trunk, which has long been recognized as a vital part of the assessment process of the rehabilitation patient, is the topic of Chapter 12. Chapter 13 reviews the spinal orthopedic and neurological evaluation methodologies that have been published, while Chapter 14 addresses the range of spinal motion. Orthopedic and range of motion testing procedures of the extremities are addressed in Chapter 15. Chapter 16 introduces the Quantitatitve Functional Capacity Evaluation (QFCE), which is a method of assessing patients before and after rehabilitation through the use of physical performance tests. The results from these tests have proven to be an excellent foundation for proving "medical necessity" when requesting rehabilitation preapproval from third-party payers. Determining a patient's work or functional capacities prior to returning the patient to the workplace may be, in many cases, the single most important determining factor for a successful outcome. The specific skills required to perform a Work Capacity Evaluation (WCE) when returning the patient to the workplace are the topic of Chapter 17. Chapter 18 completes this section on objective functional testing by discussing various low-tech methods for assessing cardiovascular and aerobic function. The many guest authors included offer a unique perspective of several of the topics presented in this section.

CHAPTER 11

Rehabilitation: High versus Low Technology

DAVID STUDE & GUNNAR ANDERSSON

▶ INTRODUCTION   ▶ NEUROMOTOR SKILL ACQUISITION

▶ HIGH-TECH EMPHASIS   ▶ DESIGN CONSIDERATIONS

▶ SPINAL BIOMECHANICS   ▶ CONCLUSION

INTRODUCTION

Interest in developing objective instrumentation for evaluating human performance, and in particular, for spinal functional performance, has been gaining critical attention since the mid-1980s. Back pain, for some time, has been recognized as an epidemic in American society (Frymoyer et al, 1989), and statistics indicate the majority of the population will have at least one disabling episode of back pain in their lifetime (Frymoyer et al, 1980; Svensson and Andersson, 1982; Biering-Sorenson, 1983; Valdenburg and Haanen, 1983; Cassidy and Wedge, 1988). In addition, although many of these episodes seem to resolve symptomatically following a previously described natural history, approximately 20% tend to become chronic and/or recurrent (Horal, 1969; Rowe, 1969; Benn and Wood, 1975; Berquiest-Ullman and Larsson, 1977). It is this group of chronic low back pain sufferers that account for the significant costs associated with evaluating and treating back pain (Pheasant, 1977; Snook, 1982; Frymoyer et al, 1983; Andersson et al, 1984; Frymoyer et al, 1985; Morris, 1985; Spengler et al, 1986). Because of this, **renewed interest in more accurately evaluating spinal function and improving methods for predicting and preventing chronicity has become an important focus for health care providers (HCPs) and researchers alike** (Klenerman et al, 1995; Cherkin et al, 1996; Hazard et al, 1996; Kendall et al, 1997; Bendix et al, 1998; and others).

The purpose of this chapter is to address practical differences between machine and nonmachine testing and training. The reason why it is important to address this area is that:

- Some investigators suggest that poor strength may be a risk factor for those who are required to perform labor-intensive tasks.
- Strength training of some sort is typically included as part of an integrated approach to treating spinal dysfunction.
- One of the best approaches to preventing back injuries is teaching workers to perform their job properly. This implies that rehabilitation programs should emphasize functional maneuvers that reflect activities of daily living (ADLs) so that there is significant overlap between the types of exercises they perform in a rehabilitation setting and those they will be expected to perform on the job or in their home.

HIGH-TECH EMPHASIS

Many specialized, high-technology evaluation protocols have been developed that appear to offer reliable information to facilitate the HCP in evaluating and making case management recommendations. With this technology, there is a current tendency to assume that there are increased benefits associated with exercise performed on machines. Computer-assisted machines seem to be thought of as more technologically advanced and so more beneficial in terms of physical outcome measures. This assumption has not yet been supported in the literature, and, on the contrary, the reverse may actually be true. **Also, the computer-aided instrumentation that is available commercially does not measure similar parameters or real-to-life movements. This commercial computer-aided instrumentation also varies with regard to subject testing position(s) and cost** (Table 11–1).

SPINAL BIOMECHANICS

To properly enhance spinal biomechanical function, whether it be through the use of active exercise, stretching, or manipulative therapy, it is necessary first of all to know how the spine functions when in an optimal state. One frame of reference that is gaining acceptance is use of the right-handed Cartesian orthogonal coordinate system (Smith and Fernie, 1987). Research evaluating spinal motion demonstrates that movement is not uniplanar (Koreska et al, 1977; Panjabi, 1982; McGill and Norman, 1985). In other words, **motion of the spine occurs in complex, coupled patterns, and these patterns differ from region to region.** Also, there is evidence to suggest that there are characteristic centers of rotation that can be used to

describe segmental motion (Gertzbein, 1984; Woltring, 1985).

The use of **machine-based exercise** (MBE) for the back would appear to restrict the ability of the spine to move about three-dimensionally. This premise is important from a practical point of view for many reasons. First, people who perform work-related tasks do so without the use of restrictive devices that are characteristic of machines. Because of this, it would then seem logical to train the person in movements that actually reflect the work they characteristically perform. This approach is applicable for the labor-intensive worker, the athlete as well as the homemaker. Since comparison studies between MBE and non-MBE have not been properly addressed through controlled clinical trials, the increased expense associated with high-technology exercise devices currently appears unsubstantiated.

Another important concept is that **the body works as a whole integrated unit rather than as independent regional entities** (Nemeth et al, 1984; Reynolds, 1984; Thorstensson et al, 1985; Nouwen et al, 1987; Paquet et al, 1994). MBE is usually associated with some degree of isolation of a part, usually exercising one primary muscle group at a time. Based on objective descriptions of whole body movements, the MBE approach seems to potentially prevent the development of three-dimensional, neuromotor skills necessary for the normal and safe accomplishment of daily tasks.

In defense of MBE, it may be necessary initially to train some individuals in a more isolated fashion, especially if the injury they sustained was severe and if whole body movements are contraindicated. This then could be used in this example as an initial training recommendation, with more complex tasks being introduced as tolerated. Also, MBE may be appropriate if it is only a portion of the entire exercise program, in order to target specific outcomes based on identified deficiencies.

Table 11–1: Comparison of Different Types and Manufacturers of Machine-based Exercise (MBE) Units

INSTRUMENT	PTM[a]	PTP[b]	PLANES TESTED[c]	COST[d]
Biodex	K	SE	S	45
Cybex	K	SE	SCT-3	160
Dynatronics-2000	M	ST or SE	ISOM	20
ISO-B-200	I	ST or SE	SCT-1	80
Isotechnologies Lift-Task	I	ST	DYNA	70
Loredan Lido-Back	K	SE	S	60
Med-X	M	SE	EXT	65
Promotron-3000	M	ST	ISOM + S	25

[a] *PTM (Principal Testing Mode):* I, isoinertial; K, isokinetic; M, isometric.
[b] *PTP (Patient Testing Position):* SE, seated; ST, standing.
[c] *Planes Tested:* SCT-1—One machine tests functional parameters simultaneously in the sagittal, coronal, and transverse planes. SCT-3—A separate machine is available for testing trunk performance parameters in each of the primary planes of motion. S—Sagittal plane. EXT—Extension plane. ISOM—Isometric whole body lift-task measurements based on NIOSH guidelines. DYNA—Multiple plane whole body lift-task measurements.
[d] Approximate cost is expressed in U.S. dollars × 1000 per machine.

Dangers in Use of MBEs

The fixed cam or fulcrum of most MBEs may actually prohibit complex joint motions, which may result in asymmetrical joint stresses such as excessive shear. This, in turn, could promote long-term joint dysfunction and may lead to instability.

MBE cannot provide or promote the kind of multiple joint motions that are typically associated with three-dimensional, nonrestrained activities. Furthermore, because most machines have a fixed cam or fulcrum, they may actually retard these complex joint motions.

NEUROMOTOR SKILL ACQUISITION

The sequence of events that occurs when an Olympic weight lifter performs a clean and jerk, although of short duration, is very complex. Similarly, when an individual is lifting boxes all day long, proper body mechanics are essential to reduce the likelihood of injury and muscular fatigue. Even though strength is considered essential to include in a rehabilitation program for spinal dysfunction, **strength deficiencies do not have predictive value in determining the likelihood of back injuries.** Strength gains are also relatively easy to achieve in an appropriate setting but strength alone does not ensure that one person will be less prone to injury than another indivdual who does not undergo specific strength training. The ability to use strength gains in an appropriate fashion may be more important than strength itself. This ability to activate appropriate musculature in order to more safely control whole body movements and activities can be termed **neuromotor skill (NMS).**

The body's ability to function in an integrated fashion relies, in part, on the communication between the musculoskeletal system and proprioceptive system. This system provides feedback about joint position, location, movement position and velocity, temperature alterations, and pain.

When initially learning a relatively complex skill, a person must remember and process many aspects cognitively, rather than being able to rely on learned reflex skills. Once an individual practices a skill repetitively, movement and position pattern habits begin to replace the need for conscious control of all activities.

MBE, at least theoretically, alters proprioceptive feedback compared to nonmachine training and, consequently, may reduce or eliminate the development of NMS that is necessary to safely perform complex tasks. Again, as mentioned earlier, the development of NMS may be a more important priority than strength for enhancing spinal functional performance. This possibility also suggests that there is an important mind–body connection required for performance of ADLs, and there is no evidence at this time to suggest that MBE enhances this relationship. On the contrary, there is evidence to suggest that MBE can prevent normal NMS development. Parkhurst and Burnett (1994) evaluated the relationship between low back injury and lumbo-pelvic proprioception in 88 working male firefighters. They found that there was a significant increase in the number of low back injuries where proprioceptive deficits were identified in spite of normal strength indices. Age was the factor that most strongly influenced proprioceptive status. Although more research is necessary in this area, it may be that age was an influential factor because there are fewer opportunities to maintain NMS with increasing chronological age, possibly due to reduced physical activity in general or to general deconditioning, or both.

Lander et al (1984) evaluated differences between performing a bench press maneuver with a free-weight barbell, compared to using an isokinetic dynamometer. Their conclusions, supported by others (Andrews et al, 1983; Hay et al, 1983), suggest that measured differences were due to the "the balancing and stabilizing efforts required in the free-weight condition, the muscle elastic property effects, and the differing baseline forces associated with the two activities" (Lander et al, 1984).

Lord and Castell (1994) evaluated the effects of a physical activity program for 44 people ranging in age from 50 to 75 years, and demonstrated that it was responsible for improving sensorimotor skills that contribute to stability. The program included non-MBE activities for 10 weeks' duration, and the control group, although not involved in the exercise component, were measured for the same physical outcomes. The exercise group was the only one to show improvements in balance, strength, reaction time, body sway on a firm surface with the eyes closed, and on a compliant surface with the eyes open and closed.

NMS development involves not only complex vertebral movement patterns, but also rotation about a joint or region. Although MBE can be useful for isolated strength development, it could be considered an incomplete training method because **machines are fixed, stable devices that do not allow these rotational movement patterns to occur through their full range of motion.** Compensatory lifting maneuvers could promote improper lifting habits when training on machines, and this could be potentially harmful since an exercise supervisor would be unable to see asymmetries clearly. Traditionally, machines do not exercise the right and left sides of an extremity or of the trunk independently. This makes it easier for an individual to twist and strain without asymmetrical deficiencies being apparent.

DESIGN CONSIDERATIONS

Because exercise machines are designed to fit the "average" person, it is impossible to accurately fit the force-position curves for movements throughout their full range of motion for most people using them. If machines were custom-made for each person in an exercise program, they might more closely approximate true force-position curves, but there is no current evidence to suggest this has been accomplished. Theoretically, an individual who is significantly larger or smaller than "average" may be at a significant disadvantage in terms of joint stress at certain ranges of motion.

Conceptual Advantages of Nonmachine-based Exercise

- Cost and maintenance are relatively low.
- It provides an opportunity for infinite exercise method variability.
- Asymmetrical training patterns can be recommended, if appropriate.
- Asymmetrical training patterns can be more easily detected by a supervisor, and corrected, if appropriate.
- Whole-person movement patterns can be incorporated with associated proprioceptive demands.
- It more closely parallels ADLs and so the potential carry-over effect is greater.
- Variations in movement velocity are greater.
- It offers increased opportunities to promote patient self-sufficiency, as this method can be more easily performed at home.
- Coupled, vertebral spinal movement patterns can occur in the absence of machine-based restraints.
- A lot of specialized, expensive equipment is not required; thus, it is more accessible to the general public at large.

Conceptual Disadvantages of Nonmachine-based Exercise

- Because it largely involves whole-person, three-dimensional movements, it presents a higher potential risk for injury. This emphasizes the need for professional supervision.
- If an individual presents with severe dysfunction, restrained and limited movements may be necessary during the early phases of a rehabilitation program.
- Automatic adjustment to maintain constant velocity, thereby reducing the potential for injury, is difficult, if not impossible (ie, isokinetic training mode).
- Uniform resistance throughout the full range of motion is more difficult to achieve, and so addressing the "weak link" may be more challenging.
- Small, subtle, but very critical alterations in the performance of an exercise maneuver could produce latent pain symptoms and, subsequently, further damage and delay in achieving a positive outcome. This may be less likely in a restrained and, therefore, more controlled environment.

Conceptual Disadvantages of Machine-based Exercise

- Most exercise machines are built to accommodate the "average" body type. This implies that at least one third of the individuals who use them do not fit them properly.
- Most machines are fixed instruments that restrain a person's activity, and therefore, restrict the multi-planar movements that are associated with ADLs.
- Since individual machines are required that each promote limited movement potential, many machines are necessary to address all major muscle groups adequately. Therefore, the costs associated with purchase and maintenance are considerable, relative to non-MBE.
- Most machines have weight increments from 2.5 to 10.0 pounds, and this may be too much of an increase for some people.
- Most machines do not allow individuals to train opposite sides independently. Therefore, training may be incomplete. Also, an individual could recruit more effort from the "good" side and an imbalance could be created. A supervisor would also have more difficulty detecting asymmetrical differences.
- Very few machines are easily accessible to the general public that adequately address the trunk musculature.
- Most machines require that individuals exercise in a recumbent or seated posture, and most ADLs are performed while standing.
- There is significantly less training variability available with a program that is dedicated only to a MBE environment.
- MBE is more restricted and, therefore, controlled and so the potential benefits associated with intensive exercise are proportionately reduced (ie, it may be safer since the potential risk for injury with MBE is relatively less).

Conceptual Advantages of Machine-based Exercise

- Machines are large and heavy so security is not a problem.
- It does restrain movement activity and so may be beneficial for patients with severe spinal dysfunction and in need of restricted activity during the early phases of their program.
- Since it promotes restrained activities, it is potentially safer in that it eliminates movements that could produce injury. However, there is the potential to promote subtle long-term damage by preventing normal complex joint movements, and thereby introducing aberrant joint stressors.
- Less supervision is typically required of machines.
- Using machines to assist an HCP in the evaluation process may prove to be a reliable way for gathering specific information regarding the presence or absence of physical deficiencies, providing an objective method for re-evaluation of these identified elements.

One study has been conducted (Timm, 1994) that evaluated the differences between passive and active treatment interventions in a chronic low back pain population. Comparisons were also made between two different forms of active exercise, specifically, the MBE and non-MBE approach.

The patients participating in this study (n = 250) were all employed for an automobile manufacturing plant and were working for at least 6 months prior to the initiation of the study. Each individual complained of chronic low back pain (68 females, 182 males), following an L5 laminectomy performed at least 1 year prior to the initiation of the study. Table 11–2 summarizes the characteristics of the subjects included in the study.

Subjects were divided into one of five experimental groups (Table 11–3) and the treatment sessions were scheduled for eight weeks at a frequency of three times per week. The relative costs associated with various treatment interventions are summarized in Table 11–4 (not including objective baseline and comparison measurements for the high-technology group).

The results of Timm's study suggest the following conclusions:

- Active approaches to managing chronic low back pain are more effective than passive interventions. However, the fact that passive modalities were not used in combination with other interventions may have influenced the results. Also, the choice for spinal manipulation techniques may also not have been the most effective choice for this form of mechanical dysfunction.

Table 11–2: Description of Subjects Included in the Study

Number	250
Age range	34–51 years
Males enrolled	182
Females enrolled	68
Surgical history	L5 laminectomy
	133 (53.2%) right-sided laminectomy
	117 (46.8%) left-sided laminectomy
Lower extremity pain	Yes (but not below the knee)
Passive SLR testing	Negative

Modified from Timm, 1994.

Table 11–3: Summary Description of Experimental Groups That Participated in the Study

GROUP	N OF SUBJECTS (TOTAL)	AGE RANGE
Physical agents	50	36–47
Joint manipulation	50	35–50
Low-tech exercise	50	37–51
High-tech exercise	50	34–49
Control	50	34–51
Overall	250	34–51

Modified from Timm, 1994.

- Although both the MBE and non-MBE approaches used in this study for managing chronic low back pain were statistically superior to passive interventions, the non-MBE approach provided the longest period of pain relief and was the most cost-effective.

Table 11–4: Summary of Treatment Interventions and Their Relative Cost

TREATMENT GROUP	RELATIVE COSTS[a]
Physical agents[b]	$1,842.00/subject
	$76.75/session
Joint manipulation[c]	$1,260.00/subject
	$52.50/session
Low-tech exercise[d]	$1,392.00/subject
	$58.00/session
High-tech exercise[e]	$1,716.00/subject
	$71.50/session

[a] Costs described do not include all of the evaluation protocols that were required of all subjects.
[b] Hydrocollation, ultrasound, transcutaneous electrical nerve stimulation.
[c] Manual therapy procedures (short amplitude, high-velocity mobilization).
[d] McKenzie-based spinal loading procedures and spinal stabilization exercises (supervised and nonsupervised).
[e] Supervised program of cardiovascular, isotonic, and isokinetic exercise.
Modified from Timm, 1994.

Conclusion

The first line of defense to protect a joint complex is the muscles that surround it. If this muscle system is functioning properly, assuming neurological communication is intact and normal, it should reflexly adjust to the variety of stressors that are being placed upon it. By doing so, it can potentially prevent or retard harmful load bearing patterns from promoting destructive joint changes. There is evidence to suggest that an individual's ability to properly compensate load-bearing stressors becomes increasingly difficult with increasing muscular fatigue (Donisch and Basmajian, 1972; Farfan, 1975; Bigland-Ritchie, 1984). Therefore, subsequent increases in aberrant spinal loading, especially if prolonged, could increase the likelihood of injury.

Training patients to protect themselves involves teaching them to perform movements that recruit muscles that they will be using for extended periods of time. They will need to learn to use muscles of the trunk and limbs in a coordinated, sequential, and synergistic manner, and may need to do so for relatively extended periods of time. This principle of dynamic stabilization training has not been shown to be possible with MBE.

The muscles associated with trunk performance function by acting as prime movers and stabilizers (Morris et al, 1961; Schultz et al, 1982; Nordin and Frankel, 1989), and, therefore, act as a first line of defenses for load-bearing stress to the spine (Ortengren and Anderson, 1977). This is only possible because the muscles of the trunk are being influenced constantly by nervous system afferent pathways that communicate information to them from the environment. This afferent information is processed and transmitted to efferent communication channels, which directly influences motor function. When training a patient with a spinal injury to safely perform ADLs, it is essential to expose this person to environmental information (positional stress, alterations in gravitational forces, variations in resistance, etc) that will promote neuromotor learning to retard nondestructive load-bearing patterns. MBE, if used alone and which provides some measure of restraint, may prevent the appropriate acquisition of these neuromotor skills.

A functional rehabilitation program cannot be completed without influencing the nervous system. The afferent pathways that come from environmental influences are responsible for prescribing the action of the muscles they innervate. If the body is used to perceiving outside environmental information appropriately, then there is the potential for successful adaptation to aberrant loading. Even though spinal muscle strength may be present, lack of neuromotor control of the performance of unstrained activities might be one potential cause for aberrant spinal loading stress and subsequent injury. Trunk muscle endurance may also play a pivotal role in spinal stabilization and, therefore, should be considered an important ingredient when recommending spinal rehabilitative exercise (De Luca, 1984; Kahanovitz et al, 1987; Nordin et al, 1987; Roy et al, 1989).

REFERENCES

Andersson GBJ, Pope MH, Frymoyer JW. Epidemiology. In: Pope MH, Frymoyer JW, Andersson G, eds. *Occupational Low Back Pain*. New York, NY: Praeger; 1984:101–114.

Andrews JG, Hay JG, Vaughn CL. Knee shear forces during a squat exercise using a barbell and a weight machine. In: Masui HJ, Kobayashi K, eds. *Biomechanics VIII-B*. Champaign, Ill: Human Kinetics Publishers; 1983:923–927.

Bendix AF, Bendix T, Haestrup C. Can it be predicted which patients with chronic low back pain should be offered tertiary rehabilitation in a functional restoration program? A search for demographic, socioeconomic, and physical preditors. *Spine*. 1998;23:1775–1784.

Benn RT, Wood PH. Pain in the back: An attempt to estimate the size of the problem. *Rheumatol Rehabil*. 1975;14:121–128.

Berquiest-Ullman M, Larsson U. Acute low back pain in industry. *Acta Orthop Scan*. 1977;170(Suppl):1–117.

Biering-Sorenson FA. Prospective study of low back pain in a general population. I. Occurrence, recurrence and aetiology. *Scand J Rehabil Med*. 1983;15:71–79.

Bigland-Ritchie B. Muscle fatigue and the influence of changing neural drive. Symposium on exercise: physiology and clinical application. *Clin Chest Med*. 1984;5:21.

Cassidy JD, Wedge JH. The epidemiology and natural history of low back pain and spinal degeneration. In: Kirkaldy-Willis WH, ed. *Managing Low Back Pain*. New York, NY: Churchill-Livingstone; 1988:3–15.

Cherkin DC, Deyo RA, Street JH, Barlow W. Predicting poor outcomes for back pain seen in primary care using patients' own criteria. *Spine*. 1996;21:2900–2907.

De Luca C. Myoelectrical manifestations of localized muscular fatigue in humans. *CRC Crit Rev Biomed Eng.* 1984;11:251–279.

Donisch EW, Basmajian JV. Electromyography of deep back muscles in man. *Am J Anat.* 1972;133:25.

Farfan HF. Muscular mechanism of the lumbar spine and the position of power efficiency. *Orthop Clin North Am.* 1975;6:135.

Frymoyer JW, Pope MH, Clemonts JH, et al. Risk factors in low back pain: An epidemiological study. *J Bone Joint Surg.* 1983;65A:213–218.

Frymoyer JW, Rosen JC, Clemonts J, et al. Psychologic factors in low back pain disability. *Clin Orthop.* 1985;195:178–184.

Gertzbein S. Determination of a locus of instantaneous centres of rotation of the lumbar disk by moire fringes. *Spine.* 1984;9:409.

Hay JG, Andrews JG, Vaughn CL, Ueya K. Load, speed, and equipment affects in strength-training exercises. In: Matsue HJ, Kobayashi K, eds. *Biomechanics VIII-B.* Champaign, Ill: Human Kinetics Publishers; 1983:939–950.

Hazard RG, Haugh LD, Reid S, Preble JB, MacDonald L. Early prediction of chronic disability after occupational low back injury. *Spine.* 1996;21:945–951.

Horal J. The clinical appearance of low back pain disorders in the city of Gotenburg, Sweden. *Acta Orthop Scand.* 1969;18(suppl):1–109.

Kahanovitz N, Nordin M, Verderame R, et al. Normal trunk strength and endurance in women and the effect of exercises and electrical stimulation: Part 2—comprehensive analysis of electrical stimulation and exercises to increase trunk strength and endurance. *Spine.* 1987;12:112–118.

Kendall NAS, Linton SJ, Main CJ. *Guide to Assessing Psychosocial Yellow Flags in Acute Low Back Pain: Risk Factors for Long-term Disability and Work Loss.* Wellington, New Zealand: Accident Rehabilitation & Compensation Insurance Corporation of New Zealand and the National Health Committee; 1997.

Klenerman L, Slade P, Stanley I, et al. The prediction of chronicity in patients with an acute attack of low back pain in a general practice setting. *Spine.* 1995;20:478–484.

Koreska J, Robertson D, Hills R, Gibson D, Albisser A. Biomechanics of the lumbar spine and its clinical significance. *Orthop Clin North Am.* 1977;8(1):121–133.

Lander J, Bates B, Sawhill J, Hamill J. *A Comparison Between Free-Weight and Isokinetic Bench Pressing.* Eugene, Ore: Biomechanics/Sports Medicine Laboratory, University of Oregon, 1984:344–352.

Lord S, Castell S. Physical activity program for older persons: Effect on balance, strength, neuromuscular control, and reaction time. *Arch Phys Med Rehabil.* 1994;75:648–652.

McGill S. Norman R. Dynamically and statically determined low back moments during lifting. *J Biomech.* 1985;18:877–885.

Morris A. Identifying workers at risk to back injury is not guesswork. *Occup Health Saf.* 1985;55:16–20.

Morris JM, Lucas DB, Bresler B. The role of the trunk in the stability of the spine. *J Bone Joint Surg.* 1961;43A:327.

Nemeth G, Ekholm J, Arborelius UP. Hip load moments and muscular activity during lifting. *Scand J Rehabil Med.* 1984;16:103–111.

Nordin M, Frankel VH. Biomechanics of tendons and ligaments. In: Frankel VH, Nordin M, eds. *Basic Biomechanics of the Skeletal System.* Philadelphia, Pa: Lea and Febiger; 1989:59–60.

Nordin M, Kahanovitz N, Verderame R, et al. Normal trunk strength and endurance in women and the effect of exercises and electrical stimulation: Part 1—normal endurance and trunk muscle strength in 101 women. *Spine.* 1987;12:105–111.

Nouwen A, Van Akkerveeken PF, Versloot JM. Patterns of muscular activity during movements in patients with chronic low back pain. *Spine.* 1987;12:777–782.

Ortengren R, Anderson GBJ. Electromyographic studies of trunk muscles with special reference to the functional anatomy of the spine. *Spine.* 1977;2:44.

Panjabi MM. Error in kinematic parameters of planar joint. *J Biomech.* 1982;15:537.

Paquet N, Malouin F, Richards C. Hip-spine movement interaction and muscle activation patterns during sagittal trunk movements in low back pain patients. *Spine.* 1994;19(5):596–603.

Parkhurst T, Burnett C. Injury and proprioception in the lower back. *JOSPT.* 1994;19(5):282–293.

Pheasant HC. The problem back. *Curr Pract Orthop Surg.* 1977;7:89–115.

Reynolds H. Stereoradiographic measurement and analysis of three-dimensional body movement. International Conference on *Concepts Mech Neuromusc Funct.* 1980:42–46.

Rowe ML. Low back pain in industry. *J Occup Med.* 1969;11:161–169.

Roy S, De Luca C, Casavant D. Lumbar muscle fatigue and chronic lower back pain. *Spine.* 1989;14:992–1001.

Schultz A, Anderson GBJ, Ortengren R, et al. Analysis and quantitative myoelectric measurements of loads of the lumbar spine when holding weights in standing postures. *Spine*. 1982;7:390.

Smith TJ, Fernie GR. Functional biomechanics of the spine. Symposium on Biomechanical Testing; September 1987; Vancouver, Canada.

Snook SH. Low back pain in industry. In: White AA, Gordon SL, eds. *Symposium in Idiopathic Low Back Pain*. St. Louis, Mo: CV Mosby; 1982.

Spengler DM, Bigos SJ, Martin NA, et al. Back injuries in industry: A retrospective study. I. Overview and cost analysis. *Spine*. 1986;11:241–245.

Svensson HO, Andersson GBJ. Low back pain in 40–47-year-old men. I. Frequency of occurrence and impact on medical services. *Scand J Rehabil Med*. 1982;14:47–53.

Thorstensson A, Oddsson L, Carlson H. Motor control of voluntary trunk movements in standing. *Acta Physiol Scand*. 1985;125:309–321.

Timm K. A randomized-control study of active and passive treatments for chronic low back pain following L5 laminectomy. *JOSPT*. 1994;20(6):276–285.

Valdenburg HA, Haanen HCM. The epidemiology of low back pain. *Clin Orthop*. 1983;179:9–22.

Woltring HJ. Finite centroid and helical axis estimation. *J Biomech*. 1985;18:379.

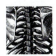

CHAPTER 12

Strength and Endurance Testing

Hannu Alaranta

INTRODUCTION

Musculoskeletal disorders are characterized by dysfunction such as impaired joint mobility (Alaranta et al, 1994a), decreased muscle strength or endurance (Andersson, 1991), and deficits of motor skill and coordination (Alaranta et al, 1994c; Fig. 12–1). The problem of the strength measurements in patients with musculoskeletal pain is that there is a large individual variation in the relationship of muscle performance capacity and musculoskeletal disorders. However, there is some evidence that musculoskeletal dysfunctions could be a cause, as well as a consequence, of certain musculoskeletal disorders (Andersson, 1991). Muscle strength due to neurogenic atrophy is usually classified manually using the 0-to-5 scale (Kendall et al, 1975). There are both simple isometric and more sophisticated isokinetic dynamometers (Härkönen et al, 1993; Hurri et al, 1995). Muscular strength and endurance can also be measured using nondynamometric performance tests (Alaranta et al, 1994b).

The high cost of dynamometric methods for trunk muscles has raised questions about the real benefits of the complicated test machines (Schoene, 1991). Rissanen et al (1994) investigated the correlations of nondynamometric and isokinetic tests with the perceived disabilities (Million Index) of 185 patients with low back pain. Unexpectedly, the arch-up and sit-up tests had an even stronger association to the perceived disability than the isokinetic tests. **The nondynamometric tests are still useful in clinical practice in spite of the development of more accurate muscle strength evaluation methods.**

Poor static back endurance strength was found to be linked to an increased risk of low back pain during a follow-up of 1 year (Luoto et al, 1995). Adjusted for age, sex, and occupation, the odds ratio of new low back pain in those with poor endurance was 3.4 (95% confidence interval, 1.2–10.0) compared to those with medium or good performance.

This chapter focuses on nondynamometric performance tests of muscular strength and endurance of trunk. The nondynamometric tests included in this chapter include (1) the repetitive sit-up, (2) the repetitive arch-up, (3) the repetitive squat, and (4) the static back endurance tests. Why choose only these tests over others that are available? Strength testing of the trunk and antecedent rehabilitation are important aspects of obtaining resolution for many individuals struggling with low back pain. Although high tech methods are available to measure trunk strength, low tech testing may be more accessible to a greater number of health care providers (HCPs) due to cost and/or availability. However, regardless of the strength measuring method chosen, it is appropriate to consider the following criteria when choosing a test: safety, reliability, validity, practicality, and utility (Yeomans and Liebenson, 1996).

The normative values for the strength and endurance tests referred to in this chapter are based on a sample of 508 male and female white-collar and blue-collar employees aged 35 to 54 years (Alaranta et al, 1994b). The subjects were evaluated clinically to determine the reliability of repetitive sit-ups, repetitive arch-ups, repetitive squatting, and static back endurance tests. The instruction of repetitions with a peaceful but constant pace was chosen. The purpose—not to choose the tests with maximum velocity—was intentional to avoid aggravating possible low back pain by the high-speed test procedure. The 1-year intraobserver reproducibility of the muscular measurements showed fairly high coefficient values ranging from .63 to .87 (Table 12–1; Alaranta et al, 1994b). **The highest values were noted for repetitive sit-ups and squatting.** None of the tests showed statistically significant shifts between the two measurements. The interobserver reliability coefficients were also fairly good or excellent, ranging from .66 to .95 (Table 12–2; Alaranta et al, 1994b). Repetitive squatting had the highest value. The back endurance test was the only one that showed a statistically significant shift between the two measurements.

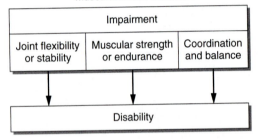

Figure 12–1. The biomechanical components of musculoskeletal impairment that affect disability.

(From Alaranta et al,1994c, Figure 1, p. 338.)

PRACTICAL ASSESSMENTS

REPETITIVE SIT-UP TEST

The patient is placed in a supine position with knees flexed at 90 degrees and is fixed by the tester in the ankle region. The patient approximates the thenar pads of the hands to the superior pole of the patella. The patient completes the cycle by curling the upper trunk back down to the supine position, touching the head to the horizontal surface. A rate of one repetition per 2 to 3 seconds is utilized during the test. The movement is repeated as many times as possible at a peaceful but constant pace. **If the motion becomes clearly jerky or asymmetrical, the test should be stopped.** The maximum number of repetitions is 50 (Fig. 12–2).

REPETITIVE ARCH-UP TEST

The patient lies in a prone position with the arms positioned along the sides and the ankles are supported by the tester. The inguinal region of the pelvis is placed at the edge of the test table and the upper trunk is flexed downward to 45 degrees. The patient raises the upper trunk upwards to horizontal position followed by returning back down to 45 degrees to complete a cycle. The repetition rate is one repetition per 2 to 3 seconds. The movement is repeated as many times as possible at a peaceful but constant pace. If the motion becomes jerky or asymmetrical, or does not reach the horizontal level, the test should be stopped. The maximum number of repetitions is 50 (Fig. 12–3).

Table 12–1: Intraobserver Reproducibility by the Same Tester 1 Year Apart Among Subjects Without Low Back Pain (n = 93)

TEST	FIRST TEST $\bar{x}$ SD	SECOND TEST $\bar{x}$ SD	p[a]	r[b]
Repetitive sit-up	23 ± 14	23 ± 15	.54	.84
Repetitive arch-up	29 ± 12	29 ± 13	.61	.65
Repetitive squatting	30 ± 14	30 ± 15	.47	.87
Static back endurance (sec)	96 ± 51	99 ± 58	.60	.63

SD, standard deviation; $\bar{x}$, mean of all measurements.
[a] Statistical significance of systematic shift (paired t-test).
[b] Reliability coefficient.

Table 12–2: Interobserver Reliability by Two Testers 1 Week Apart Among Subjects Without Low Back Pain (n = 17 subjects; 34 measurements)

TEST	$\bar{x}$	r	D$\bar{x}$	DSD	t	p
Repetitive sit-up	27	.91	.35	6.53	.32	.75
Repetitive arch-up	33	.83	2.06	7.16	1.68	.10
Repetitive squatting	32	.95	−.33	4.99	.38	.71
Static back endurance (sec)	109	.66	23.44	41.83	3.27	.003

DSD, deviation of DX; D$\bar{x}$, mean difference (1. − 2.); p, statistical significance of systematic shift; r, reliability coefficient; t, paired t-test (df = n − 1); $\bar{x}$ = mean of all measurements (2 × n).

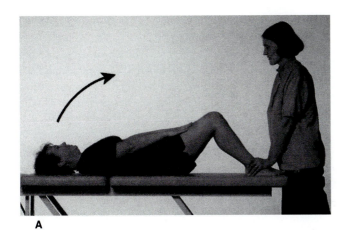
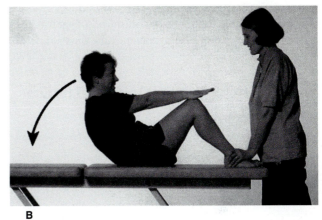

Figure 12–2. Repetitive sit-up test.

(Courtesy of the National Association of the Disabled, Finland.)

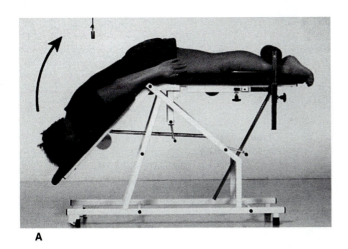
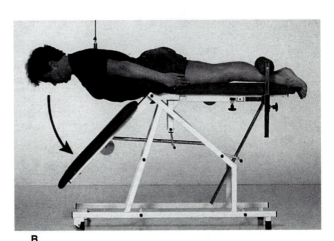

Figure 12–3. Repetitive arch-up test.

(Courtesy of the National Association of the Disabled, Finland.)

REPETITIVE SQUATTING TEST

In the initial position, the patient stands with the feet 15 cm apart. Slight finger touching is allowed without otherwise interfering with the test performance. The patient squats until the thighs are horizontal and then returns to a standing position. The repetition rate is one repetition per 2 to 3 seconds. Slight trunk flexion inclination and heel raising are allowed during downward motion. The movement is repeated as many times as possible at a peaceful but constant pace. The maximum number of repetitions is 50 (Fig. 12–4).

STATIC BACK ENDURANCE TEST

The patient lies in prone position, fixed in the ankle region, and the upper limbs are held along the sides. The upper trunk is supported horizontally with the inguinal region placed at the edge of the test table. The number of seconds the patient is able to maintain the horizontal position is recorded. The test should be discontinued if aggravated by pain or muscle spasm. The maximum time duration is 240 seconds (Fig. 12–5).

GUIDELINES FOR CONDUCTING THE TEST

It is appropriate for the HCP to discuss in detail why the muscular performance capacity will be tested. If the patient

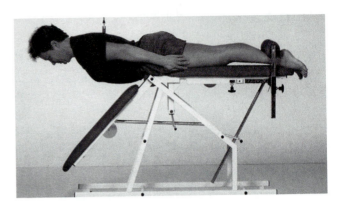

Figure 12–5. Static back endurance test.
(Courtesy of the National Association of the Disabled, Finland.)

thoroughly understands the purpose of the testing, his or her motivation will be enhanced.

It is recommended that a patient warm up his or her muscles by using a bicycle ergometer for approximately 5 minutes prior to beginning any testing. If the several muscular tests are retested, the order of the single tests should be similar. Also, back muscle testing should not be performed immediately after each other. There should be at least a 1-minute interval between each test. The tester may count repetitions aloud but should remain as neutral as possible, not encouraging or motivating the patient in any

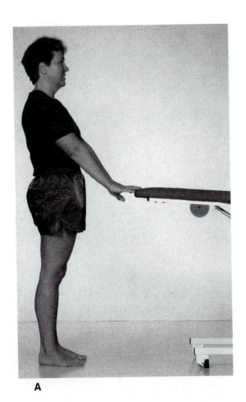
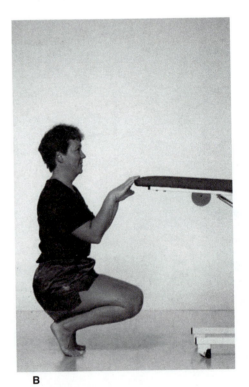

A   B

Figure 12–4. Repetitive squatting test.

(Courtesy of the National Association of the Disabled, Finland.)

Pain as an Indicator

The pain that a patient experiences before the test is not an absolute contraindication of the test, nor is a mild degree of pain during the test an indication to terminate it. If the test significantly increases pain or creates unpleasant feelings or symptoms, it should not be continued. The HCP should document whether or not the reason for terminating the test was due to fatigue or pain.

specific way. The patient will be told only one time to correct his or her trunk motion or position. If that does not normalize the trunk motion or position, the test should be terminated. The patient should be informed about the mild painful feelings in tested muscle groups during the couple

of days following the maximal test. If the tests are performed peacefully, the risk of complications due to the test are uncommon.

A physiotherapist or another HCP is the best person to administer the test. He or she should interview the patient carefully. If the patient has a history of cardiac disorder, asthma, diabetes, severe arthritis, or any other severe disease or disorder, the HCP should consult the patient's physician about whether or not to perform the tests before proceeding.

NORMATIVE VALUES

Mean values and standard deviations of repetitive sit-up, arch-up, squatting, and static back endurance tests according to sex, age, and occupation groups are presented in Table 12–3 (Alaranta et al, 1994b). Arbitrary scoring from

Table 12–3. Mean Values and Standard Deviations of Repetitive Sit-up, Arch-up, and Squatting Tests, and Static Back Endurance Test

| | MALES | | | | | | FEMALES | | | | | |
| | Blue Collar | | White Collar | | All | | Blue Collar | | White Collar | | All | |
AGE	$\bar{x}$	SD	$\bar{x}$	SD	$\bar{x}$	SD	$\bar{x}$	SD	$\bar{x}$	SD	$\bar{x}$	SD
Repetitive sit-up-test												
35–39	29	13	35	13	32	13	24	12	30	16	27	14
40–44	22	11	34	12	27	13	18	12	19	13	19	12
45–49	19	11	33	15	24	14	17	14	22	15	19	14
50–54	17	13	36	16	23	16	9	10	20	13	11	11
35–54	23	13	35	13	27	14	17	13	24	15	19	14
Repetitive arch-up-test												
35–39	26	11	34	14	29	13	28	13	27	11	27	12
40–44	23	12	36	14	28	14	25	14	20	11	23	13
45–49	24	13	34	16	28	15	25	15	31	16	27	15
50–54	21	11	35	17	26	15	18	14	26	14	19	14
35–54	24	12	35	15	28	14	24	14	26	13	24	14
Repetitive squatting test												
35–39	39	13	46	8	42	12	24	11	27	12	26	12
40–44	34	14	45	9	38	13	22	13	18	8	20	12
45–49	30	12	40	11	33	13	19	12	26	13	22	13
50–54	28	14	41	11	33	14	13	10	18	14	14	11
35–54	33	14	43	10	37	13	20	12	23	12	21	12
Static back endurance test (sec)												
35–39	87	38	113	47	97	43	91	61	95	48	93	55
40–44	83	51	129	57	101	57	89	57	67	51	80	55
45–49	81	45	131	64	99	58	90	55	122	73	102	64
50–54	73	47	121	56	89	55	62	55	99	78	69	60
35–54	82	45	123	55	97	53	82	58	94	62	87	59

SD, standard deviation; $\bar{x}$, mean of all measurements.
From Alaranta et al, 1994b. Reprinted with permission.

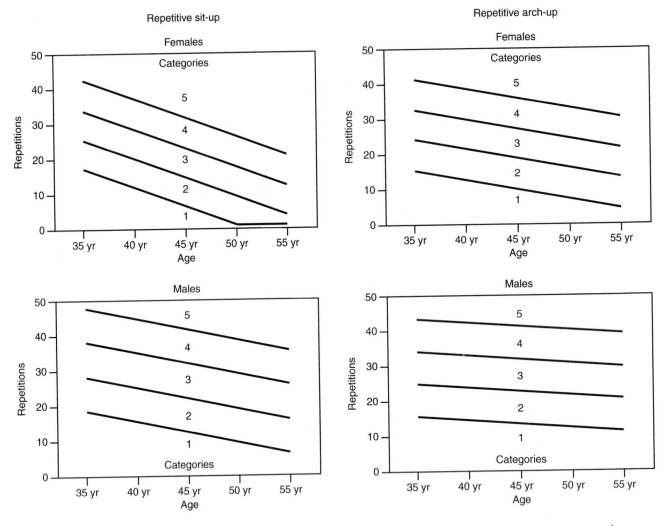

Figure 12–6. Repetitive sit-up test results.
(Courtesy of the National Association of the Disabled, Finland.)

Figure 12–7. Repetitive arch-up test results.
(Courtesy of the National Association of the Disabled, Finland.)

1 to 5 of the tests are presented in Figures 12–6 to 12–9 according to sex and age groups. Descriptions of the five categories follow:

- Category 5: Extremely good (better than mean +1 SD)
- Category 4: Good (better than mean + 1/3 SD)
- Category 3: Moderate (mean +/– max. 1/3 SD)
- Category 2: Poor (weaker than mean –1/3 SD)
- Category 1: Extremely poor (weaker than mean –1 SD)

Using the scoring lines from 1 to 5, it is also possible to interpolate normative values for subjects younger or older than those evaluated in this normative study.

EVALUATING THE RESULTS OF THE TESTS

The HCP should provide for enough time to evaluate the outcomes for the patient. The results will be rather individual and, therefore, must be individually tested. **It is essential not to draw any major conclusions because of one poor test result.** The test should be repeated after a couple of weeks. If a repeated test is still clearly below the mean values, it is an indication that training is needed.

The health care provider performing the test should obtain sufficient knowledge to counsel reasonable training (Basmajian and Wolf, 1990). If some training is recommended, the muscular capacity should be retested after 2 to 3 months. This will provide the HCP an opportunity to evaluate the adequacy of the rehabilitation training recommendations.

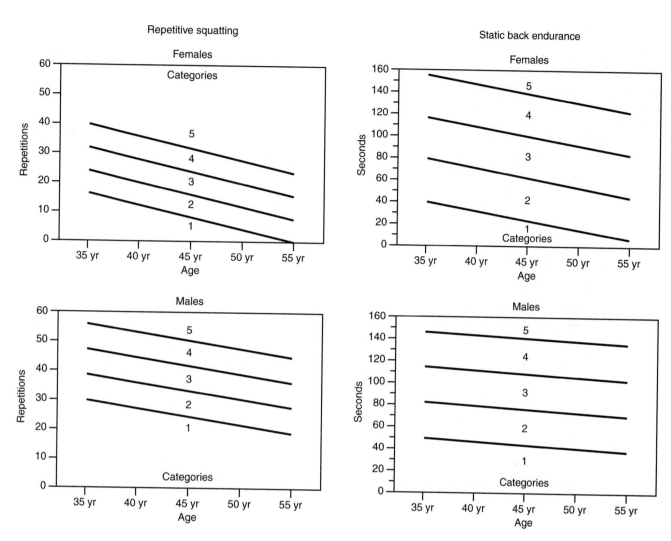

Figure 12–8. Repetitive squatting test results.
(Courtesy of the National Association of the Disabled, Finland.)

Figure 12–9. Static back endurance test results.
(Courtesy of the National Association of the Disabled, Finland.)

CASE STUDY 12–1
SAMPLE TEST RESULTS AND CONCLUSIONS

Hypothetical test results and conclusions utilizing a 45-year-old male, white collar worker:

Test	Patient Result	Normative Data	Category
Repetitive sit-up	15	33 ± 15	1 (extremely poor)
Repetitive arch-up	33	34 ± 16	3 (moderate)
Repetitive squatting	24	40 ± 11	1 (extremely poor)
Static back endurance	120	131 ± 64	3 (moderate)

The most significant weakness is noted in the repetitive sit-up and repetitive squat tests. Therefore, rehabilitation for this patient should focus on muscular training of abdominal and lower extremity regions.

Conclusion

The nondynamometric tests described in this chapter have been found to be valid, reliable, safe, practical, and responsive measures of trunk strength and endurance. The utility of these tests is particularly attractive as a low-tech/low cost method of assessing trunk strength and endurance in a primary care setting, resulting in meaningful data that can help identify weak trunk muscle strength. The same tests can then be repeated after instituting a rehabilitation training program to determine the endpoint of rehabilitation when muscle strength and endurance is regained. Because of the importance of trunk strength in the management of a number of disorders, particularly low back pain, adding these tests and subsequent rehabilitation to the treatment plan of the low back pain patient is particularly helpful in obtaining a successful treatment outcome.

REFERENCES

Alaranta H, Hurri H, Heliövaara M, Soukka A, Harju R. Flexibility of the spine: Normative values of goniometric and tape measurements. *Scand J Rehab Med.* 1994a;26:147–154.

Alaranta H, Hurri H, Heliövaara M, Soukka A, Harju R. Non-dynamometric trunk performance tests: Reliability and normative data. *Scand J Rehab Med.* 1994b;26:211–215.

Alaranta H, Moffroid M, Elmqvist L-G, Held J, Pope M, Renström P. Postural control of adults with musculoskeletal impairment. *Clin Rev Phys Rehab Med.* 1994c;6(4):337–370.

Andersson GB. Evaluation of muscle function. In: Frymoyer JW, ed. *The Adult Spine: Principles and Practice.* New York, NY: Raven Press; 1991:241–274.

Basmajian JV, Wolf SL. *Therapeutic Exercise.* Baltimore, Md: Williams and Wilkins; 1990.

Härkönen R, Piirtomaa M, Alaranta H. Grip strength and hand position of the dynamometer in 204 Finnish adults. *J Hand Surgery Br.* 1993;18B:129–132.

Hurri H, Hupli M, Alaranta H. Strength and mobility measurements in assessing outcome of an intensive back rehabilitation program. *Eur J Phys Med Rehabil.* 1995;5:160–164.

Kendall HO, Kendall FP, Wadsworth GE. Muscles—testing and function. Baltimore, Md: Williams and Wilkins; 1975.

Luoto S, Heliövaara M, Hurri H, Alaranta H. Static back endurance and the risk of low-back pain. *Clin Biomechanics.* 1995;10:323–324.

Rissanen A, Alaranta H, Sainio P, Härkönen H. Isokinetic and non-dynamometric tests in low back pain patients related to pain and disability index. *Spine.* 1994;19:1963–1967.

Schoene M, ed. Back machines: A waste of money? *The Back Letter.* 1991;5:8.

Yeomans SG, Liebenson C. Quantitative functional capacity evaluation: The missing link to outcomes assessment. *Top Clin Chiro.* 1996;3(1):32–43.

CHAPTER 13

Spinal Orthopedic and Neurological Testing

STEVEN G. YEOMANS

INTRODUCTION

The use of outcomes based objective testing is an important aspect of the clinical assessment of a patient. Just as the subjective tools such as questionnaires help the health care provider (HCP) track change over time, it has been assumed that physical examination tools can accomplish this task objectively. The same criteria that apply to the pen-and-paper tools are also applicable with objective tests. That is, validity, reliability, responsiveness, practicality, utility, and safety are necessary criteria to fulfill if one is to obtain confidence in the test. A unique feature found in some quantitative objective tests is the inclusion of normative data which, when available, allows for baseline comparisons to the patient's results. The goal of this chapter is to look beyond the definition and description of the many provocative orthopedic tests, which have been thoroughly addressed elsewhere (Mazion, 1980; Cipriano, 1991; Evans, 1994; and others). This chapter focuses instead on differentiating among provocative tests, neurological tests, and physical performance tests, and explores how they relate to each other. Methods for improving the clinical utility of provocative and physical performance testing are also included.

Objective outcomes can include many different types of tests of both high- and low-tech varieties. Low-tech objective testing can be accomplished inexpensively and, therefore, has good utility and practicality for use in a clinical setting. **When necessary, high-tech tests are available; however, these are usually reserved for triaging conditions to determine the next therapeutic decision.** A partial list of objective testing can include the following:

• Provocative tests (for extremities, see Chap. 15)
• Neurological tests

163

- Physical performance tests (see Chap. 16)
- Routine physical examination
- Nonorganic tests (see Chap. 16)
- Range of motion procedures (see Chap. 14 for spinal; Chap. 15 for extremity)
- Functional or work capacity tests (see Chap. 18)
- Aerobic capacity tests (see Chap. 17)
- Strength and endurance tests (see Chaps. 11, 12, and 16)
- Electrodiagnostic testing (electromyography [EMG], somatosensory evoked potential [SSEP], current perception threshold [CPT], and vibrometry)
- Doppler testing devices
- Laboratory tests (cells and fluids; eg, tissue, blood, urine, etc)
- Radiological tests
- Special imaging tests such as nuclear bone scanning, magnetic resonance imaging (MRI), computed tomography (CT) scanning, diagnostic ultrasound, positive emission tomography (PET), thermography, videofluoroscopy, and others

This list is not meant to represent the entire spectrum of objective testing. It does, however, illustrate many different varieties of objective tests that HCPs can access. For purposes of this chapter, discussion will be limited to only the first three categories listed: provocative tests, neurological tests, and physical performance tests. Those who wish to pursue further investigation of some of the other tests listed should refer to the other chapters referenced. Deyo et al (1994) also discuss some of these topics in an article that summarizes the design recommendations for studies concerning diagnostic tests in low back pain and radiculopathy populations.

When reviewing the literature or when considering conducting a study of diagnostic test validity and reliability, Deyo et al (1994) recommend several key study design features, as follows:

- Independent comparison of the diagnostic test results with an appropriate "gold standard"
- Blinded assessment of the new test and the gold standard or competing tests
- The reproducibility and interpretation of the test being examined
- Sensitivity and specificity of the test against the final gold standard diagnosis

Similarly, Breen (1992) discusses four issues that are central to the validation of a testing procedure, as follows:

- Calibration against a known standard
- Test–retest reliability
- Internal consistency
- Observer variability

Although a strong quantitative element is desired in testing, achieving this in practice is difficult for the following reasons:

- There are few, if any, standards against which calibration can be done.
- Test–retest reliability is difficult because the biological material changes with each test.
- Internal consistency is difficult to assess as the tests used to compare the procedure being evaluated are not often valid.
- Observer variability often leads to surprising results.

CORRELATING OBJECTIVE TESTS TO THE DIAGNOSIS

There is a wide gap between the reliability of musculoskeletal examination procedures and their clinical usefulness. Similarly, agreement of a specific diagnosis is poor due to the inability of **objective** provocative tests to adequately discriminate between different types of spinal conditions.

For example, low back pain such as facet syndrome (Carette et al, 1991; Jackson, 1992), sacroiliac joint pain (Dreyfuss et al, 1996), the piriformis syndrome, and degenerative disc disease as a cause of instability (Fager, 1984; Nachemson, 1985; Hanley, 1993) cannot be adequately differentiated from each other by provocative testing. However, by broadening the diagnoses into categories such as those suggested by the Quebec Task Force (QTF) (Spitzer et al, 1987), agreement of the diagnostic category is more likely to occur compared to agreement of the specific conditions/diagnoses that are popular and currently in use.

Three broad diagnostic categories for **spinal conditions** can be derived from the QTF, which include (1) mechanical, (2) nerve root, and (3) red flags. In the example cited previously, it is more likely to find consensus agreement that the conditions cited are all included in the mechanical low back pain category. Therefore, as HCPs, we try first and foremost to rule out "red flags" which, for low back pain, include cauda equina syndrome, cancer, infection and fracture (Deyo et al, 1992, Bigos et al, 1994). Refer to Chapter 19 for a discussion of the red and yellow flags. Next, we must offer the presenting patient reassurance followed by pain relief, functional restoration, and reinforcement. The latter consists of teaching long-term, self-help concepts with the understanding that the patient must be an active participant in his or her own care and that activity restoration be the primary focus, not pain reduction.

PROVOCATIVE TESTS

LUMBAR SPINE

Understanding the pitfalls to **provocative** testing is necessary in order to appreciate its strengths and deficiencies. For example, the wide biological variables that exist in the musculoskeletal system reduce the reliability of some provocative testing approaches. However despite this, **objective testing remains an essential part of the evaluation process as it helps determine the anatomical location of the lesion, regardless of the specific diagnosis.** It also may give clues to the indicated and/or contraindicated forms of treatment and allow for outcomes assessment at a later date, which will help determine treatment effect/benefit. As a result, endpoints of care can be established. Lastly, the current reimbursement system in which HCPs practice demands accountability for "supporting the patient's subjective complaints with objective findings." Therefore, documenting provocative test results will continue to be a requirement until a more valid and reliable substitute becomes the standard.

Palpation

Probably the most commonly performed provocative test is that of palpation. Palpation includes the use of manual touch consisting of varying degrees of pressure applied to an injured region with the intention to provoke a pain response from the patient. **The goal of palpation is to localize and define the area of complaint.** In addition, the response observed by the patient can give the HCP clues as to the amount of tissue injury as, usually, the more sensitive the area, the greater the degree of tissue disruption. However, since pain is a subjective phenomenon, it is not logical that pain can be objectively assessed. For more information regarding the subjective measurement of pain, refer to Chapter 6.

In attempt to improve the **"objectivity"** of pain assessment or "harden" the reproducibility of the testing process, one can employ a pain scale that is graded by the HCP, rather than by the patient. For example, since pain behavior occurs when one is injured or "in pain," observation of the appropriateness of the pain response can be graded by using a 0-to-IV grading scale defined by the American College of Rheumatology (Wolfe et al, 1990). This is a provider-driven scoring method in which the patient's facial expression, mannerisms, and withdrawal reactions are observed and then graded (Table 13–1).

Grades I to II are clearly organic, while grade IV is clearly nonorganic and grade III is somewhere in between. Grade III responses should be carefully compared to other provocative test pain responses and, if determined to be nonorganic, an increase to a grade IV may be appropriate. **The amount of pressure exerted by the examiner should be consistent if this approach is to have any validity or reliability.** Therefore, when using this scale, the pressure applied to the injured part should be approximately 4 kg, or the amount needed to blanch the fingernail of the palpating digit. By applying this scale to any provocative diagnostic test, an "objective" pain score can be reported with each test throughout the examination. In addition, a subjective score, or one reported by the patient can be compared. Some consistency would be expected such as a numerical pain scale (VPS) of 7/10 or higher may correlate with a grade III (if organic) or grade IV (if nonorganic) objective pain score. Table 13–2 is a correlation chart that

Table 13–1: American College of Rheumatology Pain Scale (ACR-PS)

GRADE	DEFINITION
Grade I	Mild tenderness to moderate palpation
Grade II	Moderate tenderness with grimace and/or flinch to moderate palpation
Grade III	Severe tenderness with withdrawal (+ Jump Sign)
Grade IV	Severe tenderness with withdrawal (+ Jump Sign) to nonnoxious stimuli (ie, superficial palpation, pinprick, gentle percussion)[a]

[a] In noninjured tissue, this is a sign of neuropathic pain (nonorganic pain behavior).
Data compiled from Wolfe et al, 1990.

Table 13–2: Comparison of Different Pain Grading Methods

		Mild	Moderate	Severe	
A. Verbal Pain Scale (Subjective) (VPS)					
B. Numerical Pain Scale (Subjective) (NPS)	No Pain _____ / _____ / _____ Severe Pain				
		0 1 2 3 4 5 6 7 8 9 10			
C. American College of Rheumatology Pain Scale (Objective) (ACR-PS)	Grade	0 1 2 3 4 (nonorganic)			

The "objective" palpation grade (ACR-PS) should correlate with the pain scales in A and B as shown above.

compares the NPR, the American College of Rheumatology Pain Scale (ACR-PS), and a verbal pain scale (VPS) of mild, moderate, and severe. Several studies have referred to an NPS of 7/10 or greater as representative of "severe pain" (Blankenship, 1991; Von Korff et al, 1992), which has been identified as a risk factor of chronicity (see Chaps. 10 and 21) (Haldeman et al, 1993; Von Korff et al, 1993; Burton et al, 1995).

Other studies have investigated the reliability of palpation. For example, McCombe et al (1989) found tenderness to be an unreliable sign when palpation is performed over the paravertebral or buttock soft tissues, whereas palpation over a bony prominence was "potentially reliable" or "reliable." Others have reported similar results (see Appendix I–1 and I–2). The ability to identify specific anatomical points utilizing static palpation methods revealed discrepancies between observers as well as within the same observer (Keating et al, 1990; Byfield et al, 1991). Motion palpation of the sacroiliac joints showed higher intrarater and inter-rater correlations (Herzog et al, 1989) than did lumbar spine motion palpation (Keating, 1989). One explanation may be the difficulty in locating and naming the involved specific lumbar spinal segments versus the more easily palpable sacroiliac joint (Harvey and Byfield, 1991). Others have postulated that the overlying soft tissues make precise identification of bony landmarks difficult, especially in the obese person (Strender et al, 1997b).

Orthopedic Tests

The primary goal of provocative orthopedic testing utilizes movements and/or positions that reproduce pain. **The purpose of orthopedic tests is to identify the anatomical location or source of pain.** Studies investigating the validity and reliability of provocative testing have been published in many sources (Troup, 1981; Mayer et al, 1985; Gatchel et al, 1986; Cibulka et al, 1988; Leboeuf et al, 1989a, 1989b; McCombe et al, 1989; Thelander et al, 1992; McCarthy, 1994; Dreyfus et al, 1996; Wachter et al, 1996; Donelson et al, 1997; Strender et al, 1997a, 1997b; and others).

McCombe et al (1989) utilized three examiners—two orthopedic surgeons and one physiotherapist—who examined two independent groups of patients. The first group consisted of 50 patients with an average age of 44.3 years (+/− 12.2) and was comprised of 26 men and 24 women.

The two orthopedic surgeons evaluated each member of this group consecutively in the same session. The second group consisted of 33 patients (average age 46.1 +/−14.6; 26 men and 7 women) and was examined by one of the orthopedic surgeons and the physical therapist (PT). An exclusion criterion for both groups included prior spinal surgery. Eight categories of low back physical signs were performed by each evaluator and compared. The following results were reported (summarized in Table 13–3):

- **Pain pattern.** The more distal the pain, the higher the agreement between examiners. Disagreement occurred when differentiating back from buttock pain, which illustrates the importance for careful pain localization during examination.
- **Tenderness.** The least reliable signs were paravertebral and buttock soft tissue tenderness, while bony tenderness (sacroiliac, midline, and iliac crest) was "potentially reliable" or "reliable."
- **Root tension signs.** The straight leg raise and femoral nerve stretch tests were more reliable than the bowstring test or, rapid extension of the knee from a slightly flexed straight leg raise position.
- **Root compression signs.** Agreement about muscle wasting and power was good between the two surgeons but not between the surgeon and PT, as the PT found more positive signs. The authors stressed the clinical importance of these tests and warned that this should not be regarded as evidence of poor reproducibility of these signs, citing differences in training as a possible reason.
- **Inappropriate signs.** Waddell's nonorganic low back pain signs revealed no clear pattern. More specifically, the two unreliable signs (superficial tenderness and abnormal regional sensory or motor disturbance) appear to require more subjective judgment than pain with simulation or distraction. It should be noted that this conflicts with Korbon et al (1987), who found sensory, motor, tenderness, and the straight leg raise distraction test, or "flip sign," to be the most reliable.

McCombe et al (1989) cite two prior papers that reported on the reliability of signs in low back pain: Nelson (1986) and Waddell et al (1982). Similar findings of poor reliability are described regarding low back pain signs.

Table 13–3: Three Categories of Reliability When Comparing Various Physical Signs

TEST	MOST RELIABLE	POTENTIALLY RELIABLE	POOR RELIABILITY
1. **Pain Pattern**	Thigh, leg	Buttock, foot pain	Back
2. **Posture**	Measure lordosis (cm)	NA	Spinal list measure (cm)
3. **Movement**	Flexion (Schoeber); pain on flexion; lateral bend	Extension, rotation	Extension "catch"; lateral bend (cm)
4. **Tenderness**	NA	SI, iliac crest, midline	Paravertebral, buttock
5. **SI and Piriformis**	Hip flexion (y/n)	Pain w/ER	Maitland's t.; SI compres.; SI distraction
6. **Root Tension Signs**	SLR (onset & max.)	Crossed SLR, SLR sciatic stretch test; SLR repro. symptoms	NA
7. **Root Compression Signs**	Leg numbness (y/n)	Atrophy and weakness of the quads, calf, tib. ant., peron., knee ext.; Achilles DTR	Heel/toe strength, buttock atrophy, patellar DTR
8. **Inappropriate Signs**	NA	Distraction, simulation, over-reaction	Tenderness, regional motor/sensory disturbance

Abbreviations: cm, centimeter; compres., compression; DTR, deep tendon reflex; ER, external rotation; ext, extension; max., maximum; NA, not available; n, no; peron., peronius longus and brevis; quads, quadriceps femoris; repro., reproduces; SI, sacroiliac; SLR, straight leg raise; t, test; tib. ant., tibialis anterior; w/, with; y, yes.
Modified from McCombe et al, 1989.

However, sequential refinements to the examination procedures resulted in methods that were capable of reaching acceptable agreement. They discussed the superior agreement attained by Waddell et al (1982) as possibly being due to examination procedure refinements as the study went on, resulting in examiner skill improvement in contrast to their own study where this did not occur. Similarly, Ekstrand and Gillquist (1982) observed an improvement in the coefficient of variation (CV) from 7.5 +/− 2.9 to 1.9 +/− .7 after using various physical performance tests for 2 months and making subsequent refinement, paying attention to the details regarding:

- Standardized inclinometer placement, ensuring the pendulum of the gravity type swings freely
- Stiffening up the examination table (plywood with Velcro bands)
- Identification of bony anatomical landmarks (mark on skin)
- Standardized examination bench height for each visit

McCombe et al (1989) also cite a respiratory study to compare the kappa coefficients to their results and define the highest kappa coefficient reported for reduced percussion (.52), followed by wheeze and crackles at .51 and .41, respectively (Spitteri et al, 1988). The lowest coefficient was found for displacement of the trachea (.01). If these results can be used as a benchmark for comparison, McComb et al (1989) state that the similar results they obtained in their low back study may be acceptable. They described the following conclusions:

- Be very specific about pain localization in the back or buttock and use correct anatomical terminology of bony landmarks such as lumbosacral junction, iliac crest, or buttock.
- Avoid placing much diagnostic weight on toe and heel standing as signs of muscle weakness.
- Bony tenderness carries greater validity than soft tissue tenderness.
- Sacroiliac tests, including Maitland (1977), and the compression and distraction tests "should be used with caution." Pain associated with hip flexion and external rotation of the hip, however, are reliably reproducible, although the authors point out that further evaluation of the meanings of these signs is needed.
- Record where the pain is experienced when performing any of the root tension signs (straight leg raise, femoral stretch, bowstring test).
- When assessing spinal range of motion, record when and where pain occurred during the test.
- Be careful when interpreting Waddell signs of nonorganic low back pain, including the superficial tenderness and abnormal regional sensory or motor disturbance.

It should be mentioned that the poorer results obtained by the orthopedist and PT may have resulted, at least in part, from a small sample study group (n = 33). A similar study comparing two PTs who had worked together for many years, to two physicians who had not, also showed that superior agreement was obtained by the PTs (Strender et al, 1997b). But here, also, a sample size of 50 patients was examined by the PTs and only 21 patients were examined by the physicians which may be the more likely reason why the results favored the PTs, as was similarly noted in the McCombe study. This point is illustrated in Strender et al's inability to calculate the prevalence, 95% confidence intervals, percent agreement, and kappa coefficients for 13 of the 29 physical tests evaluated. In reviewing their results and comparing them with those of the McCombe study, it may be that training variances affected results less than agreement as to how a test was done and establishing dialogue regarding the meaning of the results. Strender et al (1997b) emphasized the importance of the latter, and they concluded that a much higher degree of clinical test standardization is needed so that the tests are well understood in terms of the execution and interpretation of the results.

More recently, Michel et al (1997), investigated the association between clinical findings on physical examination and self-reported severity in back pain. In this study, a population-based approach was utilized; approximately 4000 Germans, aged 25 to 74 were randomly selected and invited for a clinical examination if they responded affirmatively to either of two questions. The two questions were "Did you have back pain today" (n = 1200) or "Have

you had back pain within the past 12 months but no back pain before" (n = 75). Thirty-four physical measurements divided into four groups were utilized. These four groups were: static measurements, dynamic measurements, neurological findings, and nonorganic physical signs. A pain questionnaire utilizing a variation of Von Korff's pain intensity and functional disability approach (Von Korff et al, 1992) and a 12-item disability questionnaire (Hannover Activities of Daily Living Questionnaire); (Kohlmann and Raspe, 1994) were utilized. Table 13–4 summarizes the tests within each of the four categories of physical measurements that corresponded best with the subjective severity of back pain and disability (Michel et al, 1997).

In Michel et al's study, the physical measurements found in Table 13–4 were placed together into one model and rough estimates of the predictive qualities of the model were calculated. The cut-off point of .46 was determined by the point where sensitivity and specificity attained its highest value. The model sensitivity was 62.84% and specificity was 83.56%. Agreement between pain and disability status as classified by the model compared with the actual outcome resulted in a kappa value of .47 (moderate agreement). Of interest, paravertebral tenderness stimulated the

Table 13–4: Physical Measures That Correlate Best With Self-reported Severity in Back Pain

TYPE OF TEST	PHYSICAL MEASUREMENTS	ODDS RATIO (95% CI)	P FACTOR
Static Measurements	Sagittal plumb line (at trochanter vs. anterior or posterior)	1.30 (1.15 – 1.47)	.000
	Presence or absence of scoliosis	2.11 (1.07 – 4.15)	.030
	Pain on percussion of the spine		
	Thoracic	1.76 (1.21 – 2.56)	.003
	Thoracolumbar	1.91 (1.18 – 3.09)	.009
	Lumbar	3.04 (2.16 – 4.27)	.000
Dynamic Measurements	Fingertip-floor distance	1.29 (1.12 – 1.48	.000
	Lateral flexion	.46 (.37 – .57)	.000
	Rotation	.72 (.58 – .90)	.004
Neurologic Measurements[a]	Positive Pseudo-Lasegue[b]	1.72 (1.25 – 2.37)	.001
	Diminished sensation (nondermatomal)	1.71 (.95 – 3.07)	.071
	Motor deficit (lower extremity)	7.25 (1.96 – 26.81)	.003
	Hand muscle strength		
	Right hand	.43 (.26 – .69)	.000
	Left hand	.63 (.39 – 1.01)	.056
Nonorganic Physical Signs	Passive rotation	2.83 (1.83 – 1.61)	.000
	Superficial tenderness	2.65 (1.31 – 5.36)	.007
	Overreaction[c]	11.87 (2.50 – 56.29)	.002

CI, confidence interval.

[a] Some neurological signs were very rare such as a positive Lasegue (n = 5) and missing or unsymmetrical patellar tendon reflex (n = 5). This resulted in a wide confidence interval and a lack of statistical significance despite the probability of a strong association.

[b] Pseudo-Lasegue test: passive straight leg raising with pain localized at the thigh or lumbosacral region.

[c] Overreaction was associated with an approximately 12 times increased risk of being in the high pain and disability class.

Data compiled from Michel et al, 1997.

most discussion between the two PTs and two physicians. This test had the lowest reliability in the PT group. Also, the three tests with the lowest reliability included those where movement was needed in the assessment process. These included (1) the springing test, (2) the sacroiliac compression test, and (3) paravertebral tenderness. One reason for the poor reliability may be the unstandardized compression used by the examiners (Michel et al, 1997).

Chris Main, PhD, offers a "Point of View" to this study that praises the study design, statistical analysis, and attempt at minimizing observer bias (Main, 1997). He points out, however, that most of the 34 measures are of unknown or undeclared reliability (and perhaps validity), and no attempt at studying their inter-rater relationships was made. Also, only six of the eight Waddell tests were studied and no offering of an analysis of a combination of nonorganic signs is included. Main cautions the approach of individual signs being used in isolation as three of the five Waddell signs were originally required to meet the necessary criteria to diagnose nonorganic pain behavior (Waddell et al, 1980). Main states that the authors have demonstrated that physical examination findings relate poorly to subjective severity. Moreover, most of the physical measurements they utilize "are of very little value." Main states that, by consensus, it is time to explore a new set of fundamental hypotheses that persistent back pain has to be considered from a biopsychosocial perspective. Main concludes, "if their study has served to discourage the continued search for needles in haystacks and 'overmedicalization' of nonspecific low back pain . . . then [it] will have been worthwhile" (Main, 1997).

Gatchel et al (1986) reported that both psychological and physical examination measures improved when patients were guided through a physical function restoration program. Both the psychological measures and the physical function measures were assessed at admission and at a 3-month follow-up. The physical measures that were found sensitive to change over time (all were P<.001) included:

- True lumbar flexion
- True lumbar extension
- Straight leg raise
- Cybex 60/sec and 120/sec extension strength

The psychological self-report measures relating to pain and disability that were found sensitive to change over time included:

- Beck Depression Inventory (BDI) (P<.001)
- Pain drawing—extremities (P<.02)
- Pain drawing—trunk (P<.001)
- Million Analogue Scale (P<.001)

Other tools utilized at baseline and 6-months postdischarge included the Million Behavioral Health Inventory (MBHI) and the Minnesota Multiphasic Personality Inventory

(MMPI). The BDI, Million Visual Rating Scale, and the Quantified Pain Drawing were assessed at admission, and again at 3 and 6 month follow-up evaluations. The results revealed that various MMPI scales that were initially clinically elevated showed a significant decrease to nonelevated levels after a successful treatment outcome. Gatchel et al (1986) stressed the importance of understanding that avoidance of assuming that a single psychological test can reliably be used as the sole predictive variable in clinical cases be practiced. The presence of these findings, in addition to the more recent studies casting shadows of doubt on the predictive capabilities of chronicity using provocative testing, support Main's recommendation that a biopsychosocial approach to patient assessment and outcomes assessment be adopted (Main, 1997).

Provocative tests commonly utilized in the diagnostic category of mechanical low back pain generally do not produce neural tension signs. Rather, they usually provoke a localized pain response in the area of injury. Included in this group are tests that reproduce low back pain arising from an articular facet joint, sacroiliac joint, and/or the surrounding soft tissues. It may also, however, include a radial or circumferential tear of the posterior annulus of the disc, which produces a localized and/or sclerotomal referred pain pattern. Studies involving direct injections into the facet joint under fluoroscopy have yielded variable results. More specifically, saline injections into the facet joint reproduced low back pain, buttock, and leg pain extending, at times, to the calf, along with reduction of deep tendon reflexes (Mooney, 1990). In spite of the variability, low back and leg pain without radiculopathy (no nerve root signs), suggests joint-related problems. It has been reported that the symptom described as an "extension catch" has "poor reliability" in reference to mechanical low back pain (McCombe et al, 1989). Lippitt (1984) found that 66% of a patient population responded favorably to facet injection when all of the following findings were present:

- Low back pain
- Hip and buttock pain
- Cramping leg pain above the knee
- Low back stiffness especially in the morning
- Absence of dysesthesia in the legs

A scoring system was then introduced assigning points for various clinical findings as follows (Lippitt, 1984):

- 30 points: Low back pain with groin or thigh pain
- 20 points: Well-localized paraspinal tenderness
- 30 points: Low back pain reproduced with extension-rotation (Kemp's test)
- 20 points: Corresponding radiographic changes (osteoarthritis)
- −10 points: Pain below the knee

This study, utilizing a 22-patient sample, revealed that those patients with scores of 60 or greater required prolonged treatment. The outcome was favorable in seven of nine patients with scores of 40 or more, but four patients with scores less than 40 points also responded to the injection therapy. In conclusion, none of the studies reviewed indicate that any one clinical finding alone was discriminatory. **Therefore, although the diagnosis is most firmly established when more than one test is positive, even then, a discriminatory assessment is unlikely.**

CERVICAL SPINE

With respect to the cervical spine physical signs, less information regarding provocative and physical performance testing is available. There have been, however, several individual studies that report validity and reliability in some physical measures including inclinometric mensurated cervical range of motion (Youdas et al, 1992; Mayer, 1994; and others) and cervical spine strength (Edwards and McDonnell, 1974; Hyde and Scott, 1983; Bohannon, 1986; Agre et al, 1987; Vernon et al, 1992; Watson and Trott, 1993). Refer to Chapter 14 for additional information and references. Selective tissue tension tests have a long history in the assessment of sciatic nerve compression/traction neuropathies and, recently, Elvey (1992) developed similar tests for the cervicobrachial plexus. These have been shown to have good reliability for differentiating upper limb nerve tension from muscle tightness (Edgar et al, 1994). They have also been able to identify a cervical component in chronic tennis elbow patients with high reliability (Yaxley and Jull, 1993). These tests differentiate between inert (nerve) and soft tissue (muscle, fascia) sources of mechanical restriction or irritation. Forward head posture and weakness of the upper cervical flexor musculature in association with cervical headaches (Kenny, 1965), EMG-based instrumentation studies (Harms-Ringdahl et al, 1988; Schuldt and Harms-Ringdahl, 1988a, 1988b; Refshauge et al, 1994), cervicothoracic kyphosis, and cervical inclination measurements in painful versus nonpainful subjects (Sandmark and Nisell, 1995) have also been reported. In addition, the validity of five common manual neck pain provocative tests was studied (Sandmark and Nisell, 1995), as follows:

1. Active rotation of the neck and upper thoracic spine with a passive manual stretch at the extreme position of ipsilateral rotation
2. Active flexion and extension of the neck and upper thoracic spine
3. Foraminal compression test
4. The upper limb tension test (combined shoulder depression and costoclavicular tests)
5. Palpation of the cervical spine facet joints

Validity criteria were met in the last three tests listed above when comparing pain provocation in 75 randomly selected men out of a population of 3144 electricians from Stockholm, Sweden. Of the 75 selected men, 22, or 29%, had neck pain/dysfunction and 53, or 71%, did not have neck pain for at least 1 year. Active rotation of the neck and upper thoracic spine with a passive manual stretch at the extreme position of ipsilateral rotation reproduced pain only in 2 of the neck pain subjects (sensitivity and specificity could not be measured) and the sensitivity was low in the second (27%). When compared to the last three tests, sensitivity was 77%, 77%, and 82% and specificity was 92%, 94%, and 79% for the last three tests, respectively. Study conclusions revealed that tests 3 and 4 (the nerve root tests) provoked localized pain due to the extreme positions of the neck and upper trunk by stretching the ligaments and muscles of the cervical spine and upper part of the back, neck, and shoulders. Since tests 3 and 4 did not provoke nerve tension signs in any of the subjects, they drew the conclusion that test 5 was the best because it did what it was designed to do, that is, provoke localized pain. The authors did, however, qualify that the small study population and absence of nerve root impingement in their sample population were probable reasons for the optimistic findings (Sandmark and Nisell, 1995).

The conclusion by Sandmark and Nisell in the latter study (1995), raises a very important issue when documenting the results of provocative tests in a patient chart. More specifically, **although a test is "negative" according to its intended definition, a *different* provocative pain response may provide important information to the evaluator—even though it may not be the defined response described in the literature.** Therefore, a description of the pain response including location, radiation, and severity will facilitate the HCP's ability to reach an accurate assessment of the patient's condition. A good example of this is increased localized pain in the cervical spine during a cervical distraction (manual traction) test. A "positive" response is defined as a decrease in neck and/or arm pain. However, if pain increases (not the intention of the test) it is *not* appropriate to describe the test as "positive." On the other hand, the term "negative" implies no pain was elicited. Therefore, **it is most appropriate to report the patient's pain response to all provocative tests rather than reporting a test as "positive" or "negative" since the latter tells nothing about the specific response that was elicited.** Moreover, it can be assumed that only a "textbook" definition applies to the patient if the term "positive," only, is reported and, similarly, no significant findings of any kind occurred when the term "negative" is utilized. Also, and perhaps most importantly, many of these tests are "prescriptive," in that a specific treatment approach is driven from the response to the test (ie, cervical traction is indicated when neck and/or arm pain reduces during a cervical distraction test but is contraindicated when pain increases). Similarly, if radicular symptoms centralize in a lumbar extension position, extension exercises are indicated and emphasized (ie, the test has prescriptive validity). Therefore, it is helpful for the HCP to be as descriptive as possible when reporting these findings for the following reasons:

CLINICAL TIP 13–1
Documenting Provocative Test Findings

Reporting "positive" or "negative" when documenting provocative test findings is inappropriate as it does not allow for test interpretation if a provocative response other than that of the defined description occurs. Also, a treatment prescription can sometimes be determined by test results, such as the indication for cervical traction when pain reduction occurs during the cervical distraction test. However, if pain worsens with a cervical distraction test (by definition, still a "negative" test), cervical traction is contraindicated and could harm the patient if utilized. Simply reporting a "negative" cervical distraction test would not alert the HCP to omit cervical traction, which clearly is contraindicated if pain increases during cervical distraction. This may have deleterious ramifications including patient discontinuing care, patient disgruntlement concerning reimbursement, and/or even malpractice implications. Thus, a description of the test result is appropriate, regardless of its technical definition.

- Optimum patient care can be administered by any HCP at any time.
- The payer has a clear picture of what is wrong with the patient and the treatment is appropriate (ie, "to get paid").
- The HCP is protected against a poor malpractice outcome that might otherwise occur simply because the records did not support the provider's actions.

Finally, documentation is thorough and complete (ie, "hard") only when a description of the test response is utilized over a simple "soft" positive or negative form of reporting.

NEUROLOGICAL TESTS

LUMBAR SPINE

Neurological examination in the neuromusculoskeletal clinical setting usually is confined to the motor and sensory evaluation of the nerve root and its peripheral nerve. The motor aspect of the examination is typically approached by the use of the deep tendon reflex (DTR) response and muscle strength. The sensory aspect of the examination is often performed by the use of a pinwheel, light touch, but may include vibration, two-point discrimination, and Semmes–Weinstein monofilaments. Special electrodiagnostic testing such as nerve conduction velocities, sensory latencies, and needle EMG are considered a "gold-standard" in the field of neurological evaluation. The discussion here is restricted to the routine approaches usually included in a "low-tech" neurological evaluation.

McCombe et al evaluated standard neurological examination procedures in a 1989 study. The root compression signs category revealed good agreement between the two examining surgeons (see Table 13–3) but not between the surgeon and PT as the PT found more positive signs. The data were plotted on a scattergram, which is an *x*, *y* axis graph divided into 4 quadrants, where the inter-rater results were categorized into most reliable, potentially reliable, and poorly reliable groups. The presence of leg numbness ("yes or no") was found to be "most reliable." Those tests included in the "potentially reliable" category included the clinical assessment of atrophy (circumferential mensuration) as well as weakness of the quadriceps femoris, gastrocnemius/soleus, tibialis anterior, peroneus longus and brevis muscles, and Achilles DTR. The heel/toe walk, buttock atrophy, and patellar DTR were classified in the "poorly reliable" category. The authors stressed the clinical importance of these tests and warned that these study results should not be regarded as evidence that these signs are worthless. More specifically, a difference in training between the PT and the surgeon was described as a possible reason for the discrepancies. Also, as previously mentioned, a smaller patient population (n = 33) was evaluated in the PT versus surgeon group compared to the surgeon–surgeon patient group (n = 50), which also may have affected the overall results.

The great majority (98%) of disc lesions are located at the L4 or L5 disc and usually affect the L5 or S1 nerve root, respectively (Kelsey et al, 1990). A frequently utilized clinical test of lower extremity motor function is performed by observing the patient walk on the tiptoes while observing for weakness of an ankle. This test has poor sensitivity, but when positive, specificity is high. Therefore, as a screen, it is an adequate test. However, a more sensitive way to assess the S1 motor nerve root is accomplished by observing the patient perform repetitive unilateral heel raises (tiptoe position) repeated five times. In this test, the patient stands on one foot and raises and lowers the heel while holding onto the wall to maintain balance. In an early stage of nerve damage or when weakness is subtle, the patient will usually perceive the weakness by the third to fifth repetition. This weakness also can usually be observable by the HCP. Similarly, repeating this in the opposite manner (repetitively raising the forefoot unilaterally times five repetitions) can facilitate assessment of an early L4/L5 weakness, or tibialis anterior motor paresis. When ankle dorsiflexion weakness occurs, it is common to find an extensor hallucis longus muscle weakness and/or sensory deficits (Blower, 1989).

It is necessary to memorize these tests is order to adequately test the presenting patient. Muscle testing is an art and must be performed to the point where the muscle is overpowered and then compared to the opposite side. When a difference in strength is detected, the two sides must be retested several times to verify the presence of weakness. Repetitive testing to fatigue the muscle facilitates localizing a subtle weakness. This testing must be performed bilaterally and each side compared to the other and repeated several times. Correlation with the history, such as pain and/or

CLINICAL TIP 13–2
Remembering Lower Extremity
Nerve Roots

An easy memorization technique of the lower extremity nerve roots can be accomplished as follows. **Rules:** Test consecutively each joint from proximal (hip) to distal (ankle) with forward movements (sagittal plane) counting consecutively upwards starting with L2/3 at the hip:

- Hip joint (flexion): L2/3
- Knee joint (extension): L3/4
- Ankle joint (dorsiflexion): L4/5
- Great toe (extension): L5
- Ankle joint (plantar flexion): S1/2

numbness extending to the lateral foot, should tip off the HCP that the S1 root must be carefully evaluated. Therefore, careful discriminative testing of the repetitive heel-raise test (5 repetitions) watching for qualitative loss of strength, compensatory movements, as well as the patient's own perception of weakness compared to the uninvolved side, adds clinical support to diagnosis of nerve root compression. Additional motor assessment includes the Achilles DTR in keeping with the above S1 example and sensibility testing of the S1/lateral distal calf and foot. If pain occurs simultaneous to the weakness, a breakaway weakness, or sudden giving up, is observed. When this occurs, true neurological loss cannot be accurately assessed without the help of an electromyogram/nerve conduction velocity (EMG/NCV) test. When breakaway weakness is observed and pain is denied, a suboptimum effort may have occurred. This may be indicative of fear-avoidance behavior such as the fear of pain, which is indicative of chronic pain behavior. Breakaway weakness without pain may also be indicative of malingering, or feigning. It is, however, very important not to jump to a conclusion of nonorganic pain if only one sign is present. As noted in Waddell et al's study (1980) and Main's "Point of View" (1997), **at least three nonorganic signs must be present before the assessment of nonorganic pain should be considered.** Refer to Chapter 16 for a detailed discussion of the Waddell Nonorganic Low Back Pain Signs.

The overall accuracy of neurological testing for disc lesions is "moderate." However, when neurological losses are found in combination and follow known neurological pathways, the reliability increases. For example, when a decreased ankle DTR and weak foot plantar flexion are present, it has been shown to have approximately a 90% sensitivity in patients with surgically proven disc herniation (Deyo et al, 1992). Similarly, surgical findings indicate that a positive straight leg raise in combination with abnormal neurological findings is reliably associated with disc herniation (Jonsson and Stromqvist, 1995).

Nerve root signs, or nerve tension signs, have been well represented in peer-reviewed literature, and may be one of the most studied of the low back provocative tests. In keeping with the diagnostic triage scheme of mechanical, nerve root, and red flag, the presence of nerve tension signs typically differentiates the mechanical from the nerve root and indicates a more serious situation. That is, conditions involving nerve root compression carry a surgical potential or have a higher prognostic risk of requiring an invasive surgical procedure than do conditions categorized as mechanical. A classic example of this is traction/compression on a nerve root such as the sciatic nerve from a herniated disk. Deyo and Tsiu-Wu (1987a) reported that the reliability of the history of sciatica carries a .95 and .88 sensitivity (true-positives) and specificity (true-negatives), respectively, for patients presenting with a herniated disk. Similarly, Deyo et al (1992) also reported that the occurrence of sciatic leg pain is considered to be high in patients with a disc lesion. The straight leg raise is typically positive for nerve root tension in the range of 15 to 30 degrees. When the straight leg raise exceeds 60 degrees, it becomes unreliable with regard to the presence of nerve tension (Kosteljanetz et al, 1984). When the straight leg raise provokes pain when performed on the asymptomatic side, sometimes referred to as the well leg raise test, it is highly specific (.90) but less sensitive (.25) for disc herniation (Hakelius and Hindmarsh, 1972; Spangfort, 1972; Deyo et al, 1992). The straight leg raise, well leg raise, and bowstring tests were found to be "potentially reliable" when assessing the sciatic nerve (McCombe et al, 1989). Similarly, the femoral nerve stretch test, sometimes referred to as Ely's test, performed by passive heel to buttock approximation of the prone patient, was also found to be "potentially reliable" (McCombe et al, 1989). Higher lumbar disc lesions are more rare. When present, symptoms may include low back pain, proximal leg pain such as anterior hip or thigh numbness (which is more prominent than calf symptoms), patellar DTR reduction, weakness of the hip flexors (psoas muscles) and/or quadriceps muscles, as well as hypesthesia of the anterior and lateral upper leg and, more rarely, medial foot.

The range of the straight leg raise test is not dependent on the size or position of the disc herniation (Thelander et al, 1992). More specifically, when patients were evaluated before nonoperative care, the straight leg raise was equally restricted in blunt versus sharply pointed herniated discs. After 3 months, the sharply pointed herniated discs were found to be associated with less pain. At 24 months, the straight leg raise tended to normalize, though a decrease in the herniated disc size over time, regardless of the shape, did not statistically correlate with a concomitant improvement in the straight leg raise. Because of this, Thelander et al (1992) speculate that additional factors such as inflammatory nerve root pain may be a significant participant in the radicular process, not just the mechanical pressure created by the herniated disc. In another study, the straight leg raise test was described as correlating with the severity of symptoms in lumbar disc herniation (Jonsson and Stromqvist, 1995). More specifically, a linear correlation was almost achieved when comparing the positive straight leg raise and pain at rest, at night, with coughing, and reduction of walking capacity. It was also noted that the regular use of analgesics was associated with more significantly reduced straight leg raises (< 30 degrees). In addition, a positive straight leg raising test in the early postoperative period correlated with inferior postsurgical outcomes (Table 13–5A–C) (Jonsson and Stromqvist, 1995).

Peripheral entrapment of the sciatic nerve by the adjacent piriformis muscle may occur and clinically mimic a nerve root lesion. An accurate differential diagnosis relies on a careful history and examination. More specifically, historical findings of this syndrome usually include little to no low back pain and buttock pain is the chief complaint in the absence of true sciatica. The physical examination reveals a positive straight leg raising test, and hip internal rotation results in a pain onset that occurs at a lower angle but reproduces primarily localized pain that rarely extends below the level of the knee. Pain is noted with resisted hip external rotation, the latter of which was found to be "potentially reliable" (McCombe et al, 1989) and palpation typically reveals a trigger point in the involved piriformis.

The neurological examination is typically negative, but caution is advised in assuming this since intervertebral disc syndrome and piriformis syndrome are often frequently concurrent disorders (Steiner et al, 1987). Table 13–6 reveals a summary of some of the most commonly used provocative and neurological tests associated with herniated disc, including their sensitivity, specificity, and associated reference(s) (Bigos et al, 1994).

CLAUDICATION: NEUROGENIC VERSUS VASCULAR

Differential diagnosis with other conditions that create leg pain, such as vascular disorders and spinal stenosis, must be considered as diagnostic possibilities. In spinal stenosis, the history often reveals an individual over 55 years old with a chronic history of low back pain and claudicating leg pain. A hallmark of spinal stenosis is the historical description of difficulty walking beyond a specific distance or time factor. After a brief rest, often 5 to 10 minutes, the patient describes the ability to walk again for a similar specified distance or time, and this process is ongoing. The spinal stenotic patient is usually most comfortable in flexion and

Table 13–5: Correlation of SLR Test Results With Preoperative and Postoperative Surgical Findings

A. RESULTS OF THE SLR TEST AS A PERCENTAGE OF EACH CATEGORY PREOPERATIVELY AND AT 4 MONTHS AND 1 YEAR POSTOPERATIVELY

		Postoperatively	
SLR test	Preoperatively	4 Months	1 Year
0–30 degrees	42%	1	0
30–60	26	6	9
60–90	18	15	9
Negative	14	78	82

B. PERCENT INCIDENCE OF PAIN RELATED TO THE PREOPERATIVE SLR TEST RESULTS

	Positive SLR			Negative SLR
SLR test	0–30	30–60	60–90	
Pain at rest	95%	79	77	71
Pain at night	89	74	50	47
Pain on coughing	82	68	58	62

C. PERCENT INCIDENCE OF PAIN RELATED TO POSTOPERATIVE SLR TEST RESULTS

	Positive SLR			Negative SLR
SLR test	0–30	30–60	60–90	
Pain at rest	100%	67	41	13
Pain at night	100	67	50	14
Pain on coughing	100	56	41	16

SLR, straight leg raise
Modified from Jonsson and Stromqvist, 1995.

Table 13–6: Estimated Accuracy of Physical Examination for Lumbar Disc Herniation Among Patients With Sciatica

REFERENCES	TEST	TRUE POSITIVE RATE (SENSITIVITY)	TRUE NEGATIVE RATE (SPECIFICITY)	COMMENTS
Hakelius and Hindmarsh (1972); Kosteljanetz et al 1984	Ipsilateral SLR	.80	.40	Positive result: leg pain at <60 degrees
Hakelius and Hindmarsh (1972); Spangfort (1972)	Crossed SLR	.25	.90	Positive result: reproduction of contralateral pain
Hakelius and Hindmarsh (1972)	Ankle dorsiflexion weakness	.35	.70	HNP usually at L4–L5 (80%)
Hakelius and Hindmarsh (1972); Kortelainen et al (1985)	Great toe extensor weakness	.50	.70	HNP usually at L5–S1 (60%) or L4–L5 (30%)
Hakelius and Hindmarsh (1972); Spanfort (1972)	Impaired ankle reflex	.50	.60	HNP usually at L5–S1; absent reflex increases specificity
Kortelainen et al (1985); Kosteljanetz et al (1984)	Sensory loss	.50	.50	Area of loss poor predictor of HNP level
Aronson and Dunsmore (1963)	Patellar reflex	.50	NA	For upper lumbar HNP only
Hakelius and Hindmarsh (1972)	Ankle plantar flexion weakness	.06	.95	
Hakelius and Hindmarsh (1972)	Quadriceps weakness	<.01	.99	

Note: Deyo, Rainville, and Kent (1992) calculated sensitivity and specificity. Values represent rounded averages where multiple references were available. All results are from surgical case series.
HNP, herniated nucleus pulposus; NA, not available; SLR, straight leg raising.
Reprinted with permission from Bigos et al, 1994.

worse in extension. Nerve tension signs are rarely present. In the early stages, the time and distance may vary considerably, making diagnosis by history difficult. The history may include the inability of the patient to walk more than one block or 5 minutes. In general, the shorter the time period or the distance tolerated by the patient, the worse the condition and, the condition is usually slowly progressive. The clinical examination of the claudicating patient must include a circulatory assessment in which the peripheral pulses (popliteal, dorsalis pedis, posterior tibial arteries) and capillary filling function are assessed, comparing left to right. When normal lower extremity pulses are present after walking to a point of claudication and a longer recovery time period is required for a reduction of lower extremity paresthesia, neurogenic claudication is favored over vascular claudication. It has been observed that cycling or walking are sensitive diagnostic tests. Also, reduced pain with increased walking or cycling time is noted when lumbar forward flexion is maintained (Dong and Porter, 1989). However, this test has not been found to be reliable in differentiating vascular from neurogenic claudication, although only a small patient sample of 19 subjects was used

(Dong and Porter, 1989). When neurogenic claudication is present, it has a 60% sensitivity for the diagnosis of spinal stenosis but the diagnostic specificity is probably higher "though not reported" (Dong and Porter, 1989).

CLINICAL UTILITY OF PHYSICAL PERFORMANCE TESTING

Moffroid (1994) reported that most low back pain patients are treated without adequate subclassifications. When the 53 National Institute of Occupational Safety and Health (NIOSH) low back pain tests were assessed, only 23 tests could successfully discriminate between subjects with low back pain and those without it. The seven strongest tests together had a sensitivity of 87% and specificity of 93%. These include tests that measure symmetry, strength, passive mobility, and dynamic mobility. Refer to Chapter 16 (Table 16–6) for a complete discussion of this study. These tests measure physical performance rather than pain provocation. This distinction is important as these tests assess strength and movement. Therefore, unlike provocative testing, these tests are not utilized to elicit a pain response but, rather, to assess functional losses or impairment. Because of the discriminative power of physical performance tests, perhaps this type of objective testing protocol should be adopted rather than the provocative tests more popularly utilized. Moreover, **these tests are favored in a case where the provocative tests are no longer pain reproducing but the patient still describes symptoms and dysfunction.** In this scenario, the comment "the subjective complaint is not supported by the objective findings" may result in claim closure. However, had physical performance tests been carried out, objective findings would very likely show some degree of functional loss. And, until that functional pathology is addressed in some form of active care program, resolution of the complaints is less likely. Therefore, **these types of tests work very well in the pre- and postrehabilitation setting when the functional losses can be addressed and then reassessed to determine the rehabilitation outcomes.**

IMPROVING THE CLINICAL UTILITY OF QUALITATIVE TESTING

Because some provocative and physical performance tests are prescriptively useful while others are less so, it seems appropriate to utilize those tests that yield information that can be utilized in the treatment decision making process. Many of these tests are qualitative, in that a specified measurement is not required such as timing a test, counting repetitions, or measuring motion. Therefore, qualitative tests are suboptimum for measuring outcomes compared to tests that yield quantitative results. However, some qualitative tests that are able to drive treatment decisions may also be quantified by measuring time (in seconds), movement (in degrees or percent of motion), or in endurance (repetitions). More specifically, the use of a stopwatch to measure the functional impairment, such as time duration to the onset of pain, allows for future comparison and, therefore, measures outcomes. For example, when performing a cervical flexion test (Janda, 1996a), a stopwatch can be utilized to document the time at which the supine, head flexed patient's chin protracts forward and/or the head drops downward, which can occur because of pain and/or cervical flexor muscle weakness. By timing the response, the HCP can acquire both qualitative information, identi-

fying a problem that demands a specific treatment prescription such as strengthening exercises, and quantitative information to allow for future comparison to determine if the treatment is helping the patient. Similarly, the shoulder abduction test, which is designed to offer the HCP important information regarding the coordination of scapulo-humeral rhythm, can be measured using a standard goniometer. More specifically, as the patient abducts the shoulder, the range of motion measurement is recorded at the point where the shoulder shrugs upwards (point of upper trapezius muscle contraction). An abnormal test is described as scapulo-humeral elevation prior to 60 degrees (Janda, 1996b).

These two examples change a previously qualitative test into a quantitative outcomes-oriented test (Hazard et al, 1996). Techniques such as this allow for mensuration and, therefore, quantification of an otherwise strictly qualitative test. Refer to other tests described elsewhere in this text and try to apply a quantitative approach when possible (Table 13–7). Of course, until all the criteria that make up a good test are properly evaluated (validity, reliability, responsiveness, practicality, safety), the issue of the sensitivity and specificity of improvised methods of mensuration described in Table 13–7 may be challenged. If, however, the measurement techniques appear to be useful clinically and "make sense," one can certainly argue that the test has face or content validity (Vernon, 1996; see Chap. 2). Also, if one finds the measuring method sensitive to detecting change over time (assessing outcomes), the responsiveness of the technique can be argued. Moreover, if all tests are excluded that lack randomized, double-blinded research backing, one would have to exclude most of the tests that are considered standard in the current physical examination approach of the patient. Also, it would not be possible to provide ideas for future study of examination methods or concepts that are clinically useful. Most importantly, not being able to improvise with techniques would remove the creativity or "art," which is the heart and soul of diagnosis and treatment.

The tests found in Tables 13–6 and 13–7 are by no means meant to represent a complete list of tests that can be quantified or drive treatment decisions. The point is that all tests should be looked at from a quantitative and prescriptive standpoint so that useful information can be obtained when performing provocative and/or physical performance tests. Since some of the above tests may not be familiar to all readers, a description of each test is offered (Table 13–8).

Table 13–7: Measurement Options and Treatment Options for Qualitative Tests

TEST	MEASUREMENT	PRESCRIPTION
Standing tests		
1. Lunge coordination test	**Reps:** count to point of fatigue—trunk flexion or inability to reach 90 degrees of knee flexion or back knee fails to reach floor	Lunges (both on & off balance board). Wall/ball squats.
2. Extension in standing	**Inclinometer:** Measure ROM at point of lateral shift or peripheralization or centralization of radicular symptoms	Extension exercise protocols (if centralization or extension bias).
3. Flexion in standing	**Inclinometer:** Measure ROM at point of lateral shift or peripheralization or centralization of radicular symptoms	Flexion exercise protocols (if centralization or flexion bias).
4. Repeated extension in standing	**Reps:** count to point of lateral shift or peripheralization or centralization of radicular symptoms	Extension exercise protocols (if centralization or extension bias).
5. Repeated flexion in standing	**Reps:** count to point of lateral shift or peripheralization or centralization of radicular symptoms	Flexion exercise protocols (if centralization or flexion bias).
6. Sustained extension in standing	**Time:** count seconds to point of lateral shift or peripheralization or centralization of radicular symptoms (max. 30 sec.)	Extension exercise protocols (if centralization or extension bias).
7. Sustained flexion in standing	**Time:** count seconds to point of lateral shift or peripheralization or centralization of radicular symptoms (max. 30 sec.)	Flexion exercise protocols (if centralization or flexion bias).
Sitting tests		
8. Thoracolumbar rotation	**Goniometer:** measure angle of the shoulders to the frontal plane of the seated patient	Active and passive stretching into restricted side of ROM. Manipulation of fixated segments or mobilization into restricted side of ROM.
9. Shoulder abduction coordination test	**Goniometer or inclinometer:** measure angle shoulder abduction when scapula elevation or lateral rotation occurs **(and/or)** **Dynamic EMG:** measures the point of upper trapezius muscle activity (couple with ROM)	Techniques to inhibit upper trapezius muscle contraction [manual resistance techniques (MRTs), myofascial release, spray and stretch, manipulation and/or mobilization, etc]. Scapulo-thoracic mobilization.
Supine tests		
10. Hip adduction	**Goniometer:** Measure angle hip adduction with knee flexion and extension	Active, passive, resistive, stretching of adductors.
11. Trunk flexion coordination/strength test (Measure ONLY if unable to complete 1 rep; use repetitive sit-up test if able to perform 1 or more reps— see QFCE regarding repetitive sit-up test)	**Tape measure:** measure vertical distance from T1 spinous process to table/floor **(and/or)** **Inclinometer:** place in sagittal plane on sternum and measure angle **(and/or)** **Dynamic EMG:** measure point of maximum contract and measure with an inclinometer if unable to do one rep.	Abdominal strengthening. Pelvic stabilization. (Utilize both floor and gym ball methods to enhance coordination and sensory-motor training.)

Table 13–7: (cont.)

TEST	MEASUREMENT	PRESCRIPTION
12. Head/Neck flexion coordination test	**Time:** count in seconds the time prior to chin poking or dropping of head back **(and/or)** **Pressure gauge:** Inflate BP cuff to 30 mm Hg, place behind head, pre-position chin-tucked head and count in seconds the point where head falls back and pressure increases.	Deep anterior neck flexor muscle strengthening exercises: Isometric, isotonic, isokinetic. Inhibit tight SCM's.
Sidelying test 13. Hip abduction coordination test	**Goniometer or inclinometer:** measure angle of hip abduction when hip hiking, pelvis rotation, hip external rotation (ER), or hip flexion occurs	MRT's: Facilitate involved synergists; inhibit involved antagonists; (consider: over-active QL if hip hiking; weak Gme if difficulty abducting or pelvic rotation; overactive piriformis if ER occurs or tight TFL if hip flexion occurs)
Prone tests 14. Hip extension coordination test	**Dynamic EMG:** electrodes placed on the Gma, (H), and QL, bilaterally. Determine firing sequence: Gma and H 1st, contralateral QL 2nd, homolateral QL 3rd.	Facilitation techniques to the GM. Inhibition to the TFL, iliopsoas, QL, piriformis &/or hamstrings. Lower kinetic chain assessment & correction: subtalar instability (gait analysis); tight gastrocnemius soleus muscles; lower extremity joint impairments.
15. Repeated extension in lying	**Reps:** count reps to point of lateral shift or peripheralization or centralization of radicular symptoms (max. 30 sec.)	Extension exercise protocols (if centralization or extension bias).
16. Sustained extension in lying (Prone press-up)	**Time:** count seconds to point of lateral shift or peripheralization or centralization of radicular symptoms (max. 30 sec.)	Extension exercise protocols (if centralization or extension bias).

ER, external rotation; Gma, gluteus maximus; Gme, gluteus medius; H, hamstrings; max., maximum; MRT's, manual release techniques; QL, quadratus lumborum; TFL, tensor fascia lata; Reps, repetitions.

Cibulka MT, Delitto A, Koldehoff RM. Changes in innominate tilt after manipulation of the sacroiliac joint in patients with low back pain: An experimental study. *Phys Ther.* 1988;68:1359–1363.

Cipriano JJ. *Photographic Manual of Regional Orthopaedic and Neurological Tests.* 2nd ed. Baltimore, Md: Williams & Wilkins; 1991.

Coste J, Delecoeuillerie G, Cohen de Lara A, Le Parc JM, Paolaggi JB. Clinical course and prognostic factors in acute low back pain: An inception cohort study in primary care practice. *Br Med J.* 1994;308:577–580.

Delitto A, Cibulka MT, Erhard RE, et al. Evidence for use of an extension-mobilization category in acute low back syndrome: A prescriptive validation pilot study. *Phys Ther.* 1993;73:216–228.

Delitto A, Shulman AD, Rose SL, et al. Reliability of a clinical examination to classify patients with low back syndrome. *Phys Ther Practice.* 1992:1:1–9.

Deyo RA, Haselkorn J, Hoffman R, Kent DL. Designing studies of diagnostic tests for low back pain or radiculopathy. *Spine.* 1994;19:2057S–2065S.

Deyo RA, Rainville J, Kent DL. What can the history and physical examination tell us about low back pain? *JAMA.* 1992;268(6):760–765.

Deyo RA, Tsui-Wu YJ. Descriptive epidemiology of low-back pain and its related medical care in the United States. *Spine.* 1987a;12(3):264–268.

Deyo RA, Tsui-Wu YJ. Functional disability due to back pain: A population based study indicating the importance of socioeconomic factors. *Arthritis Rheum.* 1987b;30:1247–1253.

Donelson R, Aprill C, Medcalf R, Grant W. A prospective study of centralization of lumbar and referred pain. *Spine.* 1997;22:1115–1122.

Dong GX, Porter RW. Walking and cycling tests in neurogenic and intermittent claudication. *Spine.* 1989;14:965–969.

Dreyfuss P, Michaelsen M, Pauza K, McLarty J, Bogduk N. The value of medical history and physical examination in diagnosing sacroiliac joint pain. *Spine.* 1996;21:2594–2602.

Edgar D, Jull G, Sutton S. The relationship between upper trapezius muscle length and upper quadrant neural tissue extensibility. *Aust J Physiother.* 1994;40:99–103.

Edwards RHT, McDonnell M. Hand-held dynamometer for evaluating voluntary muscle function. *Lancet.* 1974;2:757–758.

Ekstrand J, Gillquist J. The frequency of muscle tightness and injuries in soccer players. *Am J Sp Med.* 1982;10:75–78.

Elvey R. The investigation of arm pain. In: Grieve G (ed): Modern manual therapy of the vertebral column. Edinburgh: Churchill Livingstone, pp. 530–535.

Evans RC. *Illustrated Essentials in Orthopedic Physical Assessment.* St. Louis, Mo: Mosby-Year Book; 1994.

Fager CA. The age old back problem: New fad, same fallacies. *Spine.* 1984;9:326–328.

Gatchel RJ, Mayer TG, Capra P, Diamond P, Barnett J. Quantification of lumbar function. Part 6: The use of psychological measures in guiding physical functional restoration. *Spine.* 1986;11:36–42.

Gatchel RJ, Polatin PB, Kinney R. Predicting outcome of chronic back pain using clinical predictors of psychopathology: a prospective analysis. *Health Psychology.* 1995;14:415–420.

Hakelius A, Hindmarsh J. The comparative reliability of preoperative diagnostic methods in lumbar disc surgery. *Acta Orthop Scand.* 1972;43:234–238.

Haldeman S, Chapman-Smith D, Peterson DM Jr. *Guidelines for Chiropractic Quality Assurance and Practice Parameters.* Gaithersburg, Md: Aspen; 1993.

Hanley EN. Lumbar spine fusion: Matching expectations and outcomes. *AAOS Bull.* 1993;April:6–7.

Harms-Ringdahl K, Ekholm J, Schuldt K, Nemeth G, Arborelius UP. Load moments and myoelectric activity when the cervical spine is held in full flexion and extension. *Clin Biomech.* 1988;3:129–136.

Harvey D, Byfield D. Preliminary studies with a mechanical model for the evaluation of spinal motion palpation. *Clin Biomech.* 1991;6:79–82.

Hazard RG, Haugh LD, Reid S, Preble JB, MacDonald L. Early prediction of chronic disability after occupational low back injury. *Spine.* 1996;21:945–951.

Herzog W, Read LJ, Conway PJW, Shaw LD, McEwen MC. Reliability of motion palpation procedures to detect sacroiliac joint fixations. *J Manipulative Physiol Ther.* 1989;12:86–92.

Hyde SA, Scott OM, Goddard CM. Myometer: Development of a clinical tool. *Physiotherapy.* 1983;69:424–427.

Jackson RP. The facet syndrome: myth or reality? *Clin Orthop.* 1992;279:110–121.

Janda V. Evaluation of muscular imbalance. In: Liebenson C, ed. *Rehabilitation of the Spine: A Practitioner's Manual.* Philadelphia, Pa: Williams & Wilkins; 1996a:102,106 (Chin flexion test).

Janda V. Evaluation of muscular imbalance. In: Liebenson C, ed. *Rehabilitation of the Spine: A Practitioner's Manual.* Philadelphia, Pa: Williams & Wilkins; 1996b:102,107 (Shoulder abduction test).

Jonsson B, Stromqvist B. The straight leg raise test and the severity of symptoms in lumbar disk herniation. *Spine*. 1995;20:27–30.

Keating J Jr. Interexaminer reliability of motion palpation of the lumbar spine: A review of quantitative literature. *Am J Chiropractic Med*. 1989;2:107–110.

Keating JC, Bergmann TF, Jacobs GE, Finer BA, Larson K. Interexaminer reliability of eight evaluative dimensions of lumbar segmental abnormality. *J Manipulative Physiol Ther*. 1990;13:463–470.

Kelsey JL, Golden AL, Mundt DJ. Low back pain/prolapsed lumbar intervertebral disc. *Rheum Dis Clin North Am*. 1990;16:699–712.

Kenny WR III. Development and comparison of electrical strain dynamometer and cable tensiometer for objective muscle testing. *Arch Phys Med Rehabil*. 1965;46:793–803.

Kohlmann TH, Raspe HH. Die patientennahe Diagnostik von Funktionseinschrankungen im Alltag. *Psychomed*. 1994;6:21–27.

Korbon GA, DeGood E, Schroeder ME, et al. The development of a somatic amplification rating scale for low-back pain. *Spine*. 1987;12(8):787–791.

Kortelainen P, Puranen J, Koivisto E, Lahde S. Symptoms and signs of sciatica and their relation to the localization of the lumbar disc herniation. *Spine*. 1985;10:88–92.

Kosteljanetz M, Expersen JO, Halaburt H, Miletic T. Predictive value of clinical and surgical findings in patients with lumbago-sciatica. A prospective study (Part I). *Acta Neurochir (Wien)*. 1984;73(1–2):67–76.

Leboeuf C, Gardner V. Chronic low back pain: Orthopaedic and chiropractic test results. *J Am Chiro Assoc*. 1989a;19:9–15.

Leboeuf C, Gardner V, Carter A, Scott TA. Chiropractic examination procedures: A reliability and consistency study. *J Aust Chiro Assoc*. 1989b;19:101–104 (SI tests).

Lippitt AB. The facet joint and its role in spinal pain: Management with facet joint injections. *Spine*. 1984;9:746–750.

Main C. Point of view. *Spine*. 1997;22:303–304.

Maitland GD. Vertebral manipulation, 2nd ed. London: Butterworths; 1977:65–67.

Mayer TG, Gatchel RJ, Keeley J, Mayer H, Richling D. A male incumbent worker industrial data base. *Spine*. 1994;19:755–761.

Mayer TG, Gatchel RJ, Kishino N, et al. Objective assessment of spine function following industrial injury: A prospective study with comparison group and one-year follow-up. *Spine*. 1985;10:482–493.

Mazion JM. *Illustrated Manual of Neurological and Orthopedic Tests for Office Procedures*. 2nd ed. Orlando, Fla: Daniels Publishing Co; 1980.

McCarthy KA. Improving the clinician's use of orthopedic testing: An application to low back pain. *Top Clin Chiro*. 1994;1:42–50.

McCombe PF, Fairbank CT, Cockersole BC, Pynsent PB. Reproducibility of physical signs in low-back pain. *Spine*. 1989;14:908–918.

McKenzie RA. *Mechanical Diagnosis and Therapy of the Lumbar Spine*. Waikanae, New Zealand: Spinal Publications; 1981.

Michel A, Kohlmann T, Raspe H. The association between clinical findings on physical examination and self-reported severity in back pain. *Spine*. 1997;22:296–304.

Moffroid MT. Distinguishable groups of musculoskeletal low back pain patients and asymptomatic control subjects based on physical measures of the NIOSH Low Back Atlas. *Spine*. 1994;19(12):1350–1358.

Mooney V. Facet syndrome. In: Winstein J, Wiesel S, eds. *The Lumbar Spine*. Philadelphia, Pa: Saunders; 1990.

Nachemson AL. Fusion for low back pain and sciatica. *Acta Orthop Scand*. 1985;56:285–286.

Nelson MA. The identification of back pain syndromes. In: Hulkins DW, Hullholland RC, eds. *Back Pain, Methods for Clinical Investigation and Assessment*. Manchester, England: Manchester University Press; 1986:13–15.

Polatin PB, Kinney RK, Gatchel RJ, Lillo E, Mayer TG. Psychiatric illness and chronic low back pain: The mind and the spine: Which goes first? *Spine*. 1993;18:66–71.

Porter RW, Trailescu IF. Diurnal changes in straight leg raising. *Spine*. 1990;15:103–106.

Refshauge K, Goodsell M, Lee M. Consistency of cervical and cervicothoracic posture in standing. *Aust J Physiother*. 1994;40:235–240.

Sandmark H, Nisell R. Validity of five common manual neck pain provoking tests. *Scand J Rehab Med*. 1995;27:131–136.

Schuldt K, Harms-Ringdahl. Cervical spine position vs. e.m.g. activity in neck muscles during maximum isometric neck extension. *Clin Biomech*. 1988a;3:129–136.

Schuldt K, Harms-Ringdahl K. EMG/moment relationships in neck muscles during isometric cervical spine extension. *Clin Biomech*. 1988b;3:58–65.

Spangfort EV. The lumbar disc herniation. *Acta Orth Scand.* 1972;142(suppl):1–95.

Spitteri MA, Clark SW, Cook DG. Reliability of eliciting physical signs in examination of the chest. *Lancet.* 1988;1:873–875.

Spitzer WO, Le Blanc FE, Dupuis M, et al. Scientific approach to the assessment and management of activity-related spinal disorders: A monograph for clinicians. Report of the Quebec Task Force on Spinal Disorders. *Spine.* 1987;12(suppl 7):S1–S59.

Steiner C, Staubs C, Ganon M, Buhlinger C. Piriformis syndrome: Pathogenesis, diagnosis and treatment. *J Am Osteopathic Assoc.* 1987:318–323.

Strender LE, Lundin M, Nell K. Interexaminer reliability in physical examination of the neck. *J Manipulative Physiol Ther.* 1997a;20:516–520.

Strender LE, Sjoblom A, Sundell K, Ludwig R, Taube A. Interexaminer reliability in physical examination of patients with low back pain. *Spine.* 1997b;22:814–820.

Thelander U, Fagerlund M, Friberg S, Larsson S. Straight leg raising test versus radiologic size, shape, and position of lumbar disc hernias. *Spine.* 1992;17:395–399.

Troup JDG. Straight-leg raising (SLR) and the qualifying tests for increased root tension. *Spine.* 1981;6:526–527.

Vernon H. Pain and disability questionnaires in chiropractic rehabilitation. In: Liebenson C, ed. *Rehabilitation of the Spine: A Practitioner's Manual.* Philadelphia, Pa: Williams & Wilkins; 1996:60.

Vernon HT, Aker P, Aramenko M, Battershill D, Alepin A, Penner T. Evaluation of neck strength with a modified sphygmomanometer dynamometer: Reliability and validity. *J Manipulative Physiol Ther.* 1992;15:343–349.

Von Korff M, Deyo RA, Cherkin D, Barlow W. Back pain in primary care: Outcomes at 1 year. *Spine.* 1993;18:855–862.

Von Korff M, Ormel J, Keefe F, Dworkin SF. Grading the severity of chronic pain. *Pain.* 1992;50:133–149.

Wachter KC, Kaeser HE, Guhring H, Ettlin TM, Mennet P, Muller W. Muscle damping measured with a modified pendulum test in patients with fibromyalgia, lumbago, and cervical syndrome. *Spine.* 1996;21:2137–2142.

Waddell G, Feder G, McIntosh A, Lewis M, Hutchinson A. Low back pain evidence review. London, England: Royal College of General Practitioners; 1996.

Waddell G, Main C, Morris E, et al. Normality and reliability in the clinical assessment of backache. *Br Med J.* 1982;284:1519–1523.

Waddell G, McCulloch JA, Kummel E, Venner RM. Nonorganic physical signs in low-back pain. *Spine.* 1980;5:117–125.

Watson DH, Trott PH. Cervical headache: An investigation of natural head posture and upper cervical flexor muscle performance. *Cephalgia.* 1993;13:272–284.

Wolfe F, Smythe HA, Yunnus MB, et al. The American College of Rheumatology 1990 criteria for classification of fibromyalgia. *Arthritis Rheum.* 1990;33:160–172.

Yaxley GA, Jull G. Adverse tension in the neural system. A preliminary study of tennis elbow. *Aust J Physiother.* 1993;39:15–22.

Youdas JW, Grant TR, Suman VJ, Bogard CL, Hallman HO, Carey JR. Normal range of motion of the cervical spine. An initial goniometric study. *Phys Ther.* 1992;72:770–780.

CHAPTER 14

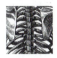

Spinal Range of Motion:
Is This a Valid Form
of Outcomes Assessment?

STEVEN G. YEOMANS

INTRODUCTION

Range of motion (ROM) assessment has long been considered a standard procedure included in a physical examination of patients presenting with orthopedic-related problems. **The importance of performing an accurate assessment of ROM is emphasized by the fact that it is often utilized in the process of rating permanent impairment at a point of plateau in healing, short of full resolution.** This chapter includes a review of the literature as it relates to normative data, impairment rating, a review of various methods of assessing ROM, and the use of ROM to discriminate between those with and those without low back pain. The proper use of inclinometers and a list of many variables that should be appreciated when using inclinometry is included.

In the assessment of mobility, a variety of methods are available. Probably the *least* valid but, paradoxically, the *most* utilized approach is that of visual estimation, perhaps because it demands the least amount of work. In this approach, the health care provider (HCP) simply watches the patient move through the range and records an estimated ROM based on a visual estimation. Because of its poor reliability and validity (Youdas et al, 1991), the visual estimation method should not be used as an objective outcome assessment tool.

RANGE OF MOTION EXAMINATION AS A PROVOCATIVE TEST

SUBJECTIVE

If one were to utilize ROM assessment only as a pain-generating test or as a screen, visual estimation might be adequate. More specifically, the ROM examination often prompts a response from the patient (ie, subjective) regarding pain associated with certain movements, which can then be specifically located and quantified by grading it on a numerical scale such as 0–4, 0–10, and so on. The astute evaluator will also pay attention to the *quality* of movement and report additional information such as "sharp pain graded at 3/4 @ 20; motion very slow and cautious; unable to reverse the lumbar lordosis." This type of reporting "tells a story" rather than just reporting a number that represents the ROM.

OBJECTIVE

In addition to having the patient grade his or her pain subjectively, the HCP can also grade the patient's pain behavior "objectively" and quantify it based on a modification of a palpation pain scale described by Wolfe in assessment of fibromyalgic patients (Wolfe et al, 1990). This scale, in its original form, is described in greater detail in Chapter 13 (see Table 13–1). In this modification of the objective pain grading scale, the evaluator assigns one of the following grades:

- Grade 0: No pain behavior and no pain reported when verbally prompted
- Grade I: Mild pain behavior noticed by observation, and when verbally asked
- Grade II: Moderate pain behavior with observable grimace and/or flinch, and verbal expression of pain may occur without prompting
- Grade III: Severe response with compensatory movement or list, withdrawal, flinch, prompt cessation of movement, usually with a verbal expression of pain
- Grade IV: Severe response with withdrawal to a nonnoxious stimulus (nonorganic pain behavior); this may include fear-avoidance behavior and/or exaggerated responses both verbally and visually observed

The ideal approach to examination and documentation is to evaluate both the actual ROM using dual inclinometry and the pain grade from the patient's as well as the HCP's perspective. By including all three approaches, a subjective assessment of the patient's perception of pain coupled with an objective evaluation of the patient's pain behavior and a quantitative determination of the ROM yields very useful information that can help the HCP monitor the treatment effects (ie, track outcomes).

CERVICAL SPINE

METHODS OF MENSURATION

Various techniques of measuring the active ROM of the cervical spine have been introduced by many researchers through the years. A partial list of these techniques includes the following:

- Electrogoniometers (Alund and Larsson, 1990)
- Bubble goniometers (Buck et al, 1959; Bennett et al, 1963)
- Protractors (Kittke and Blanchard, 1953; Ferlic, 1962)
- Radiographs (Mayer et al, 1984; Lind et al, 1989; Mimura et al, 1989; Penning, 1990; Portek et al, 1993)
- Hydrogoniometers (O'Driscoll and Tomenson, 1982)
- Magnetic compasses (Lind et al, 1989; Alund and Larsson, 1990; Youdas et al, 1991, 1992; Nilsson et al, 1996a, 1996b)
- Computed tomography (Penning and Wilmink, 1987)

With the exception of Ferlic (1962), Lind et al (1989), and O'Driscoll and Tomenson (1982), most researchers used small subject samples of the same gender or with narrow ranges of age (Leighton, 1956; Buck et al, 1959; Bennett et al, 1963; Defibaugh, 1964; Penning and Wilmink, 1987; Mimura et al, 1989). Similarly, many reported the range of motion as the total excursion or global movement in one plane rather than starting at a neutral "0" position. Thus, there was no separation of flexion from extension in the sagittal plane and right from left rotation and lateral flexion in the frontal and transverse planes, respectively (Ferlic, 1962; Defibaugh, 1964; O'Driscoll and Tomenson, 1982; Penning and Wilmink, 1987; Lind et al, 1989; Mimura et al, 1989; Alund and Larsson, 1990). As a result, comparing data between the various studies is difficult due to the different approaches and equipment utilized in prior studies.

Inclinometry

The use of the gravity-dependent goniometer is not a recently discovered technique (Leighton, 1956; Defibaugh, 1964; Loebl, 1967). However, the use of inclinometry did not gain popularity until the late 1980s and early 1990s, at which time the third edition of the AMA *Guides to the Evaluation of Permanent Impairment* (hereafter referred to as the AMA *Guides*) (Engelberg, 1988) recommended that impairment ratings based on the ROM model utilize inclinometry rather than the previously accepted two-arm goniometer. Further, HCPs were given until 1990 to acquire the skills needed to utilize inclinometry and, after that date, any impairment rating using the inclinometer method would be favored over a rating not utilizing inclinometry. The gravity-dependent goniometer is utilized to measure cervical sagittal (flexion-extension) and frontal plane (lateral flexion) active ROMs, usually with the patient seated. A chair with a firm, upright back works well to stabilize the trunk. It is also easier to manually control and read the inclinometers with the patient seated. The inclinometer can be used to measure rotation or transverse plane active ROM by laying the patient supine so that the pendulum can swing freely. Refer to Chapter 16, Figure 16–2, for illustration of the cervical ROM inclinometer evaluation. The following text offers an explanation of the proper technique.

Flexion/Extension—Cervical Spine

1. One inclinometer is placed so that a line drawn at the T1 spinous process (SP) is straddled by the midline of the inclinometer.
2. A second inclinometer is placed at the midpoint of the convex calvarium. **Care must be taken not to place the T1 inclinometer too high as it may collide with the posterior occiput or the cranial incli-** nometer when measuring cervical extension. Hence, the inclinometer can be moved laterally from the T1 SP to avoid inclinometer displacement.
3. The inclinometers are then set to "0" and the patient is asked to flex the head/neck forward, while holding the lumbar and thoracic spine firmly against the back of a straight-backed chair. This may be preceded by warm-up stretching by completing 5 repetitions prior to the tested repetition (Mayer et al, 1994). If the AMA *Guides* are being used, following the specific protocol is necessary where the highest of three consecutive trials that fall within 5 degrees or 10% of the average of the three trials is recommended (Engelberg, 1988). The inclinometers are then carefully read and the result reported after subtracting the T1 from the cranial inclinometric measurement to obtain the true cervical flexion angle.
4. The patient then returns to the neutral position to either repeat this process three times (AMA *Guides* approach) or prepares for the measurement of cervical extension.

Lateral Flexion—Cervical Spine

1. The inclinometers are next placed in the frontal plane so that the base lines up with the line drawn at the T1 SP and the other at the vertex of the calvarium. The T1 inclinometer must be held vertically and not pressed flush against the back, so that the gravity-dependent pendulum swings freely.
2. After positioning the two inclinometers so that the needle is hanging on the "0" mark, the patient laterally flexes to one side keeping the thoracolumbar spine against the chair.

CLINICAL TIP 14–1
Securing the Inclinometer

If the base of the inclinometer is unusually long or flat, less accurate readings are likely due to the "rocking" or wobbling effects that can occur. Therefore, extra care must be practiced to keep the inclinometer in a secure, stable position; for example, by cupping the palmar surface of the hand and placing the thenar and hypothenar pads on the convex spine or occiput while holding the inclinometer between the thumb and index fingers. If using the ROM as an outcome assessment device, it may be best to place the caudal inclinometer onto a flat area of the upper thoracic spine, below the C7/T1 junction to avoid the rocking effect that can occur at this transitional motor unit. When this is done, accurately report the upper end of the inclinometer with the specific spinous process (such as, "cephalad end of T1 inclinometer at T2") so that exact inclinometer placement can be reproduced at the time of the next reexamination.

CLINICAL TIP 14–2
"Re-zeroing" the Inclinometer

Although it is not mentioned specifically in the *Guides* or in Mayer et al's article (1994), **do not** re-zero the inclinometers when returning to neutral after each repetition of flexion prior to assessing extension. Failure to return to the exact same starting point will result in an altered measurement than that which is truly present. This is especially important when repeating each movement three times. Also, if the inclinometers are not re-zeroed when assessing sagittal plane motion, the results of flexion and extension can be added together and compared to normative data reported in global motion in sagittal plane or data that did not utilize a neutral starting point. The latter appear, by literature review, to be more valid and reliable than breaking up flexion/extension into two separate movements.

Table 14–2: Normative Data for Cervical Spine ROM According to Various Sources

	AMA *GUIDES* (1993)	LIND (1989)[a] (X-RAY)	MAYER ET AL (1984, 1994) Male	YOUDAS ET AL (1992) (DEGREE CHANGE/ DECADE)	YOUDAS ET AL (1992) (MEAN RANGE[b]) Male	Female
Flexion	50°	—	50°	3°	64.0–36.4°	
Extension	60°	—	63°	5°	85.6–52.3°	85.6–50.3°
Right lateral flexion	45°	45°	45°	3°	44.9–22.2°	48.9–22.6°
Left lateral flexion	45°	45°	45°	3°	46.3–22.0°	46.6–22.6°
Right rotation	80°	71°	85°	3°	74.1–44.2°	74.9–51.8°
Left rotation	80°	71°	85°	4°	72.3–45.2°	71.6–50.5°

[a] Rotation measurement utilized a compass, by radiography; flexion and extension were combined when measured. No gender difference.
[b] Mean figures and the range in ROM due to age variances are reported for males and females utilizing the CROM instrument.

published. This method parallels the technique recommended and described in the AMA *Guides* (Doege, 1993). Because data was broken down by age (35 to 54 years old), gender, and also by work class (blue vs white collar), the normative data can be used and is preferred over data that is not segregated by these factors (see Table 14–4).

FACTORS AFFECTING RANGE OF MOTION MENSURATION

Cervical Range of Motion: Active versus Passive Assessment

There is a significant difference when assessing active versus passive ROM. More specifically, **passsive ROM tends to be less reliable than active ROM because the examiner determines the endpoint based on end-feel, whereas active ROM relies only on the examiner reading the goniometer** (Nilsson et al, 1996a). Intra- and inter-examiner reliability

of measuring active ROM have been reported (Kadir et al, 1981; Tucci et al, 1986; Zachman et al, 1989; Alund and Larsson, 1990; Capuano-Pucci et al, 1991; Mior et al, 1991; Youdas et al, 1991; Rheault et al, 1992), but only a few studies are available that utilized passive ROM (Dvorak et al, 1992; Wong and Nansel, 1992; Nilsson, 1995; Nilsson et al, 1996b). In two of these studies, only the assessment of global planar motion was found to be interexaminer reliable (Nilsson et al, 1996a; Dvorak et al, 1992). Utilizing a CROM device, Nilsson et al (1996a) found that assessing six separate directions from a neutral zero was less acceptable (Pearson's r = .39–.70) versus global measurements (r = .61–.88). Similarly, utilizing a CA 6000 Spine Motion Analyzer (from Orthopaedic Systems Inc., Hayward CA), Dvorak et al (1992) found reliability acceptable measuring global passive ROM assessments in the three planes (r = .64–.85).

In the initial study, Nilsson (1995) indicated that they were unable to determine if the reason for poor inter-

Table 14–3: Normative Data for Lumbar Spine ROM According to Various Sources

	AMA *GUIDES* (1993)	HASTEN[a] (1995) Male	Female	KEELEY ET AL (1986) Male	Female	MAYER ET AL (1994) Male	MAYER ET AL (1984) Both
Flexion	60°	48.3°	44.1°	65.0° ± 8.2°	64.4° ± 8.2°	65°	55° ± 9.2°
Extension	25°	22.2°	24.3°	26.6° ± 10.8°	27.3° ± 8.5°	30°	27° ± 12.8°
Right lateral flexion	25°	14.9°	17.9°	—	—	25°	—
Left lateral flexion	25°	15.5°	17.8°	—	—	25°	—
Right rotation	—	—	—	10.4° ± 3.14[ob]	—	—	—
Left rotation	—	—	—	10.6° ± 3.03[ob]	—	—	—

[a] Hasten et al assessed healthy subjects (16 males, 18 females), 17 to 35 years in age, mean 22.8 years (±4.9).
[b] Not clinically significant due to method utilized.

> ! **CLINICAL ALERT 14–4**
>
> **Caution!** Compare data only if the same assessment method was utilized as that reported.

examiner reliability was caused by the relative inexperience of one of the examiners or some inherent problem in measuring passive ROM. Nilsson's second study (1996a) allowed for two examiners to become familiar with the CROM device prior to assessing 35 asymptomatic volunteers (17 men, 18 women, aged 20 to 28 years). Despite this, results only met acceptable inter-rater reliability when global planar passive ROM was assessed. However, this follow-up study found the less optimum interexaminer reliability for global passive ROM in the earlier study (Nilsson, 1995) to be caused by examiner inexperience. **Nilsson stresses the importance of inter-examiner reliability over that of intra-examiner reliability as normative data from a procedure can only be of value if it can be reliably shared between HCPs.**

Effects of Aging and Gender on Range of Motion Assessment

Many researchers have studied the effects of age and gender, reporting that women, in general, are more flexible than men and that a linear decrease in ROM occurs as age advances (Schoening and Hannan, 1964; Youdas et al, 1991, 1992; Dvorak et al, 1992; Good and Michelson, 1992; Kulman, 1993; and others). More specifically, Nilsson et al (1996b) reported normative data of cervical passive ROM based on age and gender using the CROM device. They reported that women, in general, are more flexible than men after age 40, but men are more flexible between the ages of 20 and 40 years, except for lateral flexion, where men are more flexible regardless of age. Statistically significant differences were found between the two genders, as a decreased passive ROM with age was reported.

Lind et al (1989) reported similar results utilizing digitized x-rays in the frontal and sagittal planes in a group of 35 men and 35 women, segregated in age by decade. More specifically, sagittal, frontal, and axial ROM decreased with age. However, the decrease did not become statistically significant ($P < .01$) until the third decade. This study also indicates that extension contributed the greatest to the loss of sagittal plane motion.

The cervical ROM in elderly subjects was compared to that in younger subjects to establish normative cervical ROM values for the elderly (Kuhlmann, 1993). A breakdown in data was offered by gender, and two groups of subjects, the first of which included 42 subjects (17 men, 25 women) between the ages of 70 and 90 years. The second group of 31 subjects (16 men, 15 women) included the younger subjects aged between 20 and 30 years. Instrumentation included a single, gravity-dependent inclinometer magnetically attached to an adjustable head halter with chinstraps. The metal platform to which the inclinometer was attached allowed for three planes to be assessed, including sagittal, frontal, and transverse for flexion-extension, lateral flexion, and rotation, respectively. The results revealed a significantly reduced ROM as age increased ($P < .001$) in all six movements, with the following data reported:

- 12% less flexion
- 32% less extension
- 22% less lateral flexion
- 25% less rotation

Women were reported to have a greater cervical ROM than men in both groups studied. The variability in the range of movement was significantly higher in the elderly group, with exception of cervical flexion in females, and the standard deviation was correspondingly higher in five of the six motions. The difference in mean ROM values for cervical extension was significant between women and men in the younger group ($P < .001$), but not in the elderly

Table 14–4: Normative Data of Cervical Rotation[a]

| AGE (YRS) | MALES (N = 242) | | | | | | FEMALES (N = 233) | | | | | |
| | Blue Collar | | White Collar | | All | | Blue Collar | | White Collar | | All | |
	x	SD	x	SD	x	SD	x	SD	x	SD	x	SD
35–39	77°	7°	78°	6°	77°	6°	77°	6°	78°	8°	77°	7°
40–44	75°	9°	75°	7°	75°	9°	75°	8°	73°	7°	74°	8°
45–49	71°	12°	77°	4°	73°	10°	74°	9°	75°	7°	74°	8°
50–54	72°	7°	74°	7°	72°	7°	67°	9°	74°	7°	68°	9°
35–54	74°	9°	76°	6°	75°	8°	73°	9°	75°	7°	74°	8°

[a] The normative data using one inclinometer, measured in the supine position for cervical rotation, is reported. Note the last row is an average of all subjects aged 35 to 54 years. SD, standard deviation.
Compiled from data in Alaranta et al, 1994.

group ($P = .893$). The amount of extension loss was significant when comparing the older to the younger groups (19.4% men, 29.2% women) compared to only 6.2% less flexion (women) and 10.9% (men). Study limitations include the following:

- The author actively assisted or guided each subject's head during the six measurements, which may have influenced the study results. This was found to be necessary with geriatric subjects, however, due to the high variability observed in the elderly.
- Because rotation is measured supine, the ROMs can be expected to be greater compared to sitting assessments due to the compressive forces of the head being removed (Kottke and Blanchard, 1990). I have observed similar findings.
- The use of the headgear the inclinometer was mounted to demanded a starting point that may vary, depending on the shape of the subject's head.
- The neutral starting position was reported to be between 10 degrees of flexion and 9 degrees of extension in order to maintain a horizontal with the plane of the lower surface of the upper teeth (Defibaugh, 1964).
- Because a second inclinometer was not utilized at the upper thoracic region, the data obtained in this study may be larger than studies using two inclinometers or those using x-ray analysis.
- Inaccuracies may have occurred in the reading of the goniometer as well as the perceptions of the end range of motion by both the subject and the evaluator.
- The difference between active and passive ROM measurements was found to be significant with approximately 10% more passive motion noted (Wong and Nansel, 1992). Also, a greater variance in the ROM measurements was noted when the assessment was performed with the subject's eyes open vs. closed (Nansel and Peneff, 1990).

Normative data was reviewed in a 1994 literature search that included the years 1966 to 1992, which resulted in a review of 59 articles and two textbooks (Bussieres, 1994). Normative data derived from healthy male and female subjects of the same age reveals females have a greater active ROM than males for all active ROMs except neck flexion (Youdas et al, 1992). Also, females have approximately 5 degrees greater cervical extension and 2 to 4 degrees greater lateral bending and rotation than males of the similar age. When testing flexion and extension together, Fouse et al (1973) reported the mean and standard deviations as follows:

- Ages 18 to 24: 137.2 ± 14.8 degrees in the young adults
- Ages 35 to 44: 115.5 ± 17.4 degrees in the middle age group (15.9% decrease)

- Ages 62 to 74: 96.5 ± 16.2 degrees in the elderly age group (16.5% decrease)

This represents a 15.9% decrease in the ROM between age groups 18 to 24 and 35 to 44 and a 16.5% decrease between age groups 35 to 44 and 63 to 74 years. A 29.7% decrease is noted when comparing the 18 to 24 and 62 to 74 year old groups. Hence, in summary, Fouse et al reported approximately a loss of 30% sagittal plane motion when comparing the youngest (18 to 24) to the oldest (62 to 74) age groups.

Mayer et al (1994) reported the cervical ROMs measured with dual inclinometry in a group of 160 male railroad workers, mean age 35.1 years (SD = 7.5); mean height 64.9 inches (SD = 2.6), and mean weight 187 pounds (SD = 28.6). Surprisingly, they reported a greater cervical ROM in the railroad workers than that found in a previously "normal" study (Mayer et al, 1984) regarding normative cervical ROM, as follows:

Cervical ROM: Railroad Workers	Percent of Norm (Normal)
Flexion: 53 ± 12.1 SD	105.6 (50)
Extension: 71 ± 14.1 SD	112.6 (63)
Right lateral flexion: 49 ± 7.2 SD	109.6 (45)
Left lateral flexion: 50 ± 7.8 SD	112.0 (45)
Right rotation: 88 ± 10.6 SD	103.3 (85)
Left rotation: 90 ± 9.6 SD	105.5 (85)

In this article, the authors discuss the lack of disability derived from cervical spine injuries when compared to the low back. Normative data was presented using a group of workers employed in a high-risk work environment. Results suggest that there are no significant differences in the data between the incumbent railroad workers and a normative population. Hence, no discriminatory behaviors between the two groups were observed, nor does a concern need to be considered when returning workers back to work or when pre-employment screening is done.

Using both radiographic and clinical examination approaches, Lind et al (1989) similarly reported that a linear reduction in all cervical ROMs occurred after the third decade with the exception of flexion. Of interest however, Lind et al did not find a statistically significant gender difference in motion. Several studies found that a 40% reduction in cervical ROM across genders can be expected over a lifetime, with a loss of about 25% for males and 13% for females by early-middle age (Lysell, 1969; Foust et al, 1973; Youdas et al, 1992; Penning, 1990). It is consistently reported that flexion loss with age is significantly less than that of extension. Generally, with each 10-year change in age, both males and females will lose about 5 degrees of neck extension and about 3 degrees of active ROM for each of the five other movements (Youdas et al, 1992).

Other factors have been reported that also affect the measurement process of ROMs regardless of the mensuration (measurement) technique utilized. For example, when passive ROMs are assessed, not only are the ROMs significantly greater than the active ROMs, but in 22- to 38-year-old, pain-free subjects displaying significant passive end range asymmetries, the reductions in active movement toward the most versus least restricted side of end range were not of equal proportion (Wong and Nansel, 1992). More specifically, **the restriction in active end range was found to be approximately twice as much toward the side of greatest passive end range capability than it was for movement toward the side of most restricted passive end range.** The compensatory reduction in active motion toward the side of greatest potential end range capability appears to be an attempt to preserve symmetry at the expense of reducing the overall ROM. This finding suggests that when only the active range is assessed, less consistent and, therefore, potentially less reproducible results may be obtained. This may be especially true in a population experiencing pain. Therefore, consideration should be given to the assessment of the passive end ranges so that detection of potential end range asymmetries will not be missed and, as a result, left untreated.

LUMBAR SPINE

REVIEW OF NOTABLE RANGE OF MOTION STUDIES

Two landmark studies were introduced in the mid-1980s which seemed to stimulate the change from less accurate ROM measurement systems to that of inclinometry (Mayer et al, 1984; Keeley et al, 1986). More specifically, in 1984, Mayer et al measured lumbar range of motion (LROM) in normal subjects and those with chronic low back pain. Two different inclinometer methods of evaluating LROM were compared. These included the standard dual inclinometer method generally attributed to Loebl (1967) and Troup et al (1968), and a single inclinometer method described as a modification of the method described by Loebl (1967, 1973). Mayer et al (1984) used an inexpensive hardware-type device to assess LROM at the T12 segment in the dual inclinometer approach, as well as in the single inclinometer method. The sacral measurement of the dual in-

clinometer approach was assessed using a more expensive mechanical inclinometer where the scale was graduated in .5° increments over the 360° range and was affixed to either a straight edge base or two-point contact base. **The two-point contact based inclinometer is favored over the sacrum due to its convex surface.** The T12 inclinometer spans the T12–L1 spinous process, and importance of identifying bony landmarks was emphasized. Accuracy of readings was decreased in obese subjects due to bony landmark identification difficulties. Measurements taken at the sacrum were subtracted from those taken at T12 to determine true lumbar flexion. Similar techniques were performed in extension. In the single inclinometer approach, the less expensive hardware variety inclinometer was initially placed at the T12 position and, at the point of full flexion, moved to the pelvis area. However, rather than moving the inclinometer to the sacrum, the device was placed on the examiner's index finger, which was positioned parallel to the floor on the iliac crest in the neutral starting position and remained fixed on the iliac crest in flexion. No significant difference in accuracy was reported by the authors as the findings were as follows:

- Dual inclinometer: mean pelvic flexion—63° ± 14.8
- Single inclinometer: mean pelvic flexion—63° ± 15.1 (Mayer et al, 1984)

In the single inclinometer approach, it was observed that to read the inclinometer resting on the index finger located over the lateral iliac crest, a second person is required to report the amount unless the inclinometer endpoint can be locked. However, this would require stopping between each trial, removing the instrument, and recording the motion, which is not ideal if multiple readings are required (Mayer et al, 1984).

Normative Data

Normative data measured utilizing the dual inclinometer approach is summarized in Table 14–5. Note that the arbitrary neutral starting point for flexion and extension range was the subject's fully erect position, where 10° to 20° of extension inclination was present at T12–L1. The following paragraphs describe how various studies arrived at this data.

Table 14–5: Sagittal Lumbar ROM Normative Data Using the Dual Inclinometer Approach

	FLEXION	EXTENSION	TOTAL
Gross motion: T12 motion	122° ± 15.6°	45° ± 14.6°	167° ± 22.4°
True lumbar motion	55° ± 9.2°	27° ± 12.8°	82° ± 18.1°
Pelvic–hip motion	66° ± 14.3°	18°	84°
Straight leg raise mean	—	—	82° ± 19.9°

N = 13 (7 males, 6 females), mean age 31 years, range 19 to 51 years. Results represent degree ± standard deviation.
Compiled from data in Mayer et al, 1984.

In 7 of the 13 normal subjects, Mayer et al (1984) reported that motion measured at T12–L1 and sacrum were individually assessed at 15- to 30-degree increments during lumbar flexion in an attempt to assess the amount of participation at the two sites during the flexion arc. The results revealed an almost linear increase with T12–L1 motion exceeding that of sacral–hip flexion through much of the range until after approximately 90 degrees of flexion, where the majority of motion occurs at the sacrum/pelvis. More specifically, the ratio of the slopes between T12–L1 and sacral–hip flexion motion is 1.72 (slopes = .63 and .37, respectively) up to 90 degrees of gross flexion and .17 between 90 and 120 degrees as the lumbar spine flexes only 4.3 compared to sacral–hip flexion of 25.7. Gracovetsky et al (1995) reported a 50:50 ratio of T12–L1 to sacral–hip flexion using a computerized method of assessment, but the selection criteria for the two studies were markedly different and the motion assessment method differences were described as possible reasons for the difference in ratios reported.

Mayer et al (1984) also compared radiographic flexion-extension motion taken at the T12 inferior end plate and the superior surface of S1, with dual inclinometry in 12 patients. The inclinometric mean lumbar motion of 60.5 ± 16.7 was measured at the time the x-ray study was conducted. The x-ray motion of flexion-extension was measured at 58.5 degrees, revealing no significant difference in the two measuring techniques ($P \leq .01$). Due to the radiation exposure, the dual inclinometry approach is preferred, although if clinically necessary, the x-ray assessment can be used to compare if suboptimal effort is suspected. More commonly, flexion-extension radiography is used to assess lumbar stability. Thus, if this were performed prior to LROM inclinometry, the latter might be considered inappropriate if instability were present, as excessive loading of the unstable motion segment a second time could be avoided.

More recently, Saur et al (1996) reported very close correlation of lumbar range of motion measurements taken with and without radiological verification of inclinometer placement ($r = .93$; $P < .001$). More specifically, flexion alone demonstrated close correlation ($r = 95$; $P < .001$) whereas extension was less reliable ($r = .82$; $P < .001$). Total lumbar range of motion ($r = .94$; $P < .001$) and flexion ($r = .88$; $P < .001$) were closely related but, again, exten-

sion showed less correlation ($r = .42$; $P < .05$). A near linear correlation existed for measurements of the total lumbar range of motion ($r = .97$; $P < .001$) and flexion ($r = .98$; $P < .001$), whereas extension ($r = .75$; $P < .001$) again correlated less well. The authors concluded that **noninvasive inclinometer techniques proved highly reliable and valid but the extension measurement requires further refinement** (Saur et al, 1996). The data derived from a patient population (n = 38, 25 males, 13 females; mean age 34 years, range 20 to 59 years) in Saur's study is summarized in Table 14–6. Mayer et al (1984) criticize the use of global measurement of thoracolumbar motion to rate impairment with no attempt to differentiate the spinal movement from the sacral–hip motion and reference the American Academy of Orthopedic Surgeons (Mayer et al, 1984; AAOS, 1965). This same criticism led to the change made from the second to the third editions of the AMA *Guides to the Evaluation of Permanent Impairment* (Engelberg, 1988), where inclinometry was considered the preferred method of evaluating spinal ROM rather than the previously utilized two-arm goniometer.

Sacral–Hip Flexion Movement

The sacral–hip flexion movement was reported to be approximately 20% less than the tightest straight leg raise (SLR) in the cooperative individual (Mayer et al, 1984). More specifically, Mayer reported an average of 82 degrees SLR in normal subjects, which is 24% or 16 degrees greater compared to the normal pelvic flexion measurement of 66 degrees. In the patient population, a 56-degree average SLR was reported, which is 33% or 14 degrees greater compared to the pelvic flexion measurement of 42 degrees (Mayer et al, 1984). Symptom magnifiers may yield wider discrepancies than patients limited only by pain. The validity screen of the SLR compared to sacral–hip motion as it is currently described in the AMA *Guides* was initially reported by Keeley et al, in 1986. More specifically, **as the tightest SLR reaches its passive ROM limit, further elevation forces the pelvis to tilt anteriorward until the hyperextension limit of the contralateral hip is reached.** This limit of contralateral hip extension equals the total of hip flexion plus hip extension. A 15-degree allowance is recommended for the difference between active and passive hamstring stretch.

Table 14–6: Sagittal Lumbar ROM Patient-derived Data

	FLEXION	EXTENSION	TOTAL
Gross motion: T12 motion	$65° \pm 24°$	$19° \pm 13°$	$84°$
True lumbar motion	$28° \pm 14.1°$	$9° \pm 9.5°$	$37° \pm 21.6°$
Pelvic–hip motion	$42.2° \pm 18.5°$	—	—
Straight leg raise mean	—	—	$56° \pm 15°$

N = 38 (25 males, 13 females), mean age 34 years, range 20 to 59 years. Results represent degree ± standard deviation. NA, not available.
Compiled from data in Saur et al, 1996.

Lumbar Rotational Assessment Method

Keeley et al (1986) also report ROM data for two study groups. The first consisted of both normal and patient subjects. Two PTs evaluated the LROM using dual inclinometer methods and, after each subject, compared results and discussed technique "thus permitting a learning curve to be established across subjects." The second group, also consisting of both normal subjects and patients, was evaluated using the same method but excluding the comparison of data. This blinded group was then compared to the "nonblinded" group and the inter- and intra-rater reliability were assessed and compared. Results revealed a definite reduction in reliability of the hip measurement where the correlation coefficient for measuring the controls compared to the patients was lower or, better. More specifically, the following ranges of correlation coefficients were reported (Keeley et al, 1986):

- Group I ("nonblinded"): normal subjects .90 (gross motion) to .99 (left SLR)
- Group I ("nonblinded"): patient subjects .92 (gross motion) to .98 (left and right SLR)
- Group II ("blinded"): normal subjects .74 (hip motion) to .94 (right SLR)
- Group II ("blinded"): patient subjects .82 (hip motion) to .96 (left SLR, and gross motion)

Keeley et al (1986) concluded that the convex sacrum, a fat pad covering of variable thickness, and poor definition of bony landmarks lead to the errors reported in the nonblinded subject group II. These factors also result in "wobble" of the inclinometer and, although both PTs developed methods that were reliable within themselves (intra-rater), the methods may not be comparable. Therefore, care must be taken when applying adequate digital pressure over the fat pad for consistent positioning of the inclinometer on the sacrum.

Keeley et al reports normative data utilizing 28 subjects, segregating data into male and female gender groups, as summarized in Table 14–7. The gender differences in this study were noted in pelvic flexion and SLR, where

women performed better than men. This may be due to true gender differences or possibly due to the age variance between the two groups, and further study with more careful control of age was recommended prior to drawing any gender-based conclusions. The difference in the extension ROM was found to be greater in this study than in Mayer et al's 1984 study. This is described as being possibly due to the fact that five repetitions of each ROM were performed as a warm-up prior to testing in this study, but not in Mayer et al's 1984 study.

The rotational measurement assessment method reported by Keeley et al (1986) was described as "encouraging." This method is performed by having the subject bend forward at the waist to 90 degrees (verified using an inclinometer placed at T12–L1 in the sagittal plane and stopping forward flexion process at 90). The knees are locked in extension to control pelvic rotation (verified by a sacral inclinometer placed in the frontal plane), and the arms are crossed over the chest. The subject then performs maximum rotation by twisting slowly with the inclinometer placed over the T12–L1 interspace in the frontal plane. Right rotation is defined as lowering the left and raising the right shoulder (clockwise when viewed from behind). Results revealed symmetrical motion in the normal subjects but not in the patient group. Also, there was less motion in the normal group compared to the motion reported in the patient group, as noted in Table 14–8. The gender of the subjects studied was not reported.

In Keeley et al's 1986 study, the measurements were performed one time by each PT and results compared. The following are possible reasons for the suboptimal results in assessing rotation lumbar ROM:

- Small subject sample (8 patients, mean age 42.0 years; 12 normal subjects, mean age 33.3 years)
- "Nonblinding" of the subject data obtained from the evaluating PTs
- Inability to maintain a 90 degree T12–L1 flexed position with the knees locked straight
- Use of a patient-driven estimation of the neutral starting point rather an inclinometric measure

Table 14–7: Sagittal Lumbar ROM Normal-derived Data

	FLEXION (DEGREE ± SD)		EXTENSION (DEGREE ± SD)	
	Males	Females	Males	Females
Gross motion: T12 motion	118.6° ± 14.1°	123.2° ± 12.6°	40.4° ± 11.6°	41.4° ± 8.9°
True lumbar motion	65.0° ± 8.2°	64.4° ± 8.2°	26.6° ± 10.8°	27.3° ± 8.5°
Pelvic–hip motion	53.6° ± 10.8°	58.9° ± 10.5°	13.7° ± 4.4°	14.1° ± 5.9°
SLR—mean right	73.6° ± 9.6°	82.9° ± 7.1°	—	—
SLR—mean left	72.7° ± 8.7°	83.4° ± 8.1°	—	—

N = 28 (14 males, mean age 40.1 years; 14 females, mean age 30.1 years). SLR, straight leg raise.
Compiled from data in Keeley et al, 1986.

Table 14–8: Transverse Plane Lumbar ROM Normal-derived and Patient Group Data

	NORMAL GROUP (N = 12)		PATIENT GROUP (N = 8)	
	Left Rotation	**Right Rotation**	**Left Rotation**	**Right Rotation**
Therapist 1	10.4° ± 3.14°	11.0° ± 3.67°	15.1° ± 6.02°	12.2° ± 5.16°
Therapist 2	10.4° ± 3.03°	10.6° ± 3.03°	15.2° ± 7.96°	12.6° ± 4.15°

Normal groups: n = 12, mean age 33.3 years; patient group: n = 8, mean age 42.0 years. Results represent degree ± standard deviation. *Compiled from data in Keeley et al, 1986.*

- "Locking" of the facet joint as a result of forward trunk flexion

This single inclinometer method of mensurating lumbar rotation was not included in the AMA *Guides*. Rather, dual inclinometry utilized in the sagittal and frontal plane lumbar spine ROM are the described methods. A version similar to this was described in the measurement of thoracic rotation. Also, a technique using two inclinometers, one placed at T12–L1 and the other at T1 to measure thoracic rotation has been described (Engelberg, 1988), but reliability and validity of this technique is unknown.

As reported with respect to the cervical ROM of rotation data published by Alaranta et al (1994; previously reviewed), lumbar flexion ROM using dual inclinometry in a manner consistent with the AMA *Guides* is also available. The patient was evaluated in the standing position and inclinometer placement included T12, which was located by counting down from C7, and the superior foot of the inclinometer was placed at the spinous process (SP) of T12. The superior foot of the second inclinometer was placed just below a line connecting the posterior superior iliac spine (PSIS) and maximal flexion was recorded. Extension was measured from a prone position, and rotation was also measured. Lateral flexion was measured with a tape measure between the start and endpoints of hand down lateral thigh movement. Hence, only flexion ROM is comparable to the impairment rating charts currently in use, as noted in Table 14–9.

Reliability of Lumbar Range of Motion

The reliability of LROM was also studied using 14 examiners who were not familiar with the three instruments utilized, so as to resemble a clinical type of practice (Brand and Lehman, 1983) and remove instrument bias from the examiner (Mayer, 1995). Using three instruments, 18 healthy subjects were measured in full flexion twice in a randomized sequence and were blinded from the readings. The results revealed mean test–retest reliability was 4.9 degrees and the probability that an error would be made of 5, 10, and 15 degrees or larger was computed as 44%, 12%, and 2%, respectively. The intra-examiner reliability did not differ significantly and was reliable. There was, however, a statistically significant variance between examiners, which averaged 7.9 degrees across the three instruments. The probability of error occurring at 5, 10, or 15 degrees was 59%, 28%, and 11%, respectively, confirming that large errors are more likely when different examiners are compared. These findings resulted in the conclusion that **ROM measurements must be interpreted with caution in clinical use, disability evaluations, and research.** The most likely explanation for the poor inter-examiner reliability was reported to be difficulty in locating the bony landmarks. The comment that careful training of the inclinometer technique may yield more reliable results correlates well with another study, in which the examiners compared data and techniques, resulting in improved inter-examiner reliability results (Keeley et al, 1986). However, the majority of studies found inter-examiner reliability to be poor, especially when compared to intra-examiner reliability.

Study Results of a Computerized Goniometer

A study utilizing a computerized goniometer was compared to other physical examination methods, including dual inclinometry in 120 healthy subjects to establish normative data (Dopf et al, 1994). The computerized instrument was reported to be more reliable in all LROMs except flexion, where the differences were not significant. Although the normative data for the low-tech dual inclinometer is not included, several interesting observations are reported. These include:

- Females are reported to have a greater LROM in left and right lateral flexion, left rotation, and global frontal plane motion (right lateral flexion plus left lateral extension).
- All LROMs decreased as age increased, except rotation. However, this was described as a very weak correlation suggesting the age group studied of 20 to 35 year olds is a fairly homogenous group.

CLINICAL TIP 14–5
Standardizing the Assessment Approach

The sequence in which the ROM is gathered may also play a significant role in ROM measurements. Recommendations for standardizing the assessment approach are clearly necessary in order to obtain valid and reliable results, especially in a patient-based population.

Table 14–9: Lumbar Flexion ROM[a] Normative Data

AGE (YRS)	MALES (N = 242)						FEMALES (N = 233)					
	Blue Collar		White Collar		All		Blue Collar		White Collar		All	
	x	SD	x	SD	x	SD	x	SD	x	SD	x	SD
35–39	52°	8°	50°	9°	51°	9°	51°	8°	46°	12°	48°	10°
40–44	47°	10°	50°	8°	48°	10°	44°	9°	40°	11°	43°	10°
45–49	46°	8°	47°	9°	46°	9°	42°	9°	43°	12°	43°	10°
50–54	46°	10°	45°	10°	45°	10°	41°	10°	44°	8°	44°	10°
35–54	48°	10°	49°	9°	48°	9°	41°	10°	44°	8°	44°	10°

[a] The normative data using two inclinometers, measured in the standing position for lumbar flexion, is reported. Note the last row is an average of all subjects aged 35 to 54 years. SD, standard deviation.
Compiled from data in Alaranta et al, 1996.

- The dominant hand does not significantly affect spine motion.
- Measuring the arc of motion or global motion in each plane has better reliability or less variability than measuring the motions individually.
- Attempts to duplicate submaximal motion have significantly more variability than repeated attempts of maximal motion.
- Lumbar rotation is substantially diminished with forward flexion (Dopf et al, 1994).

High-Resolution Motion Analysis System

The Workers' Compensation Board of Quebec funded and supervised a study with the goal of establishing a normative database for a high-resolution motion analysis system (Gracovetsky et al, 1995). Patterns of spinal movement were assessed as a function of load, age, and gender by the use of motion detecting skin markers and a high-resolution three-dimensional camera system with simultaneous paraspinal muscle surface electromyography. Measurements were assessed for consistent, specific patterns recognizable as normal lumbar spine skin motion and correlates with normal lumbar spine function. These findings were then compared to radiographic studies to confirm the correlation between the motion of skin markers and lumbar spine function. The results revealed:

- There was consistent and minimal variation with various applied loads (0 vs 4.5 kg).
- Gender had no significant effect except in the first 20 degrees of movement.
- Older subjects had less mobility but similar coordination during movement.
- The contribution of the pelvis to the motion increased as the lumbar spine stiffened with age.
- The younger spine had a significantly greater intersegmental motion at lower lumbar levels (L4–5,

L5–S1) in all LROMs compared to the thoracolumbar motion.
- Consistent findings were noted with previous radiological investigations for sagittal and frontal plane motion (Gracovetsky et al, 1995).

Inter-rater Reliability of Three Different Lumbar Range of Motion Methods

The inter-rater reliability was assessed using three different methods of LROM assessment, including single inclinometry, dual inclinometry, and back ROM inclinometry methods (Rondinelli et al, 1992). Two experienced evaluators tested eight healthy subjects, and three replicates of lumbar flexion were obtained from each evaluator using the previously mentioned approaches and a B200 assessment. The median range of error was 8.5 degrees using the single inclinometer, 10.5 degrees using the double inclinometer and 16 degrees using the back ROM method. As previously noted, the intra-rater reliability was generally greater than inter-rater reliability and the intermethod reliability was low in most cases, reflecting poor cross-validity across the three inclinometer techniques and the B200. The authors concluded that even with a "controlled" setting using experienced observers, standard examination techniques in asymptomatic healthy subjects, significant measurement error was noted. They question the reliability of assessing impairment utilizing these methods.

LUMBAR RANGE OF MOTION INCLINOMETRIC TECHNIQUE

It is evident that, if inclinometric assessments are performed with accuracy, staying focused on the shortcomings of the technique, useful information regarding outcomes assessment can be obtained. Refer to Chapter 16, Figure 16–4, for lumbar spine ROM inclinometry evaluation. When measuring flexion of the lumbar spine, following these steps will help yield accurate results:

Flexion/Extension—Lumbar Spine

1. One inclinometer is placed so that a line drawn at the T12 SP is straddled by the midline of the inclinometer.
2. A second inclinometer is placed at the midpoint of the convex sacrum. Care must be taken not to place the sacral inclinometer too high as it may be displaced when measuring lumbar extension. Hence, it is recommended that a line be drawn at the apex of the convex sacrum so that the lower inclinometer straddles the line. Note that if the base of the inclinometer is unusually long, less accurate readings are likely. Also, a flat-based inclinometer is less optimal due to the "rocking" or wobbling effects that can occur. Therefore, extra care must be practiced to keep the inclinometer in a secure position, such as by cupping the ulnar side of the hand holding the inclinometer and securing the hand onto the part being evaluated.
3. The inclinometers are then set to "0" and the patient is asked to flex forward keeping the knees locked to a maximum flexion position. This may be preceded by warm-up stretching by completing five repetitions prior to the tested repetition (Mayer et al, 1994). If the AMA *Guides* are being used, following the specific protocol is necessary where the highest of three consecutive trials that fall within 5 degrees or 10% of the average of the three trials is reported. The inclinometers are then carefully read and the result reported after subtracting the sacral–hip motion from the T12 measurement to obtain the true lumbar flexion angle.
4. The patient then returns to the neutral position to either repeat this process three times (AMA *Guides* approach) or prepare for the measurement of extension LROM.

CLINICAL TIP 14–6
Tips for Increasing Inclinometer Effectiveness

It helps to instruct the patient to run the hand down the lateral thigh toward the knee to minimize the possibilities of flexion during the lateral flexion measurement. It was also recommended that the measurement be obtained with the patient facing a wall to help minimize flexion (Mellin et al, 1991). Mellin et al also recommend that the exact distance between the lines drawn at T12 and at the sacral convex apex be measured using a tape measure from the spinal level adjacent to the highest iliac crest (eg, from the L4 spinous process). This mesurement can then be used as a reference point at the time of the next reexamination to compare to the palpation location of T12 and sacrum line.

5. **Straight leg raise (SLR) validity test:** Once the flexion and extension ROM are completed, the SLR validity test can be performed by comparing the tightest SLR to the sum of sacral–hip movements of flexion plus extension. The total sacral–hip motion should be within 15 degrees of the tightest SLR. The normative data for the SLR was reported at 75 degrees. Therefore, if the tightest SLR is 60 degrees, the sum sacral–hip motion cannot be less than 45 degrees or else the test would be invalidated. This validity test should not be used if the total sacral–hip motion exceeds 55 degrees for men or 65 degrees for women (Doege, 1993).

Lateral Flexion—Lumbar Spine

1. The inclinometers are next placed in the frontal plane so that the base lines up with the line drawn at the T12 SP and the midsacral convexity drawn line. The T12 inclinometer must be held upside down and not pressed flush against the back, so that the gravity-dependent pendulum swings freely.
2. After positioning the two inclinometers so that the needle is hanging on the "0" mark, the patient laterally flexes to one side, keeping the knees straight.
3. The sacral–hip measurement is subtracted from the T12 inclinometric measurement to obtain the final result.
4. The process is then repeated on the opposite side.

FACTORS AFFECTING RANGE OF MOTION MENSURATION

Various factors affecting ROM mensuration and previously described regarding the cervical spine also affect the results of LROM. In addition, other factors are involved that are unique to the lumbar spine.

Subject Position

Subject position with respect to the effects on measurments of flexion, extension, and lateral flexion of the spine was investigated (Mellin et al, 1991). Inclinometric mensuration techniques were utilized to evaluate thoracic and lumbar forward flexion, extension, and lateral flexion. No significant differences in repeatability and ROM were found between measurements in the different positions. From a convenience of performance standpoint, the following positions were recommended:

- Forward flexion from sitting
- Extension while lying on an examination table with arms braced ahead (prone press-up)
- Lateral flexion close to and facing a wall

Diurnal Variations

Another factor to consider when assessing LROM is the variability in ROM with time of day or the diurnal variations that have been reported (Wing et al, 1992; Ensink et al, 1996). In addition to ROMs being affected by **diurnal changes,** other researchers have reported similar variance with other aspects of orthopedic testing such as the SLR orthopedic test, where the SLR was found to be tighter in the morning (Porter and Trailescu, 1990). Wing et al (1992) utilized stereophotography and standard clinical examinations performed in the evenings and after a minimum of 8 hours of bed rest and reported an average increase in height of 20 mm. Approximately 40% of the increase occurred in the lumbar spine, but this was not due to a change in lordosis. Another 40% occurred in the thoracic spine due to a reduction in kyphosis. The remaining 20% could not be accounted for, although the cervical spine lordosis was not studied. The flexion ROM of the spine and SLR are reported as decreased in morning, whereas extension, rotation, and femoral stretch testing were not as significantly affected by diurnal variation. Similarly, Ensink et al (1996) reported mean lumbar flexion using dual inclinometry was 42.20 degrees (SD = 10.3 degrees), 49.9 degrees (SD = 11.9 degrees), and 53.3 degrees (SD = 14.5 degrees) in the morning, at noon, and in the afternoon, respectively. Extension was 12.10 degrees (SD = 6.6 degrees), 13.3 degrees (SD = 8.0 degrees), and 15.0 degrees (SD = 7.0 degrees), respectively, between morning, noon, and afternoon. Hence, flexion increased significantly greater than extension diurnally, similar to that reported by Wing et al (1992).

INCLINOMETRY: SOURCES OF ERROR

The accuracy and sources of error with computerized inclinometer measurements have also been investigated (Mayer et al, 1995; Mayer et al, 1997). Similar deficiencies exist in identifying sources of error leading to variability for other human performance measurements such as strength, endurance, lifting capacity, and so on (O'Driscoll and Tomenson, 1982; Carlson, 1986; Penning, 1987; Mimura et al, 1989; Carman et al, 1990; Cowell, 1990; Granberry et al, 1990; Paquet et al, 1991). However, because ROM carries important clinical applications in monitoring outcomes and assessing impairment, specific investigation of this technique was performed. In one study of lumbar sagittal mobility using 38 healthy individuals, after bench testing the device for device error the following procedure was utilized (Mayer et al, 1997):

1. Untrained test administrators with no control of human performance or procedural variables
2. Identical tests by well-trained test administrators controlling human performance variability by monitoring and controlling total motion
3. Test by procedurally trained adminstrators without controlling for human performance variability

Results revealed the accuracy of the methodology progressively deteriorated by the various sources of error, with device error being reported as negligible. **Lack of training and the magnitude of the measured quantity were the primary reasons for test degradation.** The most accurate

measurement was combined gross lumbar flexion (> 95%), and pelvic extension was worst (> 36%). Mayer et al (1997) concluded that lumbar sagittal motion assessment sources of error are, in order of importance:

A. Test administrator training
   1. Locating bony landmarks (especially T12 spinous process)
   2. Motion of the skin mark at T12 as the subject flexed or extended
   3. "Rocking" or "wobbling" of the inclinometer on the convex sacrum
   4. Misplacing the inclinometer sensor back to T12 after subject movement
   5. High placement of the inclinometer on the sacrum (at L5 or above)
B. Human/device interface error
   1. Residual error related to bony landmark not correctable by training (eg, obesity, short stature)
   2. Improper instruction to subjects (posture, warm-up, etc)
   3. Lack of firm, two-point positioning on underlying bony prominence (may be due to lack of two-point contact, stick-on skin attachment, use of abdominal belts, etc)
C. Small motion magnitude (eg, sacral extension)
D. Device error
E. Human performance variability (ie, age, gender, motivation) (Mayer et al, 1997)

These authors point out that "a test may be criticized for being difficult to perform, but is not inaccurate simply because investigators failed to learn the proper technique" (Mayer et al, 1997). Studies critical of the use of inclinometry due to problems of interpreting the clinical research findings were reported (Whaley, 1973; Winer, 1984; Battie et al, 1990; Dillard et al, 1991; Newton and Waddell, 1991; Portek et al, 1993; Dopf et al, 1994; Rainville et al, 1994; Mayer et al, 1995). These problems coexist in other functional performance tests as well.

Therefore, the problem lies in following the experimental design rather than with inclinometry itself, as faulty bony landmark identification may be the primary issue. Usual factors of human variability include age, gender, morphology, and motivation. Additional factors may accompany a patient population and, therefore, add to the degradation of accuracy, as patient values may be lower than normal/nonpatient values. These factors may include pain, poor motivation, and disincentives for optimum effort. In general the smaller the magnitude of mobility (smaller angle), the lower the percentage of accuracy. This is exemplified by the lower accuracy reported for pelvic extension. Again, this is a factor common to all human performance testing. However, in spite of the low magnitude of motion that occurs at the pelvis in extension, the difference between the magnitude in a patient versus the normal may be sufficient to allow for discrimination between the two.

Mayer et al (1997) conclude that **HCPs should correct the common errors, including careful identification of bony landmarks, rocking inclinometers, and relocating the T12 segment when returning the "sensor" to T12** (specific for the Cybex EDI-320). Perhaps an argument can be made for favoring dual inclinometry over the EDI-320 since there is no moving of the sensors with dual inclinometry. However, if mechanical inclinometers are used, care must be exercised in reading the inclinometer accurately. Using the same technique pre- and post-treatment will allow for accurate outcomes assessment, which is perhaps more important than comparing the patient's ROM to normative data, especially if the normative data is not age and gender specific.

OTHER METHODS OF MEASURING LUMBAR RANGE OF MOTION

Many methods of measuring the ROM of the low back have been reported, which include:

- Finger-to-floor distance (Macrae and Wright, 1969)
- Modified Schober tests (Macrae and Wright, 1969)
- Radiographs (Mayer et al, 1984)
- Flexicurves (Anderson and Sweetman, 1975; Burton et al, 1989)
- Protractors (Troup et al, 1968)
- Goniometers (Fitzgerald et al, 1983)
- Inclinometers (Loebl, 1967; Burdett et al, 1986; Keeley et al, 1986; Mellin, 1986; Chiarello and Savidge, 1993)

Merritt et al (1986) studied three clinical methods of assessing trunk flexibility in 50 normal subjects. This group consisted of 25 men and 25 women in age categories of 18 to 25, 26 to 35, 36 to 45, 46 to 55, and 56 to 65 years old, with five subjects per category. The mean coefficient of variation (CV) for inter-examiner and intra-examiner reproducibility, respectively, and range, mean, and standard deviation revealed the following:

Test	CV	Range (degrees)	Mean ± SD
Fingertip-to-floor	83% and 76.4%	0–40	4.0 ± 6.9
Flexion–Schober/ Moll	6.3% and 6.6%	4.3–10.3	7.2 ± 1.2
Right lateral flexion—Moll	11.9% and 8.9%	2.5–10.8	6.4 ± 1.8
Left lateral flexion—Moll	10.2% and 9.5%	2.3–20.0	6.5 ± 1.8
Lumbar extension—Moll	9.5% and 7.3%	6.8–19.0	14.3 ± 2.7
Lumbar flexion—Loebl	9.6% and 13.4%	13–49	31.0 ± 6.6
Lumbar extension—Loebl	65.4% and 50.7%	0–201	9.1 ± 17.5

Poor reliability is noted with fingertip-to-floor and Loebl extension methods, but all other tests studied had good reproducibility. The authors report discrepancy rates of up to 30% (Nelson et al, 1979; Wolf et al, 1979) by simple "observation," which is inadequate for determining trunk mobility. Goniometry did not improve these rates, as CVs of up to 53% with the use of a goniometer were reported (Fitzgerald et al, 1983). The Schober and Moll tests were recommended to be added to the routine examination of the back. Inclinometry was reported as showing promise but requires more time, training, and calculations to perform the technique. Table 14–10 includes a description of the previously mentioned tests (see also Figs. 14–1 to 14–4).

In a similar study, four methods—the fingertip-to-floor distance, modified Schober, dual inclinometer, as well as a photometric technique of assessing lumbar motion—were examined (Gill et al, 1988). In this study, 10 subjects, 5 men and 5 women, aged between 24 and 34 years, were examined in full flexion, full extension, and the erect position, both standing and sitting. Findings revealed poor repeatability with the fingertip-to-floor method in all postures, probably due to the effect of many more vertebrae as well as the variability in flexion of the upper extremity joints, including the fingers, hand, wrist, elbow, and shoulder. Also, the inclinometer placement at T12 in the standing, full flexion position showed the greatest variability. Similar to the findings reported by Merritt et al (1986), the most repeatable approach was that of the modified Schober method of determining lumbar spinal motion and, therefore, this approach was recommended as a routine, noninvasive, clinical evaluation for assessing lumbar spine motion. Gill et al (1988) also state that the Schober method and dual inclinometer method are both repeatable and reliable in quantifying the functional improvement. The advantage of the dual inclinometer method is that flexion and extension are assessed in degrees making assessment of impairment feasible, whereas the modified Schober method can only be used as an outcome tool, since there is no correlation between the units measured, or degrees versus centimeters. The photometric approach was not reliable or repeatable due to difficulty in placing markers on the chest wall and variability in position on the pelvis. The authors recommend more electrodes be placed in the lumbar spine to improve reliability and repeatability. Table 14–11 compares the reliability between these two studies.

The difference between the reported coefficient of variation between the two authors is described as difficult to explain. Possibly investigator error and/or differences in time between the trials are reported (Gill et al, 1988). Small sample size may also be a reason for the difference.

Alaranta et al (1994) reported a 594-subject normative study in which subjects were categorized by age (35 to 54 years old), gender, and work class (white vs blue collar). Flexibility of the spine utilizing dual inclinometry of cervical ROM included flexion combined with extension, lateral flexion, and cervical rotation (supine, one inclinometer). Lumbar flexion and extension were assessed by the

Table 14–10: Description of Mobility Tests[a]

TEST	DESCRIPTION
Fingertip-to-floor (Macrae and Wright, 1969)	A forward flexed position is held for 15 sec, with feet shoulder-width apart and arms and knees straight. The distance from the tip of digit 3 to the floor is measured to the nearest .5 cm (measure second trial).
Flexion (Schober, 1937; Moll and Wright, 1971)	Skin markings are made at the midpoint between the two PSISs (S1), and additional marks are made 10 cm above and 5 cm below the S1 mark. The subject is then asked to bend forward, with knees straight, and the distance between the two points 15 cm apart is remeasured and 15 cm subtracted.
Lateral flexion (Moll et al, 1972a)	The subject places hands behind the head and two skin marks are made. The lower mark is placed at the top of the iliac crest in the midaxillary line (MAL) and the second is made 20 cm above it in the same MAL. The subject then laterally flexes without rotating, the distance between the two marks is measured, and 20 cm subtracted.
Extension (Moll et al, 1972b)	The end of the string of a pendulum (string with a weight) is held at the upper point 20 cm above the iliac crest, previously made for measuring lateral flexion. The subject extends backwards, hands held out in front, feet hooked behind a belt, and ischium leaning against a tabletop. The distance from the lower spot to the string on a horizontal is measured with a rigid tape in cm. If hip contractures or abnormal hip laxity is present, "modifications to recalibrate the neutral lumbar position would have been necessary."
Flexion and extension (Loebl, 1967)	Due to difficulty in identifying the T12 SP, a point 15 cm above S1 is marked with the patient standing erect. Flexion is measured from a seated position and extension from a prone position. The measurements are made with a single engineer's inclinometer (gravity pendulum).

PSIS, posterior superior iliac spine; SP, spinous process.

[a] The procedure required for each test studied by Merritt et al (1986) is described. A modification of the original test is noted where applicable.

dual inclinometry method. Trunk rotation was measured in a seated position in a chair without a backrest, and the subject was secured by a safety belt to the chair. A bar was held behind the neck, while monitoring the rotation motion in front of a mirror, keeping the head pointed straight forward. A water scale with adjustable arms and compass inclinometer was attached to the inferior level of the scapulae, keeping the compass as close to the spine as possible. Trunk side bending was measured with the subject against a wall, feet 15 cm apart, and the movement of the index fingertip against the lateral thigh was marked and measured from the starting point to a mark representing the finish. Unfortunately, a different statistical analytical approach was used, and the inter-rater reliability was tested at a 1-week time interval. The mean value of all measurements, reliability (r) factor, change in the mean, deviation of the change of the means, paired t-test (df = n − 1), and P-factor representing the statistical significance of systematic shift were reported. The intra-rater reliability was reported at a 1-year time interval and showed acceptable data for cervical flexion-extension motion, cervical lateral flexion, and trunk side bending. The following conclusions were made:

- Spinal flexibility decreased with advancing age (especially in blue-collar workers).
- Males predominated in lumbar flexion and rotation while females predominated in cervical flexion-extension.
- Spinal flexibility was negatively related to those experiencing disabling pain with the strongest correlation with cervical flexion-extension and neck pain and between trunk side bending and low back pain during the preceding year.
- The inter-rater reliabilities were found to be generally good for all measurements, with trunk side bending showing the highest reliability coefficients.
- The intra-rater reliability (measured at 1 year) was found to be acceptable only for cervical flexion-extension, cervical side bending, and trunk side bending (Alaranta et al, 1994).

Normative data charts are presented that include data broken down by age, gender, and class. These represent excellent resources of information to compare patients pre- and post-treatment (see the discussion of "Quantitative Functional Capacity Evaluation" in Chap. 16).

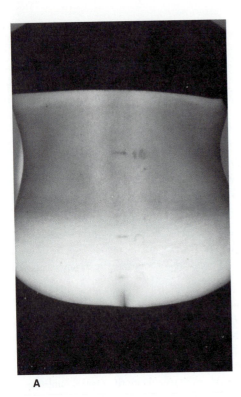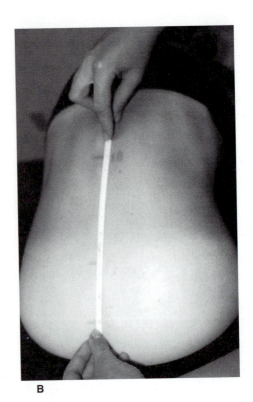

A   B

Figure 14–1. The modified Schober flexion method (Schober, 1937; Moll and Wright, 1971). **A.** A line is drawn between the PSIS and a point located in the midline marks the "0" reading. A second horizontal line is placed 10 cm above the line and a third, 5 cm below the "0" point. **B.** The change in distance between the top and bottom points in full flexion.

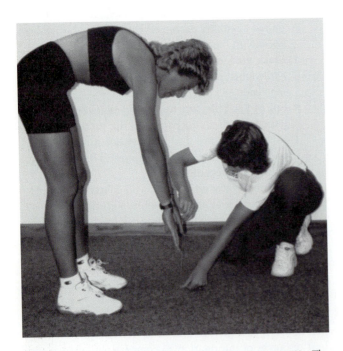

Figure 14–2. Fingertip-to-floor test (Macrae, 1969). The fingertip-to-floor distance can be directly measured in centimeters (cm).

HIGH- VERSUS LOW-TECH METHODS OF ASSESSING LUMBAR RANGE OF MOTION

Shirley et al (1994) compared high-tech equipment that included a SPINETRAK spinal motion analysis system (Motion Analysis Corporation, Santa Rosa, CA), a MedX lumbar extension testing, and a MedX rehabilitative exercise machine (MedX Corporation, Gainesville, FL) to the low-tech approach using liquid dual inclinometers. Total lumbar sagittal motion was measured using each device in a group of 9 female and 35 male patients with chronic low back pain arising from work-related injuries. Subjects were asked to move five times from full flexion to full extension. Results indicated that the **motion analysis system correlated significantly with the liquid inclinometer method and mildly with the MedX.** The inclinometer and MedX also correlated significantly, and the individual measures did not significantly differ (49.6 degrees ± 16.9 SD; and 52.1 degrees ± 16.5 SD, respectively), whereas the SPINE-TRAK yielded significantly lower measurements (36.0 degrees ± 15.6 SD). This may be because the SPINETRAK averaged the five repetitions and, therefore, does not report

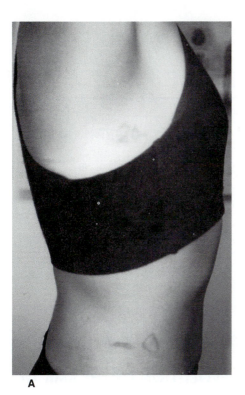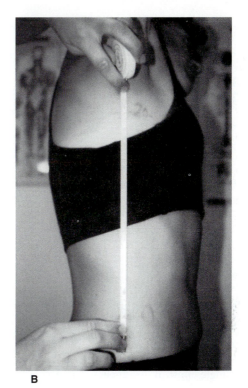

A   B

Figure 14–3. Lateral flexion (Moll et al, 1972a). The assessment of lateral flexion is similar to the Schober method of assessing flexion. Lines are drawn at the top of the iliac crest in the midaxillary line ("0" position) 20 cm apart, and the change in distance is measured in full lateral flexion. The measurement taken in neutral, upright position **(A)** is then subtracted from the larger measurement taken in full flexion **(B)** to yield a "net" range of motion (ROM), reported in centimeters.

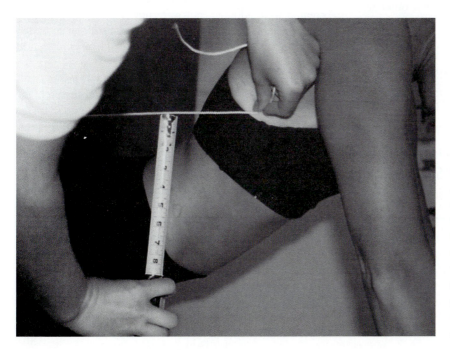

Figure 14–4. Lumbar extension (Moll et al, 1972b). The skin markings during lateral flexion are utilized to measure extension. Extension is measured in centimeters at the end range of motion (ROM) by suspending a line with a weight from the upper mark. Using a steel tape, the distance between the string bottom mark used in Figure 14–3 is measured. No subtraction is required, as it is a direct measurement.

Table 14–11: Comparison of Inter-rater and Intrarater Reliability[a]

STUDY	MERRITT (N = 50)[b]		GILL (N = 10)[c]	
	Inter-rater (%)	Intrarater (%)	Inter-rater (%)	Intrarater (%)
Modified Schober flexion	6.3	6.6	NA	.9 (poor)
Dual inclinometry—Full flexion	9.6	13.4	NA	33.9
Dual inclinometry—Full extension	65.4	50.7	NA	3.6
Fingertip-to-floor	83	76.4 (poor)	NA	14
Photometric assessment	NA	NA	NA	Poor
Right lateral flexion—Moll	11.9	8.9	NA	NA
Left lateral flexion—Moll	10.2	9.5	NA	NA
Extension—Moll	9.5	7.3	NA	NA

NA, not available.

[a] Data listed are coefficients of variation.

[b] Data from Merritt et al, 1986.

[c] Data from Gill et al, 1988.

the patient's best single effort. It also included an acceleration and deceleration component, which may lower the patient's "comfort zone," resulting in smaller measurements. The authors recommend a larger study to determine reliability and calculate a "correction factor" so the results could be utilized for impairment rating as, currently, the results differ from inclinometry, the recommended ROM approach for rating permanent impairment (Doege, 1993).

Hasten et al (1995) reported similar results utilizing the Applied Rehabilitation Concepts (ARCON) computerized system with standard dual inclinometry assessing flexion, extension, lateral flexion, and SLR. In a two-part study, the two methods lacked repeatability, as consistent differences were seen for some of the measurements, although a high degree of correlation with each other was noted. In part two, improved stabilization techniques resulted in a higher reliability for the ARCON. The conclusion was similar in that **the ARCON should not be used for rating impairments based on standard inclinometry** (Hasten et al, 1995).

IMPAIRMENT RATING AND RANGE OF MOTION: APPROACHES AND CONTROVERSIES

When rating permanent impairment, several approaches have been reported (McBride, 1962; Clark et al, 1988; Doege, 1993). Though any of these systems can be utilized, the AMA *Guides to the Evaluation of Permanent Impairment* was mentioned as one of the most commonly utilized and relied-upon approaches (Lowery et al, 1992), which is consistent with my own experience.

EVOLUTION OF THE AMA *GUIDES*

Four editions of the AMA *Guides* have been published. The first edition, published in 1971, was essentially a collection of articles that appeared in the *Journal of the American Medical Association* between 1959 and 1970. Because there was little to no guidance in the first edition for the reader to follow, John Mazion and Stanley Kaplan, both chiropractors, developed different formulas—essentially, a system for using the *Guides*. This approach was taught in the postgraduate orthopedics course initially through National College of Chiropractic and, later, through many other chiropractic colleges. The second edition was printed in 1984, 13 years later. In this edition, many of the formulas and aspects of the system that Drs Kaplan and Mazion created were adopted, but were not appropriately cited or referenced. As a result, the *Guides* became easier to understand and utilize, since the need for outside text references was reduced.

The third edition of the AMA *Guides* was printed only 4 years later in 1988 due to the vast influx of research and information that was reported during this period. In the third edition, the use of dual inclinometry for rating spinal ROM impairment was introduced, and providers rating spinal permanent impairment were given until 1990 to learn how to perform dual inclinometry (Engelberg, 1988). After 1990, an impairment rating utilizing dual inclinometry would take precedence over one using a two-arm goniometer. The 1988 AMA *Guides* also introduced a table combining specific diagnoses with the ROM impairment rating. This set the stage for the Diagnostic-Related Estimates (DRE) model introduced in the latest (fourth) edition, printed in 1993, which represents perhaps the greatest change in spinal rating of impairment since the *Guides* were first introduced. More specifically, the method of rating permanent impairment by a diagnosis rating method rather than by assessing loss of function ("impairment") was preferred. Until the most recent (fourth) edition, the *Guides* relied heavily on the use of the ROM model in the rating of spinal impairment. Although the method of using the inclinometer-based ROM model is still recommended and included in the *Guides*, its use is restricted to special circumstances, such as a tiebreaker when the DRE category cannot be decided or agreed upon. The DRE model was introduced, in part, due to criticisms of the lack of age- and gender-specific normative data utilized in the ROM tables as well as the technical skill required to perform inclinometry. Although the DRE model is the preferred model when an injury has occurred, it is necessary to utilize the ROM model, especially if the following scenarios are present:

- As a tiebreaker if the specific DRE impairment grade cannot be agreed upon
- If a past impairment rating using the ROM or functional model was previously utilized, and a comparison to that method is needed
- If impairment results that is not caused by a specific injury

Mayer (1987) also discusses controversies or problems associated with rating impairment. For example, the lack of standardized approaches to the rating of spinal impairment when compared to an impairment evaluation of an extremity is described. The variation between state and federal laws, in addition to the fact that a back injury is considered an injury to the "whole person" rather than a

smaller unit, results in impairment or disability evaluations that can differ, at times, tenfold between different evaluators. Couple this with injuries that are superimposed on a pre-existing disabling degenerative process that is not appropriately apportioned out (*if* pre-existing disability accompanied the degenerative process), and variations in impairment and/or disability evaluations are likely. Another controversy concerns the fact that the impairment rating process involves a one-time evaluation and assumes that the disability (intolerance to activities of daily living) associated with the impairment (loss of function such as ROM, strength, sensation; ie, a clinically measurable entity) is a static rather than a dynamic process. More specifically, pain associated with an injury more often than not results in decreased activity or activity intolerance on the part of the patient. This may be "organic" or real due to the extent of the injury, or "nonorganic" such as fear-avoidant behavior that accompanies pain. In either case, the activity intolerance leads, in turn, to disuse and deconditioning, which play a major role in contributing to impairment. Therefore, the process is usually ongoing, or dynamic, rather than static, especially if reactivation into activities through a rehabilitation program is not included in the treatment approach.

A third controversy in rating impairment lies in the fact that "disability behaviors" due to the imbalance between incentives and disincentives associated with litigation can exist. Often, the HCP views this as a negative factor and, as a result, reduces the measurement of impairment. The HCP's objectivity may be further impaired by the absence of objective measures to counter the claimant's allegations and physical "nonorganic signs" (Waddell et al, 1980). Since there is no contralateral side with which to compare function in spinal injuries, further difficulty faces the evaluator when rating impairment. The lack of objective measures commonly utilized in the evaluation process often leads to frustration on the part of the evaluator. The acute signs and symptoms are usually well resolved by the time of an impairment evaluation, and the physical examination methods commonly accepted as being "objective" are not sensitive or specific enough to disclose the underlying physical impairment. Mayer (1987) discusses the flaws associated with goniometric ROM evaluation compared to inclinometric ROM assessment approaches. It should also be mentioned that many evaluators of impairment still rely on visual estimation of spinal ROM, which has been clearly found to be inaccurate and, therefore, inappropriate for use when evaluating permanent impairment (Merritt et al, 1986; Gill et al, 1988; Rainville et al, 1994; Youdas et al, 1992; Doege, 1993).

Mayer (1987) discusses four major concepts as solutions to the problem associated with lumbar spine impairment examination. These are:

1. The back is a musculoskeletal unit with low back symptoms related to dysfunction.
2. When permanent neurological deficits exist, extremity deficits/dysfunction result.

CLINICAL TIP 14–7
ROM versus DRE Models

The ROM model is also very helpful when apportionment is required. I have noted at times that the DRE model fails to adequately reflect the total impairment, especially when a pre-existing condition is present and apportionment, or subtracting the pre-existing impairment is necessary. For example, if a mechanical low back condition results from an injury and a DRE category II is utilized, a 5% impairment is generated using the DRE injury model. However, if a less disabling form of mechanical low back pain was present before the accident, and apportionment is being considered, subtracting 5% for a pre-existing DRE category II condition would result in a 0% rating. The latter would be appropriate only if the residual effects of the second injury fully resolved back to the pre-second injury condition. However, if the current condition is worse or, the pre-second injury status could not be reached, the ROM model is often more practical since a pre-existing level of impairment can be calculated based on pre-second injury records and subtracted out of the most recent calculation of impairment. The resulting "apportioned" impairment rating will, therefore, reflect the residual injuries sustained from the second injury.

3. Because the low back is a "functional unit," its functional capacity can be objectively measured similar to a sports medicine assessment of an extremity.
4. The absence of visual feedback **makes quantitative assessment a necessity,** especially since there is no contralateral comparison. Moreover, **normal databases must be developed to compare patient capabilities against standardized population norms.**

Mayer then notes that an "important corollary concept is emerging" with respect to functional restoration or rehabilitation designed for the lumbar spine and guided by functional capacity measures to address the deconditioning syndrome (1987). Even though patients harboring impairment may suffer from a complex having both physical as well as psychosocioeconomic issues, the physical issues should be quantitatively assessed and attended to. Identifying the loss of function (physical performance) can greatly complement the diagnostic process of impairment evaluation in the lumbar spine.

Mayer (1987) includes a method for evaluating and quantifying lumbar function utilizing the following approaches:

- ROM measures (dual inclinometry)
- Isolated trunk strength measurement: extension/flexion and rotation (Cybex dynamometer)
- Cardiovascular fitness measures (bicycle ergometry)

CLINICAL TIP 14–8
Role of Physical Performance Testing

Physical performance/functional capacity testing is a much more sensitive and specific examination approach for identifying impairment, although it does not result in an "impairment rating," per se. Many tests available for evaluators to utilize have been reported in peer-reviewed literature as being safe, valid, reliable, reproducible, of good utility, *and* for which normative data is also included. Normative data can be compared to the patient's physical performance and a percentage of normal calculated. In my experience, it is common to find abnormal physical performance by the use of these tests in patients where classic provocative orthopedic testing is negative. By performing physical performance tests, functional pathologies can be identified *and* compared to normative data, when normative data exists. In a sense, impairment, which means loss of function, is proven to be either present or absent by the use of physical performance tests. Therefore, physical performance testing is a missing link in a standard disability/impairment evaluation. Refer to Chapter 16 for more information regarding a collection of physical performance tests called the quantitative functional capacity evaluation (QFCE).

- Lifting capacity measurement (Cybex lifttask—isokinetic lifting device)
- Measurement of activities of daily living (obstacle course—stations include pulling/pushing, shoveling, reaching overhead, bending into a bin, lifting at various levels, climbing, squatting, and twisting/bending; gait speed—stopwatch and measured course)
- Global effort rating (made by therapist using "effort factors" built into each functional capacity test; these are quantified and reported in summary as poor, fair, good, or excellent)

Much of what Mayer recommends necessitates the use of expensive, high-tech assessment equipment. However, a low-tech alternative approach that includes valid and reliable physical performance tests with normative data for comparative quantitative assessment includes the following tests, respectively:

- ROM measures (dual inclinometry) (ie, no change)
- Isolated trunk strength measurement: static back endurance test (back extensor muscles) (Alaranta et al, 1994); repetitive sit-up test (abdominal musculature) (Alantara et al, 1994); side bridge (quadratus lumborum musculature) (McGill, 1998)
- Cardiovascular fitness measures (3-minute step test) (Golding et al, 1989)
- Lifting capacity measurement (Matheson and Mooney, California functional capacity protocols) (Mooney et al, 1994)
- Measurement of activities of daily living (spinal function sort) (Mooney et al, 1994)
- Global effort rating (internal consistency and effort is evaluated in the spinal function sort); Waddell nonorganic low back pain signs (Waddell et al, 1980)

For a more complete description, please refer to Chapter 18 for cardiovascular fitness tests and Chapter 16 for quantitative functional capacity evaluation (QFCE)/physical performance tests, and spinal functional sort.

Mayer (1987) concludes with a discussion of future assessment approaches, stating that the "deconditioning syndrome" must be dealt with prior to concluding permanency. The "major caveat" described is that correction of these functional deficits requires the *"active participation"* on the part of the patient. However, the psychosocial barriers often accompanying long-term pain may prevent compliance. In spite of this, patients deserve the opportunity to help themselves become reintegrated into the workforce and return to a nondisabled status. Mayer describes as the "crux of the future medical–political conundrum" these questions:

- Will the additional rehabilitation costs facing the third-party payer be accepted for the willing and complying patient?
- What is to become of the patient who, because of psychosocioeconomic resons, does not comply or

actively participate in the rehabilitation role? Are such patients penalized, for example, by failing to continue ongoing disability payments or other rewards for their role? Similarly, should cardiac rehabilitation patients be penalized for smoking and/or failing to comply with a strict diet?

Mayer concludes: "the fact that we are in a position to begin to ask such questions demonstrates the new opportunity and challenge involved in spinal disability determination through lumbar quantitative assessment of function" (1987).

CERVICAL SPINE IMPAIRMENT RATING

In review of the cervical spine impairment rating charts found in the AMA *Guides*, the cutoff measurements for a nonimpairing ROM are as follows:

- 80 degrees of rotation ROM
- 45 degrees of lateral flexion ROM
- 50 degrees of flexion ROM
- 60 degrees of extension ROM (Doege, 1993)

In other words, a 0% impairment would result if a patient's ROM were at or greater than the measurements listed.

Creating a normative data ROM charting system that accurately reflects age and gender factors would allow for a more reliable way of rating impairment. Alaranta et al (1994) published age, gender, and work-type specific normative data for cervical rotation, which can be compared to the AMA *Guides* as the same one-inclinometer ROM methodology was practiced. This normative data was previously reported in Table 14–4. Because the most restricted cervical rotation ROM is 67 degrees, which represents the normative range for blue-collar females at ages 50 to 54 years a .5% impairment would result when utilizing the impairment rating figures currently in use (Doege, 1993). More specifically, 60 degrees is rated at 1% and 80 degrees represents 0% impairment. Therefore, extrapolating between the two, or 70 degrees, would yield a .5% impairment as it relates to the whole person, which would then be added to the impairments derived from the other cervical ROMs, yielding the total cervical ROM impairment. Using the same rationale and applying it to the remaining Alaranta ROM normative data (Table 14–4), any ROM between 65 and 75 degrees would be assigned a .5% impairment rating for rotation. In a review of the Table 14–4 data, this would include:

- Blue-collar males and females between the ages of 45 to 49 years (71 to 75 degrees)
- White-collar males and females over the age of 50 years (74 degrees)
- White-collar females between the ages of 40 to 44 years (73 degrees)

Because the worst impairment rating in rotation is .5%, one could argue that a small rating of .5% is in a sense, "close enough" and argue in favor of leaving the cervical rotation impairment rating chart the way it is as it results in less than 1% impairment for all the subjects tested.

Although only one inclinometer was utilized for lateral flexion in Alantara et al's study, it has been my experience that very little movement, such as 0 to 3 degrees, occurs at the T1 inclinometer during lateral flexion, especially if the shoulders are carefully held firmly against a chair back. The description of the technique used in measuring lateral flexion by Alaranta et al specifically states that similar care was taken, in addition to being seated in front of a mirror to further aid in avoiding trunk movement. If a conservative approach is used, such as reducing the Alaranta normative data by 5 degrees to represent the T1 inclinometer measurement (which should more than satisfy the trunk motion), a comparison of Alaranta et al's normative data and that of the AMA *Guides* can then be accomplished. Table 14–12 depicts Alaranta et al's normative data minus 5 degrees.

Considering the AMA *Guides'* impairment rating charts for cervical lateral flexion, the following represents the impairment and the corresponding measurement:

Table 14–12: Adjusted Normative Data for Cervical Lateral Flexion[a]

AGE (YRS)	MALES		FEMALES	
	Blue Collar	White Collar	Blue Collar	White Collar
35–39	34°	32°	35°	34°
40–44	32°	32°	33°	32°
45–49	27°	32°	32°	32°
50–54	28°	29°	28°	31°
35–54	31°	31°	31°	33°

[a] The normative data using one inclinometer measured in the seated position for cervical lateral flexion is reported. A 5-degree subtraction was utilized to compensate for the lack of a T1 inclinometer. Note the last row is an average of all subjects aged 35 to 54 years.
Modified from Alaranta et al, 1994.

- 0 degrees = 4% impairment whole person
- 15 degrees = 2%
- 30 degrees = 1%
- 45 degrees = 0%

Since 45 degrees represents 0% impairment and 30 degrees represents 1% impairment, for the majority of the normative data reported in Table 14–12, regardless of whether the male, female, white-collar, or blue-collar data is considered, the impairment rating is 1% for lateral flexion. Of interest, if the 5 degrees had not been subtracted from Alaranta et al's normative data, the impairment rating would still be .5% to 1%, depending on age, gender, and work type. Again, an argument could be made that a .5% to a 1% impairment for lateral flexion may be too small to consider changing the impairment rating charts.

Unfortunately, Alaranta et al combined flexion with extension and reported the global sagittal ROM using one inclinometer. However, utilizing normative data derived from the cervical ROM (Youdas et al, 1992), using only one inclinometer, the normative data for cervical flexion in both males and females between 10 and 90 year old ranges between 64.0 and 36.4 degrees, respectively. Of interest, there were no significant gender differences found with cervical flexion. Again, little movement occurs at T1 if the technique is performed on a seated patient who is carefully maintaining his or her back against the seat back. Therefore, assigning a value of 5 to represent T1 inclinometer motion allows for comparison to the AMA tables as previously reported for rotation. Doege (1993) reports that the cutoff between impairment and no impairment in cervical flexion is as follows:

- 50 degrees = 0%
- 30 degrees = 2%
- 15 degrees = 4%
- 0 degrees = 5%

A revised normal range of flexion is 59 to 31.4 degrees and, hence, a 0% to 2% impairment rating for cervical flexion would exist, as 50 degrees represents 0% and 30 degrees represents 2%, as noted.

In extension, the cervical ROM normative data for individuals 10 and 90 years of age ranges between 85.6 and 52.3 degrees for males and 85.6 and 50.3 degrees for females. Again, subtracting 5 degrees of ROM for T1 inclinometer movement, the ranges are reduced to 80.6 to 47.2 degrees and 80.6 to 45.3 degrees for males and females, respectively. The impairment percentages would, therefore, range between 0% and 1.5%, as 60 degrees represents 0% and 40 degrees reperesents 2% for both genders.

To complete the cervical spine impairment rating, ROM impairments in the same region are added together. Therefore, using the *least* normal ROM for each cervical motion, the maximum possible impairment rating is calculated as shown in Table 14–13. The smallest ROM was taken from the normative tables, 5 degrees was subtracted to compensate for the lack of a second inclinometer placed at the T1 area, and impairment of the whole person calculated. The total impairment figure reveals the maximum possible cervical spinal impairment using the most restricted ROM of the normative data. The measurements are derived from the data for 70- to 89-year-old males or females, depending on which was the lowest ROM.

Table 14–14 represents the impairment rating based on several authors' normative data utilizing the AMA *Guides* (Doege, 1993). Note that the normative data reported by Youdas et al (1992; right hand column) is reported in the range where the highest number represents the 10-year-old mean ROM, and the lowest number represents the 97-year-old mean. Hence, the impairment rating is also reported in a range from low to high impairment, respectively, and is gender specific.

Calculating the impairment leaving the impairment rating charts as they are, the percent impairment would

Table 14–13: Calculation of ROM Impairment Rating[a]

	ROM[a]	% IMPAIRMENT[a]	ROM[b]	% IMPAIRMENT[b]
Flexion	NA (39.2)	NA (1)	39.2°	1
Extension	NA (49.4)	NA (1)	49.4°	1
Right lateral flexion	28°	1	23.8°	1.5
Left lateral flexion	28°	1	22.6°	1.5
Right rotation	67°	.5	46.4°	1
Left rotation	67°	.5	46.8°	1
Total		5 (using Youdas data for flexion and extension impairment)		7

NA, not available.
[a] From Alaranta et al, 1994: Normative data using the least ROM to calculate the highest possible impairment rating. Since flexion and extension were combined, the 5% rating reflects an amount adding the Youdas et al data for greatest sagittal plane impairment.
[b] From Youdas et al, 1992.

Table 14–14: Cervical ROM Impairment Rating Based on the AMA *Guides*

	AMA *GUIDES* (ROM = IR%) (1993)	ALARANTA ET AL (1994)[a]		MAYER ET AL (1994)	YOUDAS ET AL (1992) (DEGREE CHANGE/ DECADE)	YOUDAS ET AL (1992) (MEAN RANGES AND IR%)	
		Male	Female	Male		Male	Female
Flexion	50° = 0%			50°	3°	64.0–36.4°	
	30° = 2%	(42.3–40.5°)[b] 1% IR	44.5–36 1–1.5% IR	0% IR		0%–.5%	
Extension	60° = 0%			63°	5°	85.6–52.3°	85.6–50.3°
	40° = 2%	(63.2–54.9°)[b] 0–1% IR	(73–60.3°)[b] 0% IR	0% IR		0–1% IR	0–1% IR
Right lateral flexion	45° = 0%	27–34°	28–35°	45°	3°	44.9–22.2°	48.9–22.6°
	15° = 2%	1% IR	.5–1% IR	0% IR		0–1.5 IR	0–1.5% IR
Left lateral flexion	45° = 0%	27–34°	28–35°	45°	3°	46.3–22.0°	46.6–22.6°
	15° = 2%	1% IR	.5–1% IR	0% IR		0–1.5% IR	0–1.5% IR
Right rotation	80° = 0%	71–78°	67–78°	85°	3°	74.1–44.2°	74.9–51.8°
	40° = 2%	0–.5%	0–.5%	0% IR		.5–2% IR	.5–1.5% IR
Left rotation	80° = 0%	71–78°	67–78°	85°	4°	72.3–45.2°	71.6–50.5°
	40° = 2%	0–.5%	0–.5%	0% IR		.5–1.5% IR	.5–1.5% IR
Total % impairment whole person	0–12%	4–5% IR[b] 3%[c]	2–4.5% IR[b] 1–3%[c]	0% IR	NA	.5–8% IR	.5–7.5% IR

IR, impairment rating; NA, not available.

[a] Normative data range is combined blue and white collar/gender groups between the ages of 35 and 54 years.

[b] Flexion and extension measurements were globally assessed by Alaranta et al and, hence, not comparable. Substituting the Youdas et al adjusted normative data, the impairment of flexion and extension increase the total by 1–2% for males (M) and 1–1.5% for females (F) aged 30–59 years.

[c] Partial impairment due to lack of flexion and extension normative data.

range between 1% in the 10- to 19-year-old bracket and 8% in the male 70- to 79-year-old bracket. Utilizing the normative data charts derived from Mayer et al (1994), where dual inclinometry was utilized as specifically described in the AMA *Guides,* the data can be modified to accommodate aging effects. More specifically, utilizing the information reported by Youdas et al (1992) where degrees are subtracted for each decade of aging, Table 14–15 reflects the adjusted ROM and associated impairment rating.

The results reported in Table 14–15 are very similar to the impairment ratings calculated in Table 14–14 using the data published by Alaranta et al (1994) and Youdas et al (1992) and by modifying it to compare more closely to the technique specifically described in the AMA *Guides* (Doege, 1993). The data reported in Table 14–15 represents the modified ROM after subtracting the degrees per decade of increasing age (Youdas et al, 1992). Previously, the question of leaving the impairment rating tables as they are since the ratings for each individual movement is small was raised. As one can see, the percent impairment calculated in Tables 14–14 and 14–15 illustrates the need for formulating tables modified to reflect the normal aging process and subsequent normal reduction in ROM, since the impair-

ment rating adds up as the effects of aging are introduced. When applying a reduction of degrees per decade to previously reported normative cervical spine data, the impairment rating charts shown in Tables 14–16 through 14–22 accommodate for the age and gender differences that result.

In order to determine "normative data" for lateral flexion, Youdas et al (1992) stated that the difference between genders was 2.0 degrees for left and 2.7 degrees for right lateral flexion. Therefore, taking the mean of 2.35 degrees, and rounding off to the nearest whole number, a 2-degree difference can be utilized to represent the difference between males and females. Since a 3-degree average loss was noted between decades, Tables 14–19 and 14–20 describe the adjusted normative data. Note that the normative data as reported by Mayer et al (1984) is increased by 3 degrees for the female group to represent the increased ROM noted in several of the studies for females (Mayer et al, 1984; Youdas et al, 1992).

LUMBAR SPINE IMPAIRMENT RATING

An argument similar to that raised earlier—regarding individual ROM movement impairments being so small that perhaps the impairment rating lumbar ROM charts should

Table 14–25: Adjusted Lumbar ROM Impairment Rating: Males

	32 YRS[a]	DEGREE CHANGE/ DECADE	40–49 YRS	50–59 YRS	60–69 YRS	70–79 YRS	80–89 YRS
Gross lumbar flexion motion	122° ± 15.6°	—	—	—	—	—	—
True lumbar flexion	65° (55°)[b] 0% (1–4%)[c]	2°	53° 1–4%	51° 2–4%	49° 3–4%	47° 3–5%	45° 4–5.5%
Gross lumbar extension	45° ± 14.6°	—	—	—	—	—	—
True lumbar extension	30° (25°)[d] 0%	3°	22° 1%	19° 2%	16° 3%	13° 4%	11° 5%
Right lateral flexion	25° (1994) 0%	2°	23° .5%	21° 1%	19° 1%	17° 1.5%	15° 2%
Left lateral flexion	25° (1994) 0%	2°	23° .5%	21° 1%	19° 1%	17° 1.5%	15° 2%
Total % impairment whole person	1–4	NA	3–6	6–8	8–9	10–12	13–14.5

NA, not available.

[a] This column represents Mayer et al's normative data, with modifications as indicated by footnotes b, c, and d.

[b] Although Mayer et al reported a 65 degree normal for true lumbar flexion, previously published normative data suggests this to be high. Therefore, based on previously published normative data as well as personal experience in rating impairment and collecting normative data, a 55 degree starting point for normal was utilized. A 2-degree reduction per decade was chosen based on personal experience that flexion is fairly well preserved in the elderly, although a significantly higher percentage of motion takes place at the sacral–hip region compared to a younger population where lumbar (T12–L1) motion is greater (Mayer et al, 1984; personal observation).

[c] Represents a range of impairment depending on the amount of sacral–hip motion. The low number of impairment represents the sacral–hip motion of 45 degrees or greater while the high number represents the sacral–hip motion of 40 to 44 degrees.

[d] Although Mayer et al reported a 30-degree normal for 32-year-old male railroad workers, Keeley et al (1986) reported 26.6 degrees and 27.3 degrees for males and females, respectively, and Mayer et al (1984) published an average of 27 degrees between males and females. Hence, a 25-degree amount was chosen to represent the normal.

RANGE OF MOTION MODEL OF IMPAIRMENT RATING: FACTORS TO CONSIDER

Factors previously discussed that can affect the ROM measurement results must also be considered when utilizing the ROM model for rating permanent impairment of the spine. More specifically, if only the active ROM is utilized, the rating of impairment may result in an excessively high figure since passive ROMs are generally greater by approximately 10% (Wong and Nansel, 1992). The AMA *Guides* are not clear as to the recommended ROM inclinometric mensuration approach to use. The *Guides* specifically recommend using inclinometry "firmly applied to the subcutaneous skeletal structure while the structure is moving through the entire range of motion" (Doege, 1993). However, no instructions or recommendations such as active, passive, or actively assisted forms of ROM mensuration are described in the *Guides*. Therefore, confusion exists as to whether one should measure active, passive, or actively assisted ROM when rating permanent impairment using the ROM model. Since ROM is generally performed actively in activities of daily living, one might assume that rating impairment in a functional or ROM model should be done by measuring the active ROM. Although this is how students are generally instructed in postgraduate courses, the *Guides* are not specific on this issue. This point, coupled with the fact that the ROM impairment rating charts are not broken down into age and gender categories and do not mention whether the eyes are to remain open or closed (Nansel and Peneff, 1990), may further lead one to suspect the validity of rating impairment using the ROM model.

The use of spinal ROM in determining impairment was specifically studied in 81 healthy subjects by two orthopedic surgeons using the dual inclinometer method (Lowery et al, 1992). In this study, the impairment ranged between 2% and 38.5% with a mean value of 10.8%. The SLR validity screen was included in the lumbar ROM impairment assessment where the tightest SLR must be within 15 degrees of the sum of flexion and extension sacral–hip measurements. In the latter, 40 of the 81 subjects (49.4%) were invalidated using this approach. The

Table 14–26: Modified Lumbar Flexion Impairment Rating[a]

SACRAL–HIP FLEXION ANGLE (DEGREES)	TRUE LUMBAR SPINE FLEXION ANGLE (0 DEGREES)						% IMPAIRMENT WHOLE PERSON
	(≤ 39 yrs)	40–49 yrs	50–59 yrs	60–69 yrs	70–79 yrs	80–89 yrs	
	55°+	50°+	45°+	40°+	35°+	30°+	0
	45°	41°	37°	33°	29°	25°	2
45°+	30°	27°	24°	21°	18°	16°	4
	15°	14°	12°	11°	9°	8°	7
	0°	0°	0°	0°	0°	0°	10
	50°+	45°+	40°+	35°+	30°+	25°+	0
30–45°	40°	36°	32°	28°	24°	20°	4
	20°	18°	16°	14°	12°	10°	7
	0°	0°	0°	0°	0°	0°	10
	40°+	35°+°	30°+	25°+	20°+	15°+	2
0–29°	30°	26°	22°	18°	14°	11°	5
	15°	13°	11°	9°	7°	6°	8
	0°	0°	0°	0°	0°	0°	11

[a] In the first row, 55 degrees was chosen based on Alaranta et al (52 degrees; 1994), Mayer et al (55 degrees; 1984), and personal experience in collecting normative data. A 5-degree per decade reduction over age 40 was chosen based on normative data of Alaranta et al, who reported data based on age, gender, and work-class (true lumbar flexion of 41–46 degrees for 50–54 year olds). Ratios were established to calculate the percent change between the ≤ 39-year-old column, which remained unchanged from the AMA *Guides* except for lowering the starting measurement to 55 degrees. An additional rating of 0% was assigned to the 30–45 degree sacral–hip (SH) row, since true lumbar flexion, regardless of the ROM, would yield an impairment if the SH measurement was < 45 degrees and the existing ROM table were not modified.

Table 14–27: Modified Lumbar Extension Impairment Rating[a]

≤ 39 YRS	40–49 YRS	50–59 YRS	60–69 YRS	70–79 YRS	80–89 YRS	% IMPAIRMENT WHOLE PERSON
0°	0°	0°	0°	0°	0°	7
10°	9°	8°	7°	6°	5°	5
15°	14°	12°	10°	8°	7°	3
20°	18°	16°	13°	11°	9°	2
25°	22°	19°	16°	13°	11°	0

[a] Extension is from a neutral (0 degree) position. A 3-degree decrease in ROM was chosen based on Alaranta et al's normative data of 14–20 degrees for 34–39 year olds (1994). The original data published in the AMA *Guides* was retained, as a normative data of 27 degrees was consistently reported by Mayer et al (1984), Keeley et al (1986), Hasten (1995) (22 degrees, males; 24 degrees, females), and personal experience in gathering normative data and rating impairment.

Table 14–28: Modified Lumbar Lateral Flexion Impairment Rating[a]

≤ 39 YRS	40–49 YRS	50–59 YRS	60–69 YRS	70–79 YRS	80–89 YRS	% IMPAIRMENT WHOLE PERSON
0°	0°	0°	0°	0°	0°	5
10°	9°	8°	7°	6°	5°	3
15°	14°	12°	11°	10°	8°	2
20°	18°	16°	14°	13°	11°	1
25°	23°	21°	19°	17°	15°	0

[a] Lateral extension is from a neutral (0 degree) position.

mean cervical impairment was 7.8 degrees ± 2.96 SD, for men and 8.17 degrees ± 4.08 SD, for women. The mean lumbar impairment was 2.91 degrees ± 2.73 SD for men and 3.33 degrees ± 4.29 SD for women. The mean total impairment was 10.45 degrees ± 4.64 SD and 11.12 degrees ± 6.92 SD for men and women, respectively. A linear relationship between age and percent impairment was also found as the level of impairment increased with age for cervical, lumbar, and total impairment percentages ($P = .0001$). Lowery et al (1992) concluded that an overestimate of impairment of up to 38% was possible and recommended using an alternate method of rating impairment that accounts for age-related differences in spinal motion.

One of the primary objectives of the AMA *Guides* is to obtain similar impairment rating results when different HCPs evaluate impairments using similar methods (Doege, 1993). Therefore, utilizing the most reliable examination approach makes the most sense. The "injury model" may better accomplish this goal, as no age- or gender-specific spinal ROM impairment rating charts are available to utilize.

Results reported by Rainville et al (1994) in a prospective chronic low back pain study that compared total lumbar flexion (T12 measurment only) to true lumbar flexion, correlated better with self-reported disability (using the Million Visual Analogue Scale, and other measures of pain, depression, and impairment) after completion of an intensive rehabilitative program. More specifically, prior to rehabilitation, both measurements accounted for similar amounts of the variance in disability scoring. However, after treatment/rehabilitation, total flexion correlated higher with self-reported disability ($r = -.62$ vs $r = -.43$). Dual inclinometry has been criticized as being too time consuming (Merritt et al, 1986), requiring skilled examiners to obtain reliable measurements (Chiarello and Savidge, 1993), and any error made in a single measurement is compounded when a second measurement is made (Rondinelli et al, 1992). Rainville et al (1994) reported that the total flexion and true lumbar flexion correlated well both before and after treatment ($r = .88$, and $r = .84$, respectively). However, total lumbar flexion correlated best with disability scores after treatment, as true lumbar flexion did not change as significantly. Waddell et al (1992) studied 70 normal and 120 subjects with chronic mechanical low back pain and reported similar findings. More specifically, they reported that the total lumbosacral flexion motion measured at T12–L1 explained the greatest proportion of the variance of disability scores of any other physical examination measure, including true lumbar flexion (Waddell et al, 1992). Rainville et al (1994) reports that total lumbosacral motion correlates closely with true lumbar flexion both before and after rehabilitation and, therefore, substitution may be possible for assessing impairments of the lumbar spine using total lumbosacral flexion.

In summary, the following factors affect validity and reliability when measuring ROM:

- Time of day or diurnal ROM variances (Wing et al, 1992; Ensink et al, 1996)
- Mouth open versus closed affects cervical flexion/extension range (Alaranta et al, 1994)
- Eyes open versus closed (Nansel and Peneff, 1990)
- Active versus passive ROM (Wong and Nansel, 1992)
- Psychological factors (Whaley, 1973)
- Age- and gender-specific variances (O'Driscoll and Tomenson, 1982; Keeley et al, 1986; Youdas et al, 1991, 1992; Good and Mikkelson, 1992; Dvorak et al, 1992; Kuhlman, 1993; Bussieres, 1994)
- Data derived from different technologies are not interchangeable (Youdas et al, 1991)
- Maximum effort cannot be guaranteed and the type of instructions given to the patient during isokinetic trunk strength testing affects effort (Matheson et al, 1990); this similarly was reported for ROM testing (Mayer et al, 1994)
- Accuracy of technique between evaluators is less reliable (Mayer et al, 1995, Nilsson et al, 1996a) and the type of inclinometer utilized may affect accuracy; these technical accuracy factors include:
  - difficult-to-read dials
  - increments of greater than 1 degree (such as 2- or 5-degree increments)
  - pendulum "hang-up" (unless the pendulum swings freely, it can get caught on the inside of the inclinometer)
  - inclinometer base shape (flat bases rock or wobble on convex surfaces); the best shape is an inclinometer with "feet" at the ends of the base so that a two-point contact can be achieved
  - accurate placement of the inclinometer, as bony landmarks can be difficult to locate, especially in obese individuals; this demands careful identifi-

---

CLINICAL TIP 14–9
Viable Inclinometer Alternatives

Any inclinometer "qualifies" as being appropriate for assessment of ROM impairment. Therefore, one can perform accurate ROM assessments very inexpensively with hardware store types of inclinometers. Often, modifications to these instruments can be made so that the face/dial rotates rather than remaining fixed, which allows for a true-zero position to be obtained in nonhorizontal or nonvertical starting points (eg, sacral base, T12, and T1). In my experience, dual inclinometry such as that shown in Figures 16–14 (LROM) and 16–22 (CROM) allows for minimal error and ease of application, as there is no moving of the inclinometer master or slave during the procedure. Also, the LED readout extrapolates the math or subtraction of the two inclinometer figures, and it is not attached to a base unit where the cord might get in the way.

cation of the inclinometer placement so that close to the same placement can be repeated in future assessments

- re-zeroing of the inclinometer is not recommended as failure to return to identical starting points adds error to the measurement, especially when comparing individual motion such as flexion/extension to global sagittal motion data
- the most accurate approach is dual inclinometry, as it avoids the need for movement of the single-inclinometer method, which only adds to the potential for error

RANGE OF MOTION AS A DISCRIMINATOR OF LOW BACK PAIN

In several studies, ROM mensuration and other forms of physical performance tests have been reported to be able to discriminate between those with and without low back pain (Haas and Nyiendo, 1992; Hamalainen et al, 1993; Tsai and Wrendmark, 1993; Moffroid et al, 1994; Moffroid and Haugh, 1995; Thomas, 1998). Moffroid and Haugh (1995) discuss a classification schema for both acute and subacute low back pain, stating that biases must be minimized when attempting to validate criteria used in researching for a reliable approach. In attempting to offer terminology that can be embraced by both HCPs and those in research, Harper et al (1992) offered the following three major categories:

1. *Primary impairments:* pain and movement loss
2. *Secondary impairments:* activity intolerance due to movement restrictions, including work, sexual activity, recreation, home management, self-care, and transportation; and secondary disabilities, including problems associated with feelings of well-being, role adaptation, thinking, emotions, and quality of life
3. *Tertiary handicaps:* related to self-sufficiency, family membership, social interactions, and occupation

McKENZIE SYNDROME CLASSIFICATION SYSTEM

McKenzie classified low back pain patients based on ROM movement patterns and the presence or absence of rapidly centralizing, peripheralizing, or abolishing low back and radiating pain into one of three syndromes, entitled (1) derangement, (2) dysfunction, and (3) postural syndromes (McKenzie, 1981). These syndromes, in brief, are analogous to (1) disc injury, (2) mechanical shortening of soft tissues, and (3) constant static postural forces placed on tissues, respectively (Moffroid and Haugh, 1995). The clinical phenomenon known as "centralization" was first described by McKenzie in 1981. This is the finding in which

the most distal extent of referred or radicular symptoms rapidly recedes to the midline of the spine by using singular or repeated end-range lumbar movements. The midline pain may also be abolished by the same testing procedure. Although this can occur in any spinal region, it is often discussed in context with lumbar spine and sciatic nerve complaints. Because agreement on lumbar diagnoses is so variable (Spitzer et al, 1987), the chosen treatment regimens may be aimed at a faulty diagnosis and may, therefore, lead to a resulting poor treatment response. The situation is often further augmented by the confusion that establishing a diagnosis often becomes dependent on high-tech assessment methods such as computed tomography (CT) or magnetic resonance imaging (MRI) scanning. However, the previously reported high rates of false-positives (Boden et al, 1990; Jensen et al, 1994) and false-negatives (Kornberg, 1988; Zuchermann et al, 1988) support the inadequacies of relying on these expensive and sometimes misleading tests (Bigos et al, 1994). Hence, the importance of establishing an accurate diagnosis of lumbar radiculopathy has been a topic of shared concern for some time.

Donelson et al (1997) compared, prospectively, the McKenzie protocol with discographic pain provocation and annular competency. **Centralization of referred pain has been reported as a very common occurrence during the McKenzie assessment and treatment of patients with discographic pain** (Donelson et al, 1990, 1991a, 1991b; Delitto, 1993; Erhard, 1994; Long, 1995). The Donelson et al study set out to prove or disprove whether any relationship between disc arrangement as assessed by discography with patient responses of centralization and peripheralization exists. Commonly used lumbar test movements performed repeatedly in both loaded and unloaded positions will determine the presence of a directional preference based on whether referred pain can be centralized or midline pain abolished. The commonly used lumbar tests movements include the following:

- Flexion in standing (toe-touches): single and repeated
- Extension in standing (leaning backward while supporting the low back with the hands): single and repeated
- Slide-gliding while standing (with or without overpressure): right and left, single and repeated
- Extension while lying (prone press-up): single and repeated
- Flexion while lying (double knee-to-chest from a supine position): single and repeated
- Flexion/rotation with overpressure (patient supine, knees and shoulders moved in opposite directions) (Donelson et al, 1997)

Of these positions, extension is the most common position that centralizes radicular symptoms (Donelson et al, 1991a; McKenzie, 1981), **whereas side-gliding or laterally**

directed movements are less common. In McKenzie's 1981 text, he proposed that the direction of bending that centralizes the pain correlates precisely with the direction in which the nucleus pulposus migrates, thus placing mechanical pressure upon a nerve root, resulting in referring symptoms into the lower extremity. **In the normally hydrated disc, an offset load on the disc in the lesion-specific direction of the spinal movement can reduce the pressure of the nucleus of the disc onto the nerve root, thus allowing centralization and/or reduced low back pain. The position that abolishes symptoms is called the "directional preference" or position biased (such as extension bias).** Generally, if multiple positions peripheralize or worsen radicular symptoms and no directional preference can be found, the annulus is considered to be incompetent and the hydrostatic mechanism nonfunctional. This study utilized 63 patients, 41 men and 22 women (average age 39.6 ± 11.1 years) all complaining of low back pain of at least 3 months (median 15.3 ± 12.2 months) with varying degrees of lower extremity altered sensation and pain. Results revealed that the McKenzie assessment process reliability differentiated those with dicogenic pain from those without discogenic pain ($P < .001$). Also, differentiation between those with—versus those without—a competent annulus in symptomatic discs was accomplished with McKenzie protocols ($P < .042$), and **was superior to magnetic resonance imaging in distinguishing painful from nonpainful discs** (Donaldson et al, 1997).

CLINICAL TIP 14–10
Surgical Criteria for Lumbar Disc Injury

I have noticed that, when centralization occurs, the prognosis is far more favorable than when pain does not centralize. Although this prognostic factor may seem obvious, the ability to determine a poor prognosis on day 1 when evaluating the sciatic-presenting patient is clinically very important as the need for aggressive therapy for the more difficult patient may be identified and administered immediately. This immediate response may improve results and/or allow for a more prompt diagnostic workup (CT, MRI, EMG, etc) and surgical consultation. The following surgical criteria for lumbar disc injury were developed after interviewing three orthopedic surgeons and three neurosurgeons in preparation for a presentation:

- Pain must exceed the level of the knee
- Neurological losses (motor and/or sensory) must be objectively identified
- Patients must have failed to respond to nonsurgical care for at least 6 weeks
- Progressive neurological losses, bowel/bladder weakening, and/or acute foot drop constitute medical emergencies
- ***Most Important:*** the patient consents to and, wants to proceed with surgery

---

Riddle and Rothstein (1993) offer a less optimistic result regarding McKenzie protocols. More specifically, 363 patients with low back pain were evaluated by randomly paired physical therapists (PTs; 16 total) in 8 different clinics. A dual purpose of the study included, first, assessment of the inter-tester reliability of the McKenzie method, and second, determination if the training level of the PTs affects reliability. With respect to the latter, some of the PTs had prior training while others had less training. In this study, the kappa value on agreement of patient classification was .26, suggesting poor reliability, and agreement on which syndrome was present was 39%. Riddle and Rothstein (1993) concluded that **assessments of the syndrome present in patients with low back pain appear to be unreliable when using the McKenzie system.** This paper includes an appendix where an excellent description of the McKenzie protocol is summarized from the original 1981 text. More specifically, the lumbar spine evaluation includes the following:

A. History
B. Examination
   1. Posture standing
   2. Posture sitting
   3. Leg length discrepancy
   4. Neurological examination
C. Assessment of movement loss
   1. Flexion
   2. Extension
   3. Side-gliding
D. Effects of test movements on the patient's pain (see previously described test movements) (Riddle and Rothstein, 1993)

A physical examination form for the various McKenzie tests can be found in Appendix Form E–1.

Refer to Chapter 16 regarding quantitative function capacity evaluation for further discussion on discriminative tests. More optimistic were the findings of Kilby and associates (1990), who reported that therapists trained in McKenzie techniques were able to classify patients successfully using the three McKenzie groups.

ASSOCIATION BETWEEN SPINAL RANGE OF MOTION AND LOW BACK PAIN

The association between low back pain and spinal mobility in a primary care setting was investigated as a possible discriminator for differentiation between subjects with low back pain and those without (Thomas et al, 1998). The study included 344 participants with low back pain who were compared to 118 subjects who denied ever having back pain. Various methods of ROM assessment were utilized, including right and left lateral flexion, standing extension, modified Schober's test, finger-to-floor distance, and right and left knee extension (modified SLR). A statistically significant reduction in all planes of motion was reported in those with low back pain. Modified Schober's test, standing extension, and left knee extension were the most discriminatory tests, with likelihood ratios of approximately 5 for the optimal cutoff. Three of the seven movements were observed in 50% of the low back pain cases and in less than 5% of the pain-free participants. There was no significant stratification noted by the presence of radiating leg pain (Thomas et al, 1998).

The numerous patient classification approaches previously discussed illustrate the need for establishing clear criteria in order to understand the pathological process and cause, establishing optimum management and treatment strategies, and predicting outcomes. No clear agreement exists as to which factors should be used, either singularly or as a group, to establish patient classification; thus, the quest for this answer remains at large until more concise research addresses these issues.

Conclusion

ROM assessment has a long history of representing one of the "standard" physical examination tests in patients presenting with neuromusculoskeletal complaints. Various reported technologies that can be utilized from a low-tech, low-expense standpoint have been reviewed in this chapter, and where available, normative data included and compared. Age and gender factors as well as a host of other factors affecting ROM mensuration have been presented. In the medical–legal arena, the ROM model has historically been a basis for rating permanent impairment. Therefore, a section of this chapter model has historically been a basis for rating permanent impairment. Therefore, a section of this chapter devoted to this subject was included as well as a historical view of the AMA *Guides to the Evaluation of Permanent Impairment* from the 1950s to present. Modified impairment rating charts for cervical and lumbar spinal impairment rating, including age- and gender-specific factors where applicable, were introduced in an attempt to provide a more accurate alternative to the present tables available in the AMA *Guides.* Perhaps the most important use of ROM reviewed was its ability to discriminate between various assessment and treatment outcomes in a population with low back pain. Future research may shed further light on how well ROM assessment approaches will be able to predict surgical and nonsurgical outcomes, similar to the Quebec Task Force Classification method (Atlas, 1996).

Although there are controversies associated with spinal ROM testing, clinically practical information is derived from its assessment, and as a result, it has continued to survive these criticisms and remains an important examination procedure. Further investigation may change the approach to the use of technologies that have been reported to assess ROM. For example, comparing ROM to disability scores before and after rehabilitation, global ROM such as gross lumbar flexion measured from T12 inclinometry exclusively correlated best with disability scores after treatment, as true lumbar flexion did not change as significantly (Rainville et al, 1994). Perhaps alternative noninclinometric methods of assessing lumbar flexion, such as the modified Schober method, will become the standard. Future research will help shed further light on the most valid and reliable method of spinal ROM assessment so that HCPs can continue to modify their approaches accordingly. The use of ROM as an objective outcome assessment tool has proven itself, in my experience, as well as the many referenced materials reviewed in this chapter.

REFERENCES

Alaranta H, Harri H, Heliovaara M, Soukka A, Harju R. Flexibility of the spine: Normative values of goniometric and tape measurements. *Scand J Rehab Med.* 1994;26:147–154.

Alund M, Larsson S-E. Three-dimensional analysis of neck motion: A clinical method. *Spine.* 1990;15:87–91.

AAOS. *Joint Motion: Method of Measuring and Recording.* Chicago, Ill: American Academy of Orthopaedic Surgeons; 1965.

Anderson JAD, Sweetman BJ. A combined flexi-rule/hydrogoniometer for measurement of lumbar spine and its sagittal movement. *Rheumatol Rehabil.* 1975;14:173–179.

Atlas SJ, Deyo RA, Patrick DL, Convery K, Keller RB, Singer DE. The Quebec Task Force Classification for Spinal Disorders and the severity, treatment, and outcomes of sciatica and lumbar spine stenosis. *Spine.* 1996;21:2885–2892.

Battie M, Bigos S, Fisher L, et al. The role of spinal flexibility in back pain complaints within industry: A prospective study. *Spine*. 1990;15:768–773.

Bennett JG, Bergamanis LE, Carpenter JK, Skowlund HV. Range of motion of the neck. *J Amer Phys Ther Assoc*. 1963;43:45–47.

Bigos SJ, Bowyer RO, Braen RG, et al. *Acute Low Back Problems in Adults*. US Dept of Health and Human Services, Public Health Service, Agency for Health Care Policy Research publication 95-0642.

Boden SD, Davis DO, Dina TS, Patronas NJ, Wiesel SW. Abnormal magnetic-resonance scans of the lumbar spine in asymptomatic subjects: A prospective investigation. *J Bone Joine Surg [Am]*. 1990;72:403–408.

Brand RA, Lehmann TR. Low back impairment rating practices of orthopaedic surgeons. *Spine*. 1983;8:75–81.

Buck CA, Dameron FB, Dow MJ, Skowlund HV. Study of normal range of motion in the neck utilizing a bubble goniometer. *Arch Phys Med Rehabil*. 1959;40:390–392.

Burdett RG, Brouwn KE, Fall MP. Reliability and validity of four instruments for measuring lumbar spine and pelvic positions. *Phys Ther*. 1986;66:677–684.

Burton AK, Tillotson KM, Troup JDG. Variation in lumbar sagittal mobility with low-back trouble. *Spine*. 1989;14:584–590.

Bussieres A. A review of functional outcome measures for cervical spine disorders: Literature review. *J CCA*. 1994;38:32–40.

Capuano-Pucci D, Rheault W, Aukai J, Bracke M, Day R, Pastrick M. Intratester and intertester reliability of the cervical range of motion device. *Arch Phys Med Rehabil*. 1991;72:338–340.

Carlson A. *Communication Systems*. 3rd ed. New York, NY: McGraw-Hill; 1986:180–185.

Carman D, Brown R, Birch J. Measurement of scoliosis and kyphosis radiographs: Intra-observer and interobserver variation. *J Bone Joint Surg [Am]*. 1990;72:319.

Chiarello CM, Savidge R. Interrater reliability of the Cybex EDI-320 and fluid goniometer in normals and patients with low back pain. *Arch Phys Med Rehabil*. 1993;74:32–37.

Clark WL, Haldeman S, Johnson P, et al. Back impairment and disability determination: Another attempt at objective, reliable rating. *Spine*. 1988;13:332–341.

Cole TM, Tobis JS. Measurement of musculoskeletal function: Goniometry. In: Kottke FJ, Stillwell GK, Lehman JF, eds. *Krusen's Handbook of Physical Medicine and Rehabilitation*. 3rd ed. Philadelphia, Pa: Saunders; 1982:19–33.

Cowell H. Editorial: Radiographic measurements and clinical decisions. *J Bone Joint Surg [Am]*. 1990;72:319.

Defibaugh JJ. Measurement of heat motion. *J Am Phys Ther Assoc*. 1964;44:157–168.

Delitto A, Cibullia MT, Erhard RE, et al. Evidence for use of an extension-mobilization category in acute low back syndrome: A prescriptive validation pilot study. *Phys Ther*. 1993;73:216–228.

Dillard J, Trafimow J, Andersson G, Cronin K. Motion of the lumbar spine: Reliability of two measurement techniques. *Spine*. 1991;16:321–324.

Doege TC, ed. *Guides to the Evaluation of Permanent Impairment*. 4th ed. Chicago, Ill: American Medical Association; 1993.

Donelson R, Aprill C, Medcalf R, Grant W. A prospective study of centralization of lumbar and referred pain: A predictor of symptomatic discs and annular competence. *Spine*. 1997;22:1111–1122.

Donelson R, Grant W, Kamps C, Medcalf R. Pain response to sagittal end-range spinal motion: A multi-centered, prospective, randomized trial. *Spine*. 1991a;16:S206–S212.

Donelson R, Grant W, Kamps C, Medcalf R. Pain response to end-range spinal motion in the frontal plane: A multi-centered, prospective trial. Presented at the International Society for the Study of the Lumbar Spine, Heidelberg, Germany, May 1991b.

Donelson R, Silva G, Murphy K. The centralization phenomenon: Its usefulness in evaluating and treating referred pain. *Spine*. 1990;15:211–215.

Dopf CA, Mandel SS, Geiger DF, Mayer PJ. Analysis of spine motion variability using a computerized goniometer compared to physical examination: A prospective clinical study. *Spine*. 1994;19:586–595.

Dvorak J, Antinnes JA, Panjabi M, Loustalot D, Bonomo M. Age and gender related normal motion of the cervical spine. *Spine*. 1992;17:S393–S394.

Engelberg AL, ed. *Guides to the Evaluation of Permanent Impairment*. 3rd ed. Chicago, Ill: American Medical Association; 1988:71–94.

Ensink F-BM, Saur PMM, Frese K, Seeger D, Hildebrandt J. Lumbar range of motion: Influence of time of day and individual factors on measurements. *Spine*. 1996;21:1339–1343.

Erhard RE, Delitto A, Cibullia MT. Relative effectiveness of an extension program and a combined program of manipulation and flexion and extension exercises in patients with acute low back syndrome. *Phys Ther*. 1994;29:1093–1100.

Ferlic D. The range of motion of the "normal" cervical spine. *Bull Johns Hopkins Hosp*. 1962;110:59–65.

Fitzgerald GK, Wynveen KJ, Rheault W, Rothschild B. Objective assessment with establishment of normal values for lumbar spinal range of motion. *Phys Ther*. 1983;63:1776–1781.

Foust DR, Chaffin BC, Snyder RG, Baum JK. Cervical range of motion and dynamic response and strength of cervical muscles. *SAE Transactions*. 1973;82:3222–3234.

Gill K, Krag MH, Johnson GB, Haugh LD, Pope MH. Repeatability of four clinical methods of assessment of lumbar spine motion. *Spine*. 1988;13:50–53.

Golding LA, Myers CR, Sinning WE, eds. *Y's Way to Physical Fitness*. 3rd ed. Champaign, Ill: Human Kinetics; 1989.

Good CJ, Mikkelsen GB. Intersegmental sagittal motion in the lower cervical spine and discogenic spondylosis: A preliminary study. *J Manipulative Physiol Ther*. 1992;15:556–564.

Gracovetsky S, Newman N, Pawlowsky M, Lanzo V, Davey B, Robinson L. A database for estimating normal spinal motion derived from noninvasive measurements. *Spine*. 1995;20:1036–1046.

Granberry W, Noble P, Woods W. Evaluation of an electrogoniometric instrument for measurement of laxity of the knee. *J Bone Joint Surg [Am]*. 1990;72:1316–1322.

Haas M, Nyiendo J. Lumbar motion trends and correlation with low back pain. A roentgenological evaluation of quantitative segmental motion in lateral bending. *J Manipulative Physiol Ther*. 1992;15:224–234.

Hamalainen O, Vanharanta H, Bloigu R. Determinants of +Gz-related neck pain—a preliminary survey. *Aviat Space Environ Med*. 1993;64:651–652.

Harper AC, Harper DA, Lambert LJ, et al: Symptoms of impairment, disability and handicap in low back pain: A taxonomy. *Pain*. 1992;50:189–195.

Hasten DL, Johnston A, Lea RD. Validity of the Applied Rehabilitation Concepts (ARCON) System for lumbar range of motion. *Spine*. 1995;20:1279–1283.

Jensen MC, Brant-Zawadski MN, Obuchowski N, Modic MT, Malkasian D, Ross JS. Magnetic resonance imaging of the lumbar spine in people without back pain. *N Engl J Med*. 1994;331:69–73.

Kadir N, Grayson MF, Goldberg AAJ, Swain MC. A new neck goniometer. *Rheumatol Rehabil*. 1981;20:219–226.

Keeley J, Mayer TG, Cox R, Gatchel RJ, Smith J, Mooney V. Quantification of lumbar function. Part 5: Reliability of range-of-motion measures in the sagittal plane and an in vivo torso rotation measurement technique. *Spine*. 1986;11:31–35.

Kilby J, Stignant M, Roberts A. The reliability of back pain assessment by physiotherapists using a McKenzie algorithm. *Physiotherapy*. 1990;76:479–583.

Kornberg M. Discography and magnetic resonance imaging in the diagnosis of lumbar disc disruption. *Spine*. 1988;14:1368–1372.

Kottke FJ, Blanchard RS. A study of degenerative changes of the cervical spine in relation to age. *Bull Univ Minn Hosp*. 1953;24:470–479.

Kuhlman KA. Cervical range of motion in the elderly. *Arch Phys Med Rehabil*. 1993;74:1071–1079.

Leighton JR. Flexibility characteristics of males ten to eighteen years of age. *Arch Phys Med Rehabil*. 1956;37:494–499.

Lind B, Sihlbom H, Norwall A, Malchau H. Normal range of motion of the cervical spine. *Arch Phys Med Rehabil*. 1989;70:692–695.

Loebl WY. Measurement of spinal posture and range of spinal movement. *Ann Phys Med*. 1967;9:103–110.

Loebl WY. Regional rotation of the spine. *Rheumatol Rehabil*. 1973;12:223.

Long AL. The centralization phenomenon: Its usefulness as a predictor of outcome in conservative treatment of chronic low back pain (a pilot study). *Spine*. 1995;20:2513–2521.

Lowery WD, Horn TJ, Boden SD, Wiesel SW. Impairment evaluation based on spinal range of motion in normal subjects. *J Spinal Disord*. 1992;5:398–402.

Lysell E. Motion in the cervical spine: An experimental study on autopsy specimens. *Acta Orthop Scand*. 1969;Supp 123:61.

Macrae IF, Wright V. Measurement of back movement. *Ann Rheum Dis*. 1969;28:584–589.

Matheson L, Mooney V, Jarvis G, et al. Progressive lifting capacity with masked weights: Reliability study. International Society for the Study of the Lumbar Spine. Boston, MA, June, 1990.

Mayer RS, Chen I-H, Lavender SA, Trafimow JH, Andersson GBJ. Variance in the measurement of sagittal lumbar spine range of motion among examiners, subjects, and instruments. *Spine*. 1995;20:1489–1493.

Mayer TG. Assessment of lumbar function. *Clin Ortho Rel Res*. 1987;August (221):99–109.

Mayer TG, Gatchel RJ, Keeley J, Mayer H, Richling D. A male incumbent worker industrial database. *Spine*. 1994;19:755–761.

Mayer T, Kondraske G, Beals S, Gatchel R. Spinal range of motion. Accuracy and sources of error with inclinometric measurement. *Spine.* 1997;22:1976–1984.

Mayer TG, Tencer AF, Kristoferson S, Mooney V. Use of noninvasive techniques for quantification of spinal range-of-motion in normal subjects and chronic low-back dysfunction patients. *Spine.* 1984;9:588–595.

McBride ED. Disability evaluation. *J Bone Joint Surg.* 1962;44A:1441–1446.

McGill S. LACC Rehabilitation class notes. Denver, Colo, March, 1998.

McKenzie RA. The lumbar spine: Mechanical diagnosis and therapy. Waikanae, New Zealand: Spinal Publications; 1981.

Mellin G. Measurement of thoracic lumbar posture and mobility with a Myrin inclinometer. *Spine.* 1986;11:759–762.

Mellin G, Kiiski R, Weckstrom A. Effects of subject position on measurements of flexion, extension, and lateral flexion of the spine. *Spine.* 1991;16:1108–1110.

Merritt JL, McLean TJ, Erickson RP, Offord KP. Measurement of trunk flexibility in normal subjects: Reproducibility of three clinical methods. *Mayo Clin Proc.* 1986;61:192–197.

Mimura M, Moriya H, Wantanabe T, et al. Three-dimensional motion analysis of the cervical spine with special reference to the axial rotation. *Spine.* 1989;14:1135–1139.

Mior SA, Gluckman J, Fournier G, Vernon H. A comparison of two objective measures in assessing cervical range of motion. *Proceedings of the 1991 International Conference on Spinal Manipulation.* Washington, DC: Foundation for Chiropractic Education and Research; 1991:79–81.

Moffroid MT, Haugh LD. Classification schema for acute and subacute low back pain. In: Managing Acute Low Back Pain in the New Health Care Environment. Part I. *Orthop Phys Ther Clin North Am.* 1995;4(2):179–191.

Moffroid MT, Haugh LD, Henry SM, Short B. Distinguishable groups of musculoskeletal low back pain patients and asymptomatic control subjects based on physical measures of the NIOSH low back atlas. *Spine.* 1994;19:1350–1358.

Moll JMH, Liyanage SP, Wright V. An objective clinical method to measure lateral spinal flexion. *Rheum Phys Med.* 1972a;11:225–239.

Moll JMH, Liyanage SP, Wright V. An objective clinical method to measure lateral spinal extension. *Rheum Phys Med.* 1972b;11:293–312.

Moll JMH, Wright V. Normal range of spinal mobility: An objective clinical study. *Ann Rheum Dis.* 1971;30:381–386.

Mooney V, Matheson LN. Objective measurement of soft tissue injury: Feasibility study. *Examiner's Manual.* October 1994:4.

Nansel D, Peneff A. Short communication: effects of eye closure on goniometrically-assessed cervical lateral-flexion passive end-range capability. *J Manipulative Physiol Ther.* 1990;13:350–351.

Nelson MA, Allen P, Clamp SE, De Dombal FT. Reliability and reproducibility of clinical findings in low-back pain. *Spine.* 1979;4:97–101.

Newton M, Waddell G. Reliability and validity of clinical measurement of the lumbar spine in patients with chronic low back pain. *Physiotherapy.* 1991;77:796–800.

Nilsson N. Measuring passive cervical motion: a study of reliability. *J Manipulative Physiol Ther.* 1995;18:293–297.

Nilsson N, Christensen H, Hortvigsen J. The interexaminer reliability of measuring passive cervical range of motion, revisited. *JMPT.* 1996a;71:302–305.

Nilsson N, Hortvigsen J, Christensen H. Normal ranges of cervical motion for women and men 20–60 years old. *J Manipulative Physiol Ther.* 1996b;19:306–309.

O'Driscoll SL, Tomenson J. The cervical spine. *Clin Rheum Dis.* 1982;8:617–630.

Ordway NR, Seymour R, Donelson RG, Hojnowski L, Lee E, Edwards T. Cervical sagittal range-of-motion analysis using three methods: Cervical range of motion device, 3Space, and radiography. *Spine.* 1997;22:501–508.

Paquet N, Malouin F, Richards C, Dionne J, Comeau F. Validity and reliability of a new electrogoniometer for the measurement of sagittal dorsolumbar movements. *Spine.* 1991;16:516–519.

Penning L. Functional pathology of the cervical spine. Amsterdam: Excerpta Medica; 1968. In: White AA III, Panjabi MM, eds. *Clinical Biomechanics of the Spine.* 2nd ed. Philadelphia, Pa: Lippincott, 1990:118.

Penning L, Wilmink JT. Rotation of the cervical spine: A CT study in normal subjects. *Spine.* 1987;12:732–738.

Portek I, Pearcy M, Reader G, Mowat A. Correlation between radiographic and clinical measurement of lumbar spine movement. *Br J Rheumatol.* 1993;22:197–205.

Porter RW, Trailescu IF. Diurnal changes in straight leg raising. *Spine.* 1990;15:103–106.

Rainville J, Sobel J, Hartigan C. Comparison of total lumbosacral flexion and true lumbar flexion measured by a dual inclinometer. *Spine*. 1994;19:2698–2701.

Rheault W, Albright B, Byers C, et al. Intertester reliability of the cervical range of motion device. *J Orthop Sports Phys Ther*. 1992;15:147–150.

Riddle DL, Rothstein JM. Intertester reliability of McKenzie's classifications of the syndrome types present in patients with low back pain. *Spine*. 1993;18:1333–1344.

Rondinelli R, Murphy J, Esler A, Marciano T, Cholmakjian C. Estimation of normal lumbar flexion with surface inclinometry. A comparison of three methods. *Am J Phys Med Rehabil*. 1992;71:219–224.

Saur P, Ensink F, Frese K, Seeger D, Hildebrandt J. Lumbar range of motion: reliability and validity of the inclinometer technique in clinical measurement of trunk flexibility. *Spine*. 1996;21:1332–1338.

Schober P. Ledenwirbelsaule und Kreuzschmerzen. *Munch Med Wochenschr*. 1937;84:336–338.

Schoening HA, Hannan V. Factors related to cervical spine mobility: Part I. *Arch Phys Med Rehabil*. 1964;45:602–609.

Shirley FR, O'Connor P, Robinson ME, MacMillan M. Comparison of lumbar range of motion using three measurement devices in patients with chronic low back pain. *Spine*. 1994;19:779–783.

Spitzer WO, LeBlanc FE, Dupuis M, et al. Scientific approach to the assessment and management of activity-related spinal disorders. *Spine*. 1987;12:7S.

Thomas E, Silman AJ, Papagerorgiou AC, Macfarlane GJ, Croft PR. Association between measures of spinal mobility and low back pain. *Spine*. 1998;23:343–347.

Troup JD, Hood CA, Chapman AE. Measurements of sagittal mobility of the normal lumbar spine and hips. *Ann Phys Med*. 1968;9:308–321.

Tsai L, Wredmark T. Spinal posture, sagittal mobility, and subjective rating of back problems in former female elite gymnasts. *Spine*. 1993;18:872–875.

Tucci SM, Hicks JE, Gross EG, Campbell W, Dahoff J. Cervical motion assessment: A new, simple and accurate method. *Arch Phys Med Rehabil*. 1986;67:225–230.

Waddell G, McCulloch JA, Kummel E, Venner RM. Nonorganic physical signs in low-back pain. *Spine*. 1980;5:117–125.

Waddell G, Somerville D, Henderson I, Newton M. Objective clinical evaluation of physical impairment in chronic low back pain. *Spine*. 1992;17:617–628.

Whaley, D. Psychological Testing and the Philosophy of Measurement. Kalamazoo, Mich: Behaviordelia; 1973:35–43.

Winer B. *Statistical Principles in Experimental Design*. New York, NY: McGraw-Hill; 1984.

Wing P, Tsang I, Gabnon F, Susak L, Gagnon R. Diurnal changes in the profile shape and range of motion of the back. *Spine*. 1992;17:761–766.

Wolf SL, Basmajian JV, Russe CTC, Kutner M. Normative data on low back mobility and activity levels. *Am J Phys Med*. 1979;58:217–229.

Wolfe F, Smythe HA, Yunnus MB, et al. The American College of Rheumatology 1990 Criteria for Classification of Fibromyalgia. *Arthritis Rheum*. 1990;33:160–172.

Wong A, Nansel D. Comparisons between active vs. passive end-range assessments in subjects exhibiting cervical range of motion asymmetrics. *J Manipulative Physiol Ther*. 1992;15:159–163.

Youdas JW, Carey JR, Garrett TR. Reliability of measurements of cervical range of motion—Comparison of three methods. *Phys Ther*. 1991;71:98–104.

Youdas JW, Garrett TR, Suman VJ, Bogard CL, Hallman HO, Carey JR. Normal range of motion of the cervical spine: An initial goniometric study. *Phys Ther*. 1992;72:770–780.

Zachman ZJ, Traina AD, Keating JJ, Bolles ST, Braun PL. Interexaminer reliability and concurrent validity of two instruments for the measurement of cervical ranges of motion. *J Manipulative Physiol Ther*. 1989;12:205–210.

Zuckerman J, Derby R, Hsu K, et al. Normal magnetic resonance imaging with abnormal discography. *Spine*. 1988;13:1355–1359.

CHAPTER 15

Outcome Measures for the Upper and Lower Extremities

JEFFREY M. WILDER

INTRODUCTION

Over the course of the last several years, health care providers (HCPs) have been introduced to a new concept that is radically changing the manner in which patients are examined and treated. Not only is the HCP expected to treat the patient's malady and restore that patient to a healthy condition, but there is a new expectation (primarily driven by the third-party payment system) that the HCP must somehow *measure* the patient's complaint and response to treatment. Depending on the patient's complaint, it may be appropriate to measure pain, loss of function, loss of strength, range of motion restrictions, or other factors.

This pretreatment measurement of the patient's condition is used to establish a baseline. The patient's response to treatment can also be measured, and can be retrospectively compared to the baseline measurements to determine if the patient really did improve with the provided treatment. Figure 15–1 shows an example of simple disability measures, such as the Oswestry Low Back Pain Disability Questionnaire or the Neck Disability Index (NDI), used to track the progress of a hypothetical patient as treatment is provided. In this example, the disability indices are measured each month, and the relative progress over time is easily understood.

In essence, the HCP is now expected by many outside observers to be able to demonstrate that:

- The patient had a significant, *measurable* health care problem.
- The patient had *measurable* improvement with the provided clinical care.

If these two elements are not documented, the payer may claim that there was insufficient "medical necessity" to require treatment, or that the treatment provided was ineffective in improvement of the condition. Given that significant differences exist in the recommended treatment and outcomes by their training and specialty (Solomon et al, 1997), it is critical for each HCP to constantly self-scrutinize his or her own rationale for clinical decision making.

Throughout most of the history of health care, the patient and the HCP determined whether the patient was making satisfactory improvement through simple conversation. Much of the idea of not only treating the patient, but also attempting to measure the patient's malady or the success of the provided treatment, is quite new. **The HCP who wishes to meet these new challenges is faced with the very difficult decisions of determining which specific clinical aspects of the individual patient's case are best suited to measurement.**

Measurement of neuromusculoskeletal complaints and the effects of treatment is especially complex. Pain is the primary complaint for 80% of all office visits to physicians each year in the United States (National Center for Health Statistics, 1986). Yet pain is, by definition, a subjective measurement at best, and as we will see in this chapter, may not be the best choice for measuring outcomes.

The HCP who wishes to conscientiously research the use of outcome measurements for the treatment of various extremity conditions is faced with a dizzying array of information. The MEDLINE database currently indexes 3784 biomedical journals and contains over 9 million studies, with unlimited search capabilities at the touch of a computer button. However, it must be readily admitted that science's ability to *collect* this information is far advanced over our ability to effectively *use* the information. This chapter shows that much of the information in the current biomedical literature base is conflicting, and in the final analysis the HCP must choose the most appropriate measurement device for each specific patient. In many cases, the information available is so specific that it may actually be difficult to use effectively in a clinical setting. For example, does the latest study on common shoulder problems in elite 25-year-old volleyball players (Kugler et al, 1996) directly apply to other types of overhead sports injuries to the shoulder?

Many studies in the biomedical literature that investigate potential outcome measurements suffer from common errors, such as small sample size or poor study design, which limit the validity of their key findings. As an example, a division of the US Department of Health and Social Services known as the Agency for Health Care Policy and Research (Bigos et al, 1994) completed a review of the literature on acute low back pain. Over 10,000 peer-reviewed, published studies were initially included, but the multidisciplinary panel felt that less than 900 of the studies had sufficient validity to use in the development of clinical guidelines. The acute low back pain guidelines that were eventually published made clinical recommendations based on this evidence; only two relevant studies were needed to qualify for its top evidence category of "strong research-based evidence" and only one relevant study was necessary to qualify for "moderate research-based evidence." Gabriel et al (1997) pointed out that many larger scale studies use current diagnostic coding groups, which do not capture important factors such as injury acuity, severity, or diagnostic uncertainty. Studies that have these limitations, especially for diagnostic information, are likely to suffer from biases that can skew results in unpredictable ways. Therefore, the conclusions drawn from such studies are likely to be flawed.

The purpose of this chapter is to investigate the literature, especially of the past several years, and determine if there is a gold standard for use with some common extremity problems. Where there is not a gold standard, the chapter makes recommendations, or suggests relevant and interesting studies, methods, or clinical pearls. Armed with this information, interested HCPs can measure the clinical outcomes of patients. As more and more HCPs utilize similar methods of measurement, the resulting information will become more consistent, more precise, and more in conformity with that of other specialists around the world. The chapter places special emphasis on describing outcome measurements for the extremities that are low-tech, low-cost, and relatively simple to administer in a primarily nonsurgical ("conservative") clinical environment.

Efficacy of nonsurgical or conservative treatment has been demonstrated in many conditions that traditionally have been regarded as "surgical" cases. There is increasing awareness of the ability of conservatively oriented HCPs to successfully treat extremity conditions such as thoracic outlet syndrome (Novak et al, 1995); carpal tunnel syndrome (Katz, 1994; Sucher, 1994; Valente and Gibson, 1994); adhesive capsulitis of the shoulder (Polkinghorn, 1995; Mao et al, 1997); cervical disc herniation with radicular pain (Ericsen, 1998); impingement syndrome, rotator cuff tendinitis, and frozen shoulder (Hjelm et al, 1996); acromioclavicular dislocation (Rawes and Diao, 1996); and all the shoulder girdle disorders (Winters et al, 1997b). In addition, conservative treatment has been shown to be beneficial in cases that have often traditionally been treated via medication, such as fibromyalgia (Blunt et al, 1997).

The HCP should attempt to utilize existing outcome measures, such as those presented in Part II of this text and in this chapter, **if he or she feels the outcome measure is appropriate for the clinical parameter to be measured for a particular patient.** This will allow for precise communication with any other HCP who is familiar with that outcome assessment device. However, it is quite possible that none of the available outcome measurements meet the individual needs of the patient. The HCP should always be allowed to extrapolate the best available information to fit the clinical circumstance that he or she is treating. It should always be accepted as proper to adapt "established" or "published" scales or measurement devices if it is necessary to

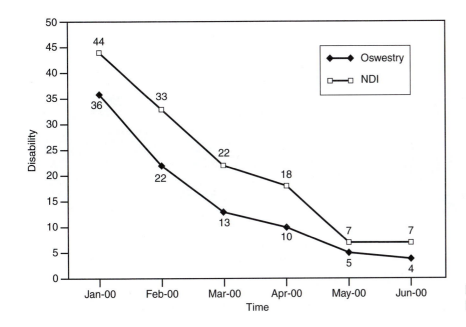

Figure 15–1. Outcome measures in a hypothetical patient.

fit the unique needs of individual patients, or groups of unique patients within a specialized practice.

The description of outcome measures for trauma or resulting joint arthroplasty are well studied and numerous. Readers who are interested in outcome measures primarily for traumatic cases (fractures and dislocations) are referred to Pynsent's text, *Outcome Measures in Trauma*. In contrast, the outcome measurements for nonsurgical extremity cases, which have not yet been compiled in a single source, are discussed thoroughly in this chapter.

ALL EXTREMITIES

A variety of techniques to measure the degree of symptoms or the impact of these symptoms upon a patient's function have been proposed. The most commonly encountered techniques that are used for the assessment of extremity conditions are described in the paragraphs that follow.

RANGE OF MOTION

Range of motion (ROM) is an important, measurable variable in the examination and proper treatment selection of the extremity complaints. Increased ROM is often listed as a primary goal of treatment for neuromusculoskeletal conditions. However, ROM measurement is not as straightforward as some HCPs assume. Studies of the reliability of basic ROM measurement, including goniometry, have been surprisingly limited in number and scope.

Goniometry

Widely used in clinical practice, goniometry is the measurement of ROM in a joint. A variety of instruments can be used for goniometry, including simple plastic protractors called goniometers (Fig. 15–2), inclinometers (Fig. 15–3), electronic inclinometers (Fig. 15–4), or more complex computer-assisted stations. Many variables have been described in the literature that can decrease accuracy and limit validity. Some of the many types of variables that have been reported to reduce accuracy in goniometry include:

- Different type of instrumentation
- Varying procedures and protocols for measurement
- Differences among joint actions and body regions
- Passive versus active measurements
- Intra-tester versus inter-tester measurements
- Different patient types (Gajdosik and Bohannon, 1987)
- Age: No significant differences in extremity ROM have been shown to be attributable to increasing age. Furthermore, physical activity, as assessed by a questionnaire and a rating scale, has not been shown to be related to specific changes of joint range. There does not appear to be an accurate database of normative ROM values for extremities in older individuals (Walker et al, 1984).
- Geographical and cultural differences: Ahlberg et al (1988) compared 50 Saudi Arabian men 30 to 40 years of age without present or previous history of injury or disease to a similar study from Scandinavia for measurement of the ROM in the basic planes of hip, knee, and ankle joint. There was a highly significant difference in external rotation of the hip, flexion of the knee, and dorsiflexion of the ankle. Cultural differences in the activities of daily life were suggested to explain the differences in the range of motion.
- Type of goniometer: The three major types of goniometers in current use include the universal goniometer, the fluid goniometer, and the electrogoniometer. It has been shown that interchangeable use of different types of goniometer in a clinical set-

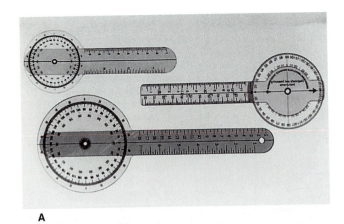

A

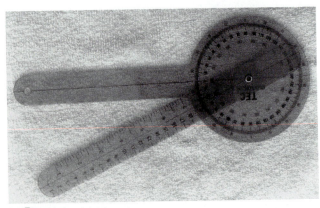

B

Figure 15–2. Simple plastic protractors, or goniometers.

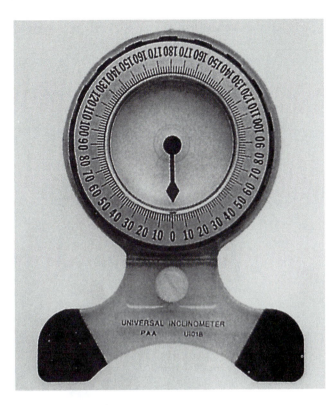

Figure 15–3. Inclinometer.

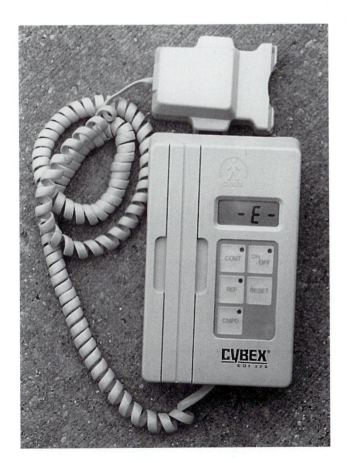

Figure 15–4. Inclinometer.

ting is inadvisable, and increases the amount of intrinsic error in the testing procedures. Goodwin et al (1992) demonstrated significant differences between the goniometers used, the testers, and the replications. Significant interaction effects also exist between the goniometers and the occasion, the goniometers and the testers, and the testers and replications.

- Right- or left-handedness: Gunal et al (1996) measured the active and passive arcs of motion of the shoulder, elbow, forearm, and wrist in 1000 healthy male subjects who were right-hand dominant and who ranged in age from 18 to 22 years. The ROMs on the right side were significantly smaller than those on the left. The authors concluded that the contralateral, normal side may not always be a reliable control in the evaluation of restriction of motion of a joint.

When care is taken to minimize as many variables as is clinically possible, goniometry has been shown to provide acceptable validity and reliability. Intra-tester and inter-tester variability and reliability of goniometric measurements on upper and lower extremity motions of normal male subjects were reviewed by Boone et al (1978). The authors offered these findings:

- In general, **inter-tester variation was less for the upper extremity** motions than for those of the lower extremity.
- When the same tester measures the same movement, **increases in joint motion of at least 3 to 4 degrees determine improvement** for either the upper or lower extremity.
- When more than one tester measures the same movement, increases in joint motion which are deemed to determine **improvement should exceed 5 degrees for the upper extremity and 6 degrees for the lower extremity.**

Mayerson and Milano (1984) showed that repeated goniometric measurements of the upper and lower extremities under controlled conditions can confidently be expected to fall within approximately 4 angular degrees of each other. It was suggested that 4 angular degrees be construed as global upper limit estimates of applied goniometric reliability. However, the significance of this study is lessened by the use of only one subject; all joint measurements were made on the same patient.

Visual Assessment
Assessment of hypermobility and hypomobility of the extremities is frequently performed visually with all its reported limitations. Critics charge that the ability of the human to estimate angular measurement is universally poor, yet proponents of visual measurement often counter that experienced HCPs can easily tell normal from abnormal without detailed measurements. Dijkstra et al (1994) sug-

gested that an individual's general joint mobility could by measured by a screening procedure used as a standardized joint mobility measurement method (see Fig. 15–5). The screen developed by Dijkstra and colleagues consisted of the following movements:

1. Maximal range of motion of passive hyperextension of the fifth digit (measured in degrees).
2. Passive apposition of the thumb to the wrist (measured in millimeters).
3. Active hyperextension of the elbow and knee (measured in degrees).

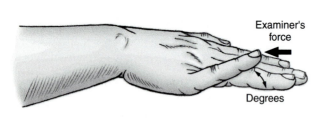

A. Maximal ROM of passive hyperextension of fifth digit.

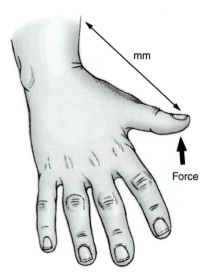

B. Passive apposition of thumb to wrist.

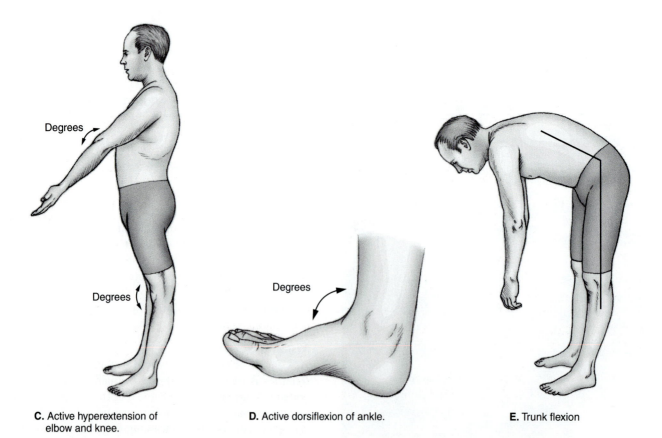

C. Active hyperextension of elbow and knee.

D. Active dorsiflexion of ankle.

E. Trunk flexion

Figure 15–5. Dijkstra's method of measuring joint mobility.

4. Active dorsiflexion of the ankle (measured in degrees).
5. Trunk flexion (measured in degrees).

Using experienced observers, it was concluded that the ability to visually estimate these motions was reliable and accurate, and was within the range of error for goniometric measurement.

STRENGTH TESTING

Strength testing is a commonly used clinical method for determining outcome. However, strength testing is also prone to a number of clinical variables and differing literature opinions that cloud the interpretation. Several different camps have voiced very strong opinions on the most "proper" methods to measure clinically significant variations in muscle strength.

Manual Muscle Testing

Manual muscle testing is most commonly reported using the "Lovett" scale. This 0-to-5 point scale assigns a numerical score to muscle grades in the manner shown in Table 15–1. There is a great deal of variation among HCPs who attempt to grade the strength of muscles that are felt to fall between number grades. The most common of these applies a plus or minus sign to the numerical muscle grades 2, 3 or 4 to signify an increase or decrease from the numerical muscle grade. Using this scheme, 4+ represents a muscle that is stronger than 4 which, in turn, is stronger than 4–. Alternately, some HCPs choose to use a 0-to-10 scale, a 0-to-100 scale, or name grades (such as poor, fair, good, and normal). Kendall (1993) developed a chart that compares various muscle grading systems, which is reproduced in Table 15–2.

Beasley (1956) showed long ago that manual muscle testing, even with experienced HCPs, is often insensitive to strength losses of 20% to 25%. Manual muscle testers typically overestimate muscle strength, assuming strength to be normal, and may neglect to observe clinically important losses in muscle strength. For example, Dvir (1997) measured estimated anti-gravity static muscular moments (MGM) at the shoulder, elbow, hip, and knee joints and compared them with published data relating to

the isokinetic strength (MIM) of the same muscle groups. (MGM and MIM correspond to grades 3 and 5 in manual muscle testing.) The study found that muscles commonly measured to be grade 4 may generate as low as 10% of normal (in elbow and knee) to 20% to 30% of normal (in the shoulder and hip). Coupled with the very limited human precision in sensing of force, the author pointed out that these findings indicate that where accuracy in muscle testing is required (such as setting targets in muscle strength conditioning or when measuring permanent impairment), grade 4 cannot and should not serve as a valid criterion.

Dynamometry

Strength and power assessment is a difficult task. Proposed reasons for this difficulty include the fledgling status of research within the area, our limited understanding of the mechanisms underpinning strength and power performance and development, and limitations associated with various forms of dynamometry. Therefore, opinions on the most accurate or most meaningful method for strength measurement are widely varied. Currently, isometric, isoinertial, and isokinetic dynamometry are employed in assessment of muscular strength. Each form of dynamometry has its supporters and detractors. Proponents of isokinetic and isometric dynamometry emphasize the apparently high internal validity, while critics point out the apparently low external validity. In general, the converse relationship exists for isoinertial dynamometry, with low internal validity and high external validity. It appears that all three methods of dynamometry can have acceptable reliability, if utilized with consistent methodology (Abernethy et al, 1995).

Satisfactory test–retest reliability of handheld dynamometry when practiced by a single experienced tester was demonstrated by Kilmer (1997) and Bohannon (1986). Good to high inter-tester agreement for hand-held dynamometry has also been shown (Bohannon and Andrews, 1987; Bohannon et al, 1965). Inter-instrument reproducibility (reliability and variability) between fixed isokinetic equipment and handheld dynamometers has been shown to be comparable. Thus, under limited circumstances these instruments may be interchangeable. The handheld dynomometer is less expensive, more portable

Table 15–1: Muscle Strength Testing Grades

NUMERICAL GRADE		DESCRIPTION
0	Zero:	No contraction
1	Trace:	Muscle palpably tightens, but does not move the joint
2	Poor:	Joint movement is produced only with gravity eliminated
3	Fair:	Ability to produce joint movement against gravity only
4	Good:	Full contraction, producing joint movement against some external resistance
5	Normal:	Full contraction, producing joint movement against external resistance without notable fatigue

Table 15–2: Key to Muscle Grading

	Function of the Muscle	Grade Symbols		
No Movement	No contraction felt in the muscle	Zero	0	0
	Tendon becomes prominent or feeble contraction felt in the muscle, but no visible movement of the part	Trace	T	T
Test Movement	**MOVEMENT IN HORIZONTAL PLANE**			
	Moves through partial range of motion	Poor–	P–	1
	Moves through complete range of motion			
	Moves to completion of range against resistance or Moves to completion of range and holds against pressure	Poor+	P+	3
	ANTIGRAVITY POSITION			
	Moves through partial range of motion			
Test Position	*Gradual* release from test position	Fair–	F–	4
	Holds test position (no added pressure)	Fair	F	5
	Holds test position against slight pressure	Fair+	F+	6
	Holds test position against slight to moderate pressure	Good–	G–	7
	Holds test position against moderate pressure	Good	G	8
	Holds test position against moderate to strong pressure	Good+	G+	9
	Holds test position against strong pressure	Normal	N	10

Reproduced with permission from Kendall FP, 1993.

and simpler to use, and may be a practical alternative for the clinical measurement of muscle strength (Bohannon, 1990), provided the assessor's strength is greater than that of the specific muscle group being measured (Stratford and Balsor, 1994). See Figures 15–6 and 15–7.

Study data by Agre et al (1987) showed that although the handheld dynamometer is reliable for testing upper extremity muscle groups, it is unreliable for testing lower extremity muscle groups. It is quite possible that the reliability of handheld units is simply limited by the upper extremity strength of the examiner to hold the device steady against the patient's much stronger lower extremity muscle groups. Hsieh and Phillips (1990) concur with the concept that the HCP must have superior strength to the muscle group of the patient being tested, and believe that manual dynamometry is an acceptable procedure only when utilizing the patient-initiated method and is not acceptable for the HCP-initiated method. Additional reasons for variability in dynamometry include:

- Test–retest variability
- Time of day (Coldwells et al, 1994)
- Strength of the tester (Stratford and Balsor, 1994)
- Patient-initiated versus HCP-initiated methods of testing (Hsieh and Phillips, 1990)

When dealing with conditions in which spasticity is present, care must be taken to select a velocity that is low enough not to evoke a stretch reflex (to isolate nonreflex components) and another that is high enough to elicit a

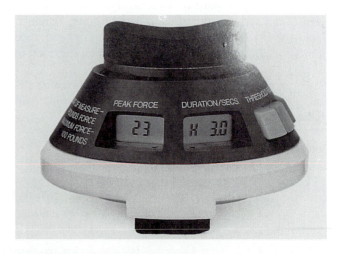

Figure 15–6. A handheld dynamometer for manual muscle testing.

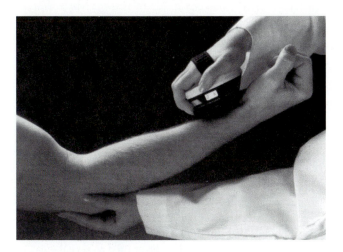

Figure 15–7. Example of handheld dynomometry.

reflex response, so that it becomes possible to differentiate the reflex and nonreflex components involved in spasticity. Such a distinction is important for the choice of treatment procedures (Boiteau et al, 1995). In a large percentage of older men and women, great intersubject variability is expected, and at least two tests may be necessary to determine isokinetic peak torque (Frontera et al, 1993).

PREDICTORS OF INJURY AND RISK FACTORS

Some studies attempt to isolate specific factors that can be shown to put an individual at risk for the development of a particular type of illness or injury. Obviously, evaluation of possible risk factors is important in determining activities that can lead to future pain and disability. Shoulder pain, for example, is perceived as common in competitive swimmers. A study to identify the incidence of interfering shoulder pain in this population (McMaster and Troup, 1993) showed that the prevalence of current shoulder pain is positively correlated with the number of years spent in competitive swimming. Therefore, the number of years the athlete is involved in competitive swimming is itself a risk factor for the development of shoulder pain. In those athletes with a painful shoulder, weight training, use of hand paddles, kickboard use, stretching, and various resistance activities aggravated the painful shoulder.

Unfortunately, other studies have failed to demonstrate significant patterns for the prediction of injury, even when common sense suggests to us that a pattern *should* exist. For example, Jackson et al (1978) measured joint flexibility and laxity among 2300 West Point cadets and high school and collegiate football teams. The study showed that there was no statistical relationship between flexibility or joint laxity and joint injuries sustained in general athletic competition involving the ankle, knee, shoulder, or elbow.

SELF-REPORTED QUESTIONNAIRES

In general, self-reported questionnaires and similar measurement tools are somewhat controversial among authors of various studies involving neuromusculoskeletal symptoms. Proponents of patient self-report describe many practical advantages: low cost, increased speed of obtaining assessments, and the potential for assessing a wide range of complex functional dimensions. Criticisms of the self-reported questionnaire center around the degree to which the data are a reliable and valid reflection of patient function (Jette, 1987), and the degree to which the patient's biases in reading, understanding or answering the questions will ultimately bias the study results. **As a result of this lack of agreement, there are many differing versions of similar questionnaires, with each author attempting to improve slightly on the purpose of the questionnaire, claiming to diminish these biases, and therefore, to improve on reliability and validity.**

It has been shown (Haapanen et al, 1997) that the agreement between self-reported diseases in a questionnaire survey and data from medical records of Finnish men and women was poor for musculoskeletal conditions, such as lower back disorder, hip and knee arthrosis, and claudication. In a 1996 study by Viikari-Juntura et al, it was demonstrated that validity of self-reported physical workload and musculoskeletal symptoms by questionnaire assessments by 2756 men in the forest industry was not good for studying quantitative exposure-effect relationships. The authors believed that the subject's perception of musculoskeletal pain may bias the self-assessment of workload.

The Health Assessment Questionnaire (HAQ) has been used to measure a variety of health related variables, such as pain and loss of function. Several studies have used the HAQ as the primary or sole outcome measure of their study (Pearlmutter et al, 1995). However, there are many experts who hold a contrary viewpoint. In a study of the effects of exercise upon joint mobility, muscle strength, and physical condition, the reliability of the HAQ as an outcome measure in short-term exercise trials was shown to be poor. The HAQ has been shown to be an inappropriate instrument to detect changes in physical impairments due to short term exercise therapy (van den Ende et al, 1997).

Many other health status questionnaires and measurement devices have been proposed for use in neuromusculoskeletal assessment. Some authors feel it is only appropriate to use a test that has been validated for a specific purpose, such as using only validated knee scales to test knee function. Other authors have no problem with "borrowing" a test from another area of health care if it serves the needs of their study. Some of these health status questionnaires have been used and permutated in many different ways, with each author making changes (sometimes subtle, sometimes bold), to the questionnaire. The following are health status instruments that have been used to measure outcome in extremity, arthritic, or rheumatic conditions. Most tests are referenced with a brief description of the original purpose of the instrument:

- **Stanford Child Health Assessment Questionnaire (CHAQ).** This questionnaire was designed to allow children to self-report their symptoms in rheumatic and arthritic conditions and has been adapted for use in many languages. Its proponents claim excellent measurement when using parents or children more than 9 years old as responders (Andersson et al, 1993; Feldman et al, 1995).
- **Juvenile Arthritis Functional Status Index (JASI).** This questionnaire was developed to assess a variety of daily living and functional mobility tasks in children with juvenile rheumatoid arthritis. JASI Part I consists of 100 functional items divided into five activity categories (self-care, domestic, mobility, school, extracurricular). A 7-point degree of difficulty rating scale is used for responses. JASI Part II is a priority function section within which the child identifies and scores important activities for improvement (Wright et al, 1996).
- **Disability Rating Index (DRI).** This is an instrument for assessment of physical disability, mainly intended for clinical settings. Most of the patients of the original study displayed neck, shoulder, and low back pain, but some were arthritis patients waiting for hip or knee replacement surgery, or wheelchair patients with multiple sclerosis. The DRI proved to be a robust, practical clinical and research instrument with good responsiveness and acceptability for assessment of disability caused by impairment of common motor functions (Salen et al, 1994).
- **Sickness Impact Profile (SIP).** This is a behaviorally based measure of health status with 136 items in 12 categories. It was originally tested on patients with hyperthyroidism, rheumatoid arthritis, and hip replacements to assess reliability and validity (Bergner et al, 1981).
- **Coping Strategy Questionnaire (CSQ).** This questionnaire attempts to identify specific coping strategies as they relate to functioning. Jensen et al (1992, 1994) compared composite with individual coping scale scores in the prediction of adjustment among chronic pain patients. The individual scales provided more information than the composite measures regarding the relationship between coping and adjustment to chronic pain. The results also suggested that individual scale scores may be more useful than composite scores in identifying the conditions under which coping efforts have their greatest effects on adjustment.
- **Multidimensional Pain Inventory (MPI).** Patients with chronic headaches of diverse causes were administered the MPI for measuring the cognitive, behavioral, and affective dimensions of pain. Results suggest that the MPI is a valid measure of the cognitive, behavioral, and affective aspects of pain (Walter and Brannon, 1991).
- **Questionnaire on Musculoskeletal Disorders of the Japanese Committee on Occupational Cervicobranchial Disorders.** This instrument was shown to be valid by Laubli et al (1991). The standardized illustrated questionnaire is composed of 37 items about the occurrence of symptoms in 12 distinct body regions. The questionnaire was judged to be a valid instrument for studying musculoskeletal disorders at the workplace.
- **Keitel Index.** This instrument is composed of 24 questions, focusing on both anatomical ability and functional performance of the upper and lower extremities (Eberl et al, 1976).
- **Signals of Functional Impairment Index (SOFI).** A self-administered hand test used to reveal evidence of hand impairment. It is especially easy to use because of its picture-based format (Eberhardt et al, 1988).
- **Lee Index.** This instrument consists of 17 questions, primarily simple functional questions; for example, Can you lift a teapot? (Lee et al, 1973).
- **Convery Index.** This instrument was designed and evaluated for the functional evaluation of patients with polyarticular disease. A single assessment can be done in approximately 15 minutes (Convery et al, 1977).
- **Independent Measure of Functional Capacity.** An extensive, 96-question, 10-page questionnaire, with some emphasis on positive/negative change after beginning medication (Helewa et al, 1982).
- **Functional Status Index (FSI).** Originally tested for validity in patients with hip fracture, 18 questions ask patients if they experience pain, require assistance, or have difficulty when performing simple activities of daily living (Jette, 1987).
- **Arthritis Impact Measurement Scales (AIMS).** This is a multidimensional index that measures the health status of individuals with arthritis. The AIMS is a combination of health status scales that assess physical, emotional, and social well-being. The self-administered AIMS questionnaire has been pilot tested in a mixed arthritis population (Meenan et al, 1980).
- **Arthritis Impact Measurement Scales 2 (AIMS2).** A revised version of the original AIMS, which has been modified to be more comprehensive and sensitive. Three new scales were added to evaluate arm function, work, and social support. Sections were also added to assess satisfaction with function, attribution of problems to arthritis, and self-designation of priority areas for improvement. This is an extensive study; patients' questionnaire completion times averaged 23 minutes (Meenan et al, 1992).
- **McMaster Toronto Arthritis Preference Disability Questionniare (MACTAR).** The purpose of this tool was to quantify the functional priorities of the patient. Comparison against global improvement

suggests that this instrument has the potential to detect small clinically important changes in function (Tugwell et al, 1987).

- **Dougados Functional Index.** This is an index of functional impairment and a system of scoring joint tenderness for use in the assessment of ankylosing spondylitis. The functional index consists of 20 questions and the articular index is based on the scoring of a total of 10 joint responses after movement or firm digital pressure. These changes were highly correlated with patients' overall assessment of their own clinical condition (Dougados et al, 1988).

- **Rapid Assessment of Disease Activity in Rheumatology Questionnaire (RADAR).** This is a brief, self-administered questionnaire of disease signs and symptoms in patients with rheumatoid arthritis. The 2-page RADAR questionnaire produces valid estimates of joint involvement and clinical status that are sensitive to change (Mason et al, 1992).

- **Fibromyalgia Impact Questionnaire (FIQ).** This is a brief 10-item, self-administered instrument developed to assess the current health status of women with the fibromyalgia syndrome. It measures physical functioning, work status, depression, anxiety, sleep, pain, stiffness, fatigue, and well being (Burckhardt et al, 1991).

Interestingly, **many questionnaires that are longer, take more time to complete, and are more difficult to score have not been shown to be more valid than shorter, less difficult questionnaires.** Katz et al (1992b) studied health status measurements of varying complexity and concluded that the brief health measurements were equally or more responsive than longer questionnaires.

The remainder of this chapter details a region-by-region evaluation of some of the current outcome measures that are in use today by various HCPs.

UPPER EXTREMITY

QUESTIONNAIRES AND PERFORMANCE TESTS

Some outcome measurement instruments have been constructed specifically for the upper extremity as a unit, rather than separate measurement of the shoulder, elbow, wrist, and hand. One such measurement is the joint initiative of the American Academy of Orthopedic Surgeons (AAOS), the Council of Musculoskeletal Specialty Societies (COMSS), and the Institute for Work and Health (Toronto, Ontario) in the development of the Disabilities of the Arm, Shoulder, and Hand (DASH) questionnaire (Hudak et al, 1996a). This questionnaire began with a review of 13 outcome measurement scales currently in use

and hopes to combine the best elements of each into a brief, easy to complete questionnaire.

A recent upper extremity functional test for geriatrics is the Upper Extremity Performance Test for the Elderly, known as the TEMPA (after the original French description Test d'Evaluation des Membres Superieurs de Personnes Agees by Desorsiers et al in 1995). This test asks the senior to perform various common tasks, such as the opening of a jar, shuffling and dealing playing cards, or the application a postage stamp. These tasks are timed, and normative data is provided to allow assessment of sensorimotor parameters, which are known to decline with increasing age.

PREDICTORS OF INJURY AND RISK FACTORS

Several studies which seek to identify risk factors of developing dysfunction have been aimed not at specific upper extremity joints, but rather at the entire upper extremity as a unit. Examples of peer-reviewed studies in this area include:

- Poor matching of desk height with chair height has been shown to be related to neck pain and arm pain in a study of Japanese clerical workers (Ignatious et al, 1993). In this study, workers' finger pain and arm pain were directly related to the period of time they had worked as typists.

- Age, gender, and duration of symptoms have been shown to bear no relation to a subject's current ability to work. The best predictors of current work hours in a recent study were, in descending order, the Fibromyalgia Impact Questionnaire (FIQ), Modified Stanford Health Assessment Questionnaire (SHAQ), weeks of absence from work, passive wrist flexion angle of the affected arm, neck pain or stiffness on movement, and grip strength in the affected arm. FIQ and SHAQ scores were significantly correlated with objective measures of upper extremity function (Friedman, 1997).

- Screening tools have been proposed for the detection of cumulative trauma disorder (CTD) in the workplace, using combinations of questionnaires and physical examination methods. The specific goals of one such study were to detect employees who might be at risk of sustaining a CTD injury and to identify trends of CTD at their specific workstations. One company utilizing such a screening procedure for its workers noted that employee complaints of upper extremity discomfort have significantly decreased (Muffly-Elsey and Flinn-Wagner, 1987).

Jerosch-Herold (1993) showed that almost all of the commonly used upper extremity sensory tests are not able to predict patients' ability to use their hands in everyday activities, thus indicating that patients are able to compensate for sensory deficit through the use of vision and bilateral use of the hands. **Therefore, an assessment of outcome for the upper extremity should include an additional measure of performance on activities of daily living.**

SHOULDER

INCIDENCE

The shoulder is a commonly involved joint, and patients with shoulder pain and disability are seen frequently in nonsurgical clinical practice. Yet precise diagnosis of all but the most severe and obvious cases is often circumspect. An episode of recurring or disabling shoulder symptoms lasting more than a month occurs in 5% of all adult Americans every year (Bjelle, 1989). Estimates of incidence for current shoulder pain range from 7% to 20% of the adult population in Great Britain (Pope et al, 1996). A recent Dutch study (van der Windt et al, 1995b) suggests the cumulative incidence of shoulder complaints in general practice was estimated to be 11.2 per 1000 patients per year (95% confidence limits 10.1 to 12.3). Rotator cuff tendinitis was the most frequently recorded disorder, comprising 29% of the shoulder problems evaluated.

Hasvold and Johnsen (1993) described the prevalences of reported neck/shoulder pain as unspecified complaints in over 20,000 adult Danish subjects aged 20 to 56 years. They found that 15.4% of the men and 24.9% of the women complained of neck/shoulder conditions that were self-described as rendering the subject unfit for work. The prevalences of reported neck or shoulder pain increased significantly with age. The authors concluded many people in the general population live with disabling complaints, and that only a proportion of these sufferers were seeking professional help.

PREDICTORS OF SHOULDER INJURY AND RISK FACTORS

Many separate factors have been identified which predispose an individual toward future bouts of shoulder dysfunction. Subjects with kyphosis and rounded shoulders had an increased incidence of interscapular pain, and those with a forward-head posture had an increased incidence of cervical, interscapular, and headache pain (Griegel-Morris et al, 1992). In another study, no differences were observed when comparing age or anthropometric measurements between workers with and without shoulder/neck complaints. Significantly weaker shoulder muscles were found in workers with shoulder/neck complaints than in those without. A higher median strain on the shoulders in the working situation of workers with shoulder/neck complaints than in the group with no complaints was suggested by the authors

after biomechanical analysis of the worker's different work tasks (Bjelle et al, 1987).

Kugler et al (1996) demonstrated that volleyball players known as "attackers" (and presumably other athletes playing overhead sports, such as tennis and baseball players) have a different muscular and capsular pattern at the playing shoulder compared to the opposite shoulder. Their playing shoulder is depressed, the scapula lateralized, and the dorsal muscles and the posterior and inferior part of the shoulder capsule shortened and tightened. These differences were of greater significance in volleyball attackers with shoulder pain than in volleyball players without shoulder pain. These anatomical differences have been proposed as a mechanism for producing the player's shoulder symptoms. Following are other factors associated with the likelihood of the development of shoulder problems.

- Internal rotation restriction—the minimum difference achieved between the tip of a thumb and the spinous process of C7 (Pope et al, 1996).
- Forward head position (Griegel-Morris et al, 1992; Greenfield et al, 1995).
- Scapular protraction and rotation (Greenfield et al, 1995).
- Passive humeral elevation (Greenfield et al, 1995).
- Kyphosis and rounded shoulders (Griegel-Morris et al, 1992).
- Weak shoulder muscles (Bjelle et al, 1987)

The following factors were unassociated with increased likelihood of developing shoulder problems:

- Restriction of external rotation (Pope et al, 1996).
- Age, anthropometric measurements (Bjelle et al, 1987).

RANGE OF MOTION

ROM of the shoulder has been measured using various methods by different investigators. It must be noted that there is substantial variation among various authors in their opinion of what constitutes "normal" ROM of the shoulder (see Table 15–3). Notice that not all authors agree on even the basic anatomical nomenclature used to describe the motions of the shoulder, the relative importance of the measurements, or the manner in which those motions should be measured. For example, Hoppenfeld (1976) is representative of authors who measure shoulder flexion starting from the horizontal plane and, therefore, recognizes a full amount of shoulder flexion as approximately 90 degrees. The majority of authors choose to measure shoulder flexion beginning with the arm held at the side; therefore, shoulder flexion approximates 160 to 180 degrees.

Matsen et al (1994) feels that internal rotation is best measured, not in degrees, but rather in the ability of the highest vertebral level which can be reached by the patient's thumb. Other authors feel that this maneuver is not

Table 15–3: Range of Motion of the Shoulder from Various Sources

SHOULDER	HOPPENFELD (1976)	AMA *GUIDES* (1993)	MAGEE (AROM) (1992)	MATSEN ET AL (1996)[a]	SOUZA (1994)	KAPANDJI (1980)
Abduction	180°	180°	170–180°	M: 160° ± 8° F: 167° ± 7°	180°	180°
Adduction	45°	50°	50–75°	—	75°	30–45°
Flexion	90°	180°	160–180°	—	180°	180°
Extension	45°	50°	50–60°	—	60°	45–50°
Internal (medial) rotation	55°	90°	60–100°	M: reach to T6 ± 2 F: reach to T5 ± 2	80° with arm at side; 50° with arm abducted	95°
External (lateral) rotation	40–45°	90°	80–90°	M: 72° ± 13° F: 78° ± 15°	60° with arm at side; 50° with arm abducted	80°
Elevation through the plane of the scapula	—	—	170–180°	—	—	170–180°
Horizontal adduction/ abduction	—	—	130°	—	130°	—
Circumduction	—	—	200°	—	—	—

AROM, acute range of motion.

[a] Based on a study of 81 normal subjects, 60 to 70 years old.

strictly measuring internal rotation, but may be including shoulder adduction, scapulothoracic or elbow movement as well. Mallon et al (1996) used computed tomographic scans of the shoulder in differing positions, scapular lateral radiographs, and posteroanterior radiographs to analyze elbow flexion at the limits of internal rotation behind the back, and found that maximal internal rotation behind the back occurs in approximately a 2:1 ratio between the glenohumeral joint and the scapulothoracic articulation. However, the scapulothoracic articulation was more significant in placing the arm behind the back, whereas the glenohumeral joint performed most of the internal rotation in front of the body. The scapulothoracic articulation assists in this motion by both extension and internal rotation of the scapula on the thorax. The limits of internal rotation behind the back are reached with a significant contribution from elbow. Mallon et al concluded that measuring shoulder internal rotation by the maximal vertebral level reached by the patient's thumb greatly oversimplifies the concept of internal rotation and that limitations in this motion may not be strictly due to a loss of internal rotation at the glenohumeral joint (1996).

Other points of interest in measuring the ROM of the shoulder:

- Goniometric passive range of motion (PROM) measurements for the shoulder appear to be highly

reliable when taken by the same tester, regardless of the type of the goniometer used. The degree of inter-tester reliability for these measurements appears to be ROM-specific (Riddle, 1987).
- In a study of glenohumeral rotational ROM in 39 members of the United States Tennis Association National Tennis Team, loss of internal rotation appeared to increase progressively with longer periods of play. This loss of internal rotation of the shoulder is an absolute loss of motion because total rotation also decreases (Kibler et al, 1996).
- PROM of the shoulder has been used in attempts to measure the anterior capsular ligament, which Hjelm et al (1996) feel can be a direct, primary cause of shoulder pain, ranging from frozen shoulder to impingementlike symptoms.
- Schenkman et al (1997) advocate the measurement of shoulder protraction and thoracolumbar rotation, and state that these motions can be measured with adequate between-rater and within-rater reliability.
- Ellenbecker et al (1996) demonstrated the importance of active internal rotation as a measurement of shoulder function. In a study of elite junior tennis players, external rotation was found to have no significant difference from dominant to nondominant arm. However, the analysis of active internal

rotation differences showed significantly less active internal rotation on the dominant arm for both males and females. Significantly less dominant arm total rotational ROM was also found in both males and females. The apparent loss of dominant arm active internal rotation has clinical application for both the development of rehabilitation and preventative flexibility/ROM programs.

- Pope et al (1996) believes that reduced ROM in external rotation is the most specific finding for shoulder symptoms, but notes that it is necessary to examine movement in multiple planes to assess the true burden of shoulder pain in the community.

Attempts to significantly improve upon the accuracy of visual or commonly used goniometric measurements of shoulder ROM have been frustrating. The scapulohumeral goniometer (SHG) is a relatively new device designed to measure scapular and glenohumeral rotation during active arm elevation in the scapular plane. Measurements of active ROM of scapular and glenohumeral rotation made by the same physical therapist during arm elevation in the scapular plane were shown to be clinically unacceptable when obtained with the current techniques for positioning the SHG (Youdas et al, 1994). The authors advised that these measurements should be approached with caution, because of the high degree of variability associated with this procedure.

Scapular Range of Motion

Scapular position, measured at rest and throughout its movement during shoulder ROM, is vital to the investigation of many types of shoulder conditions. In particular, the scapula which can only rest in an elevated and abducted position has a high correlation with shoulder girdle dysfunction. The most frequently used methods to measure scapular motion are:

- Lennie test: scoliometer and caliper
- Kibler: tape measure
- DiVeta: tape measure

The Lennie test has been found to have moderate to high inter-tester reliability and to provide an accurate measurement of the anatomical location of the scapulae based on x-ray verification. The classic tape measurement method of Kibler was preferred over that of DiVeta et al (1990) upon review by T'Jonck et al (1996).

Smooth motion of the scapula and humerus with respect to the thorax is essential for shoulder function, and abnormalities may be indicative of clinical shoulder syndromes. In general, the available tests for measuring scapular position, including posterior scapular displacement, scapular winging, and scapular tipping, have been reported as reliable and valid (Sobush et al, 1996; Plafcan et al, 1997). However, the inter-tester reliability of these tests has been disputed by at least one author (Gibson et al, 1995).

Does Range of Motion Matter?

Several authors have directly challenged the conventional wisdom that ROM is accurately measurable in the shoulder, and that such a measurement provides a meaningful outcome of shoulder function. Mayer et al (1994a, 1994b) reported that ROM of the shoulder shows a wide variation and does not possess high validity. Shoulder ROM has been reported by Bartolozzi et al (1994) as a factor which, although measurable, does not influence clinical outcome. Most people with self-reported shoulder pain do not have widespread restriction of movement. Restriction in at least one plane of motion has been shown to be present in 77% of those individuals with shoulder pain in one study, but was also present in half of those without pain. Bak and Magnussen (1997) demonstrated that both symptomatic and nonsymptomatic competitive swimmers exhibited increased external ROM and reduced internal ROM compared with normalized data. However, these changes in shoulder ROM were not significantly related to the occurrence of "swimmer's shoulder" pain.

Many exercise and treatment protocols are based upon the logical concept that increased strength and/or stretching techniques will lead to increased ROM of the shoulder. However, Nelson and Cornelius (1991) were not able to prove the hypothesis that increased maximum voluntary isometric contraction (MVIC) used with flexibility techniques would be able to provide greater ROM in the shoulder.

Girouard and Hurley (1995) demonstrated that rehabilitation of shoulder complaints with the use of flexibility techniques (without strength techniques) was successful in increasing ROM in shoulder abduction. However, the use of concurrent strength and flexibility techniques eroded much of the ROM gains.

SPECIFIC SHOULDER CONDITIONS

There is currently great debate in clinical circles concerning the interrelationships between instability, impingement, and rotator cuff tears or dysfunction. Impingement syndrome and moderate anterior glenohumeral instability have some significant overlap of clinical signs and symptoms. Warner et al (1990) make the following observations:

- Asymptomatic shoulder: Internal rotation strength is usually significantly (30%) stronger in the dominant shoulder when there are no shoulder symptoms.
- Glenohumeral instability: Patients with both anterior and multidirectional instability have excessive external rotation as well as increased capsular laxity in all directions. Sixty-eight percent of the patients with instability had significant impingement signs in addition to apprehension and capsular laxity.
- Impingement syndrome: There is usually marked limitation of shoulder motion, but minimal laxity on drawer testing.

Glenohumeral Instability

Thorough descriptions of specific physical examination tests used to determine glenohumeral instability are lacking in the scientific literature. The physical examination of a patient whose history suggests subtle glenohumeral joint instability may be extremely difficult for the HCP due to the normal amount of capsular laxity commonly present in most individuals. An essential component of the physical examination is a through and meticulous subjective history, which includes the mechanisms of injury and/or dysfunction, chief complaint, level of disability, and aggravating movements. The physical examination must include an assessment of motion, static stability testing, muscle testing, functional capacity evaluation, and a neurological assessment. A comprehensive understanding of various stability testing maneuvers is important for the HCP to appreciate (Wilk et al, 1997). Some additional points to consider in glenohumeral instability are as follows:

- Most clinical instability of the shoulder occurs with the shoulder in 90 degrees of abduction. The anterior and posterior band of the inferior glenohumeral ligament complex has recently been shown to be the primary anterior–posterior stabilizer of the abducted shoulder (O'Brien et al, 1995). This has led to a relatively new test for labral tears by O'Brien et al (1998), known as the "active compression test." The patient is asked to actively forward flex the arm to 90 degrees with the elbow in full extension, then adduct the arm medial 10 to 15 degrees, and finally to internally rotate the arm, pointing the thumb down. The patient attempts to press upward, while the examiner pushes downward (Fig. 15–8). Pain or painful clicking is a positive finding for the first ma-

neuver and can often be localized to the shoulder (likely positive for labral tear) or to the acromioclavicular joint. A positive test will usually show reduction of pain if the test is repeated with the patient's forearm supinated (by turning the thumb up).

- Anterior–posterior (AP) translation of the shoulder joint has been measured with reported validity and reliability by positioning a device known as a "knee laxity tester" horizontally over the shoulder girdle, while the AP translation was measured after applying a standardized sagittal force (Jorgenson and Bak, 1995).

Impingement Syndrome

Impingement syndrome remains a difficult clinical entity to diagnose with precision. An optimum testing position for impingement syndrome has recently been described that may assist HCPs with this diagnosis. Using magnetic resonance imaging (MRI) and gadolinium-impregnated markers, it has been shown that impingement of the distal aspect of the supraspinatus tendon between the acromion and the greater tuberosity of the humerus was well visualized during forward flexion and abduction of more than 30 degrees. Shoulder impingement was best seen at 60 degrees forward flexion, 60 degrees abduction, and internal rotation; see Figure 15–9 (Brossmann et al, 1996). This data demonstrates that primary change in the normal internal rotator/external rotator ratio of the shoulder is an etiological factor implicated in impingement (Leroux et al, 1994).

Shoulder pain in swimmers has in general been regarded as synonymous with coracoacromial impingement (anterior shoulder pain due to rotator cuff tendinitis), but new knowledge suggests that a concomitant glenohumeral instability plays an additional and important role (Bak, 1996). One of the most commonly accepted treatments for swimmer's shoulder is strengthening of the external rotators. One study (Bak and Faunl, 1997) indicates that in cases with loss of strength of the shoulder and resulting pain, lost ROM of the internal rotators was found to be the most statistically significant factor for the development of swimmer's shoulder. Rehabilitation protocols should therefore include strengthening of internal as well as external rotators.

STRENGTH TESTING

Strength testing for the shoulder muscles currently lacks standardization. Various schools of thought have proposed various anatomical "starting points" for the testing of muscle strength around the shoulder. It has been reported that measurement of shoulder strength is extremely sensitive to even small changes in positioning (Tis and Maxwell, 1996). The recent literature has shed some additional light on this topic, and optimal positions for testing the strength of shoulder muscles are summarized in Table 15–4. The use of these constant, optimal positions will enable HCPs to

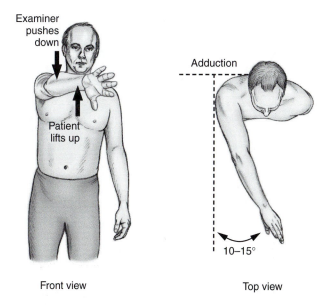

Figure 15–8. O'Brien's test for labral tears.

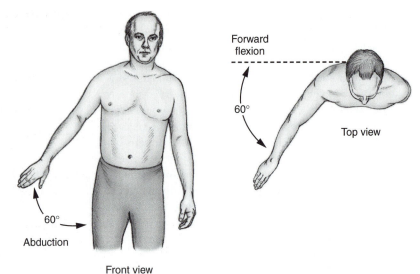

Figure 15–9. Optimal position for demonstration of shoulder impingement.

more accurately measure shoulder strength. See Figures 15–10 through 15–13.

Many authors have developed studies that attempt to isolate various significant factors relative to the measurement of shoulder strength. The HCP may wish to consider the following opinions during assessment of shoulder strength:

- Arm dominance: Two major studies showed essentially opposite results in determining whether arm dominance is a factor that must be considered in the isokinetic assessment of shoulder muscle strength. Ivey et al (1985) demonstrated no statistical difference was found between dominant and nondominant shoulders, even though there was a consistent pattern of greater strength in the dominant shoulder throughout six planes of motion. A more recent study (So et al, 1995) showed that significant bilateral differences did exist during shoulder testing of flexion and extension. Therefore, the authors feel it is inappropriate to use the uninjured extremity to predict the preinjured strength of the injured side without adjustment. Models have been developed relating the expected maximal isokinetic measurement of the dominant shoulder to the nondominant shoulder measurements.

- Muscle strength ratio: Reporting agonist/antagonist ratios has been touted as more clinically applicable than reporting absolute strength values of single muscle groups. The HCP should be aware that shoulder strength ratios are dependent on position and that the scapular plane may be advantageous in some cases for testing and treatment (Tata et al, 1993). Perhaps due to these position dependent errors, Kramer and Ng (1996) noted high variability with ratio data, and recommend HCPs exercise caution when making treatment-related decisions using ratio data.

- Normal strength ratios: The asymptomatic shoulder functions with an expected balance among the major muscle groups. The normal shoulder will usually show adduction strength as the greatest, followed by extension, flexion, abduction, internal rotation, and external rotation (Ivey et al, 1985).

- Isometric, isotonic, and isokinetic methods of measurement of shoulder strength each seem to have

Table 15–4: Optimal Positions for Testing Strength of the Shoulder Muscles (Determined via Electromyography)

POSITION	DESCRIPTION
Supraspinatus	Elevation at 90° of scapular elevation and +45° (external rotation) of humeral rotation (Kelley et al, 1996)
Infraspinatus	External rotation at 0° of scapular elevation and −45° (internal rotation) of humeral rotation (Kelley et al, 1996)
Subscapularis	Best achieved with Gerber (1991) push-off test (Kelley et al, 1996)
	Arm abducted to 90°, 30–45° anterior to the coronal plane, with arm midpoint between full internal and full external rotation (Jenp et al, 1996)
Infraspinatus and teres minor	Arm flexed to 90°, with forearm midpoint between neutral position and full external rotation (Jenp et al, 1996)

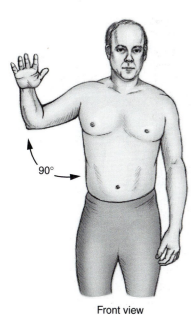
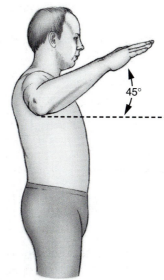

Front view   Side view

Figure 15–10. Optimal position for testing strength of supraspinatus.

their opponents and detractors. Perhaps because of the relatively high cost of the measurement devices, isokinetic equipment appears to be more controversial than isometric or isotonic measurements, as evidenced by the studies highlighted below:

- Mayer et al (1994a, 1994b) reported peak torque and angle at peak torque have been found to have relatively low reproducibility in the shoulder. The shoulder is generally much less reliably measured using these techniques than other joints, such as the knee.
- However, the Biodex isokinetic dynamometer has been shown to be reliable for the test–retest measure of peak torque for glenohumeral medial and lateral

rotator muscles, using the isokinetic eccentric mode of the Biodex (Frisello, 1994).
- Review of popular isometric strength testing devices has shown the Biodex isokinetic dynamometer, and Isobex 2.0 to have high intra-examiner and inter-examiner reliability for measurement of internal rotation, external rotation, and abduction strength in normal subjects. The Nicholas Manual Muscle showed high intra-examiner reliability and moderate inter-examiner reliability, and benefits from the shortest time to complete testing (Leggin et al, 1996).
- Kuhlman et al (1992) emphasized the importance of standardization of the positions for testing the strength of motions of the shoulder and recommend

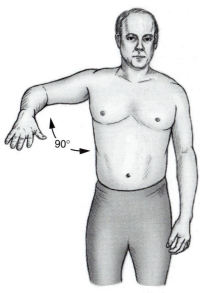
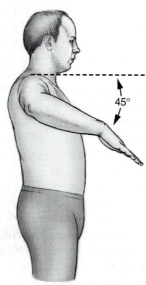

Front view   Side view

Figure 15–11. Optimal position for testing strength of infraspinatus.

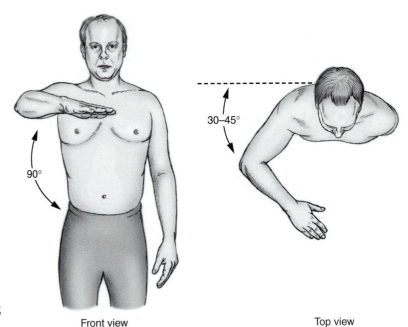

Figure 15–12. Optimal position for testing strength of subscapularis.

Front view

Top view

the following: isometric strength of external rotation should be measured in the scapular plane with the shoulder in 45 degrees of abduction and 45 degrees of internal rotation; isometric strength of abduction, in the scapular plane with the shoulder in 45 degrees of abduction; and isokinetic strength of external rotation and abduction, in the scapular plane at 90 degrees per second. When tested in this method, both isokinetic and isometric testing in the scapular plane are valid methods for measurement of the strength of external rotation and abduction of the shoulder (Kuhlman et al, 1992).

- Isokinetic and isometric reliability appear to be higher for involved shoulders than uninvolved shoulders. The implication of these findings is that there appears to be greater variability with eccentric than concentric or isometric testing of shoulder rotation (Malerbaa et al, 1993).

Bohannon et al (1997) published the most extensive data yet for handheld dynamometry. This data includes subjects from 20 to 79 years, is expressed in newtons and as a percentage of body weight, and is organized by gender, decade of age, and dominant side.

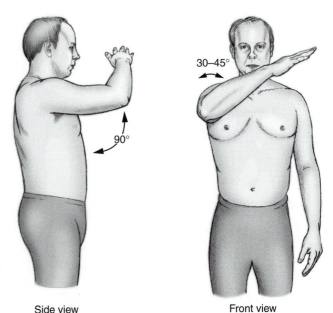

Figure 15–13. Optimal position for testing strength of the infraspinatus and teres minor.

Side view

Front view

DIAGNOSTIC AND PROVOCATIVE TESTS

The literature on the shoulder is replete with many different provocative or "diagnostic" tests. These tests are often named for their originator, or for the anatomical purpose of the test. There is little consensus as to which tests are the most effective, sensitive, or specific for the diagnosis of various shoulder conditions. As Tables 15–5 through 15–8 show, the sensitivity and specificity of various common provocative shoulder tests diverges widely upon investigation by various authors. In addition, there appears to be great variation in the nomenclature of the various provocative tests as utilized by various specialties and professions.

Leroux et al (1995) compared the results of three clinical tests for detecting shoulder impingement syndrome (Neer's, Hawkins–Kennedy, and Yocum's tests) and

Table 15–5: Dynametric Normal Values for Lateral Rotation of the Shoulder (newtons ± standard deviation)

AGE	MEN DOMINANT	MEN NONDOMINANT	WOMEN DOMINANT	WOMEN NONDOMINANT
20–29	206.8 ± 39.6	205.0 ± 33.5	108.4 ± 18.8	97.0 ± 19.3
30–39	188.2 ± 43.0	181.1 ± 48.9	115.4 ± 23.1	105.5 ± 23.2
40–49	189.9 ± 36.9	175.7 ± 23.6	115.6 ± 23.2	113.6 ± 24.4
50–59	166.7 ± 42.7	152.3 ± 36.4	107.9 ± 19.0	107.7 ± 23.3
60–69	150.4 ± 36.5	134.3 ± 28.6	87.2 ± 19.5	86.5 ± 22.0
70–79	140.1 ± 29.0	134.1 ± 30.0	81.8 ± 10.8	79.3 ± 16.2

From Bohannon RW et al, 1997.

Table 15–6: Dynametric Normal Values for Extension of the Shoulder (newtons ± standard deviation)

AGE	MEN DOMINANT	MEN NONDOMINANT	WOMEN DOMINANT	WOMEN NONDOMINANT
20–29	396.5 ± 75.2	385.1 ± 68.2	205.6 ± 39.2	192.2 ± 37.9
30–39	402.5 ± 88.3	376.4 ± 93.5	207.4 ± 48.0	196.9 ± 50.0
40–49	400.1 ± 78.6	409.4 ± 71.6	210.9 ± 41.1	202.0 ± 44.7
50–59	332.1 ± 60.0	303.4 ± 54.3	194.5 ± 37.4	191.0 ± 47.2
60–69	270.9 ± 59.7	272.2 ± 55.2	154.1 ± 37.5	160.9 ± 34.7
70–79	276.0 ± 45.6	259.4 ± 53.1	143.9 ± 34.9	136.5 ± 26.8

From Bohannon RW et al, 1997.

Table 15–7: Dynametric Normal Values for Abduction of the Shoulder (newtons ± standard deviation)

AGE	MEN DOMINANT	MEN NONDOMINANT	WOMEN DOMINANT	WOMEN NONDOMINANT
20–29	258.4 ± 61.0	246.3 ± 43.9	153.2 ± 28.8	135.3 ± 21.2
30–39	249.2 ± 60.2	237.2 ± 69.6	138.5 ± 25.2	135.5 ± 28.4
40–49	245.5 ± 37.5	244.9 ± 43.1	139.0 ± 33.1	129.1 ± 26.2
50–59	240.4 ± 57.6	222.5 ± 47.5	137.2 ± 24.7	134.9 ± 29.9
60–69	203.0 ± 45.1	195.8 ± 44.7	112.1 ± 25.1	103.7 ± 16.1
70–79	191.8 ± 31.5	187.9 ± 33.7	95.9 ± 21.9	101.6 ± 21.3

From Bohannon RW et al, 1997.

Table 15–8: Comparison of Commonly Performed Shoulder Tests: Specificity and Sensitivity

TEST	ATTRIBUTES
Subscapularis test (Gerber's lift-off test)	*Specificity:* Good; maximizes electromyographic activity of subscapularis (Kelly et al, 1996) Poor; does not correlate with surgically observed rotator cuff lesions (Leroux et al, 1995)
Jobe's (supraspinatus)	*Sensitivity:* Acceptable *Specificity:* Poor (Leroux et al, 1995) *Sensitivity:* 85% for type II impingement; 100% for rotator cuff tear (Ure et al, 1993)
Neer's, Hawkins', Yocum's, Patte's, palm-up (long head of biceps)	*Sensitivity:* Acceptable *Specificity:* Poor (Leroux et al, 1995) Hawkins' test for impingement was more sensitive than Neer's test (Bak, 1997)
Yergason's	*Sensitivity:* Poor; only 50% of patients with known primary biceps involvement had positive test (Post, 1994)
Leffert	Best of the instability tests; predictive in 73% of cases
Abduction external rotation (AER) test	*Sensitivity:* Sensitive to neck and shoulder disorders but also, to some extent, to the carpal tunnel syndrome (Toomingas et al, 1991)

four tests for determining the location of the rotator cuff lesion [Jobe's test (supraspinatus), Patte's test (infraspinatus), lift-off test (subscapularis), and palm-up test (long head of the biceps brachii] to intraoperatively observed anatomical lesions in 55 consecutive patients who had surgery for Neer's syndrome. These tests were found to be satisfactorily sensitive, but the specificity of the tests was poor. Of special interest is that the severity of functional impairment during Jobe's and Patte's maneuvers was not correlated with the size of the tear. See Figures 15–14 and 15–15.

These findings were partially contradicted by the work of Ure et al (1993), who compared the results of clinical shoulder examination including 20 special tests as compared with subsequent arthroscopic findings in 45 patients. The highest sensitivity for stage II impingement was found for the supraspinatus test (85%) and the lift-up test (92%); the sensitivity of these tests for rotator cuff tears was 100% and 89%, respectively. Differentiation between impingement syndrome with and without rotator cuff tear by one of these tests alone was not possible because of their low positive predictive values (26% and 56%). In contrast, in 90% of patients with negative rotator tests the rotator cuff was complete, while the negative predictive value of the supraspinatus test was 100%. Instability was confirmed in only 53% of cases; the Leffert test had the highest positive predictive value (73%). The authors concluded the clinical diagnosis of a shoulder lesion cannot reliably be achieved by single tests; rather overall evaluation by an experienced clinician is necessary.

Additionally, Yergason's test has been shown to be unlikely to be able to detect weakness or dysfunction of the biceps, which is the stated purpose of the test (Post, 1987).

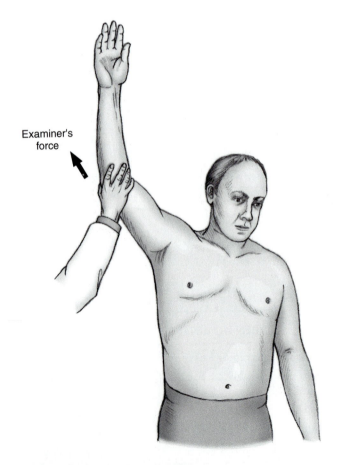

Examiner's force

Figure 15–14. Neer's test for shoulder impingement.

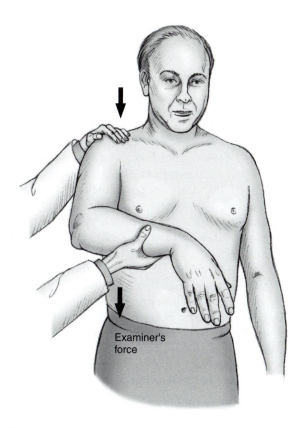

Figure 15–15. Hawkins–Kennedy test for shoulder impingement.

James Cyriax's approach to diagnosis and treatment of soft tissue disorders is frequently used by orthopedic and sport physical therapists. This method requires the HCP to assess the quality of motion at the last portion of joint ROM, sometimes called "end-feel." Pellecchia et al (1996) noted that the Cyriax evaluation can be a highly reliable schema for assessing patients with shoulder pain, listing "almost perfect" agreement among examiners. Chesworth et al (1998) essentially agreed, finding that assessment of joint "end-feel" was highly reliable. However, Winters et al (1997a) are in opposition to these opinions. Using cluster data analysis of a large patient base, Winters et al present an opinion that the more detailed shoulder classifications, such as the Cyriax methodology, may not be suitable for the diagnosis of patients with shoulder complaints in general practice.

MEASURING NECK AND SHOULDER PAIN

Other measurement devices that have been used to measure neck and shoulder pain include:

- Doliometry: The dolorimeter is a small, handheld device which is designed to measure the amount of tolerance to pressure, and expresses the patient's sensitivity to pain. This is also known as pressure al-

gometry. The dolorimeter (or algometer) typically has a dial that reads the pressure threshold reading in kg/cm^2. The dolorimeter is steadily pressed against the desired muscle by the examiner with a steadily increasing force of 1 kg/sec. Published values exist for the pressure threshold at which various muscle groups become painful, known as the "abnormal pressure threshold" (Rachlin, 1994). For example, the upper trapezius has a abnormal pressure threshold of 2.0 to 4.0 kg/cm^2 for females and 2.9 to 4.7 kg/cm^2 for males. The repeatability of the dolorimeter has been reported to be good, but sensitivity and specificity for neck/shoulder symptoms are poor. The dolorimeter is a good device for measurement of cervicobrachial tenderness when the subject acts as his or her own control (Levoska et al, 1993).

- Facial action coding system: The results of one study support the validity and generality of facial expression as a measurement of glenohumeral joint pain, show that they yield graded sensitive information, and suggest that facial expressions encode information about the psychosocial context of pain problems. Facial actions that have been shown to be related to pain indices include eyebrow lowering, narrowing and closing of the eyes, lip pulling, nose wrinkling, and mouth opening. Facial actions during clinical tests showed consistent relationships with sensory and affective pain scales. The theoretical implications of these findings are discussed by Prkachin and Mercer (1989).

- Shoulder pain score: This outcome measurement tool is comprised of six pain symptom questions selected from the literature, together with a 101-Numerical Rating Scale (NRS-101). The score was tested in a follow-up study of 101 patients with shoulder complaints. The shoulder pain score gave a reliable impression of the pain experienced and proved to be a useful instrument for following the course of the disorder over time and giving an indication of when a patient feels cured (Winters et al, 1996).

PREDICTORS OF SHOULDER PAIN AND RISK FACTORS

There is great interest in accurately demonstrating predictive factors for future shoulder problems; the most logical approach to treating tomorrow's shoulder condition is to avoid known risk factors today. Poor posture of the head, neck, and shoulders has been cited by many studies as an important factor in the development of upper extremity and shoulder conditions. Clinical assessment of posture, however, tends to be rather subjective in nature. Recent studies that detail both new uses for common tools and also the use of new technology have begun the process of measuring postural deviations. These studies include the following:

- The use of a computer-assisted slide digitizing system has been proposed by Braun and Admundson (1989) who found that postural elements were reproducible, and found the reliability of the system was adequate for postural analysis.
- A method of measuring sagittal plane postural alignment of the head and shoulder in relationship to the lateral malleolus was developed using a carpenter's trysquare with a line level attached to the horizontal arm and a goniometer with a line level attached to the horizontal arm. Horizontal measures were taken with the trysquare from a vertical reference point to the tragus of the ear, to the shoulder axis, and to the lateral malleolus. Angular measures were taken with the goniometer of C7-tragus from a horizontal reference point and tragus-corner of the eye from a horizontal reference point. Harrison et al (1996a) demonstrate a reliable and practical method for taking postural measurements in the clinic and describe a pilot study for comparing a patient with a nonpatient sample.
- Using a variety of task-specific measurement techniques, scapular protraction and rotation, forward head position, midthoracic curvature, and passive humeral elevation in the plane of the scapula were measured randomly in standing. Forward head position was significantly greater in patients with shoulder complaints, and humeral elevation was significantly greater in normal shoulders. Scapular protraction, rotation, midthoracic curvature, and scapular symmetry were not found to be significant (Greenfield et al, 1995).
- Forward shoulder posture has been described as measurable using four objective techniques: the Baylor square, the double square, the Sahrmann technique, and scapular position. The researchers demonstrated clinical reliability for each technique; however, validity compared with radiographic measurement could not be established. These techniques may have clinical value in objectively measuring change in a patient's shoulder posture as a result of a treatment program (Peterson et al, 1997).

PROGNOSTIC FACTORS

Shoulder pain is common in primary health care. Nevertheless, information on the outcome of shoulder disorders is scarce, especially for patients encountered in general practice. In one study (van der Windt et al, 1996), 23% of all patients showed complete recovery after 1 month; this figure increased to 59% after 1 year. Unfortunately, this means 41% percent of shoulder patients still had significant symptoms after a full year of treatment; this is an embarrassingly high figure for HCPs who consider themselves efficacious. A speedy recovery has been shown to be related to preceding overuse or slight trauma and early presentation. A high risk of persistent or recurrent complaints was found for patients with concomitant neck pain and severe shoulder pain during the day at original clinical presentation.

Patient characteristics and prognostic factors that have been shown to be associated with an unfavorable clinical outcome include a rotator cuff tear greater than 1 cm^2, a history of pretreatment clinical symptoms for greater than 1-year duration, and significant functional impairment at initial presentation. Factors not associated with clinical outcome include patient age, occupation, gender, associated instability, dominance, chronicity of onset, active ROM, or specific treatment modalities. Early operative intervention is recommended for patients with poor prognostic factors to avoid a protracted clinical course (Bartolozzi et al, 1994).

The best independent prognostic factors in patients with rotator tendinosis (stage II impingement syndrome) of the shoulder are the following: participating in active treatment, working (not being on sickness leave), and avoiding regular medication. The influence of regular medication was particularly high in those who had no disease apart from the painful shoulder. The authors of one study recommended that HCPs should attempt to limit prescription of medication and sick leave, and avoid polymedication (Brox and Brevik, 1996). These factors are summarized below.

Factors Associated with Favorable Prognosis

- History of slight trauma or overuse
- Early presentation
- Absence of concomitant neck pain
- Active treatment
- Not on regular medication
- Not on sick leave
- Favorable acromial morphology (type I acromion).

Factors Associated with Poor Prognosis

- Concomitant neck pain
- Severe pain during the day at presentation
- Rotator cuff tear larger than 1 cm^2
- History of pretreatment clinical symptoms for greater than 1 year
- Significant functional impairment at initial presentation
- Unfavorable acromial morphology (type III acromion)
- Lack of coordination in the scapulohumeral joint

Factors Shown to Be Unassociated with Prognosis

- Age
- Occupation
- Gender
- Associated shoulder instability
- Tenderness over the acromion
- Shoulder dominance

- Chronicity of onset
- ROM
- Specific treatment modalities (Bartolozzi et al, 1994; Brox and Bevik, 1996; van der Windt et al, 1996; Bak and Magnusson, 1997; Bak and Faunl, 1997; Morrison et al, 1997)

SHOULDER QUESTIONNAIRES

Many different types of patient questionnaires have been designed to evaluate shoulder conditions, the severity of the conditions, or the impact of the shoulder condition upon the activities of the patient. Most of these questionnaires and functional outcome tools seek to quantify dysfunction, and to express that dysfunction numerically. Several of these scales show significant overlap, or represent minor changes to existing questionnaires. The HCP should carefully assess the questionnaires to determine which devices are most appropriate for use in a given patient or a given condition. For most of these tests, reliability and validity characteristics (other than those claimed by the original authors) have not yet been thoroughly studied.

The following tests are recommended:

- **Constant Scale (also known as Constant and Murley)** (Constant and Murley, 1987). This rating system remains very popular, because it has been described for use with any diagnosis, unlike many of the other rating schemes that are dependent upon the ultimate shoulder diagnosis. It consists of five objective and two subjective items, and can be completed in approximately 5 minutes. It assigns 65 points for objective criteria (ROM and abduction strength) and 35 for subjective factors (ability to work, sleep and recreate). The Constant system therefore measures shoulder function; see Appendix Form F–1.
- **Hospital for Special Surgery (HSS) Scale** (Warren et al, 1982). This scale focuses on pain, functional limitations, ROM, impingement tests, and tenderness. It is constructed quite similarly to the Constant scale, but has different scoring elements; see Appendix Form F–2.
- **Shoulder Function Assessment (SFA) Scale.** Originally designed for patients with rheumatoid arthritis, the SFA scale is a reliable, valid, and accurate measure of shoulder function that can be completed within 3 minutes. The general format of the SFA is again similar to the Constant scale. The validity and the reliability of the SFA scale are equivalent to or better than the validity and reliability of the Constant and the HSS scales. The discriminative ability of the SFA scale was superior to both other scales (van den Ende et al, 1996); see Appendix Form F–3.
- **Croft's Shoulder-related Disability Scale.** This scale measures the frequency of problems with ac-

tivities of daily living as related to shoulder symptoms using a 22-item ("yes" or "no" questions) disability questionnaire and measures of shoulder movement. This disability questionnaire is simple to complete, very easy to score, and is useful for both general practice and population-based studies of shoulder pain (Croft et al, 1994); see Appendix Form F–4.

- **Wolfgang's Assessment Scheme for Rotator Cuff Injury.** A 5-question instrument used to assess pain, loss of abduction, strength, function, and patient satisfaction. This questionnaire is simple to use and score (Wolfgang, 1994). This questionnaire has been recently proposed for the use of conservative management of rotator cuff tears (Itoi and Tabata, 1992); see Appendix Form F–5.
- **Shoulder Pain and Disability Index (SPADI).** The SPADI is a 13-point questionnaire that measures pain and disability. This scale has been shown to be responsive to change and accurately discriminates among patients who are improved or worsened. It has been described in two different formats; using the original visual analogue scale (Roach et al, 1991) and using the numerically scaled version, which is easier to score and has been found to correlate well with the original version (Williams et al, 1995); see Appendix Form F–6.
- **Shoulder Rating Questionnaire (SRQ).** This self-administered shoulder questionnaire assesses the functional status and severity of symptoms of the shoulder. Subscales include global assessment, pain, activities of daily living, recreational/athletic activities, work, satisfaction, and areas for improvement. The SRQ was found by the authors to be valid, reliable, and responsive to clinical change (L'Insalata et al, 1997). Completion time is 5 to 10 minutes; see Appendix Form F–7.
- **Athletic Shoulder Outcome Rating Scale** (Tibone and Bradley, 1995). This 100-point rating system is intended for use in the population of athletes, where shoulder demands are higher than in the general population. Athletes are grouped according to competition levels from professional athlete in major league sports to the occasional recreational athlete. The questions are composed of subjective evaluation of pain, strength/endurance, stability, intensity, and performance; and objective evaluation of ROM; see Appendix Form F–8.
- **Simple Shoulder Test** (Matsen et al, 1995). This outcome measurement device was designed specifically to allow analysis of functional outcomes of patients without the use of a computer. This questionnaire is essentially 12 questions regarding everyday function which can be answered by the patient "yes" or "no"; see Appendix Form F–9.
- **Questionnaire on the Perceptions of Patients About Shoulder Surgery** (Dawson et al, 1996a).

This is a 12-item, multiple choice questionnaire, which is given to the patient who is considering having shoulder operations other than stabilization. This evaluation is typically performed both preoperatively and 6 months postoperatively. The questionnaire shows a high internal consistency and satisfactory reproducibility and was most efficient in distinguishing patients who said that their shoulder was much improved after surgery from all other patients. Despite the title of this scale, it has been used successfully by practitioners of nonsurgical specialties; see Appendix Form F–10.

The following tests are used with somewhat less frequency in clinical settings and are not included in this chapter. In some cases, these represent early attempts at outcome measurement, or devices designed for very specific patient groups (such as the Wheelchair User's Shoulder Pain Index). However, the use of these outcome measures should not in any way be discouraged, as they are very appropriate for specific patients:

- Subjective Shoulder Rating Scale (Kohn and Geyer, 1997). The authors developed a shoulder rating system that correlated well with the Constant–Murley Scale and was able to be completed much more quickly (average 55 seconds completion time versus 410 seconds for the Constant–Murley).
- Wheelchair User's Shoulder Pain Index (WUSPI) (Curtis et al, 1995). This questionnaire was designed to measure shoulder pain in individuals who use wheelchairs. Individual item analysis revealed that the subjects in this study experienced the most shoulder pain when wheeling up an incline or on outdoor surfaces, when lifting an object from an overhead shelf, when trying to sleep, when transferring from tub to wheelchair and when washing their backs. The final 15-item index shows high internal consistency. This instrument is useful for both clinical and research purposes to detect and monitor shoulder pain and accompanying loss of function by wheelchair users.
- Rowe Scale (Rowe et al, 1978). The Rowe system measures motion, stability and function. Originally used in the evaluation of the Bankart lesion. Several authors have been critical of the use of this scale to measure conditions other than the results of its original purpose, specifically the assessment of anterior instability of the shoulder.
- Walch–Duplay Rating Sheet for Anterior Instability of the Shoulder (Walch, 1987). This is a modification of the Rowe rating system. There is an increased focus on the return to activity, especially the return to usual sports.
- The Algofunctional Index of Patte for shoulders (Patte, 1987). The original purpose of this rating scheme was the assessment of chronically painful

shoulders that caused disability. Assessment was made for pain, function, muscle strength, and daily handicap. The scoring of this test is considered by some to be very cumbersome, and it is therefore seldom used in its original form in today's clinical practice.
- Neer Scale (Neer, 1972). The Neer Scale was developed for the investigation of outcome of anterior acromioplasty in chronic impingement syndrome. In its original form, the score was simply "satisfactory" or "unsatisfactory." Neer must be credited with one of the first attempts to quantify outcome measurements in the treatment of the shoulder.

Refer to Chapter 7 for additional discussion of the following shoulder tests:

- Self-evaluation form
- American Shoulder and Elbow Surgeons Shoulder Evaluation
- Simple Shoulder Test
- UCLA Shoulder Rating Scale

Several studies have attempted to compare the validity, reliability or applicability of these various outcome measurement devices for the shoulder. Beaton and Richards (1996) compared prospectively the validity of five questionnaires in the assessment of function of the shoulder: the Shoulder Pain and Disability Index, the Simple Shoulder Test, the Subjective Shoulder Rating Scale, the Modified American Shoulder and Elbow Surgeons Shoulder Patient Self-Evaluation Form, and the Shoulder Severity Index. In this concurrent comparison of measures of shoulder-specific outcome in the same subjects, the shoulder questionnaires performed similarly, both in describing function of the shoulder and in discriminating between levels of severity.

However, not all comparative studies showed that shoulder outcome questionnaires possess similar qualities. A comparison was also performed of the following shoulder scales: Rowe, modified-Rowe, UCLA, and the pre-1994 American Shoulder and Elbow Surgeons scale. Inter-rater reliability between the four systems was found to be poor. The study showed that generalized results of an investigation can be significantly biased based on the selection of a scoring system. The authors showed that the lack of a widely accepted scoring system for the shoulder limits comparison of management for shoulder conditions, and they described the need for a widely accepted shoulder scoring system (Romeo et al, 1996). In addition, differences in health status may be a crucial determinant in selecting the optimal management strategies for individual patients with various shoulder problems. Self-assessment questionnaires have been shown to be quite effective in characterizing these differences (Matsen et al, 1997).

In summary, it must be conceded that there is no current consensus on the "best" outcome measures to use in the evaluation and treatment of the shoulder. As outcome measurement is still in its infancy, selection criteria for the specific outcome measurement devices has not been thoroughly studied, and the decisions remain with the HCP regarding the optimum measurement device for a given patient. **It is suggested that the HCP select from the tools shown in this chapter to match the most appropriate outcome measure to the needs of the individual patient, and continue to use that outcome measure periodically throughout the treatment period.**

ELBOW

The elbow is relatively poorly studied in comparison to the shoulder and wrist among upper extremity joints. As illustrated in Table 15–9, normal ROM shows somewhat more agreement by various authors than some of the other extremities in this chapter. And yet, there remains surprising variation (as much as 25 degrees) between various proposed "normal" values of elbow motion.

Goniometric measurement of the elbow certainly seems straightforward, yet several points should be considered before measurement is attempted, as follows:

- There is no difference between the lateral and the over-the-joint methods of goniometric measurement of the elbow joint (Grohman, 1983).
- Goniometric measurements of the elbow performed in a clinical setting have been reported to be highly reliable with the use of simple, constant protocols. In one study, the use of various types of goniometers showed similar, acceptable results for each type (Rothstein et al, 1983). Intra-tester and inter-tester reliability for goniometric testing at the elbow was high.

- Petherick et al (1988), however, found nearly the opposite results, stating that the fluid-based goniometer and the standard goniometer cannot be used interchangeably. The fluid-based goniometer had high inter-tester reliability, while the standard goniometer had poor inter-tester reliability.
- The precision of the goniometric measurement of the elbow using a simple plastic goniometer appears to range from 1 to 6 degrees (Solveborn and Olerud, 1996).
- The alignment of goniometer, identification of landmarks, and variations in manual force during passive ROM are all factors that contribute to goniometric error. Relatively inexperienced raters should be able to use goniometers accurately to measure elbow position when given standardized methods to follow (Fish and Wingate, 1985).
- In some clinical studies, photography is used as a method of measuring joint movement. For example, the elbow can be photographed while in maximal flexion and maximal extension. Lines can be drawn through the midline of the forearm and upper arm, and the resulting angle can be measured with a simple plastic protractor. Fish and Wingate (1985) reported that a slightly higher degree of accuracy of elbow joint angle measurement can be obtained via photography (s +/− 2.4 to 3.4 degrees) than by standard goniometry (s +/− .7 to 1.1 degrees).

STRENGTH TESTING

Functional strength testing of the elbow has application in many conditions, ranging from epicondylitis to osteoarthritis. As with strength testing of other joints, various authors have opinions on the factors that may have an impact on the accuracy of elbow strength testing:

Table 15–9: Range of Motion of the Elbow from Various Sources

ELBOW	HOPPENFELD (1976)	AMA *GUIDES* (1993)	MAGEE (AROM) (1992)	OMBREGT (PROM) (1995)	KAPANDJI (1980)	MORREY (1993)	EVANS (1994)
Flexion	135°±	140°	140–150°	160°	AROM: 145° PROM: 160°	145°	140–150°
Extension	0–5°	0°	0–10°	0°–10°	0° normal; 5–10° in subjects with great laxity of ligaments	0°	0° normal; up to 10° of hyperextension may be seen, especially in women
Supination	90°	80°	90°	90°	90°	85°	90°
Pronation	90°	80°	80–90°	85°	85°	75°	80–90°

AROM, active range of motion; PROM, passive range of motion.

- The elbow extension strength of most subjects showed a strong dependence on both elbow and shoulder angles. Elbow extension was typically weak when the upper arm was elevated to shoulder level at the side, which unfortunately corresponds to the position often adopted by these individuals due to shoulder weakness (Kirsch et al, 1996).
- Age appears to be a factor in measuring strength at the elbow joint. Highly significant differences have been found between younger and older subjects in flexion and extension, whereas no age-related differences were found in supination and pronation. Age also appears to affect where in the ROM peak torque is produced (Gallagher et al, 1997).
- Bohannon et al (1997) recently published normal values for elbow flexion and extension arrayed by gender and age. This information is summarized in Tables 15–10 and 15–11.

PREDICTIVE FACTORS

Radial Epicondylitis

In patients with unilateral radial epicondylalgia, almost all measurements of ROM of the elbow and wrist have been found to be limited in the affected arm (Solveborn and Olerud, 1996). Stretching exercises, as well as forearm distraction bands, have been found to be successful for continuous symptom reduction. However, stretching exercises were more effective as gauged by subjective evaluation (visual analogue pain scale, tabulated pain and condition alternatives on questionnaires) and objective findings (such as palpation tenderness at the radial epicondyle, the Mills' "tennis elbow pain test," and increasing ROM) (Solveborn, 1997).

Lateral Epicondylitis

There appears to be a limited amount of quality information in the biomedical literature on outcome measures in lateral epicondylitis. In a recent study that attempted to determine the clinical course of lateral elbow pain and prognostic factors, Hudak et al (1996) reviewed 40 articles that referred to prognosis or reported use of any outcome measure. Only four studies (10%) were judged to provide

moderate strength of evidence, and no studies were graded as providing strong evidence on prognosis. The authors' conclusion is that the majority of studies on lateral elbow pain were limited by methodological weaknesses in selection and definition of the study population, length of follow-up, and analysis of prognostic factors.

Lateral epicondylitis has been shown by other studies to have some interesting prognostic factors. For example, Gerberich and Priest (1985) showed that the greater the elbow pain, the more likely that provided treatment would be able to completely resolve the condition. The following list summarizes known prognostic factors in lateral epicondylitis.

- *Indicator of good prognosis:* The greater the pain the more likely the complete success of the treatments (Gerberich and Priest, 1985).
- *Indicators of poor prognosis:* Extended duration of pain complaint (Gerberich and Priest, 1985); site of lesion and prior occurrence (Hudak et al, 1996b).

ELBOW RATING SCALES AND QUESTIONNAIRES

Unlike the shoulder, there are relatively few scales in the literature for the purpose of measuring outcome for elbow complaints. In general, the validity of these outcome devices have not yet been thoroughly investigated. The following scales are recommended:

- **Mayo Elbow Performance Index** (Morrey, 1993). This 100-point index of elbow function subtracts points for pain (45 points), limited motion (20), instability (10), and inability to perform simple daily functions (25). It is probably the most often used clinical outcome measure for elbow complaints of a nonsurgical nature. See Appendix Form F–11.
- **Elbow Functional Rating Index** (Broberg and Morrey, 1986). This rating scheme was originally described for assessment of elbow function after delayed radial head excision following old trauma. There are separate sections for range of motion (40 points), pain (35), strength (20) and stability (5).

Table 15–10: Dynametric Normal Values for Elbow Flexion Strength (newtons ± standard deviation)

AGE	MEN DOMINANT	MEN NONDOMINANT	WOMEN DOMINANT	WOMEN NONDOMINANT
20–29	285.0 ± 38.2	278.5 ± 47.8	154.9 ± 20.7	152.6 ± 21.8
30–39	268.5 ± 47.1	281.2 ± 54.3	163.8 ± 28.1	160.8 ± 31.8
40–49	268.5 ± 33.6	269.8 ± 29.7	151.3 ± 21.7	156.9 ± 25.3
50–59	286.9 ± 38.5	268.2 ± 49.6	155.3 ± 25.3	156.3 ± 22.4
60–69	259.4 ± 48.9	243.6 ± 42.7	130.6 ± 21.6	134.2 ± 19.0
70–79	237.3 ± 39.9	237.5 ± 38.1	129.9 ± 27.0	130.3 ± 28.7

From Bohannon et al, 1997.

Table 15–11: Dynametric Normal Values for Elbow Extension Strength (newtons ± standard deviation)

AGE	MEN DOMINANT	MEN NONDOMINANT	WOMEN DOMINANT	WOMEN NONDOMINANT
20–29	243.1 ± 50.5	244.5 ± 39.5	116.2 ± 20.2	115.2 ± 22.5
30–39	214.3 ± 50.8	231.1 ± 68.0	116.7 ± 31.2	118.7 ± 33.8
40–49	209.9 ± 33.4	214.1 ± 36.7	109.7 ± 21.8	112.3 ± 26.6
50–59	196.9 ± 37.2	186.1 ± 38.5	111.2 ± 19.1	106.7 ± 20.8
60–69	168.5 ± 41.6	164.7 ± 32.6	92.9 ± 20.6	95.3 ± 18.2
70–79	163.2 ± 35.2	169.5 ± 36.6	89.0 ± 17.8	88.6 ± 16.5

From Bohannon et al, 1997.

Perhaps due to the relative lack of competition, this rating scale has found utility for nonsurgical cases as well. When comparing this scale to the Mayo Elbow Performance Index, some HCPs prefer the Elbow Functional Rating Index's higher degree of specificity in the motion subscale and the addition of a subscale for strength; see Appendix Form F–12.

OUTCOME MEASURES FOR THE WRIST AND HAND

RANGE OF MOTION

There is considerable variation among the opinions of many authors regarding "normal" wrist ROM. As shown in Table 15–12, subjects can vary by as much as 25 degrees of flexion, extension, or ulnar deviation and still fall within the normal limits, depending upon the published source used to establish the meaning of "normal." Armed with the knowledge that a "normal ROM" of the wrist is a rather elusive statement, here are some additional points to consider when undertaking goniometry:

- Measurement of wrist motion by individual therapists has been shown to be highly reliable, and in-tra-rater reliability was higher than inter-rater reliability for all active and passive motions. Inter-rater reliability was generally higher among specialized therapists for unknown reasons. With the exception of pain, identified sources of error were found to have surprisingly little effect on the reliability of measurement (Horger, 1990).
- The intra-observer variation of wrist goniometry has been estimated at 5 to 8 degrees and the inter-observer variation at 6 to 10 degrees. No difference between experienced and nonexperienced observers has been found. The difference between the right and the left wrist was negligible, indicating that the opposite wrist can be used as reference when evaluating restrictions in motion (Solgaard et al, 1986).
- Radial, ulnar, and volar alignment techniques have been described to measure wrist ROM. The volar/dorsal alignment technique is the goniometric technique of choice, as it consistently has the greatest reliability (LaStayo and Wheeler, 1994).

STRENGTH TESTING

When testing strength of the wrist, use of a handheld dynamometer is often recommended. The normative data as reported by Bohannon et al (1997) is listed in Table 15–13. Even more commonly used in clinical settings are hand

Table 15–12: Normal Wrist Range of Motion from Various Sources

WRIST	HOPPENFELD (1976)	AMA *GUIDES* (1993)	MAGEE (AROM) (1992)	KAPANDJI (1980)	EVANS (1994)	GERHARDT AND RIPPSTEIN (1994)
Flexion	80°	60°	80–90°	85°	80–90°	50°
Extension	70°	60°	70–90°	85°	70–90°	60°
Ulnar deviation	30°	30°	30–45°	45°	30–45°	20°
Radial deviation	20°	20°	15°	15°	15°	30°

AROM, active range of motion.

Table 15–13: Dynametric Normal Values for Wrist Extension (newtons ± standard deviation)

AGE	MEN DOMINANT	MEN NONDOMINANT	WOMEN DOMINANT	WOMEN NONDOMINANT
20–29	184.3 ± 27.6	171.1 ± 23.6	99.6 ± 16.8	94.4 ± 19.0
30–39	169.5 ± 41.5	172.5 ± 39.9	104.6 ± 17.6	98.0 ± 19.8
40–49	185.1 ± 38.1	178.6 ± 32.2	102.1 ± 17.5	99.4 ± 21.2
50–59	148.9 ± 35.0	144.7 ± 35.9	99.7 ± 18.4	98.5 ± 17.2
60–69	138.3 ± 29.9	125.8 ± 24.4	83.2 ± 17.7	85.2 ± 19.8
70–79	130.1 ± 22.3	126.5 ± 22.1	69.8 ± 17.6	61.4 ± 17.8

From Bohannon et al, 1997.

and pinch dynamometers (see Figs. 15–16 and 15–17) of various sizes to measure grip and pinch strength. Normal values for grip strength of the hand and pinching strength of the fingers are listed in Table 15–14.

CARPAL TUNNEL SYNDROME

Carpal tunnel syndrome (CTS) is the most common focal nerve entrapment syndrome. Some patients suffering from CTS may present with a disabling musculoskeletal pain and local tenderness in the upper extremities that can persist following surgery despite resolution of neuropathic symptoms. These two symptom complexes, although both sequelae of repetitive activities, have fundamental clinicopathological differences that must be recognized because of their therapeutic, prognostic, and medico-legal implications (Lazaro, 1997).

It is important to remember that clinically symptomatic CTS is not necessarily accompanied by impaired nerve conduction values (Lazaro, 1997). Even when the patient presents with a typical clinical presentation of CTS

the diagnosis is only confirmed electrophysiologically in 61% of cases. Analysis of the sensitivity and specificity of various provocative clinical tests and diagnostic maneuvers has shown only mediocre reliability in establishing the correct diagnosis (Buch-Jaeger and Foucher, 1994). Concannon et al (1997) suggest that the positivity of electrodiagnostic studies is an artificial one, and that the clinical diagnosis of CTS is sufficient to predict the presence of the disease. According to Concannon et al, strict adherence to electrodiagnostic studies to confirm the diagnosis will exclude 13 percent of the patients with legitimate CTS from receiving appropriate therapy.

Horch et al (1997) showed the cross-sectional area of the carpal tunnel (visualized via MRI) in patients with

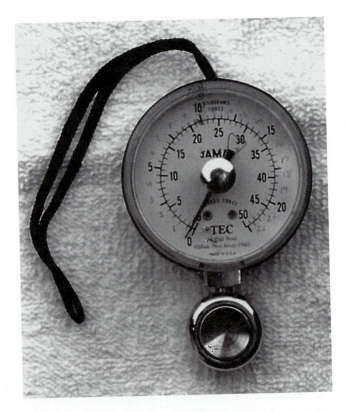

Figure 15–16. Hand dynamometer.

Figure 15–17. Pinch dynamometer.

Table 15–14: Normal Values for Grip and Pinch Strength

| | GRIP STRENGTH (KG) | | | |
| | MALES | | FEMALES | |
	Major Hand	Minor Hand	Major Hand	Minor Hand
Occupation				
Skilled	47.0	45.4	26.8	24.4
Sedentary	47.2	44.1	23.1	21.1
Manual	48.5	44.6	24.2	22.0
Average	47.6	45.0	24.6	22.4
Age Group				
<20	45.2	42.6	23.8	22.8
20–29	48.5	46.2	24.6	22.7
30–39	49.2	44.5	30.8	28.0
40–49	49.0	47.3	23.4	21.5
50–59	45.9	43.5	22.3	18.2

| | PINCH STRENGTH (KG) | | | |
| | MALES | | FEMALES | |
	Major Hand	Minor Hand	Major Hand	Minor Hand
Occupation				
Skilled	6.6	6.4	4.4	4.3
Sedentary	6.3	6.1	4.1	3.9
Manual	8.5	7.7	6.0	5.5
Average	7.5	7.1	4.9	4.7

From American Medical Association, 1993.

CTS tends to be significantly smaller than that found in nonsymptomatic volunteers. The cross-sectional area of the carpal tunnel decreases during wrist flexion at the pisiform and hamate level. During wrist extension, the cross-sectional area of the carpal tunnel decreases at the level of the pisiform. During extension, it increases at the level of the hamate. The cross-sectional area of the median nerve shows an increase at the pisiform level, a flattening of the median nerve at the hamate hook level, and palmar deviation of the flexor retinaculum at the level of the pisiform and hamate hook.

Risk Factors

Many authors have attempted to identify factors that increase the risk for developing CTS. These factors have been described as anatomical, occupational, or environmental.

Diagnostic Signs and Provocative Tests

Much has been written over the past few years regarding the specificity, sensitivity, and validity of the provocative or diagnostic CTS tests. Many authors have been quite strident in their preference of one test over another. Unfortunately, my own review fails to find a consensus for many

---

CLINICAL TIP 15–1
Risk Factors for Carpal Tunnel Syndrome

Risk factors:
- Forceful repetitive activity
- Vibration (Katz JN et al, 1994).
- Moderate to severe restriction to motion (Sucher, 1994)
- Physically small carpal tunnel (Horch et al, 1997)
- Square shaped wrist
- Median nerve hypesthesia
- Abductor pollicis brevis weakness (Kuhlman and Hennessey, 1997)
- Hand pain drawing of classic CTS
- Tinel's test positive (Katz et al, 1991)

Proven not to be a risk factor:
- Abnormal median sensory nerve conduction studies in asymptomatic workers were not predictive of future hand or finger complaints (Werner et al, 1997).

of the well-known and popular tests. This information is summarized in Table 15–15.

In general, there remains great controversy about whether CTS can be diagnosed effectively and consistently through physical or provocative signs, and whether or not electromyographic (EMG) studies have sufficient sensitivity and accuracy to serve as a "gold standard" for the diagnosis of CTS. Experts have widely varying opinions related to the ability of the HCP to diagnose CTS with clinical provocative tests, and also hold varying opinions on the necessity for EMG in CTS symptoms. Some authors are rather suspicious of the sensitivity of EMG in CTS diagnosis, and feel that CTS can exist in the absence of positive EMG findings. Many of the studies below attempt to correlate physical or provocative signs and EMG results with the ultimate diagnosis of CTS.

Table 15–15: Sensitivity and Specificity of Common Carpal Tunnel Syndrome Tests

TEST	SENSITIVITY	SPECIFICITY	SOURCE
Carpal compression test (pressure provocative test)	>Tinel/Phalen	>Tinel/Phalen	(Durkan, 1991)
	87%	95%	(Gonzalez del Pino et al, 1997)
	100%	—	(Williams et al, 1992)
	28%	—	(Kuhlman and Hennessey, 1997)
	Not useful	—	(De Smet et al, 1995)
	89% (instrumented)	96% (instrumented)	(Durkan, 1994)
Flick test	69%	High	(Megele, 1991)
	93%	—	(Pryse-Phillips, 1984)
Phalen's test	Sensitive to residual latency	—	(Glass and Ring, 1995)
	58%	—	(Buch-Jaeger and Foucher, 1994)
	Not correlated with any electrical parameters	54%	(Martinez-Abaladejo et al, 1995)
	Useful in CTS	—	(Kuschner et al, 1992)
	88%	—	(Williams et al, 1992)
	Statistically significant for severity of electrical changes	—	(Megele, 1991)
	60%: not reliable	Low	(Seror, 1988)
	51%: fair	—	(Kuhlman and Hennessey, 1997)
	—	59%: not reliable	(Heller et al, 1986)
Hoffmann–Tinel sign	Significant correlation with motor and sensory conduction velocity	—	(Martinez-Abaladejo et al, 1995)
	Not useful in CTS	—	(Kuschner et al, 1992)
	67%	—	(Williams et al, 1992)
	64%	—	(Megele, 1991)
	—	Low	(Heller et al, 1986)
	67%: not reliable	77%: not reliable	(Kuhlman and Hennessey, 1997)
	23%: poor	—	(Werner et al, 1994)
Reverse Phalen's maneuver (Wormser's) test	Better than Phalens	—	(Gunnarsson et al, 1997)
Clinical exam by experienced HCP	94%	80%	(De Smet et al, 1995)
Closed fist	—	Highly specific	(Katz and Stirrat, 1990a)
Hand diagram of classic or probable CTS	64%	73%	(Toomingas et al, 1991)
Abduction external rotation (AER) test	Some sensitivity to CTS	—	

CTS, carpal tunnel syndrome; HCP, health care provider.

Kuhlman and Hennessey (1997) investigated the sensitivity and specificity of six CTS signs: (1) the presence of a square-shaped wrist, (2) weakness of the abductor pollicis brevis, (3) median nerve hypesthesia, (4) Phalen's sign, (5) median nerve compression sign, and (6) Hoffmann–Tinel sign. The signs were not very sensitive (23% to 69%), but were fairly specific (66% to 87%) for CTS. A square-shaped wrist and abductor pollicis brevis weakness were the most sensitive signs (69% and 66%, respectively), and are recommended as part of the examination of CTS. Median nerve hypesthesia and the Phalen's sign both have fair sensitivity (51%) but good specificity (85% and 76%, respectively). The median nerve compression sign and the Hoffmann–Tinel sign both have poor sensitivity (28% and 23%, respectively), and thus are less helpful in evaluating subjects with suspected CTS.

Williams et al (1992) favor the pressure provocative test and note its 100% sensitivity and faster reaction time than Phalen's test (mean time of 9 seconds vs 30 seconds). It is described as an especially appropriate provocative test in patients with stiff or painful wrists when wrist flexion is restricted. According to Novak et al (1992), the incidence of positive pressure provocative and Phalen's tests were similar and more likely to occur in combination than separately. The Hoffmann–Tinel sign was more likely to be positive in the later stages of nerve compression. Their results suggest that the presence or absence of a provocative test is dependent upon the severity of the nerve compression.

One author (Megele, 1991) discovered Phalen's sign was highly sensitive for cervical nerve root entrapment at 74% and had medium sensitivity for Hoffmann–Tinel sign at 40%—thus implying low specificity for CTS. Only the flick sign turned out to be relatively specific for CTS—its sensitivity in cervical nerve root entrapment was around 26%—indicating its potential to function as a valid criterion for the differential diagnosis of CTS and cervical nerve root entrapment syndrome.

The use of the reverse Phalen's maneuver (sometimes known as the Wormser's test) has been postulated. This test involves wrist and finger extension held for 1 minute, with a moderate amount of pressure applied by the patient holding the dorsums of the wrist together. Werner et al (1994) demonstrated that this maneuver results in a significantly higher intracarpal canal hydrostatic pressure as compared to a traditional Phalen's or a modified Phalen's maneuver.

De Smet et al (1995) assessed the value of five provocative tests for the diagnosis of CTS. Compared to normal controls, they found that the Hoffmann–Tinel sign and the closed fist test are highly specific, but that Durkan's compression test is not useful to discriminate between symptomatic patients with and without EMG disturbances. The closed fist test is specific in these situations.

Buch and Foucher (1995) reviewed 11 CTS signs and tests (isolated or associated) and compared the outcomes of these tests with EMG examination used as "standard." None of the signs or tests reached an acceptable level of sensitivity, specificity, or predictive value. These authors recommended that positive EMG findings seems to be mandatory before deciding on surgical release of the CTS.

Durkan's original study of the instrumented carpal-compression test had an 89% sensitivity and a 96% specificity in diagnosing CTS. The instrumented device described in this study was described as lightweight and simple to use, and this instrument provides a rapid and inexpensive method of screening for carpal tunnel syndrome (Durkan, 1994).

Gellman et al (1986) reviewed the usefulness of three well-known provocative tests (wrist-flexion test, nerve-percussion test, and tourniquet test) in the diagnosis of CTS against electrodiagnostically proved CTS. The wrist-flexion test was found to be the most sensitive while the nerve-percussion test, although least sensitive, was most specific. The tourniquet test was quite insensitive and not very specific, and was not recommended to be used as a routine screening test in the diagnosis of CTS (Gellman, 1986).

With the exceptions of age, Tinel's sign, and hand pain diagram rating, findings from the physical examination and the history had limited diagnostic utility, according to Katz et al (1991). Patients under 40 years of age with possible or unlikely diagram ratings were at low risk for CTS. This finding suggests that subsets of patients may be managed without nerve conduction studies.

De Krom et al (1991) reviewed the validity of 12 provocative tests for CTS and found that all clinical diagnostic tests had a low validity. A combination of three tests with relatively high validity (paresis of abductor pollicis brevis muscle, hyperpathia, and flick sign) did not significantly change the probability of CTS. The author feels that patients with CTS symptoms should be referred directly for neurophysiological examination due to the low confidence of provocative testing.

In another study (Heller et al, 1986), EMG was performed and Phalen's and Tinel's signs were sought in 80 upper extremities clinically suspected of CTS. The two signs showed relatively low sensitivity (60% to 67%) and specificity (59% to 77%) despite a statistically significant association with the EMG findings. These two signs are not reliable as clinical criteria for carpal tunnel syndrome (Heller et al, 1986).

Katz et al (1991) feel that noninvasive tests for CTS are of limited diagnostic value (with the exceptions of age and Hoffmann–Tinel sign), and they developed a self-administered hand symptom diagram. Diagrams are rated classic CTS, probable, possible, or unlikely. Diagram ratings were compared with nerve conduction diagnoses in 110 patients with upper extremity complaints. A hand diagram rating of classic or probable CTS had sensitivity of 64% to 80%, specificity of 73% to 90%, and positive predictive value of .58. The negative predictive value of an unlikely diagram was .91. The authors concluded that the diagram is a useful diagnostic tool and may be valuable for occupational and population screening.

Sucher (1994) wrote that the presence of nocturnal wrist or hand pain, and positive provocative palpatory findings were among the most reliable physical findings in carpal tunnel syndrome diagnosis. Other tests for CTS include the following:

- Neurosentinel (NS) and NervePace (NP) electroneurometer: Compared with electrodiagnostic studies, these devices have moderate validity and similar reliability; they are probably most useful for cross-sectional or longitudinal studies of groups, but care must be taken in using them for preplacement or surveillance tests of individual workers. False-positive results may lead to discrimination, inappropriate referrals and interventions; false-negative tests can result in inappropriate reassurance and missed opportunities for intervention (Pransky et al, 1997).
- High resolution ultrasound: CTS is characterized by typical anatomical changes that its proponents believe can be shown with high-resolution sonography. To diagnose CTS, ultrasound users often consider the following patterns: median nerve changes (swelling before its entrance into the carpal tunnel and flattening in the tunnel itself), palmar bowing of the flexor retinaculum, thickening of the transverse carpal ligament, and increased depth of the carpal tunnel, as measured from the apex of the transverse carpal ligament convexity to the underlying carpal bone. High-resolution ultrasound exhibited 96% sensitivity, 95% specificity, and 93% diagnostic accuracy and may play a major role in the diagnosis of CTS (Ferrari et al, 1997). Buchberger et al (1992) showed that the results of sonography are reliable, and that the diagnosis of CTS can be established on the basis of sonographic findings.
- Vibrometry and measurement of vibrotactile thresholds: At any given level of specificity, the sensitivity of vibrometry performed after 10 minutes of wrist flexion was approximately two times that obtained before wrist flexion for detection of electrophysiologically confirmed CTS (Gerr et al, 1995).
- A diagnostic test combining the sensitivity of the Semmes–Weinstein monofilament measurement and the specificity of the wrist flexion provocational test is recommended by Korris et al (1990) as the most accurate and sensitive quantitative clinical test for median nerve compression evaluated to date.
- Tchou et al (1992) favor the use of thermography for CTS, and states that testing showed specificity that ranged between 98% and 100%. These findings would appear to confirm the value of thermography in the diagnosis of unilateral carpal tunnel syndrome.

Predictors of Outcome in Carpal Tunnel Syndrome

A number of factors that are supposed predictors of favorable or unfavorable outcome in carpal tunnel syndrome have been proposed, and are summarized in the following lists.

Predictors of Favorable Outcome

- Decrease in palpatory restriction (Sucher, 1994)
- Pain of two or more of the first four fingers
- Numbness/tingling in the second, third, and fourth fingers
- Other symptoms involving the dorsal surface of the fingers
- Pain of the upper palm
- Pain of the lower or upper arm (Bessette et al, 1997)

Predictors of Unfavorable Outcome

- Age greater than 50 years
- Duration of symptoms over 10 months
- Constant paraesthesiae
- Stenosing flexor tenosynovitis
- Phalen's test positive in less than 30 seconds (Kaplan et al, 1990)
- Numbness and tingling of the dorsum of the hand/wrist
- Numbness/tingling of the arm (Bessette et al, 1997)
- Workers' compensation recipient
- Work absence preoperatively
- Relatively poor mental health status
- Involvement of an attorney
- Milder preoperative symptom severity
- Preoperative work absence
- Exposure to hand-intensive work (Katz et al, 1997)

Kaplan et al (1990) identified five factors (noted above) that were important in predicting response to treatment: (1) age over 50 years, (2) duration of symptoms over 10 months, (3) constant paraesthesiae, (4) stenosing flexor tenosynovitis, and (5) a Phalen's test positive in less than 30 seconds. When none of these factors was present, two thirds of patients were cured by medical therapy. Failure with treatment was shown in 59.6% of patients possessing one of the factors, 83.3% with two factors, and 93.2% with

---

CLINICAL TIP 15–2
Ensuring Carpal Tunnel Syndrome Test Responsivity

No matter which provocative CTS test you prefer, be sure to have the patient hold the test long enough to truly compress the carpal tunnel. Many of the tests listed do not become responsive until 30 to 60 seconds of compression have been achieved.

three factors. No patient with four or five factors present was cured by medical management (Kaplan et al, 1990).

The use of symptom patterns on a hand diagram as predictors of outcome in CTS has been proposed. Bessette et al (1997) found that symptom patterns identified with a hand symptom diagram helped to predict the outcome of carpal tunnel release. As noted earlier, favorable indicators were: (1) pain of two or more of the first four fingers, (2) numbness and tingling in the second, third, and fourth fingers, (3) other symptoms involving the dorsal surface of the fingers, (4) pain of the upper palm, and (5) pain of the lower or upper arm. Unfavorable indicators were: (1) numbness and tingling involving the dorsum of the hand or wrist, and (2) numbness and tingling of the arm.

Some authors feel that economic and psychosocial variables have a strong influence upon both return to work and the extent of symptoms. The predominant preoperative variables associated with work absence due to CTS 6 months postoperatively were worker's compensation, work absence preoperatively, and worse mental health status. Preoperative correlates of less complete relief of symptoms included involvement of an attorney, milder preoperative symptom severity, preoperative work absence and exposure to hand intensive work (Katz et al, 1997).

Questionnaires and Self-administered Tests

The sensitivity and responsiveness of clinical outcome measures, including the use of various questionnaires and functional status scales, is generally well accepted for wrist maladies, including CTS. Several studies have shown that these outcome devices are more effective than other physical or provocative tests. This is not surprising, as the review of the physical and provocative tests shows poor sensitivity and specificity for CTS.

Self-administered symptom severity and functional status scales have been shown to be more responsive to clinical improvement than measures of neuromuscular impairment and have been recommended to serve as primary outcomes in clinical studies of therapy for CTS (Katz JN et al, 1994). Standardized questionnaires specific to wrist and CTS complaints have been shown to be more sensitive to the clinical change produced by carpal tunnel surgery than many commonly performed physical measures of outcome, such as the Medical Outcomes Study 36-item shortform health survey, the Arthritis Impact Measurement Scale, and the Brigham and Women's Hospital Carpal Tunnel Questionnaire (Amadio et al, 1996).

The following functional scales are recommended:

- **Patient-rated Wrist Evaluation** (MacDermid, 1996). This is a 15-item questionnaire that asks the patient to respond to specific questions on pain (5 questions), specific activities (6 questions), and usual activities (4 questions); see Appendix Form F–13. Several scoring options are possible within the 100 total points: total wrist score, separate pain disability and handicap scores, or separate pain and function scores.

- **Carpal Tunnel Syndrome Questionnaire (CTSQ):** A self-administered questionnaire, the CTSQ tracks both symptoms and functional status (Levine et al, 1993). This questionnaire was favorably evaluated in depth by Atroshi et al (1997a, 1997b). See Chapter 7 for a thorough discussion of this test.

- **Hand Symptom Diagram.** Bessette et al (1997) described the positive prognostic value of a hand symptom diagram in the prediction of outcome of carpal tunnel release. The patient is asked to complete a diagram, marking the location and type of symptom on a diagram of the hand and arm; see Figure 15–18. The hand symptom diagram was divided into 34 small regions (Fig. 15–19) to help visualize and categorize different symptom patterns. The presence of pain, numbness/tingling, or other symptoms is then scored on a rather complex basis to attempt prediction of likely surgical outcome.

- **Functional Disability Index for the Rheumatoid Hand.** This is a practical functional ability scale for rheumatoid hands that has also been used to assess functional handicap. The scale consists of 18 hand activity questions and has been validated in a French population (Duruoz et al, 1996); see Appendix Form F–14.

LOWER EXTREMITY

As was seen with the upper extremity, the lower extremity has been the subject of many studies that focus on the function of the entire leg, not simply the component joints (hip, knee, and ankle/foot).

RANGE OF MOTION

Many authors consider ROM in the lower extremity to be a key factor in assessing function and have proposed different methods for measurement, as well as discussions of factors that can affect the accuracy of these methods. The following list details several factors that have been reported to cause error in the measurement of lower extremity ROM:

- Measurement procedure
- Inter-individual variations (Roass and Andersson, 1982)
- Measurement device
- Inter-observer errors
- Error between different measurement sessions (Ekstrand et al, 1982)

Here are some interesting points to remember when measuring lower extremity ROM:

- There were no statistically significant differences between the ROMs of the right and left lower extremity, and it is therefore suggested that a patient's

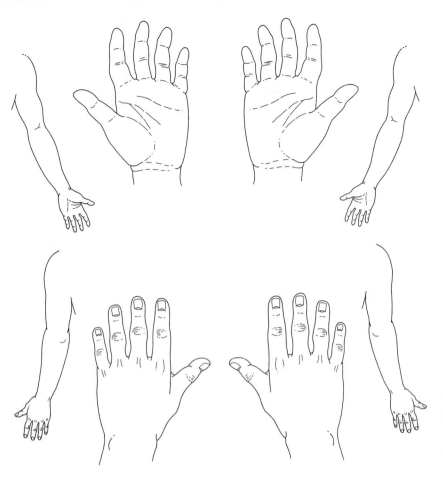

Figure 15–18. Hand symptom diagram.

(From Bessette L, Keller RB, Lew RA, et al. Prognostic value of a hand symptom diagram in surgery for carpal tunnel syndrome. J Rheumatol. 1997;24(4):726–734.)

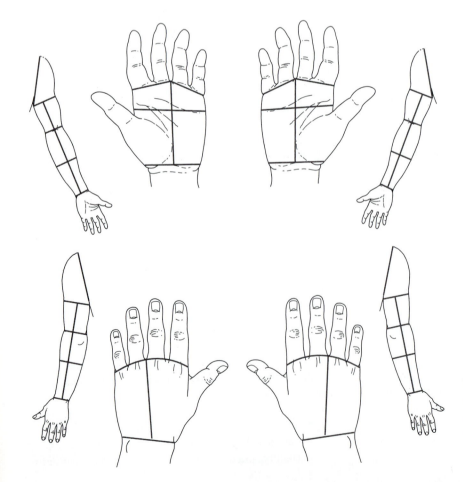

Figure 15–19. Thirty-four divisions for analysis of the hand symptom diagram.

(From Bessette L, Keller RB, Lew RA, et al. Prognostic value of a hand symptom diagram in surgery for carpal tunnel syndrome. J Rheumatol. 1997;24(4):726–734.)

healthy limb can be used for comparison with the affected side in the presence of disease or a lesion (Roass and Andersson, 1982).

- Experienced examiners have been shown to be able to measure lower extremity skeletal measures with acceptable intra-examiner and inter-examiner reliability. Specfically, femoral torsion, ankle dorsiflexion, tibial length, leg length discrepancy, genu varus/valgus, medial talonavicular joint bulge, rearfoot angle, arch angle, and foot type classification were found to be reliably measurable (Jonson and Gross, 1997).
- ROM measurements (hip flexion, hip extension, hip abduction, knee flexion, and ankle dorsiflexion with the knee extended and flexed) have been shown to be repeated accurately by the same tester with methods requiring careful measurement technique but no elaborate equipment (Ekstrand et al, 1982).

However, some investigators do not consider ROM to be an important clinical finding in the assessment or diagnosis of lower extremity injury.

- Van Mechelen et al (1992) studied runners who had sustained injury in the 12 months prior to the study. Within a group of noninjured subjects, all goniometric measurements showed no significant differences between the left and right sides of the body; similarly, for injured subjects all goniometric measurements showed no significant differences between the injured and noninjured sides of the body. These findings suggested to the authors that ROM can be characterized as a more or less stable anthropometric trait, which is not affected by dominant side nor by injury.
- Elite classical dance students have been shown to have greater hip external rotation and less hip internal rotation than controls, but similar external rotation below the hip and ankle dorsiflexion. Since external rotation below the hip joint and ankle dorsiflexion do not differ between dancers and controls, despite repeated training of these movements in ballet, there may be anatomical (bony/ligamentous) limitations to these movements (Khan et al, 1997).

PREDICTIVE FACTORS OF LOWER EXTREMITY INJURY

A variety of physical characteristics of athletes have been proposed to be related to the risk of sustaining an injury or disability in the lower extremity:

- Flexibility, anthropometric characteristics, and malalignment of the lower extremities (pelvic obliquity, rearfoot malalignment, leg length inequality, deviant footprint, knee malalignment) had no statistical effect on the risk of sustaining a sports injury (ankle sprain, muscle rupture, dislocation,

shin splints, backache). The authors of this study commented that due to the wide range of physical characteristics and the great variety of sports injuries, a comprehensive study of these factors is not practicable (Twellaar et al, 1997).

- Valgus deformity, knee instability, and obliquity have been shown to be risk factors of locomotor disability in women, but not in men (Odding et al, 1996).
- Locomotor disability is associated with female sex, low education, low income, and living in a home for the elderly. Of the signs and symptoms of the hips and knees, only pain in the hips and knees, morning stiffness, and restricted flexion of the hip were associated with locomotor disability. Radiological osteoarthritis of the hip and knee did not contribute to the explanation of locomotor disability (Odding et al, 1995).
- Tight ligaments and tight muscles have been shown to be related to injury in male college athletes, and unrelated to injury in female college athletes (Krivickas and Feinberg, 1996).

FUNCTIONAL TESTS AND QUESTIONNAIRES

HCPs routinely have used functional performance tests as an evaluation tool in deciding when an athlete can safely return to unrestricted sporting activities. They assumed that these tests provide a reliable measure of lower extremity performance; however, little research has been reported on the reliability of these measures. The following tests have been found to be reliable and useful by Bolgla and Keskula (1997) for the determination of returning an injured athlete to competition: single hop for distance, triple hop for distance, 6-m timed hop, and cross-over hop for distance. These tests were first described by Noyes et al (1991a), who used four different types of one-legged hop tests to assess limb symmetry, originally in anterior cruciate ligament–deficient knees. The hop tests were used to calculate the percentage of function of the injured leg to the noninjured leg. As athletes demonstrated increasing symmetry between injured and noninjured legs, they were thought to be ready to return to competition.

Many different questionnaires and rating systems have been studied for use in the simultaneous study of multiple joints of the lower extremity. Some of these include:

- **Lequesne's scores, Western Ontario and McMaster Universities (WOMAC) Osteoarthritis Index, and ILAS.** Sun et al (1997) believe these scores have satisfactory responsiveness to different treatment effects.
- **Nottingham Health Profile** and the **15D,** a 15-dimensional health-related quality of life (HRQOL) measure suggested for use after total hip arthroplasty and total knee arthroplasty (Rissannen et al, 1996).

- **SF-36,** which has been controversial as a lower extremity outcome measure. Kiebzak et al (1997) described the SF-36 Health Status Questionnaire as a simple, easy-to-administer, and effective instrument for monitoring improvements in patient health after total hip arthroplasty and total knee arthroplasty. The converse opinion is held by McGuigan et al (1995), who cites the poor ability of the SF-36 to predict postoperative improvement in total hip and knee arthroplasty; and therefore states this questionnaire cannot be used alone to determine treatment selection (see Appendix Form A-2).
- **Lequesne algofunctional indices** (adapted to a self-report questionnaire-format), which are not recommended due to insufficient internal consistency and questionable validity (Stucki et al, 1996b).

LEG LENGTH INEQUALITY

The examining HCP should have a high index of suspicion when evaluating patients with lower extremity and/or back pain so that the diagnosis of leg length inequality (LLI) or leg length discrepancy (LLD) is not overlooked (Baylis and Rzonca, 1988) (LLI and LLD are often used interchangeably). LLI has been known to be responsible for referral pain associated with hip or knee osteoarthritis or the groin and suprapubic areas (Rondon et al, 1992).

LLI analysis is commonly used in chiropractic, and there have been relatively few subject areas within the chiropractic profession that have led to such widespread misunderstanding, confusion, and controversy (Lawrence, 1985). Controversy persists regarding the significance of LLI, the diagnostic approach to the use of heel lifts, and the implementation of proper orthopedic support in treatment of anatomical LLIs. Through a series of measurements and pelvic assessments, an effective screening process can be accomplished before radiography (scanogram) is required (Danbert, 1988).

The precise measurement of leg length and LLDs plays an important role in the examination of the lumbar spine and lower extremities. Those real instances of LLD that may be posttraumatic or idiopathic are difficult to differentiate from LLD caused by spinal scoliosis or malposition (Krettek et al, 1994).

Many authors have contributed to our current understanding of the significance of LLI. The following are important points to consider when attempting measurement of the short leg:

- Radiographic measures such as the scanograms are recognized as the most reliable procedure for the evaluation of anatomical LLI (Manello, 1992). The scanogram is typically a radiograph of the entire leg from femoral head to ankle mortise taken alongside a radiopaque ruler. This allows for accurate measurement of each leg in comparison to an absolute linear standard. This opinion is contradicted by the work of Aspegren et al (1987), who showed that

the visual method of LLI measurement did not differ significantly from the x-ray method of measurement for leg length insufficiency.
- Inter-observer and intra-observer variation for visual measurement was shown by Rondon et al (1992) to be acceptable. This is disputed by Friberg et al (1988), who believe clinical methods have proved to be inaccurate and highly imprecise.
- Rotation, flexion, or extension of the head during visual leg length assessment is sometimes proposed as a method of determining whether there is cervical/thoracic involvement in the kinetic chain that produces functional LLI. LLI may be affected by cervical spine movements, especially cervical flexion and extension (De Witt et al, 1994). However, Falltrick and Pierson (1989) found that head rotation had no effect on LLI.
- Prone measurements for LLI were highly correlated with the standing x-ray femoral head measurement. However, despite positive correlation, prone leg length measurements for inequality are not entirely valid estimates of standing x-ray differences. The supine measurements were poorly correlated (Rhodes et al, 1995a, 1995b).
- Various modifications in measurement techniques are claimed to produce superior results in indirect measurement of LLI (DeBoer et al, 1983).
- Computed tomography is more accurate than orthoroentgenography for the measurement of LLD in patients who have a flexion deformity of the knee (Aaron et al, 1992).
- Because LLI measurement by ultrasound is more precise, accurate, and reliable than clinical methods, and is not limited by radiation hazards, ultrasound is recommended for routine use in clinical practice (Junk et al, 1992; Konermann et al, 1995; Krettek et al, 1996).
- Although there is no final agreement about the extent to which an LLD becomes clinically significant, most authors state that clinical assessment of LLD by tape measure or lengthening of the short leg with blocks of known thickness is highly unreliable (Krettek et al, 1994).

HIP

RANGE OF MOTION

With the hip, as with other joints reviewed so far in this chapter, a review of the literature shows significant discrepancies in what constitutes "normal ROM." Similar to the shoulder, leading authors do not even agree on which movements should be measured; see Table 15–16. With authors offering differing opinions on which motions should be measured, it is not surprising that there are various methods described in the literature for the performance of the actual hip ROM measurements:

Table 15–16: Normal Values for Range of Motion of the Hip from Various Sources

HIP	HOPPENFELD (1976)	STEINBERG (1991)	MAGEE (AROM) (1992)	OMBREGT (PROM) (1995)	EVANS (1994)	GERHARDT AND RIPPSTEIN (1994)
Flexion	120°	110–120°	110–120°	140°	120° knee flexed; 75–90°+ with knee extended	120°
Extension	5–10°	20–30°	10–15°	30°	15° normal; 30–40° if pelvis is not adequately fixed	15°
Abduction	45–50°	40–50°	30–50°	—	40–45°	45°
Abduction (in flexion)	—	45–60°	—	—	—	—
Adduction	20–30°	20–40°	30°	30°	20–30°	35°
Internal (medial) rotation	35°	25–45°	30–40°	45°	40°	45°
External (lateral) rotation	45°	45–50°	40–60°	60°	45°	45°

AROM, active range of motion; PROM, passive range of motion.

- The toe-touch distance (the distance from the toes that a patient can approximate with his or her fingers upon full lumbar flexion) is not a reliable indicator of either vertebral or hip mobility (Tully and Shillman, 1997). The toe-touch test is largely a measure of hamstring flexibility. Subjects with a restricted joint ROM on a clinical toe-touch test have stiffer hamstring muscles and a lower stretch tolerance (Magnusson et al, 1997).
- ROM at the hip is repeatable between HCPs using a simple plurimeter and may represent an examination that is suitable for monitoring progress and treatment (Croft et al, 1996).
- Hip flexion, extension, internal rotation, and hamstring flexibility in the men, and hip flexion and extension in women had statistically significant negative correlations with low back pain (Mellin, 1988).
- Extremes of hip ROM begin to involve maximum sacroiliac joint motion (Smidt et al, 1997).
- There is a normal range of hip instability in neonates. Patterns of hip laxity in boys and girls are identical, and in most infants, hip instability diminishes between the first and second days of life (Keller et al, 1988).

STRENGTH TESTING

Normative values for hip flexion, arrayed by gender, age and dominant side, have been recently published by Bohannon et al (1997) and are provided in Tables 15–17 and 15–18. Normative values for other hip motions do not appear in the literature at this time.

Table 15–17: Dynametric Normal Values for Hip Flexion Strength (newtons ± standard deviation)

AGE	MEN DOMINANT	MEN NONDOMINANT	WOMEN DOMINANT	WOMEN NONDOMINANT
20–29	211.7 ± 39.7	206.7 ± 41.4	139.9 ± 27.0	132.9 ± 29.6
30–39	223.6 ± 47.7	225.9 ± 58.1	119.0 ± 38.3	115.5 ± 36.5
40–49	190.7 ± 43.3	184.2 ± 37.3	124.8 ± 43.2	122.4 ± 46.9
50–59	195.2 ± 61.9	203.1 ± 58.6	116.2 ± 30.5	115.1 ± 21.6
60–69	169.1 ± 49.0	167.6 ± 47.6	103.3 ± 26.7	98.7 ± 24.6
70–79	167.4 ± 38.7	162.1 ± 39.2	92.1 ± 27.2	91.8 ± 28.9

From Bohannon RW et al, 1997.

Table 15–18: Dynametric Normal Values for Hip Abduction Strength (newtons ± standard deviation)

AGE	MEN DOMINANT	MEN NONDOMINANT	WOMEN DOMINANT	WOMEN NONDOMINANT
20–29	321.2 ± 84.7	318.8 ± 61.2	193.5 ± 37.6	189.9 ± 45.7
30–39	329.1 ± 66.6	333.3 ± 54.3	212.3 ± 58.9[a]	211.1 ± 54.6
40–49	311.1 ± 41.1	321.4 ± 66.9	218.4 ± 37.6	201.5 ± 36.1
50–59	308.9 ± 74.7	303.6 ± 69.8	214.8 ± 40.0	207.4 ± 35.1
60–69	258.9 ± 49.4	261.4 ± 67.1	172.3 ± 43.8	164.2 ± 33.9
70–79	250.8 ± 42.7	246.0 ± 42.6	152.7 ± 34.4	147.1 ± 28.5

[a] Knee extension force met or surpassed 650N and was recorded as 650N for one woman in her 30s. Reference value for this decade, therefore, may be depressed.

From Bohannon et al, 1997.

Predictive Factors of Hip Dysfunction

Hip fracture is the ultimate failure of the joint, which leads to an astonishingly high toll of morbidity and sometimes mortality. As a result, many authors have tried to identify risk factors for osteoporosis, which is ultimately detected by eventual hip fracture. These factors include anthropomorphic factors, diet, exercise, hormonal changes, and many others, as follows:

- Low body mass index, the prevalence of appendicular fractures, a higher degree of immobilization, a later age of menarche, lower exposure to sunlight, and lower indices of physical activity have all been shown to be risk factors for osteoporosis, leading to eventual hip fracture (Dequeker et al, 1991b).
- There are marked and sizeable differences in the incidence rates of hip fracture in the various countries throughout southern Europe. The reasons for these differences are not known but affect both men and women, and are likely to be related to lifestyle or genetic factors rather than to differences in endocrine status (Ellfors et al, 1994).
- Moderate excess weight and a high nutritional intake of calcium were associated with a decreased risk of hip fracture. Loss of autonomy, a higher height than normal (> 1 SD), and a history of previous fractures significantly increased the risk of fracture (Ribot et al, 1993).
- Tall women have a greater relative risk of experiencing fragility fractures of the hip (Gunnes et al, 1996).
- Late menarche, poor mental score, low body mass index and physical activity, low exposure to sunlight, and a low consumption of calcium and tea were all found to be etiological factors for osteoporotic hip fractures (Johnell et al, 1995).
- An increased number of falls in the past year, and falling while turning were much more likely to lead to a hip fracture than falling when walking in one direction (Cumming and Klineberg, 1994).

QUESTIONNAIRES

Many different types of hip questionnaires are found in the literature. Many of these outcome devices were originally constructed to attempt to measure function compared before and after total hip arthroplasty. However, as nonsurgical specialists realize the need for outcome measurement tools, they have naturally gravitated toward the known, extant outcome measurement devices for the hip. This is very logical, as several of the scales assess patient function (such as walking, standing, changing position), which are the goals of both surgical and nonsurgical treatment. Generally speaking, these devices have not been specifically tested for construct validity with a nonsurgical treatment regimen, and HCPs who use these devices presume there is satisfactory reliability. Clearly, specific studies to measure the effectiveness of these outcome measures to detect changes due to treatment in the nonsurgical hip remain to be performed.

In one study, patients' and physicians' evaluations of the results of the total hip arthroplasty were similar when the patients had little or no pain and were satisfied with the result. However, the disparity increased as the patients' ratings for pain increased and their ratings for overall satisfaction decreased (Lieberman et al, 1996). This study highlights a discrepancy between patients' and physicians' evaluations of the results of total hip arthroplasty. This discrepancy increased when the patient was not satisfied with the outcome. In other words, the physicians often tend to overestimate the success of the surgical procedure. The use of patients' self-administered questionnaires as well as traditional HCP-generated assessments may provide a more complete evaluation of the results of total hip arthroplasty (Lieberman et al, 1996).

Katz demonstrated that brief health status measures (SF-36, Functional Status Questionnaire, shortened Arthritis Impact Measurement Scales, and Modified Health Assessment Questionnaire) were equally or more responsive than the much longer and more difficult to complete Sickness Impact Profile (Katz et al, 1992b).

Presented below are a representative sample of outcome measures originally generated for the assessment of hip fractures and arthroplasty.

- **Patient-specific Index.** This instrument is used to assess the outcome of total hip arthroplasty by evaluating the preferences of the individual patient. The authors concluded that the Patient-specific Index is reliable, valid, and responsive for use with arthroplasty (Wright and Young, 1997); see Appendix Form F–15.
- **Hip–Rating Questionnaire.** This scale was originally developed for the assessment of the outcome of total hip replacement. The questionnaire uses a 100-point scale in which equal weight is given to the domains of global or overall impact of arthritis, pain, walking, and function (Johanson et al, 1992); see Appendix Form F–16.
- **MEDOS.** The Mediterranean osteoporosis study (MEDOS) questionnaire was designed to identify putative risk factors for hip fracture in a retrospective case control study applied during a prospective study of the incidence of hip fracture in 14 regions of Europe (Dequeker et al, 1991a).
- **Belfast and Newcastle Scale.** This scale seeks to provide simple prognostic scores of outcome after treatment of proximal femoral fractures (Thomas and Eastwood, 1996).
- **Total Hip Arthroplasty Outcome Evaluation Questionnaire.** This instrument is a cooperative effort of the Societe Internationale de Chirurgie Orthopedique et de Traumatologie (SICOT), the Task Force on Outcome Studies of The American Academy of Orthopaedic Surgeons, and The Hip Society to reach a consensus on the nomenclature to be used for the evaluation of the results of total hip arthroplasty (Katz et al, 1995).
- **Questionnaire on the Perceptions of Patients about Total Hip Replacement.** This is a 12-item questionnaire for completion by patients having total hip replacement. This questionnaire is short, practical, reliable, valid, and sensitive to clinically important changes (Dawson et al, 1996b).

Other self-reported questionnaires for the hip have focused primarily on changes in hip function due to osteoarthritis. Overall, knowledge about reliability and validity of clinical scores of hip and knee osteoarthritis is limited. Two well-known devices are especially well suited for the measurement of osteoarthritic severity of the hip:

- **Western Ontario and McMaster Universities (WOMAC) Osteoarthritis Index** (Bellamy et al, 1988). The WOMAC index is a multidimensional, self-administered health status instrument for patients with osteoarthritis of the hip or knee; see Appendix Form F–17. Pain, stiffness and physical function subscales fulfill conventional criteria for face,

content and construct validity, reliability, responsiveness, and relative efficiency. The index was originally designed for disease-specific evaluation of patients with lower extremity osteoarthritis, especially of the hip and knee. It asks the patient to respond to questions regarding the hip by placing an "X" along a horizontal line with "no pain or difficulty" at one end and "extreme pain or difficulty" at the other end of the line. (This is similar to the Visual Analogue Scale used in pain measurement.) The WOMAC has been shown by other investigators to have acceptable reliability and validity (Stucki et al, 1996a). McGrory and Harris (1996) stated the WOMAC can be used for evaluation of more than one joint in the same patient.

- **Lequesne Index of Severity for Hip Osteoarthritis** (Lequesne, 1991). This is a scale in which points are awarded for difficulty in performing everyday activities, with a maximum score of 32; see Appendix Form F–18. This approach is the reverse of many of the outcome measurements in this chapter, where points are awarded for ability in performing activities or for positive function.

Lequesne's scores, WOMAC, and ILAS have shown satisfactory responsiveness to different treatment effects (Sun et al, 1997). Additionally, the **Rand SF-36 Health Status Questionnaire** has been used to monitor patients with diagnosed osteoarthritis undergoing total hip and knee arthroplasty (McGuigan et al, 1995; Ritter et al, 1995).

For the HCP wishing to utilize a hip rating system in cases other than total hip arthroplasty, it is suggested that the Patient-specific Index and the Hip Rating Questionnaire are well suited for use in nonsurgical management of hip pain and dysfunction.

RADIOGRAPHIC ATTEMPTS AT MEASUREMENT

The German Society of Orthopaedic Surgery and Traumatology (DGOT) is trying to support the application of standardized and reproducible criteria in diagnosis and therapy of osteoarthritis. Observable criteria include joint space narrowing (JSN), osteophytes, sclerosis, subchondral cysts, and deformity of the femoral head. Results show that a reliable radiological classification of the severity of hip osteoarthritis is possible by assessment of certain individual radiographic features or a summary grade (Gunther et al, 1997).

No patient in whom the hip functioned well until the age of 65 years had had a center-edge angle of less than 16 degrees, an acetabular index of depth to width of less than 38 percent, an acetabular index of the weight-bearing zone of more than 15 degrees, uncovering of the femoral head of more than 31 percent, or an acetabulum in which the most proximal point of the dome had been at the lateral edge (zero peak-to-edge distance) (Murphy et al, 1995).

KNEE

Functional problems of the knee are common, and a significant portion of knee problems lead to disability. Prevalence of disability due to knee pain for U.S. men and women aged 40 to 79 years ranges from 19.3% to 28.3% (O'Reilly et al, 1996). Anterior knee pain is known to have a significantly worse outcome than any other complaint (Almekinders and Almekinders, 1994).

Overuse injuries of the knee due to repetitive motion are common in both recreational and elite athletes. In some cases, these injuries are self-limiting, but in many other cases, there is persistent pain and dysfunction. These injuries have been shown to be resistant to most of the commonly prescribed remedies: activity modification, non-steroidal anti-inflammatory drugs (NSAIDs), and stretching and strengthening exercises (Almekinders and Almekinders, 1994).

Nonoperative treatment has received little attention to date in the numerous scientific reports on knee ligament injuries. There is still tremendous controversy concerning the proper treatment of a knee with a ruptured ligament, especially the anterior cruciate ligament (ACL). Kannus and Jarvinen (1990), after an extensive review of the literature, state the indications for conservative management can be established to be all grade I and II sprains (partial tears) of knee ligaments as well as an isolated grade III sprain (complete tear) of the posterior cruciate ligament. In addition, an isolated complete rupture of an anterior cruciate or medial or lateral collateral ligament may be treated nonoperatively in an older sedentary person.

RANGE OF MOTION

As with several of the other joints reviewed in this chapter, there are significant differences (as much as 40 degrees in flexion) among the opinions of various respected authors in what comprises "normal ROM" of the knee; see Table 15–19. Note that some authors do not consider rotation to be either measurable or significant.

Many authors have published opinions on the most proper methodology for measuring ROM of the knee, among them the following:

- Goniometric measurements of the knee joint using the greater trochanter, the lateral condyle of the femur, the head of the fibula, and the lateral malleolus as bony landmarks are both reliable and valid (Gogia et al, 1987).
- Intra-tester reliability for flexion and extension of the knee was high. Inter-tester reliability was also high for other knee motions except for measurements of knee extension (Rothstein et al, 1983).
- Making duplicate or repeated measurements of the knee has not been shown to substantially increase reliability (Rothstein et al, 1983). This finding is directly contradicted by Watkins et al (1991), who recommended that HCPs should use a goniometer to take repeated PROM measurements of a patient's

Table 15–19: Normal Range of Motion of the Knee from Various Sources

KNEE	HOPPENFELD (1976)	LOGAN (1994)	MAGEE (AROM) (1992)	EVANS (1994)	SCOTT (1994)	GERHARDT AND RIPPSTEIN (1995)
Flexion	135°	120° active 140° with hip flexed 160° passive	0–135°	130–150°	110°	0–130°
Extension	0°	5–10°	0–15°	0–15°	10°	0–10°

Rotation	10° internal
	10° external
		At 0° flexion:
		  10° lateral rotation
		  5° medial rotation
		At 100° flexion:
		  15° lateral rotation
		  10° medial rotation
		At full knee flexion:
		  0° lateral rotation
		  10° medial rotation
			20–30°
			medial rotation
			of tibia on femur
			
			30–40°
			lateral rotation
			of tibia on femur
				—	—	—

AROM, active range of motion.

knee to minimize the error associated with these measurements.

- Within the first 15 degrees of knee flexion, goniometric measurement of joint excursion may be remarkably wrong. Therefore, caution should be exercised in determining movement gains or losses within the initial 15 degrees of knee flexion (Enwemeka, 1986).
- Visual estimates of knee flexion and extension are only slightly less reliable than goniometric measurements and are clinically acceptable (Watkins et al, 1991).

MEASUREMENT OF KNEE AND HAMSTRING FLEXIBILITY

Several authors have commented on the relationship between flexibility of the hamstring muscles and satisfactory ROM of the knee.

- A 30-second duration is an effective amount of time to sustain a hamstring muscle stretch in order to increase ROM. This is especially important to note prior to testing ROM (Bandy et al, 1997).
- The toe-touch test is largely a measure of hamstring flexibility. Further, subjects with a restricted joint ROM on a clinical toe-touch test have stiffer hamstring muscles and a lower stretch tolerance (Magnusson et al, 1997).
- The passive knee extension test is a simple and reliable method to measure hamstring tightness, and the associated pelvic motion is minimal (Fredriksen et al, 1997).

STRENGTH TESTING

Normative values for knee extension strength have been published and are presented in Table 15–20. Many different authors have written various studies investigating the methodology of strength measurement, and the proposed significance of those measurements to knee complaints. Their findings include the following:

- Hamstrings and quadriceps (H:Q) isokinetic strength ratio is strongly correlated to the functional ability of ACL-deficient knees in recreational athletes, and may help in the decision making process in the management of ACL-deficient knees (Lii et al, 1996).
- The evaluation of the muscle strength of knee extension revealed a decrease in torque of muscular contraction at 20 degrees of knee flexion (Kanai, 1993).
- The Genucom knee analysis system is used commonly on ACL-deficient knees. Wroble et al (1990a) reported significant day-to-day differences in individual subjects, and between examiners, which raises questions about its validity.
- The MEDmetric KT-1000 arthrometer's reliability, as investigated by Wroble et al (1990b) showed a significant difference between days for individual right and left knee translation measurements, and recommended that users report paired differences rather than individual knee measurements.
- In a study of Australian Rules Football players, hamstring muscle strain was the most prevalent injury. The subjects' injured hamstring muscles were all weaker than in the opposite leg in absolute values and hamstring-to-quadriceps muscle ratios. Flexibility (as measured by the sit-and-reach test) did not correlate with injury (Orchard et al, 1997).
- Injured knees often demonstrate lack of strength in extension. Patellofemoral pain and flexion deficit of the knee were the factors that most frequently and significantly associated with extension strength deficits. No correlation could be found between age, sex, height, weight, body mass index, length of the follow-up time, injury type, athletic activity level, immobilization method, knee stability, and the isokinetic muscular performance (Natri et al, 1996).

PREDICTORS OF KNEE DYSFUNCTION

Not surprisingly, the severity of knee pain was the strongest risk factor for self-reported difficulty performing tasks of lower extremity function (Jordan et al, 1997). Age, female

Table 15–20: Dynametric Normal Values for Knee Extension Strength (newtons ± standard deviation)

AGE	MEN DOMINANT	MEN NONDOMINANT	WOMEN DOMINANT	WOMEN NONDOMINANT
20–29	575.2 ± 92.3	578.6 ± 94.7	467.3 ± 88.8	465.7 ± 97.7
30–39	572.9 ± 76.5	572.5 ± 82.8	408.3 ± 128.8	410.8 ± 122.6
40–49	583.0 ± 73.7	588.9 ± 72.5	380.6 ± 86.5	362.7 ± 60.0
50–59	470.9 ± 92.3	467.7 ± 103.1	334.7 ± 75.8	318.7 ± 72.6
60–69	386.9 ± 94.3	376.5 ± 67.3	273.6 ± 80.0	265.9 ± 83.2
70–79	360.3 ± 72.6	365.9 ± 76.9	210.1 ± 45.6	204.7 ± 43.9

From Bohannon RW et al, 1997.

sex, obesity, and knee pain were also found to be significant risk factors for the development of osteoarthritis of the knee (Jordan et al, 1996).

Knee pain severity has been found to be more important than radiographic knee osteoarthritis severity in determining disability. Obesity is known to be independently associated with disability and compounded disability from knee pain. Future studies of disability in knee osteoarthritis should include assessment of obesity, severity of radiographic knee osteoarthritis, and severity of knee pain, as well as their interactions (Jordan et al, 1996).

QUESTIONNAIRES

Since no "standard" scoring system has been universally adopted by researchers for various knee conditions, there is limited ability for the comparison of treatment results among studies (Noyes et al, 1991b). None of these systems has found worldwide acceptance, mainly because all scoring systems attribute numerical values to factors that are not quantifiable, and then the arbitrary scores are added together for parameters that are not comparable with each other (Hefti et al, 1993). Agreement on a new system by many experienced surgeons and institutions with a large clinical volume represents a sacrifice because old rating system data will have to be discarded (Ewald, 1989). A comparison between these scoring systems is only possible after adjusting the total points, the quality and the quantity of each criterion and component of the scoring system. This can done by using a standardized rating scale like the International Knee Documentation Committee (IKDC)-score (Peters et al, 1997). At least one author (Bollen and Seedhom, 1991) has attempted to devise a "formula" for conversion from one knee rating system (Lyshom) to another (Cincinnati).

It is known that better knee rating scores will result with a patient interview, as opposed to a self-administered questionnaire. Some authors believe this is due to the presence of interview bias. The more the investigator is involved in the treatment of the patient, the greater the influence of this bias may be. To avoid such potential bias it has been suggested that a standardized self-administered questionnaire be used as the method of choice for obtaining subjective data in clinical settings (Hoher et al, 1997). It has been shown that estimates of knee pain and disability are significantly influenced by even minor changes in questionnaire content (O'Reilly et al, 1996).

While many different knee tests and questionnaires have been reported in the literature, the tools listed below are probably the most thoroughly documented:

- **International Knee Documentation Committee Questionnaire** (Hefti et al, 1993). A group of knee surgeons from Europe and America met in 1987 and founded the International Knee Documentation Committee. Their efforts resulted in the development of a common terminology and a concise one-page evaluation form. This form is claimed to be

the "standard" form for all publications on results of treatment of knee ligament injuries. The form includes seven different sections: a self-assessment of knee dysfunction upon the patient's activities, symptoms, ROM, ligament examination, compartmental findings, x-ray findings, and functional testing (a one-leg hop); see Appendix Form F–19. Critics of this questionnaire believe that scales that are partially based on joint laxity measures may artificially overestimate the disability after ACL rupture (Snyder-Mackler et al, 1997).

- **American Knee Society's Assessment System** (Insall et al, 1989). This system consists of two 100 point scales, subdivided into a knee score that rates only the knee joint itself and a functional score that rates the patient's ability to walk and climb stairs. The dual rating system is claimed to eliminate the problem of declining knee scores associated with increasing patient infirmity. The knee score has subscales for pain (50 points), stability (25), and ROM (25), and deductions are made for flexion contracture, extension lag, and malalignment. The function score grades walking (50 points) and stairs (50), with deductions for use of canes or walkers. The use of this grading system is appropriate when the HCP wishes to evaluate specific knee joint function as well as the general ability to locomote; see Appendix Form F–20.

- **Anterior Knee Pain Questionnaire.** This is a 100-point, 13-question instrument focusing on abnormal painful patellar movements, limp, pain, running, climbing stairs, and prolonged sitting with the knees flexed. As the name implies, this grading system is especially appropriate in cases of patellofemoral dysfunction (Kujala et al, 1993); see Appendix Form F–21.

- **Harrison Evaluation Tool for Patellofemoral Pain Syndrome (PFPS).** The Harrison scale is a set of 5 pain questions, 12 function questions, and 6 activity questions, with evidence of content validity for the components of anterior knee pain evaluation (Harrison et al, 1996b); see Appendix Form F–22.

- **Lequense Algofunctional Index of Severity for Knee Osteoarthritis** (Lequense, 1991). This scale consists of questions regarding knee pain (nocturnal, morning, standing, walking, sitting), the maximum distance that can be walked, and ability to perform activities of daily living; see Appendix Form F–23. Vastly divided opinions are in print on this osteoarthitis scale. The use of the Lequesne's scale has shown satisfactory responsiveness to different treatment effects (Sun et al, 1997). However, in a recent study, Singer et al (1996) state it cannot be recommended for scientific use as a reliable patient self-reporting evaluation of disease severity in osteoarthritis.

- **Cincinnati Knee Ligament Rating System** (Noyes, 1984). This outcome measurement device is intended to assess sports participation, knee function, and subjective symptomatology following ligamentous surgical procedures, especially in the assessment of athletic participation before and after treatment or surgery. The authors pointed out the need for a standard format for analysis of sports participation and knee function (Noyes et al, 1989). This scale correlates more highly with individual grading and most precisely defines outcome in athletically active patients. It may not be the best choice for low-activity-level individuals who avoid stressing their knees (Sgaglione et al, 1995).

- **Lysholm I Scale** (Tegner and Lysholm, 1985). The Lysholm scale was originally designed for assessment of ACL insufficiency. It consists of an activity grading scale and a functional score. The specificity of the Lysholm knee scoring scale for its original design of ACL loss has recently been disputed by Bengtsson et al (1996).
- **Hospital for Special Surgery Knee Rating System (HSS).** The HSS knee rating system has been described as a tool for evaluating functional performance, particularly during the postoperative period of total knee arthroplasty (Gore et al, 1986). It has also been recommended for assessment of knee function after arthroscopic meniscal repair (Stone et al, 1990).
- **Isometric and Isokinetic Scoring Scale** (Kannus and Jarvinen, 1987). This scale included four standardized knee scoring scales for subjective, objective, functional, and radiological evaluations, as well as isokinetic and isometric strength measurements.
- **Brigham, Freeman, BOA (British Orthopedic Association), and VENN Diagram.** These are four less frequently used methods for assessing total knee arthroplasty. All of these tests gave similar, satisfactory results upon review by Binazzi et al (1992).
- **Boeckstyns Instrument** (Boeckstyns, 1987). This is a simple, 10-question instrument designed to be used for the investigation of knee pain. The same author (Boeckstyns and Backer, 1989) has also studied the use of the visual analogue scale in knee conditions, and found it to be more valid than other knee pain questionnaires for determination of the patients' own opinions regarding pain.
- **Larson Method.** This utility of this scale was criticized by Singer et al (1996), who stated that it cannot be recommended for scientific use as a reliable patient self reporting evaluation of disease severity in osteoarthritis.

OTHER MEASUREMENTS OF KNEE FUNCTION

Pain threshold measurement using a pressure dolorimeter at the knee has been shown to distinguish patients with osteoarthritis from healthy controls, and has moderate relia-

bility. However, the correlations between pain threshold and measures of pain intensity were poor, and dolorimetry cannot substitute for a measure of pain intensity (Wessel, 1995).

Radiological scoring scales for the evaluation of post-traumatic osteoarthritic changes after a knee ligament injury have been proposed. One such scale is based on radiographs taken from the knee at the time of injury, and from both knees at the follow-up examination. Ten criteria were used to devise and list the scale. The scale is recommended by the authors as a method of improving the uniformity and reliability of the assessment of post-traumatic osteoarthritic changes after knee ligament injury (Kannus et al, 1988).

PROVOCATIVE TESTS

A variety of provocative tests have been proposed to determine stability of the ligamentous array of the knee. As with many of the other provocative tests in this chapter, authors hold varied opinions on the validity of the provocative tests for the knee, including sensitivity and specificity. Table 15–21 shows some of these published opinions of provocative knee testing.

The following tests have been shown to be negative in normal knees: Lachman, anterior drawer, posterior drawer, pivot-shift, external-rotation recurvatum test, and varus and valgus stress at both 0 and 30 degrees of flexion. However the reversed pivot-shift sign was present in 35% of normal knees, suggesting that it may not signify actual abnormality. The results of the posterolateral drawer test were variable, difficult to quantify, and did not always have a firm endpoint (Cooper, 1991).

Attempts to automate the decision making in anterior-posterior laxity with electrogoniometric equipment have been disappointing to date. A device known as the electrogoniometer tended to overestimate the tibial translation, tibial internal rotation, and external rotation (Granberry et al, 1990).

Anterior Instability

The diagnosis of ACL rupture is often difficult to establish, especially in recent injuries with acute hemarthrosis. The anterior drawer and Lachman tests are frequently used for determining ACL instability. The diagnostic accuracy of the Lachman test is superior to that of the anterior drawer test, while in chronic cases with third-degree instability the two tests are equally reliable (Mitsou and Vallianatos, 1988).

Clinical provocative tests of the knee are often compared to other types of testing with known validity, in the search for the elusive diagnostic "gold standard." In one such test (Lee et al, 1988), the sensitivity to detect ACL tears via MRI was 94%, compared with 78% for the anterior drawer test and 89% for the Lachman test.

The Lachman test is considered by some authors to be the most accurate provocative test, yet it is difficult to per-

Table 15–21: Sensitivity and Other Characteristics of Provocative Knee Stability Signs

TEST	FINDING
Lachman	Produced maximal tension in the majority of the ligaments (Rosenberg and Rasmussen, 1984)
	98.6% sensitive for chronic ACL (Kim and Kim, 1995)
	89% sensitive for ACL (Lee et al, 1988)
Anterior drawer	Recommended (Biushko et al, 1996)
	79.6% sensitive for chronic ACL (Kim and Kim, 1995)
	78% sensitive for ACL (Lee et al, 1988)
Posterior drawer	83% sensitivity (Staubli and Jakob, 1990)
	Absent/equivocal in 44% of straight medial instability (Hughston, 1988)
	Accuracy for detecting a posterior cruciate ligament tear was 96%, with a 90% sensitivity and a 99% specificity (Rubinstein et al, 1994)
Gravity sign	83% sensitivity (Staubli and Jakob, 1990)
Reversed pivot shift	Helpful (Staubli and Jakob, 1990)
	89.8% sensitive for ACL (Kim and Kim, 1995)
	Present in 35% of "normal" knees (Cooper, 1991)
External rotation recurvatum test	0% sensitivity (Staubli and Jakob, 1990)

ACL, anterior cruciate ligament.

form on a large person, especially by an examiner with small hands. One procedure, the alternate Lachman test, has been used with some success by examiners who have difficulty performing the Lachman test. In subjects with large thigh girth (> 43 cm), the alternate Lachman test was correct 78% of the time; the anterior drawer test was correct 59% of the time; and the Lachman test produced only 28% correct examinations. Based upon these results, the authors recommend the alternate Lachman test should be included in the regimen of manual ACL tests, especially for athletes with large thigh circumference or when performed by examiners with small hands (Draper and Schulties, 1995).

It has been shown that more accurate diagnosis in ACL deficient knees can be made by Lachman test rather than by conventional anterior drawer test in dealing with fresh injury. However, in chronic injuries, the Lachman test does not appear to show similar advantages. Positive valgus stress test on 0 degrees position suggests the possibility of ACL injury, even if the anterior drawer test is negative (Zhai, 1992).

Graham et al (1991) compared the accuracy of the Lachman test, anterior drawer test, and jerk test with the KT-1000 knee arthrometer in patients with proven ACL deficiency. Their results showed the Lachman and anterior drawer tests to be the most accurate indicators of ACL deficiency. The KT-1000 knee arthrometer was "found to be totally inaccurate, which precludes its use as an objective measure of anteroposterior laxity of the knee."

Posterior Instability
Posterior cruciate ligament (PCL) injuries are more common than has been previously reported. Recent clinical and basic science studies have helped define the important functional anatomy and biomechanics of this "forgotten" ligament and have raised questions regarding the reported benign natural history of isolated tears of the PCL. The posterior drawer test remains the "gold standard" for diagnosis of PCL instability (Miller et al, 1993).

Rubinstein et al (1994) also support the validity of the posterior drawer test, claiming the accuracy for detecting a PCL tear was 96%, with a 90% sensitivity and a 99% specificity. The examination accuracy was higher for grade II and III posterior laxity than for grade I laxity. Eighty-one percent of the time, the examiners agreed on the grade of the PCL tear for any given patient. The posterior drawer test, which included palpation of the tibia-femur step-off, was the most sensitive and specific clinical test (Rubinstein et al, 1994).

Hughston (1988) found the posterior drawer sign to be absent/equivocal in 44% of cases of straight medial instability. The phenomenon of an absent or equivocal posterior drawer test in the situation of acute straight medial instability is felt to occur when the mechanism of injury does not stress, strain, or tear the arcuate complex. If the PCL tear is not discovered and repaired, repeated stressful activity stretches the arcuate complex, and the chronically unstable knee subsequently presents with a positive posterior drawer test.

Harilainen (1987) compared clinical examination with examination under anesthesia in 350 consecutive acute knee injuries and concluded that the commonly performed tests of clinical examination are highly unreliable with many false negative findings. A summary of these findings is included as Table 15–22.

Table 15–22: Clinical Knee Tests Compared with Examination under Anesthesia

POSITIVE FINDING	PERCENTAGE OF ACTUAL POSITIVE FINDINGS DETECTED VIA CLINICAL EXAM
Valgus instability in knees with a medial collateral tear	92.5
Anterior drawer sign	50.0
Lachman	52.4
Pivot-shift test	13.8
Fresh total tears of anterior cruciate ligament	48.0
Fresh, total tears of posterior cruciate ligament	33.3
Anteromedial rotatory instability	21.3
Anterolateral rotatory instability	11.1
Posteromedial rotatory instability	0
Posterolateral rotatory instabilities	66.6

From Harilainen, 1987.

PREDICTORS OF PROGNOSIS

Because knee dysfunction is often so disabling, a number of authors have sought to isolate various factors that may help to predict the outcome of a knee condition's natural history, or factors that may have an impact on various attempts at treatment. These factors are summarized as follows.

Good Prognosis

- *PCL repair:* Bony avulsions, midsubstance or proximal ruptures, and athletic activity (Richter et al, 1996)
- *Patellofemoral pain:* The younger the patient the better the outcome; quadriceps rehabilitation is worth trying for every patient (Kannus and Niittymaki, 1994)

Poor Prognosis

- *PCL repair:* Distal ligamentous ruptures, lack of athletic activity, and temporary olecranization (Richter et al, 1996)
- *Meniscus repair:* Chronicity of injury (lasting longer than 2 weeks) (Stone et al, 1990)
- *Arthroscopic partial meniscectomy (APM):* Worker's compensation, poor baseline physical functional status, and grade III–IV cartilage damage were associated with worse postoperative function (Katz et al, 1992a)
- *Patellofemoral pain:* Age (Kannus and Niittymaki, 1994)

Not Related to Prognosis

- *Meniscus repair:* Age of the patient, sex of the patient, rim width up to 6 mm from the synovial meniscal junction, and ACL insufficiency (Stone et al, 1990)
- *Patellofemoral pain:* Patient's sex, body composition, athletic level, duration of symptoms, or biomechan-

ical malalignments in the lower extremities (Kannus and Niittymaki, 1994)

ANKLE

Rehabilitation of foot and ankle injuries is essential for full functional recovery and prevention of chronic disease which can have a devastating effect. Proper rehabilitation of the lateral ankle (inversion) sprain is critical due to its frequency and potential for chronic pain and recurrence (Losito and O'Neill, 1997).

Despite an increased focus on the prevention of running injuries, overuse injuries are still rather frequent. Of these injuries, 60% to 80% are associated with extrinsic factors, such as training errors and changes in running activities. Intrinsic factors are also common, especially malalignments, including excessive pronation and cavus foot. These changes are associated with common overuse injuries, but specific anatomical abnormalities and abnormal biomechanics of the lower extremity are not correlated with specific injuries on a predictable basis. Factors such as leg length discrepancy, poor flexibility, muscle weakness and imbalance, deficit in neuromuscular coordination, and ligamentous laxity can also cause running injuries. Acquired or secondary factors, such as kinetic chain dysfunctions, are more common than previously acknowledged. Many running injuries, especially in patients with recurrent and previous injuries, are manifestations of a dysfunction of the kinetic chain (Renstrom, 1993).

RANGE OF MOTION

Experts do not agree on which ROM measurements are most significant in the ankle, or on what the expected normal values for those measurements should be; see Table 15–23.

Table 15–23: Normal Values for Ankle Range of Motion from Various Sources

ANKLE	HOPPENFELD (1976)	LOGAN (1994)	JAHSS (1991)	MAGEE (AROM) (1992)	OMBREGT (PROM) (1995)	EVANS (1994)
Dorsiflexion	20°	20°	To an angle of 90° with the knee extended	20°	Angle between dorsum of the foot and the tibia <90°	20°
Plantar flexion	50°	30–50°	Limitation is of no clinical significance in the elderly	50°	Dorsal aspect of foot falls into line with the leg	40°
Inversion	5° subtalar	—	—	—	—	30°
Eversion	5° subtalar	—	—	—	—	20°
Supination	—	—	—	45–60°	—	—
Pronation	—	—	—	15–30°	—	—

AROM, active range of motion; PROM, passive range of motion.

Bagget and Young (1993) attempted to establish a normal range based on direct measurements and compare the standard nonweightbearing method of measuring ankle joint dorsiflexion with a weightbearing method. The normal range for ankle joint dorsiflexion was established as 0 degrees to 16.5 degrees nonweightbearing and 7.1 degrees to 34.7 degrees weightbearing. Because of poor correlation between the two measurements, the standard nonweightbearing measurement is of questionable relevance, according to the authors. That opinion is supported by Nigg and Nigg (1995), who suggest that active ROM and passive ROM measurements do not predict inversion during actual movement.

Measurement of ankle dorsiflexion ROM has been shown to be especially difficult to measure accurately; a spectrum of techniques exists to measure what appears at first glance to be a simple anatomical movement. However, information pertaining to the objective assessment of ankle joint dorsiflexion is controversial. Inter-device reliability has been shown to be poor among the universal goniometer, fluid goniometer, and electrogoniometer for measurement of ankle dorsiflexion (Rome, 1996).

Ankle dorsiflexion ROM has been shown to vary with the amount of force used to procure the dorsiflexion. Three separate methods were attempted: (1) passive ankle dorsiflexion with force adequate to encounter notable tension in the plantar flexor muscles; (2) passive ankle dorsiflexion with a maximal force; and (3) passive ankle dorsiflexion, but actively assisted by the subject. Significant differences exist among these three methods, and HCPs are reminded to use consistent techniques in all ROM measurements (Bohannon et al, 1989).

HCPs should be aware that measurements of ankle dorsiflexion ROM will differ depending on the conditions of measurement and the landmarks used. Despite the differences, measurements obtained using various combinations of conditions and landmarks will provide an indication of ankle dorsiflexion ROM (Bohannon et al, 1989).

The importance of locating and maintaining the subtalar joint in the neutral position when applying either measuring or stretching techniques is emphasized by Tiberio (1987). However, the reliability of examiners to find the subtalar neutral position has been questioned. Multiple studies have shown that while goniometric measurements of the subtalar neutral appear to be moderately reliable if taken by the same therapist over a short period of time, inter-examiner reliability is unacceptable (Elveru et al, 1988; Youdas et al, 1993).

In an easily practicable method of measuring the motion range in the ankle under load, the patient is asked to put his or her foot on a 30-cm-high stool and then lean forward as much as possible without lifting the heel from the supporting stool. The loaded plantar flexion is measured in the same position but with the heel raised as much as possible, and goniometric measurements are made. In normal daily life, at least 10 degrees are required; for performing athletics and sports activities, a loaded dorsal extension range of 20 to 30 degrees is necessary (Lindsjo et al, 1985).

Following are several variables that have been reported by various authors as important considerations in the measurement of ankle ROM:

- Weightbearing versus nonweightbearing (Baggett and Young, 1993)
- Amount of force used to elicit maximum ROM
- Anatomical landmarks used (Bohannon et al, 1989)
- Subtalar position (Tiberio, 1987)

ROM of the ankle is especially critical in the geriatric population, where diminished ROM often leads to decreased proprioceptive abilities, resulting in increased falling and subsequent disability. Various investigators have reported the effects of age and gender on ankle ROM. Several findings become apparent, as follows:

- In young adults, ROM in general is greater for women than for men.
- The ROM is about 8 degrees smaller in dorsiflexion and about 8 degrees higher in plantar flexion for women than for men in the oldest age group.
- It is speculated that physical activity and common shoe wear are factors influencing the age- and gender-dependent differences in ROM (Nigg et al, 1992).
- Passive resistive torque increases with age.
- Strength decreases with age.
- Dorsiflexion ROM decreases significantly across age groups; especially for females (Vandervoort et al, 1992a).
- Ankle joint complex ROM consistently decreases from a maximum at age 15 to 20 years to a minimum after age 60 years. The average decrement was greater for females than for males (Grimston et al, 1993).
- Passive ROM of the ankle into dorsiflexion showed decreases in the elderly, especially females, which seemed to reflect less compliant tissue structures (Vandervoort et al, 1992b).

PROVOCATIVE TESTS

Very few studies exist that describe the reliability of physical findings used to assess acute ankle injury patients. Stiell et al (1992) reported that the following factors are important in the assessment of acute ankle injuries (the variables are listed from most reliable to least):

- Ability to bear weight
- Bone tenderness at the base of the fifth metatarsal
- Bone tenderness at the posterior edge of lateral malleolus
- Bone tenderness at the tip of the medial malleolus
- Combinations of bone tenderness
- Soft tissue tenderness
- The degree of swelling of the anterior talofibular ligament
- Presence of ecchymosis
- ROM
- Bone tenderness at the proximal fibula
- Anterior drawer sign

STRENGTH TESTING

Decreased strength of the ankle joint, especially the dorsiflexors, has been implicated in ankle joint dysfunction. This is often seen in elderly populations, where the loss of ankle dorsiflexion strength is readily seen. There is com-

pelling data from both nursing home and community-dwelling subjects which indicates a strong relationship of ankle dorsiflexor strength to balance, gait, and the occurrence of falls in the elderly (Wolfson et al, 1995). Because falls resulting from ankle joint dysfunction are so debilitiating in this population, much of the current research of strength of the ankle joint comes not from athletic subjects, but from geriatric studies.

Muscle strength is usually evaluated clinically using manual muscle testing. Detection and grading of mild symmetrical muscle weakness using manual testing is difficult, in part because the examiner must take into consideration the normal variation in strength in relation to age, weight, height, and gender. In one study, manual muscle testing resulted in a significant underestimation of the frequency and severity of muscle weakness in both the ankle and the knee. In 28% to 41% of the comparisons, manual testing misclassified the strength performance by one muscle grade or more (> 25%). Misclassifications were most frequent for the ankle plantar flexors (Andersen and Jakobsen, 1997).

As a result, other types of testing for ankle muscle strength have been proposed. According to Morris-Chatta et al (1994) the use of isokinetic testing for plantar flexion and dorsiflexion tests shows high inter-rater reliability when average strength was more than about 10 Newton-meters (Nm). When average strength was less than 10 Nm, reliability was significantly less. Experienced examiners and less experienced examiners were equally reliable. Variability in strength over 6 months was no greater than variability over a few days. The authors concluded that isokinetic tests of ankle strength in older adults are highly reliable and stable when examiners are adequately trained and subjects maintain usual physical activity levels (Morris-Chatta et al, 1994). Normative data for ankle dorsiflexion is given in Table 15–24.

There is considerable age-associated loss in both voluntary and evoked strength in the plantar flexors, but the optimal angle for torque production does not appear to change significantly with age (Winegard et al, 1997). In-

---

CLINICAL TIP 15–3
Standing Heel-Rise Test

The standing heel-rise test is frequently used as a quick clinical measure to test plantar flexion function. Most texts recommend performance of this test 10 times to grade the patient's plantar flexion as normal. However, a recent study finds that many weaknesses are not detected with this method until many more repetitions are attempted. A recommendation is made to change the standard of testing plantar-flexion function, when using the standing heel-rise test, to require 25 repetitions for a grade of normal (Lunsford and Perry, 1995).

Table 15–24: Dynametric Normal Values for Ankle Dorsiflexion (newtons ± standard deviation)

AGE	MEN DOMINANT	MEN NONDOMINANT	WOMEN DOMINANT	WOMEN NONDOMINANT
20–29	385.9 ± 64.4	368.7 ± 44.2	294.9 ± 51.1	273.3 ± 45.5
30–39	372.6 ± 89.6	388.4 ± 81.5	248.7 ± 75.5	252.9 ± 55.8
40–49	376.1 ± 63.7	362.7 ± 58.5	251.0 ± 54.4	247.1 ± 51.3
50–59	323.2 ± 90.8	311.0 ± 63.3	252.9 ± 53.3	240.1 ± 48.7
60–69	269.0 ± 76.9	272.7 ± 61.2	235.7 ± 74.9	230.5 ± 57.3
70–79	240.0 ± 47.3	246.0 ± 47.6	166.2 ± 48.7	153.3 ± 36.1

From Bohannon et al, 1997.

creasing age has also shown substantial declines in abilities of healthy adults to rapidly develop ankle joint torques (Thelen et al, 1996).

Strengthening of the evertor muscles is widely advocated as a key component of lateral ankle sprain rehabilitation, but impaired invertor muscle performance has also been associated with lateral ankle ligament injury. Restoration of a normal evertor/invertor strength relationship may be accomplished through performance of an isotonic ankle strengthening program (Wilkerson et al, 1997).

Rehabilitative exercises are primarily designed to increase flexibility, ROM, strength, proprioception, and sport-specific development prior to resumption of full activity. Proper rehabilitation of the lateral ankle (inversion) sprain is critical due to its frequency and potential for chronic pain and recurrence.

PREDICTORS OF ANKLE DYSFUNCTION

Many factors are thought to cause ankle ligament injuries; various studies have been attempted to isolate factors that may predict or lead to ankle injury or dysfunction. In a study of ballet and modern dance students, the subject's age, years of training, body mass index, sex, and ankle ROM measurement had no predictive value for injury; previous injury and dance discipline both correlated with increased risk of injury, with inversion sprains being the most common injury (Wiesler et al, 1996).

Generalized joint laxity, anatomical foot and ankle alignment, ankle ligament stability, and isokinetic strength were shown to be insignificant in the prediction of future ankle inversion injuries. However, the eversion-to-inversion strength ratio and the ratio of dorsiflexion to plantar flexion strength has been shown to be significantly different for injured ankles compared with contralateral uninjured ankles. Individuals with a muscle strength imbalance as measured by an elevated eversion-to-inversion ratio have exhibited a higher incidence of inversion ankle sprains. Ankles with greater plantar flexion strength and a smaller dorsiflexion-to-plantar flexion ratio also have shown a higher incidence of inversion ankle sprains (Baumhauer et al, 1995). Unfortunately, strength in these

muscles varies widely with individual subjects, and normative values for ankle movements other than plantar flexion have not yet been published.

Lentell et al (1995) found that deficits in anatomical stability and proprioception of passive movement sensation are greater concerns than strength deficits when managing the ankle with functional instability.

SELF-REPORTED QUESTIONNAIRES

As with the other extremity joints evaluated in this chapter, several different scales exist for attempting to categorize injuries, describe the severity of dysfunction, or other uses as outcome measures in ankle conditions. Many of these scales were particularly developed for the assessment of fractures of the ankle. They include:

- **Joy Subjective Clinical Evaluation** (Joy et al, 1974). Originally designed for evaluation of reduction of severe ankle fractures, this early scale rates the ankle on a 5-point scale, from 0 (pain is incapacitating and the patient desires surgical fusion of the ankle) to 4 (normal ankle); see Appendix Form F–24.
- **Olerud and Molander Scoring System** (Orerud and Molander, 1984). This scale was also originally used for the scoring of ankle fracture. It features 100 possible points, with subscales for pain, stiffness, swelling, stair-climbing, running, jumping, squatting, supports, and work/activities of daily living; see Appendix Form F–25. The authors state that even minor subjective differences in disability experienced by the patient are significantly separated.
- **Phillips Ankle Clinical Scoring System** (Phillips et al, 1985). This is another scoring system that was intended for the evaluation of severe ankle fractures. However, this scale has questions that clearly have application for ankle maladies other than fracture (ability to walk > 10 blocks, or unlimited distances). It includes clinical, anatomical, and arthritis scores; see Appendix Form F–26.
- **Mazur Ankle Grading System** (Mazur et al, 1979). The original intended purpose of this scale is for fol-

lowing arthrodesis, but, like the Phillips scale, many questions will apply to other types of ankle maladies, from sprains to osteoarthritis. This 100-point scale features 50 points for pain, 40 points for function, and 10 points for ankle ROM; see Appendix Form F–27.

- **Kaikkonen Performance Test Protocol** (Kaikkonen et al, 1994). These authors devised a standardized test protocol and scoring scale for evaluation of ankle injuries. This test is comprised of three simple questions describing the subjective assessment of the injured ankle, two clinical measurements

(ROM in dorsiflexion, laxity of the ankle joint), ankle test measuring functional stability (walking down a staircase), two tests measuring muscle strength (rising on heels and toes), and one test measuring balance (balancing on a square beam). This test showed excellent reproducibility, and the ability to differentiate those subjects with poor or fair recovery. The scale presented is recommended for studies evaluating functional recovery after ankle injury (Kaikkonen et al, 1994); see Appendix Form F–28.

Conclusion

This chapter has reviewed hundreds of studies by authors who have attempted to add to the existing body of knowledge regarding outcomes in extremity joints. In some areas, such as ROM studies, there are wide ranges of opinions, and it is obvious that a true consensus does not exist. Strength testing is also subject to such a tremendous variety of opinions that it must be said that a critical mass of thought has yet to be reached. Many of these studies are very critical of the provocative and diagnostic clinical tests, which are still being taught in many of the finest institutions.

There are many reasons for this lack of consensus. As mentioned at the beginning of this chapter, study design is often poor, and sample sizes are small. (Some of the published, peer-reviewed studies referenced in this chapter based their findings on the measurement of only one patient subject.) It is no secret that many highly respected researchers practice in a

"publish or perish" system. It has been estimated that up to 90% of all biomedical research studies have flaws so serious that the final conclusions of the study cannot be substantiated.

However, in some areas, particularly the abundance of self-reported questionnaires and outcome tools, the HCP has several options and pathways from which to choose. One or more of the outcome measures in this chapter will probably fit the individual needs of each individual patient, perhaps with just a bit of tweaking. It is recommended that the HCP choose the outcome assessment tools that appear to be the most appropriate to the needs of the patient, and use those tools on a repeated basis to gauge patient progress. While it is true that not all HCPs agree on the the type of "yardstick" to be used to measure patient progress, all should agree that the meaningful measurement of patient progress is vital to that patient's health.

REFERENCES

Aaron A, Weinstein D, Thickman D, Eilert R. Comparison of orthoroentgenography and computed tomography in the measurement of limb-length discrepancy. *J Bone Joint Surg [Am]*. 1992;74(6):897–902.

Abernethy P, Wilson G, Logan P. Strength and power assessment. Issues, controversies and challenges. *Sports Med*. 1995;19(6):401–417.

Agre JC, Magness JL, Hull SZ, et al. Strength testing with a portable dynamometer: Reliability for upper and lower extremities. *Arch Phys Med Rehabil*. 1987;68(7):454–458.

Ahlberg A, Moussa M, Al-Nahdi M. On geographical variations in the normal range of joint motion. *Clin Orthop*. 1988;234:229–231.

Almekinders LC, Almekinders SV. Outcome in the treatment of chronic overuse sports injuries: A retrospective study. *J Orthop Sports Phys Ther*. 1994;19(3):157–161.

Amadio PC, Silverstein MD, Ilstrup DM, Schleck CD, Jensen LM. Outcome assessment for carpal tunnel surgery: The relative responsiveness of generic, arthritis-specific, disease-specific, and physical examination measures. *J Hand Surg [Am]*. 1996;21(3):338–346.

Andersen H, Jakobsen J. A comparative study of isokinetic dynamometry and manual muscle testing of ankle dorsal and plantar flexors and knee extensors and flexors. *Eur Neurol*. 1997;37(4):239–242.

Andersson Gare B, Fasth A, Wiklund I. Measurement of functional status in juvenile chronic arthritis: Evaluation of a Swedish version of the Childhood Health Assessment Questionnaire. *Clin Exp Rheumatol.* 1993;11(5):569–576.

Aspegren DD, Cox JM, Trier KK. Short leg correction: A clinical trial of radiographic vs. non-radiographic procedures. *J Manipulative Physiol Ther.* 1987;10(5):232–238.

Atroshi I, Breidenbach WC. McCabe SJ. Assessment of the carpal tunnel outcome instrument in patients with nerve-compression symptoms. *J Hand Surg [Am].* 1997;22(2):222–227.

Atroshi I, Johnsson R, Nouhan R, Crain G, McCabe SJ. Use of outcome instruments to compare workers' compensation and non-workers' compensation carpal tunnel syndrome. *J Hand Surg [Br].* 1997;22(5):882–888.

Baggett BD, Young G. Ankle joint dorsiflexion. Establishment of a normal range. *J Am Podiatr Med Assoc.* 1993;83(5):251–254.

Bak K. Nontraumatic glenohumeral instability and coracoacromial impingement in swimmers. *Scand J Med Sci Sports.* 1996;6(3):132–144.

Bak K, Faunl P. Clinical findings in competitive swimmers with shoulder pain. *Am J Sports Med.* 1997;25(2):254–260.

Bak K, Magnusson SP. Shoulder strength and range of motion in symptomatic and pain-free elite swimmers. *Am J Sports Med.* 1997;25(4):454–459.

Bandy WD, Irion JM, Briggler M. The effect of time and frequency of static stretching on flexibility of the hamstring muscles. *Phys Ther.* 1997;77(10):1090–1096.

Bartolozzi A, Andreychik D, Ahmad S. Determinants of outcome in the treatment of rotator cuff disease. *Clin Orthop.* 1994;308:90–97.

Baumhauer JF, Alosa DM, Renstrom AF, Trevino S, Beynnon B. A prospective study of ankle injury risk factors. *Am J Sports Med.* 1995;23(5):564–570.

Baylis WJ, Rzonca EC. Functional and structural limb length discrepancies: evaluation and treatment. *Clin Podiatr Med Surg.* 1988;5(3):509–520.

Beasley WC. Influence of method on estimates of normal knee extensor force among normal and post-polio children. *Phys Ther.* 1956;36:21.

Beaton DE, Richards RR. Measuring function of the shoulder. A cross-sectional comparison of five questionnaires. *J Bone Joint Surg [Am].* 1996;78(6):882–890.

Bellamy N, Buchanan WW, Goldsmith CH, Campbell J, Stitt LW. Validation study of WOMAC: A health status instrument for measuring clinically important patient relevant outcomes to antirheumatic drug therapy in patients with osteoarthritis of the hip or knee. *J Rheumatol.* 1988;15(12):1833–1840.

Bengtsson J, Mollborg J, Werner S. A study for testing the sensitivity and reliability of the Lysholm knee scoring scale. *Knee Surg Sports Traumatol Arthrosc.* 1996;4(1):27–31.

Bergner M, Bobbitt RA, Carter WB, Gilson BS. The Sickness Impact Profile: Development and final revision of a health status measure. *Med Care.* 1981;19(8):787–805.

Bessette L, Keller RB, Lew RA, et al. Prognostic value of a hand symptom diagram in surgery for carpal tunnel syndrome. *J Rheumatol.* 1997;24(4):726–734.

Bigos S, Bowyer O, Braen G, et al. Acute lower back problems in adults. *Clinical Practice Guideline, Quick Reference Guide Number 14.* Rockville, Md: US Dept of Health and Social Services, Public Health Service, Agency for Health Care Policy and Research, AHCPR Pub. No. 95-0643; 1994.

Binazzi R, Soudry M, Mestriner LA, Insall JN. Knee arthroplasty rating. *J Arthroplasty.* 1992;7(2):145–148.

Biushko VM, Malanin DA, Lomtatidze ESh, Dzakhoev ES. [The physical diagnosis and treatment of insufficiency of the anterior cruciate ligament]. *Vestn Khir Im I I Grek.* 1996;155(2):54–56.

Bjelle A. Epidemiology of shoulder problems. *Bailliere's Clin Rheumatol.* 1989;3:437–450.

Bjelle A, Hagberg M, Michaelson G. Work-related shoulder-neck complaints in industry: A pilot study. *Br J Rheumatol.* 1987;26(5):365–369.

Blunt KL, Rajwani MH, Guerriero RC. The effectiveness of chiropractic management of fibromyalgia patients: A pilot study. *J Manipulative Physiol Ther.* 1997;20:389–399.

Boeckstyns ME. Development and construct validity of a knee pain questionnaire. *Pain.* 1987;31(1):47–52.

Boeckstyns ME, Backer M. Reliability and validity of the evaluation of pain in patients with total knee replacement. *Pain.* 1989;38(1):29–33.

Bohannon RW. Test-retest reliability of hand-held dynamometry during a single session of strength assessment. *Phys Ther.* 1986;66(2):206–209.

Bohannon RW. Hand-held compared with isokinetic dynamometry for measurement of static knee extension torque (parallel reliability of dynamometers). *Clin Phys Physiol Meas.* 1990;11(3):217–222.

Bohannon RW, Andrews AW. Interrater reliability of hand-held dynamometry. *Phys Ther.* 1987;67(6):931–933.

Bohannon RW. Reference values for extremity muscle strength obtained by hand-held dynamometry from adults ages 20 to 79 years. *Arch Phys Med Rehabil*. 1997;78:26–32.

Bohannon RW, Smith J, Hull D, Palmeri D, Barnhard R. Deficits in lower extremity muscle and gait performance among renal transplant candidates. *Arch Phys Med Rehabil*. 1995;76(6):547–551.

Bohannon RW, Tiberio D, Zito M. Selected measures of ankle dorsiflexion range of motion: differences and intercorrelations. *Foot Ankle*. 1989;10(2):99–103.

Boiteau M, Malouin F, Richards CL. Use of a hand-held dynamometer and a Kin-Com dynamometer for evaluating spastic hypertonia in children: a reliability study. *Phys Ther*. 1995;75(9):796–802.

Bollen S, Seedhom BB. A comparison of the Lysholm and Cincinnati knee scoring questionnaires. *Am J Sports Med*. 1991;19(2):189–190.

Bolgla LA, Keskula DR. Reliability of lower extremity functional performance tests. *J Orthop Sports Phys Ther*. 1997;26(3):138–142.

Boone DC, Azen SP, Lin CM, Spence C, Baron C, Lee L. Reliability of goniometric measurements. *Phys Ther*. 1978;58(11):1355–1390.

Braun BL, Amundson LR. Quantitative assessment of head and shoulder posture. *Arch Phys Med Rehabil*. 1989;70(4):322–329.

Broberg MA, Morrey BF. Results of delayed excision of the radial head after fracture. *J Bone Joint Surg [Am]*. 1986;68(5):669–674.

Brossmann J, Preidler KW, Pedowitz RA, White LM, Trudell D, Resnick D. Shoulder impingement syndrome: Influence of shoulder position on rotator cuff impingement—an anatomic study. *AJR Am J Roentgenol*. 1996;167(6):1511–1515.

Brox JI, Brevik JI. Prognostic factors in patients with rotator tendinosis (stage II impingement syndrome) of the shoulder. *Scand J Prim Health Care*. 1996;14(2):100–105.

Buch N, Foucher G. [Validity of clinical signs and provocative tests in carpal tunnel syndrome]. *Rev Chir Orthop Reparatrice Appar Mot*. 1995;80(1):14–21.

Buchberger W, Judmaier W, Birbamer G, Lener M, Schmidauer C. Carpal tunnel syndrome: Diagnosis with high-resolution sonography. *AJR Am J Roentgenol*. 1992;159(4):793–798.

Buch-Jaeger N, Foucher G. Correlation of clinical signs with nerve conduction tests in the diagnosis of carpal tunnel syndrome. *J Hand Surg [Br]*. 1994;19(6):720–724.

Burckhardt CS, Clark SR, Bennett RM. The fibromyalgia impact questionnaire: Development and validation. *J Rheumatol*. 1991;18(5):728–733.

Chesworth BM, MacDermid JC, Roth JH, Patterson SD. Movement diagram and "end-feel" reliability when measuring passive lateral rotation of the shoulder in patients with shoulder pathology. *Phys Ther*. 1998;78(6):593–601.

Coldwells A, Atkinson G, Reilly T. Sources of variation in back and leg dynamometry. *Ergonomics*. 1994;37(1):79–86.

Concannon MJ, Gainor B, Petroski GF, Puckett CL. The predictive value of electrodiagnostic studies in carpal tunnel syndrome. *Plast Reconstr Surg*. 1997;100(6):1452–1458.

Constant CR, Murley AHG. A clinical method of functional assessment of the shoulder. *Clin Orthop*. 1987;214:160–164.

Convery FR, Minteer MA, Amiel D, Connett KL. Polyarticular disability: A functional assessment. *Arch Phys Med Rehabil*. 1977;58(11):494–499.

Cooper DE. Tests for posterolateral instability of the knee in normal subjects. Results of examination under anesthesia. *J Bone Joint Surg [Am]*. 1991;73(1):30–36.

Croft PR, Nahit ES, Macfarlane GJ, Silman AJ. Interobserver reliability in measuring flexion, internal rotation, and external rotation of the hip using a plurimeter. *Ann Rheum Dis*. 1996;55(5):320–323.

Croft P, Pope D, Zonca M, O'Neill T, Silman A. Measurement of shoulder related disability: Results of a validation study. *Ann Rheum Dis*. 1994;53(8):525–528.

Cumming RG, Klineberg RJ. Fall frequency and characteristics and the risk of hip fractures. *J Am Geriatr Soc*. 1994;42(7):774–778.

Curtis KA, Roach KE, Applegate EB, et al. Development of the Wheelchair User's Shoulder Pain Index (WUSPI). *Paraplegia*. 1995;33(5):290–293.

Danbert RJ. Clinical assessment and treatment of leg length inequalities. *J Manipulative Physiol Ther*. 1988;11(4):290–295.

Dawson J, Fitzpatrick R, Carr A. Questionnaire on the perceptions of patients about shoulder surgery. *J Bone Joint Surg [Br]*. 1996a;78(4):593–600.

Dawson J, Fitzpatrick R, Carr A, Murray D. Questionnaire on the perceptions of patients about total hip replacement. *J Bone Joint Surg [Br]*. 1996b;78(2):185–190.

DeBoer KF, Harmon RO Jr, Savoie S, Tuttle CD. Inter- and intra-examiner reliability of leg-length differential measurement: A preliminary study. *J Manipulative Physiol Ther*. 1983;6(2):61–66.

de Krom MC, Knipschild PG, Kester AD, Spaans F. Efficacy of provocative tests for diagnosis of carpal tunnel syndrome. *Lancet*. 1990;335(8686):393–395.

Dequeker J, Ranstam J, Valsson J, Sigurgevisson B, Allander E. The Mediterranean Osteoporosis (MEDOS) Study questionnaire. *Clin Rheumatol*. 1991;10(1):54–72.

Dequeker J, Tobing L, Rutten V, Geusens P. Relative risk factors for osteoporotic fracture: A pilot study of the MEDOS questionnaire. *Clin Rheumatol*. 1991;10(1):49–53.

De Smet L, Steenwerckx A, Van den Bogaert G, Cnudde P, Fabry G. Value of clinical provocative tests in carpal tunnel syndrome. *Acta Orthop Belg*. 1995;61(3):177–182.

Desorsiers J, Hebert R, Bravo G, Dutil E. Upper extremity performance test for the elderly [TEMPA]: Normative data and correlates with sensorimotor parameters. *Arch Phys Med Rehabil*. 1995;76:1125–1129.

De Witt JK, Osterbauer PJ, Stelmach GE, Fuhr AW. Optoelectric measurement of changes in leg length inequality resulting from isolation tests. *J Manipulative Physiol Ther*. 1994;17(8):530–538.

Dijkstra PU, de Bont LG, van der Weele LT, Boering G. Joint mobility measurements: reliability of a standardized method. *Cranio*. 1994;12(1):52–57.

DiVeta J, Walker ML, Skibinski B. Relationship between performance of selected scapular muscles and scapular abduction in standing subjects. *Phys Ther*. 1990;70(8):470–476.

Doege TC. *Guides to the Evaluation of Permanent Impairment*. 4th ed. Chicago, Ill: American Medical Association; 1993.

Dougados M, Gueguen A, Nakache JP, Nguyen M, Mery C, Amor B. Evaluation of a functional index and an articular index in ankylosing spondylitis. *J Rheumatol*. 1988;15(2):302–307.

Draper DO, Schulthies SS. Examiner proficiency in performing the anterior drawer and Lachman tests. *J Orthop Sports Phys Ther*. 1995;22(6):263–266.

Durkan JA. A new diagnostic test for carpal tunnel syndrome. *J Bone Joint Surg [Am]*. 1991;73(4):535–538.

Durkan JA. The carpal-compression test. An instrumented device for diagnosing carpal tunnel syndrome. *Orthop Rev*. 1994;23(6):522–525.

Duruoz MT, Poiraudeau S, Fermanian J, et al. Development and validation of a rheumatoid hand functional disability scale that assesses functional handicap. *J Rheumatol*. 1996;23(7):1167–1172.

Dvir Z. Grade 4 in manual muscle testing: The problem with submaximal strength assessment. *Clin Rehabil*. 1997;11(1):36–41.

Eberhardt K, Recht L, Wollheim F, Lithman T, Pettersson H, Schersten B. Detection of suspected inflammatory joint disease with a new simple self-administered hand test. *Br J Rheumatol*. 1988;27(6):457–461.

Eberl DR, Fasching V, Rahlfs V, Schleyer I, Wolf R. Repeatability and objectivity of various measurements in rheumatoid arthritis. A comparative study. *Arthritis Rheum*. 1976;19(6):1278–1286.

Ekstrand J, Wiktorsson M, Oberg B, Gillquist J. Lower extremity goniometric measurements: A study to determine their reliability. *Arch Phys Med Rehabil*. 1982;63(4):171–175.

Elffors I, Allander E, Kanis JA, et al. The variable incidence of hip fracture in southern Europe: The MEDOS Study. *Osteoporos Int*. 1994;4(5):253–263.

Ellenbecker TS, Roetert EP, Piorkowski PA, Schulz DA. Glenohumeral joint internal and external rotation range of motion in elite junior tennis players. *J Orthop Sports Phys Ther*. 1996;24(6):336–341.

Elveru RA, Rothstein JM, Lamb RL. Goniometric reliability in a clinical setting. Subtalar and ankle joint measurements. *Phys Ther*. 1988;68(5):672–677.

Enwemeka CS. Radiographic verification of knee goniometry. *Scand J Rehabil Med*. 1986;18(2):47–49.

Ericsen K. Management of cervical disc herniation with upper cervical chiropractic care. *J Manipulative Physiol Ther*. 1998;21:51–56.

Evans RC. *Illustrated Essentials in Orthopedic Physical Assessment*. St. Louis, Mo: Mosby; 1994.

Ewald FC. The Knee Society total knee arthroplasty roentgenographic evaluation and scoring system. *Clin Orthop*. 1989;248:9–12.

Falltrick DR, Pierson SD. Precise measurement of functional leg length inequality and changes due to cervical spine rotation in pain-free students. *J Manipulative Physiol Ther*. 1989;12(5):364–368.

Feldman BM, Ayling-Campos A, Luy L, Stevens D, Silverman ED, Laxer RM. Measuring disability in juvenile dermatomyositis: Validity of the childhood health assessment questionnaire. *J Rheumatol*. 1995;22(2):326–331.

Ferrari FS, Della Sala L, Cozza S, et al. [High-resolution ultrasonography in the study of carpal tunnel syndrome]. *Radiol Med (Torino)*. 1997;93(4):336–341.

Fish DR, Wingate L. Sources of goniometric error at the elbow. *Phys Ther*. 1985;65(11):1666–1670.

Fredriksen H, Dagfinrud H, Jacobsen V, Maehlum S. Passive knee extension test to measure hamstring muscle tightness. *Scand J Med Sci Sports*. 1997;7(5):279–282.

Friberg O, Nurminen M, Korhonen K, Soininen E, Manttari T. Accuracy and precision of clinical estimation of leg length inequality and lumbar scoliosis: Comparison of clinical and radiological measurements. *Int Disabil Stud*. 1988;10(2):49–53.

Friedman PJ. Predictors of work disability in work-related upper-extremity disorders. *J Occup Environ Med*. 1997;39(4):339–343.

Frisiello S, Gazaille A, O'Halloran J, Palmer ML, Waugh D. Test-retest reliability of eccentric peak torque values for shoulder medial and lateral rotation using the Biodex isokinetic dynamometer. *J Orthop Sports Phys Ther*. 1994;19(6):341–344.

Frontera WR, Hughes VA, Dallal GE, Evans WJ. Reliability of isokinetic muscle strength testing in 45- to 78-year-old men and women. *Arch Phys Med Rehabil*. 1993;74(11):1181–1185.

Gabriel SE, Amadio PC, Ilstrup D. The feasibility and validity of studies comparing orthopedists and non-orthopedists caring for musculoskeletal injuries: Results of a pilot study. *Arthritis Care Res*. 1997;10(3):163–168.

Gajdosik RL, Bohannon RW. Clinical measurement of range of motion. Review of goniometry emphasizing reliability and validity. *Phys Ther*. 1987;67(12):1867–1872.

Gallagher MA, Cuomo F, Polonsky L, Berliner K, Zuckerman JD. Effects of age, testing speed, and arm dominance on isokinetic strength of the elbow. *J Shoulder Elbow Surg*. 1997;6(4):340–346.

Gellman H, Gelberman RH, Tan AM, Botte MJ. Carpal tunnel syndrome. An evaluation of the provocative diagnostic tests. *J Bone Joint Surg [Am]*. 1986;68(5):735–737.

Gerber C, Krushell RJ. Isolated rupture of the tendon of the subscapularis muscle. Clinical features in 16 cases. *J Bone Joint Surg [Br]*. 1991;73:389–394.

Gerberich SG, Priest JD. Treatment for lateral epicondylitis: Variables related to recovery. *Br J Sports Med*. 1985;19(4):224–227.

Gerhardt JJ, Rippstein J. *Measuring and Recording of Joint Motion; Instrumentation and Techniques*. Toronto, Canada: Hogrefe and Huber; 1994.

Gerr F, Letz R, Harris-Abbott D, Hopkins LC. Sensitivity and specificity of vibrometry for detection of carpal tunnel syndrome. *J Occup Environ Med*. 1995;37(9):1108–1115.

Gibson MH, Goebel GV, Jordan TM, Kegerreis S, Worrell TW. A reliability study of measurement techniques to determine static scapular position. *J Orthop Sports Phys Ther*. 1995;21(2):100–106.

Girouard CK, Hurley BF. Does strength training inhibit gains in range of motion from flexibility training in older adults? *Med Sci Sports Exerc*. 1995;27(10):1444–1449.

Glass I, Ring H. Median nerve conduction tests and Phalen's sign in carpal tunnel syndrome. *Electromyogr Clin Neurophysiol*. 1995;35(2):107–112.

Gogia PP, Braatz JH, Rose SJ, Norton BJ. Reliability and validity of goniometric measurements at the knee. *Phys Ther*. 1987;67(2):192–195.

Gonzalez del Pino J, Delgado-Martinez AD, Gonzalez Gonzalez I, Lovic A. Value of the carpal compression test in the diagnosis of carpal tunnel syndrome. *J Hand Surg [Br]*. 1997;22(1):38–41.

Goodwin J, Clark C, Deakes J, Burdon D, Lawrence C. Clinical methods of goniometry: A comparative study. *Disabil Rehabil*. 1992;14(1):10–15.

Gore DR, Murray MP, Sepic SB, Gardner GM. Correlations between objective measures of function and a clinical knee rating scale following total knee replacement. *Orthopedics*. 1986;9(10):1363–1367.

Graham GP, Johnson S, Dent CM, Fairclough JA. Comparison of clinical tests and the KT1000 in the diagnosis of anterior cruciate ligament rupture. *Br J Sports Med*. 1991;25(2):96–97.

Granberry WM, Noble PC, Woods GW. Evaluation of an electrogoniometric instrument for measurement of laxity of the knee. *J Bone Joint Surg [Am]*. 1990;72(9):1316–1322.

Greenfield B, Catlin PA, Coats PW, Green E, McDonald JJ, North C. Posture in patients with shoulder overuse injuries and healthy individuals. *J Orthop Sports Phys Ther*. 1995;21(5):287–295.

Griegel-Morris P, Larson K, Mueller-Klaus K, Oatis CA. Incidence of common postural abnormalities in the cervical, shoulder, and thoracic regions and their association with pain in two age groups of healthy subjects. *Phys Ther*. 1992;72(6):425–431.

Grimston SK, Nigg BM, Hanley DA, Engsberg JR. Differences in ankle joint complex range of motion as a function of age. *Foot Ankle*. 1993;14(4):215–222.

Grohmann JE. Comparison of two methods of goniometry. *Phys Ther*. 1983;63(6):922–925.

Mayer F, Horstmann T, Kranenberg U, Rocker K, Dickhuth HH. Reproducibility of isokinetic peak torque and angle at peak torque in the shoulder joint. *Int J Sports Med.* 1994a;15 (suppl 1):S26–S31.

Mayerson NH, Milano RA. Goniometric measurement reliability in physical medicine. *Arch Phys Med Rehabil.* 1984;65(2):92–94.

Mazur JM, Schwartz E, Simon SR. Ankle arthrodesis. Long-term follow-up with gait analysis. *J Bone Joint Surg [Am].* 1979;61(7):964–975.

McGrory BJ, Harris WH. Can the western Ontario and McMaster Universities (WOMAC) osteoarthritis index be used to evaluate different hip joints in the same patient? *J Arthroplasty.* 1996;11(7):841–844.

McGuigan FX, Hozack WJ, Moriarty L, Eng K, Rothman RH. Predicting quality-of-life outcomes following total joint arthroplasty. Limitations of the SF-36 Health Status Questionnaire. *J Arthroplasty.* 1995;10(6):742–747.

McMaster WC, Troup J. A survey of interfering shoulder pain in United States competitive swimmers. *Am J Sports Med.* 1993;21(1):67–70.

Meenan RF, Gertman PM, Mason JH. Measuring health status in arthritis. The arthritis impact measurement scales. *Arthritis Rheum.* 1980;23(2):146–152.

Meenan RF, Mason JH, Anderson JJ, Guccione AA, Kazis LE. AIMS2. The content and properties of a revised and expanded Arthritis Impact Measurement Scales Health Status Questionnaire. *Arthritis Rheum.* 1992;35(1):1–10.

Megele R. [Diagnostic tests in carpal tunnel syndrome]. *Nervenarzt.* 1991;62(6):354–359.

Mellin G. Correlations of hip mobility with degree of back pain and lumbar spinal mobility in chronic low-back pain patients. *Spine.* 1988;13(6):668–670.

Miller MD, Johnson DL, Harner CD, Fu FH. Posterior cruciate ligament injuries. *Orthop Rev.* 1993;22(11):1201–1210.

Mitsou A, Vallianatos P. Clinical diagnosis of ruptures of the anterior cruciate ligament: A comparison between the Lachman test and the anterior drawer sign. *Injury.* 1988;19(6):427–428.

Morrey BF. *The Elbow and its Disorders.* 2nd ed. Philadelphia, Pa: Saunders; 1993:95.

Morris-Chatta R, Buchner DM, de Lateur BJ, Cress ME, Wagner EH. Isokinetic testing of ankle strength in older adults: assessment of inter-rater reliability and stability of strength over six months. *Arch Phys Med Rehabil.* 1994;75(11):1213–1216.

Morrison DS, Frogameni AD, Woodworth P. Non-operative treatment of subacromial impingement syndrome. *J Bone Joint Surg [Am].* 1997;79(5):732–737.

Muffly-Elsey D, Flinn-Wagner S. Proposed screening tool for the detection of cumulative trauma disorders of the upper extremity. *J Hand Surg [Am].* 1987;12(5 Pt 2):931–935.

Murphy SB, Ganz R, Muller ME. The prognosis in untreated dysplasia of the hip. A study of radiographic factors that predict the outcome. *J Bone Joint Surg [Am].* 1995;77(7):985–989.

Natri A, Jarvinen M, Latvala K, Kannus P. Isokinetic muscle performance after anterior cruciate ligament surgery. Long-term results and outcome predicting factors after primary surgery and late-phase reconstruction. *Int J Sports Med.* 1996;17(3):223–228.

Neer CS II. Anterior acromioplasty for the chronic impingement and syndrome in the shoulder: A preliminary report. *J Bone Joint Surg.* 1972;54A:41–50.

Nelson KC, Cornelius WL. The relationship between isometric contraction durations and improvement in shoulder joint range of motion. *J Sports Med Phys Fitness.* 1991;31(3):385–388.

Nigg BM, Nigg CR, Reinschmidt C. Reliability and validity of active, passive and dynamic range of motion tests. *Sportverletz Sportschaden.* 1995;9(2):51–57.

Nigg BM, Fisher V, Allinger TL, Ronsky JR, Engsberg JR. Range of motion of the foot as a function of age. *Foot Ankle.* 1992;13(6):336–343.

Novak CB, Collins ED, Mackinnon SE. Outcome following conservative management of thoracic outlet syndrome. *J Hand Surg [Am].* 1995;20(4):542–548.

Novak CB, Mackinnon SE, Brownlee R, Kelly L. Provocative sensory testing in carpal tunnel syndrome. *J Hand Surg [Br].* 1992;17(2):204–208.

Noyes FR, Barber SD, Mangine RE. Abnormal lower limb symmetry determined by function hop tests after anterior cruciate ligament rupture. *Am J Sports Med.* 1991a;19(5):513–518.

Noyes FR, Barber SD, Mooar LA. A rationale for assessing sports activity levels and limitations in knee disorders. *Clin Orthop.* 1989;246:238–249.

Noyes FR, McGinniss GH, Mooar LA. Functional disability in the anterior cruciate insufficient knee syndrome: Review of knee rating systems and projected risk factors in determining treatment. *Sports Med.* 1984 Jul–Aug;1(4):278–302.

Noyes FR, Mooar LA, Barber SD. The assessment of work-related activities and limitations in knee disorders. *Am J Sports Med.* 1991b;19(2):178–188.

O'Brien SJ, Pagnani JM, McGlynn SR, Wilson JB. The active compression test: a new and effective test for diagnosing labral tears and acromioclavicular joint abnormality. *Am J Sports Med.* 1998 Sep–Oct;26(5):610–3.

O'Brien SJ, Schwartz RS, Warren RF, Torzilli PA. Capsular restraints to anterior-posterior motion of the abducted shoulder: A biomechanical study. *J Shoulder Elbow Surg.* 1995;4(4):298–308.

Odding E, Valkenburg HA, Algra D, Vandenouweland FA, Grobbee DE, Hofman A. The association of abnormalities on physical examination of the hip and knee with locomotor disability in the Rotterdam Study. *Br J Rheumatol.* 1996;35(9):884–890.

Odding E, Valkenburg HA, Grobbee DE, Hofman A, Pols HA. [Locomotor disability in the elderly; the ERGO Study (Erasmus Rotterdam Health and the Elderly). ERGO Study Group]. *Ned Tijdschr Geneeskd.* 1995;139(41):2096–2100.

Olerud C, Molander H. A scoring scale for symptom evaluation after ankle fracture. *Arch Orthop Trauma Surg.* 1984;103(3):190–194.

Ombregt L, ed. *A System of Orthopaedic Medicine.* Philadelphia, Pa: Saunders; 1995.

Orchard J, Marsden J, Lord S, Garlick D. Preseason hamstring muscle weakness associated with hamstring muscle injury in Australian footballers. *Am J Sports Med.* 1997;25(1):81–85.

O'Reilly SC, Muir KR, Doherty M. Screening for pain in knee osteoarthritis: Which question? *Ann Rheum Dis.* 1996;55(12):931–933.

Patte D. Directions for the use of the severity for painful and/or chronically disabled shoulders. *Abstracts of the First Open Congress of the European Society of Surgery of the Shoulder and Elbow.* Paris; 1987:36–41.

Pearlmutter LL, Bode BY, Wilkinson WE, Maricic MJ. Shoulder range of motion in patients with osteoporosis. *Arthritis Care Res.* 1995;8(3):194–198.

Pellecchia GL, Paolino J, Connell J. Intertester reliability of the cyriax evaluation in assessing patients with shoulder pain. *J Orthop Sports Phys Ther.* 1996;23(1):34–38.

Peters G, Wirth CJ, Kohn D. [Comparison of knee ligament scores and rating systems]. *Z Orthop Ihre Grenzgeb.* 1997;135(1):63–69.

Peterson DE, Blankenship KR, Robb JB, et al. Investigation of the validity and reliability of four objective techniques for measuring forward shoulder posture. *J Orthop Sports Phys Ther.* 1997;25(1):34–42.

Petherick M, Rheault W, Kimble S, Lechner C, Senear V. Concurrent validity and intertester reliability of universal and fluid-based goniometers for active elbow range of motion. *Phys Ther.* 1988;68(6):966–969.

Phillips WA, Schwartz HS, Keller CS, et al. A prospective, randomized study of the management of severe ankle fractures. *J Bone Joint Surg [Am].* 1985;67(1):67–78.

Plafcan DM, Turczany PJ, Guenin BA, Kegerreis S, Worrell TW. An objective measurement technique for posterior scapular displacement. *J Orthop Sports Phys Ther.* 1997;25(5):336–341.

Polkinghorn BS. Chiropractic treatment of frozen shoulder syndrome (adhesive capsulitis) utilizing mechanical force, manually assisted short lever adjusting procedures. *J Manipulative Physiol Ther.* 1995;18(2):105–115.

Pope DP, Croft PR, Pritchard CM, Macfarlane GJ, Silman AJ. The frequency of restricted range of movement in individuals with self-reported shoulder pain: Results from a population-based survey. *Br J Rheumatol.* 1996;35(11):1137–1141.

Post M. Primary tendinitis of the long head of the biceps. In: Souza T, ed. Which orthopedic tests are really necessary? *Advances in Chiropractic,* Vol. 1. St. Louis, Mo: Mosby; 1994.

Pransky G, Long R, Hammer K, Schulz LA, Himmelstein J, Fowke J. Screening for carpal tunnel syndrome in the workplace. An analysis of portable nerve conduction devices. *J Occup Environ Med.* 1997;39(8):727–733.

Prkachin KM, Mercer SR. Pain expression in patients with shoulder pathology: Validity, properties and relationship to sickness impact. *Pain.* 1989;39(3):257–265.

Pryse-Phillips WE. Validation of a diagnostic sign in carpal tunnel syndrome. *J Neurol Neurosurg Psychiatry.* 1984;47(8):870–872.

Rachlin ES. Myofascial pain and fibromyalgia: Trigger point management. St. Louis, Mo: Mosby; 1994:128.

Rawes ML, Dias JJ. Long-term results of conservative treatment for acromioclavicular dislocation. *J Bone Joint Surg [Br].* 1996;78-B:410–412.

Renstrom AF. Mechanism, diagnosis, and treatment of running injuries. [Review] [62 refs]. Instructional Course Lectures. 1993;42:225–234.

Rhodes DW, Mansfield ER, Bishop PA, Smith JF. Comparison of leg length inequality measurement methods as estimators of the femur head height difference on standing X-ray. *J Manipulative Physiol Ther.* 1995;18(7):448–452.

Rhodes DW, Mansfield ER, Bishop PA, Smith JF. The validity of the prone leg check as an estimate of standing leg length inequality measured by X-ray. *J Manipulative Physiol Ther.* 1995b;18(6):343–346.

Ribot C, Tremollieres F, Pouilles JM, et al. Risk factors for hip fracture. MEDOS study: Results of the Toulouse Centre. *Bone.* 1993;14(suppl 1):S77–S80.

Richter M, Kiefer H, Hehl G, Kinzl L. Primary repair for posterior cruciate ligament injuries. An eight-year followup of fifty-three patients. *Am J Sports Med.* 1996;24(3):298–305.

Riddle DL, Rothstein JM, Lamb RL. Goniometric reliability in a clinical setting. Shoulder measurements. *Phys Ther.* 1987;67(5):668–673.

Rissanen P, Aro S, Sintonen H, Slatis P, Paavolainen P. Quality of life and functional ability in hip and knee replacements: A prospective study. *Qual Life Res.* 1996;5(1):56–64.

Ritter MA, Albohm MJ, Keating EM, Faris PM, Meding JB. Comparative outcomes of total joint arthroplasty. *J Arthroplasty.* 1995;10(6):737–741.

Roaas A, Andersson GB. Normal range of motion of the hip, knee and ankle joints in male subjects, 30–40 years of age. *Acta Orthop Scand.* 1982;53(2):205–208.

Roach KE, Budiman-Mak E, Songsirdej N, Lertratanakul Y. Development of a shoulder pain and disability index. *Arthritis Care Res.* 1991;4:143–149.

Rome K. Ankle joint dorsiflexion measurement studies. A review of the literature. *J Am Podiatr Med Assoc.* 1996;86(5):205–211.

Romeo AA, Bach BR Jr, O'Halloran KL. Scoring systems for shoulder conditions. *Am J Sports Med.* 1996;24(4):472–476.

Rondon CA, Gonzalez N, Agreda L, Millan A. [Observer agreement in the measurement of leg length]. *Rev Invest Clin.* 1992;44(1):85–89.

Rosenberg TD, Rasmussen GL. The function of the anterior cruciate ligament during anterior drawer and Lachman's testing. An in vivo analysis in normal knees. *Am J Sports Med.* 1984;12(4):318–322.

Rothstein JM, Miller PJ, Roettger RF. Goniometric reliability in a clinical setting. Elbow and knee measurements. *Phys Ther.* 1983;63(10):1611–1615.

Rowe CR, Patel D, Southmayd WW. The Bankart procedure: A long term end-result study. *J Bone Joint Surg.* 1978;60A:1–16.

Rubinstein RA Jr, Shelbourne KD, McCarroll JR, VanMeter CD, Rettig AC. The accuracy of the clinical examination in the setting of posterior cruciate ligament injuries. *Am J Sports Med.* 1994;22(4):550–557.

Salen BA, Spangfort EV, Nygren AL, Nordemar R. The Disability Rating Index: An instrument for the assessment of disability in clinical settings. *J Clin Epidemiol.* 1994;47(12):1423–1435.

Schenkman M, Laub KC, Kuchibhatla M, Ray L, Shinberg M. Measures of shoulder protraction and thoracolumbar rotation. *J Orthop Sports Phys Ther.* 1997;25(5):329–335.

Scott WN. *The Knee.* St. Louis, Mo: Mosby; 1994:660–664.

Seror P. Phalen's test in the diagnosis of carpal tunnel syndrome. *J Hand Surg [Br].* 1988;13(4):383–385.

Sgaglione NA, Del Pizzo W, Fox JM, Friedman MJ. Critical analysis of knee ligament rating systems. *Am J Sports Med.* 1995;23(6):660–667.

Singer F, Wottawa A, Hiebl S, Huber I, Wiplinger U, Wostry G. [Evaluation of 2 questionnaires with reference to their suitability for self-evaluation of patients with gonarthrosis. A contribution to quality assurance in rheumatology]. *Acta Med Austriaca.* 1996;23(4):136–141.

Smidt GL, Wei SH, McQuade K, Barakatt E, Sun T, Stanford W. Sacroiliac motion for extreme hip positions. A fresh cadaver study. *Spine.* 1997;22(18):2073–2082.

Snyder-Mackler L, Fitzgerald GK, Bartolozzi AR 3rd, Ciccotti MG. The relationship between passive joint laxity and functional outcome after anterior cruciate ligament injury. *Am J Sports Med.* 1997;25(2):191–195.

So RC, Siu OT, Chin MK, Chan KM. Bilateral isokinetic variables of the shoulder: A prediction model for young men. *Br J Sports Med.* 1995;29(2):105–109.

Sobush DC, Simoneau GG, Dietz KE, Levene JA, Grossman RE, Smith WB. The Lennie test for measuring scapular position in healthy young adult females: A reliability and validity study. *J Orthop Sports Phys Ther.* 1996;23(1):39–50.

Solgaard S, Carlsen A, Kramhoft M, Petersen VS. Reproducibility of goniometry of the wrist. *Scand J Rehabil Med.* 1986;18(1):5–7.

Solomon DH, Bates DW, Panush RS, Katz JN. Costs, outcomes, and patient satisfaction by provider type for patients with rheumatic and musculoskeletal conditions: a critical review of the literature and proposed methodologic standards. *Ann Intern Med.* 1997;127(1):52–60.

Solveborn SA. Radial epicondylalgia ('tennis elbow'): treatment with stretching or forearm band. A prospective study with long-term follow-up including range-of-motion measurements. *Scand J Med Sci Sports.* 1997;7(4):229–237.

Solveborn SA, Olerud C. Radial epicondylalgia (tennis elbow): Measurement of range of motion of the wrist and the elbow. *J Orthop Sports Phys Ther*. 1996;23(4):251–257.

Souza TA. *Sports Injuries of the Shoulder: Conservative Management*. New York, NY: Churchill Livingstone; 1994.

Staubli HU, Jakob RP. Posterior instability of the knee near extension. A clinical and stress radiographic analysis of acute injuries of the posterior cruciate ligament. *J Bone Joint Surg [Br]*. 1990;72(2):225–230.

Steinberg E, ed. *The Hip and Its Disorders*. Philadelphia, Pa: Saunders; 1991:46.

Stiell IG, McKnight RD, Greenberg GH, Nair RC, McDowell I, Wallace GJ. Interobserver agreement in the examination of acute ankle injury patients. *Am J Emerg Med*. 1992;10(1):14–17.

Stone RG, Frewin PR, Gonzales S. Long-term assessment of arthroscopic meniscus repair: A two- to six-year follow-up study. *Arthroscopy*. 1990;6(2):73–78.

Stratford PW, Balsor BE. A comparison of make and break tests using a hand-held dynamometer and the Kin-Com. *J Orthop Sports Phys Ther*. 1994;19(1):28–32.

Stucki G, Meier D, Stucki S, et al. [Evaluation of a German version of WOMAC (Western Ontario and McMaster Universities) Arthrosis Index]. *Z Rheumatol*. 1996a;55(1):40–49.

Stucki G, Meier D, Stucki S, et al. [Evaluation of a German questionnaire version of the Lequesne cox- and gonarthrosis indices]. *Z Rheumatol*. 1996;55(1):50–57.

Sucher BM. Palpatory diagnosis and manipulative management of carpal tunnel syndrome. *J Am Osteopath Assoc*. 1994;94(8):647–663.

Sun Y, Sturmer T, Gunther KP, Brenner H. Reliability and validity of clinical outcome measurements of osteoarthritis of the hip and knee—a review of the literature. *Clin Rheumatol*. 1997;16(2):185–198.

Tata GE, Ng L, Kramer JF. Shoulder antagonistic strength ratios during concentric and eccentric muscle actions in the scapular plane. *J Orthop Sports Phys Ther*. 1993;18(6):654–660.

Tchou S, Costich JF, Burgess RC, Wexler CE. Thermographic observations in unilateral carpal tunnel syndrome: Report of 61 cases. *J Hand Surg [Am]*. 1992;17(4):631–637.

Tegner Y, Lysholm J. Rating systems in the evaluation of knee ligament injuries. *Clin Orthop*. 1985;198:43–49.

Thelen DG, Schultz AB, Alexander NB, Ashton-Miller JA. Effects of age on rapid ankle torque development. *J Gerontol A Biol Sci Med Sci*. 1996;51(5):M226–M232.

Thomas M, Eastwood H. Re-evaluation of two simple prognostic scores of outcome after proximal femoral fractures. *Injury*. 1996;27(2):111–115.

Tiberio D. Evaluation of functional ankle dorsiflexion using subtalar neutral position. A clinical report. *Phys Ther*. 1987;67(6):955–957.

Tibone JE, Bradley JP. Evaluation of treatment outcomes for the athlete's shoulder. In: Matsen FA, Fu FH, Hawkins RJ, eds. *The Shoulder: A Balance of Mobility and Stability*. Rosemont, Ill: American Academy of Orthopedic Surgeons; 1995.

Tis LL, Maxwell T. The effect of positioning on shoulder isokinetic measures in females. *Med Sci Sports Exerc*. 1996;28(9):1188–1192.

T'Jonck L, Lysens R, Grasse G. Measurements of scapular position and rotation: A reliability study. *Physiother Res Int*. 1996;1(3):148–158.

Toomingas A, Hagberg M, Jorulf L, Nilsson T, Burstrom L, Kihlberg S. Outcome of the abduction external rotation test among manual and office workers. *Am J Ind Med*. 1991;19(2):215–227.

Tugwell P, Bombardier C, Buchanan WW, Goldsmith CH, Grace E, Hanna B. The MACTAR Patient Preference Disability Questionnaire—an individualized functional priority approach for assessing improvement in physical disability in clinical trials in rheumatoid arthritis. *J Rheumatol*. 1987;14(3):446–451.

Tully EA, Stillman BC. Computer-aided video analysis of vertebrofemoral motion during toe touching in healthy subjects. *Arch Phys Med Rehabil*. 1997;78(7):759–766.

Twellaar M, Verstappen FT, Huson A, van Mechelen W. Physical characteristics as risk factors for sports injuries: A four year prospective study. *Int J Sports Med*. 1997;18(1):66–71.

Ure BM, Tiling T, Kirchner R, Rixen D. [Reliability of clinical examination of the shoulder in comparison with arthroscopy. A prospective study]. *Unfallchirurg*. 1993;96(7):382–386.

Valente R, Gibson H. Chiropractic manipulation in carpal tunnel syndrome. *J Manipulative Physiol Ther*. 1994;17(4):246–249.

van den Ende CH, Breedveld FC, Dijkmans BA, Hazes JM. The limited value of the Health Assessment Questionnaire as an outcome measure in short term exercise trials. *J Rheumatol*. 1997;24(10):1972–1977.

van Den Ende CH, Rozing PM, Dijkmans BA, Verhoef JA, Voogt-van der Harst EM, Hazes JM. Assessment of shoulder function in rheumatoid arthritis. *J Rheumatol*. 1996;23(12):2043–2048.

Vandervoort AA, Chesworth BM, Cunningham DA, Paterson DH, Rechnitzer PA, Koval JJ. Age and sex effects on mobility of the human ankle. *J Gerontol*. 1992;47(1):M17–M21.

Vandervoort AA, Chesworth BM, Cunningham DA, Rechnitzer PA, Paterson DH, Koval JJ. An outcome measure to quantify passive stiffness of the ankle. *Can J Public Health*. 1992;83(suppl 2):S19–S23.

van der Windt DA, Koes BW, Boeke AJ, Deville W, De Jong BA, Bouter LM. Shoulder disorders in general practice: Prognostic indicators of outcome. *Br J Gen Pract*. 1996;46(410):519–523.

van Mechelen W, Hlobil H, Zijlstra WP, de Ridder M, Kemper HC. Is range of motion of the hip and ankle joint related to running injuries? A case control study. *Int J Sports Med*. 1992;13(8):605–610.

Viikari-Juntura E, Rauas S, Martikainen R, et al. Validity of self–reported physical work load in epidemiologic studies on musculoskeletal disorders. *Scand J Work Environ Health*. 1996;22(4):251–259.

Walch G. Directions for the use of the quotation of anterior instabilities of the shoulder. *Abstracts of the First Open Congress of the European Society of Surgery of the Shoulder and Elbow*. Paris; 1987:51–55.

Walker JM, Sue D, Miles-Elkousy N, Ford G, Trevelyan H. Active mobility of the extremities in older subjects. *Phys Ther*. 1984;64(6):919–923.

Walter L, Brannon L. A cluster analysis of the multidimensional pain inventory. Multidimensional Pain Inventory (MPI). *Headache*. 1991;31(7):476–479.

Warner JJ, Micheli LJ, Arslanian LE, Kennedy J, Kennedy R. Patterns of flexibility, laxity, and strength in normal shoulders and shoulders with instability and impingement. *Am J Sports Med*. 1990;18(4):366–375.

Warren RF, Ranawat CS, Inglis AE: Total shoulder replacement indications and results of the Neer nonconstrained prosthesis. In: Inglis AE, ed. *The American Academy of Orthopedic Surgeons Symposium on Total Joint Replacement of the Upper Extremity*. St. Louis, Mo: Mosby; 1982:56–57.

Watkins MA, Riddle DL, Lamb RL, Personius WJ. Reliability of goniometric measurements and visual estimates of knee range of motion obtained in a clinical setting. *Phys Ther*. 1991;71(2):90–96.

Werner RA, Bir C, Armstrong TJ. Reverse Phalen's maneuver as an aid in diagnosing carpal tunnel syndrome. *Arch Phys Med Rehabil*. 1994;75(7):783–786.

Werner RA, Franzblau A, Albers JW, Buchele H, Armstrong TJ. Use of screening nerve conduction studies for predicting future carpal tunnel syndrome. *Occup Environ Med*. 1997;54(2):96–100.

Wessel J. The reliability and validity of pain threshold measurements in osteoarthritis of the knee. *Scand J Rheumatol*. 1995;24(4):238–242.

Wiesler ER, Hunter DM, Martin DF, Curl WW, Hoen H. Ankle flexibility and injury patterns in dancers. *Am J Sports Med*. 1996;24(6):754–757.

Wilk KE, Andrews JR, Arrigo CA. The physical examination of the glenohumeral joint: Emphasis on the stabilizing structures. *J Orthop Sports Phys Ther*. 1997;25(6):380–389.

Wilkerson GB, Pinerola JJ, Caturano RW. Invertor vs. evertor peak torque and power deficiencies associated with lateral ankle ligament injury. *J Orthop Sports Phys Ther*. 1997;26(2):78–86.

Williams JW Jr, Holleman DR Jr, Simel DL. Measuring shoulder function with the Shoulder Pain and Disability Index. *J Rheumatol*. 1995;22(4):727–732.

Williams TM, Mackinnon SE, Novak CB, McCabe S, Kelly L. Verification of the pressure provocative test in carpal tunnel syndrome. *Ann Plast Surg*. 1992;29(1):8–11.

Winegard KJ, Hicks AL, Vandervoort AA. An evaluation of the length-tension relationship in elderly human plantarflexor muscles. *J Gerontol*. 1997;52(6):B337–B343.

Winters JC, Groenier KH, Sobel JS, Arendzen HH, Meyboom-de Jongh B. Classification of shoulder complaints in general practice by means of cluster analysis. *Arch Phys Med Rehabil*. 1997a;78(12):1369–1374.

Winters JC, Sobel JS, Groenier KH, Arendzen HJ, Meyboom-de Jong B. Comparison of physiotherapy, manipulation, and corticosteroid injection for treating shoulder complaints in general practice: Randomised, single blind study. *BMJ*. 1997;314(7090):1320–1325.

Winters JC, Sobel JS, Groenier KH, Arendzen JH, Meyboom-De Jong B. A shoulder pain score: A comprehensive questionnaire for assessing pain in patients with shoulder complaints. *Scand J Rehabil Med*. 1996;28(3):163–167.

Wolfgang GL. Surgical repair of tears of the rotator cuff of the shoulder. *J Bone Joint Surg [Am]*. 1994;56:14–26.

Wolfson L, Judge J, Whipple R, King M. Strength is a major factor in balance, gait, and the occurrence of falls. *J Gerontol*. 1995;50:64–67.

Wright FV, Kimber JL, Law M, Goldsmith CH, Crombie V, Dent P. The Juvenile Arthritis Functional Status Index (JASI): A validation study. *J Rheumatol*. 1996;23(6):1066–1079.

Wright JG, Young NL. The patient-specific index: Asking patients what they want. *J Bone Joint Surg [Am]*. 1997;79(7):974–983.

Wroble RR, Grood ES, Noyes FR, Schmitt DJ. Reproducibility of Genucom knee analysis system testing. *Am J Sports Med*. 1990;18(4):387–395.

Wroble RR, Van Ginkel LA, Grood ES, Noyes FR, Shaffer BL. Repeatability of the KT-1000 arthrometer in a normal population. *Am J Sports Med*. 1990;18(4):396–399.

Youdas JW, Bogard CL, Suman VJ. Reliability of goniometric measurements and visual estimates of ankle joint active range of motion obtained in a clinical setting. *Arch Phys Med Rehabil*. 1993;74(10):1113–1118.

Youdas JW, Carey JR, Garrett TR, Suman VJ. Reliability of goniometric measurements of active arm elevation in the scapular plane obtained in a clinical setting. *Arch Phys Med Rehabil*. 1994;75(10):1137–1144.

Zhai GH. [Diagnosis of anterior cruciate ligament injury of the knee joint]. *Chung Hua Wai Ko Tsa Chih*. 1992;30(1):10–13.

Psychosocial issues will not be specifically addressed in this chapter. Instead, the reader is referred to the chapters elsewhere in this text that deal with psychometric tools (Chaps. 7 and 8), disability prediction (Chap. 10), and identifying the high-risk for prolonged recovery patient (Chap. 21). The structural changes are most predominant early in an injury while the functional changes occur later, and often continue well past the point of healing of the structure. Therefore, tests need to be performed that not only evaluate for tissue damage, such as x-ray in a bony injury or provocative tests in a soft tissue injury, but also evaluate physical performance or functional capacity, to fully assess the effects of an injury. Failure to do so can result in the misinterpretation by the health care provider (HCP) that a complaining patient with a healed fracture or soft tissue injury whose x-ray or provocative testing results are negative must be malingering, hysterical, and/or require a psychological consult. **This misinterpretation often results in the promotion of chronic pain behavior,** which is specifically mentioned by the Agency for Health Care Policy and Research (AHCPR) as being one of the most important aspects to avoid when treating patients with low back pain (Bigos et al, 1994).

The inclusion of tests designed to measure functional impairments must become "standard" in the routine examination of patients with residual complaints following convalescence of the structural lesion. Only these types of tests will provide objective evidence to support the subjective complaints. Provocative tests will not provide useful information after the structural lesion heals, but **functional performance testing will identify "weak links" in the kinetic chain and, therefore, identify specific treatment rehabilitative protocols to address the functional impairments.** Only with the utilization of functional testing can specific rehabilitative care be identified and pursued. When deconditioning resulting from misidentification continues and pain behavior is fostered, the cycle of learned protective mechanisms will perpetuate additional compensatory movement, inactivity, and/or disuse. This, in turn, will result in a lowered threshold for failure, further reinforcing the pain cycle and deconditioning by promoting fear-avoidant behavior. Prompt identification and multidisciplinary treatment through activity restoration and psychosocial support is the only approach that can result in a successful endpoint of care in the chronically behavioral case. This approach is referred to as the **biopsychosocial model.**

CASE STUDY 16–1
FRACTURED TIBIA

A 7-year-old girl sustained a fracture of the right distal third of the tibia in October 1990. As a result of the poor blood supply that normally exists in this region, delayed union or healing occurred. A cast was worn for 10 weeks and, in spite of a residual fracture line still visible on x-ray, it was then removed, in the hope that the increased weight bearing would stimulate further healing. Gradual reduction in the girl's residual limp occurred over the ensuing 2 weeks and by early January 1991, she resumed fairly normal activity levels. The orthopedic surgeon managing the case allowed the girl to participate in a family ski trip in early February 1991 during which the tibia was re-fractured when the girl attempted to turn in deep snow, internally rotating the lower leg. Again, slow healing necessitated 12 weeks in a short leg cast and, after removal of the cast, over 8 months passed before the fracture line became difficult to visualize on the radiographs. Owing to the prolonged recovery, fear-avoidant behavior was evident in this patient

for approximately the next 2 years. Participation in normal activities was distinctly avoided. Calf muscle atrophy persisted for 4 years beyond the date of injury, probably due in part to overcompensation and disuse. A limp persisted after the re-fracture for 4 months when walking and for 12 months when running. Avoidance of certain physical activities persisted for several years.

Postfracture residuals included joint stiffness, muscle atrophy, and muscle weakness, resulting in poor physical performance that persisted well past the point of fracture healing. Because of the prolonged convalescence, dysfunctional fear-avoidant behaviors also resulted. This led to prolonged activity restrictions, which contributed further to the deconditioning process that persisted well beyond the point of fracture healing. As a result of psychosocial issues stemming from the prolonged recovery and reinjury, significant protracted disability occurred, extending the dysfunction well beyond the "natural history" of the original injury.

TERMINOLOGY: PHYSICAL MEASURES

Before addressing this area, an appreciation of the terminology associated with the evaluation of functional loss is needed. More specifically, the reader must recognize that measurement of **physical performance** and **work capacity** are distinctly different and that both are important (Yeomans and Liebenson, 1996a, 1996b). When assessing physical function, individual muscle groups of functional units—such as hamstring length, abdominal muscle strength, or cervical range of motion (ROM)—are addressed. Work capacity assessments, on the other hand, measure whole-body or "real world" movement such as bending, stooping, crawling, climbing, and reaching. Therefore, the assessment approaches for work capacity versus physical performance are different, although they are certainly related and often overlap. For example, low back repetitive arch-up physical performance testing may be weak in patients who perform poorly in work capacity testing when bending is being assessed due to back extensor muscle weakness. When compared to physical performance that identifies, for example, a "weak link" in the lumbar spine, whole-body work capacity tests have often returned to normal (Kishino et al, 1985; Curtis et al, 1994). Therefore, **physical performance testing is more sensitive in detecting subtle weaknesses compared to whole-body functional testing** (Brady et al, 1994). This is why it is necessary for patients to continue with an exercise program after discharge from rehabilitation, as it is probable that the stresses of everyday living and reduction in localized physical capacity will predispose patients to a higher risk of injury reoccurrence.

The measurement of loss of physical performance or capacity includes the **Basic Elements of Performance** (BEPs), including motion, strength, endurance, and agility (Kondraske, 1986). A measure of cardiovascular fitness may also be included and easily accomplished by use of a treadmill, bicycle ergometer, or by the use of a 3-minute step test (cardiovascular forms of testing are covered in Chapter 18). Physical performance testing has not been established in the routine physical examination of patients presenting with spinal complaints. Interestingly, however, it has been adopted to a greater extent in sports medicine in the examination of an extremity of an injured athlete. This is perhaps because, in the extremities, the injury is more easily observed and the involved limb can be easily tested against the contralateral or opposite limb with respect to strength, ROM, speed of contraction, symmetry of movement, and so forth. Research that relates trunk muscle strength to low back pain has been well established for quite some time (Mayer and Greenberg, 1942; Flint, 1955; Pederson and Staffeldt, 1972; Pederson et al, 1975; Nachemson, 1983; Biering-Sorenson, 1984, and others). In spite of this, most HCPs still inappropriately tend to pay more attention to ROM loss when examining the spine and relate this to lumbar spinal dysfunction over loss of strength.

The goal of this chapter is to introduce the reader to specific physical performance tests that meet important criteria including validity, reliability, utility, practicality, cost, and safety (see Chap. 2 for definitions). The emphasis is placed on low-tech, low-cost tests that can be implemented easily into a busy practice, have been clinically evaluated and reported in peer-reviewed literature, meet the criteria, *and* include a normative database. The importance of including a normative database cannot be overemphasized, as it allows for the patient's results to be compared directly to the normative data at the time of the initial evaluation. More specifically, by comparing the patient's physical performance determined by a specific test (such as the repetitive sit-up test for abdominal strength) to the normative data, a percentage of functional loss can be calculated. This is accomplished by dividing the patient's result by the normative data, and multiplying that number by 100 (eg, 8 sit-ups divided by an expected 22 multiplied by 100 equals 36% of normal). When completed at the time of the initial evaluation prior to beginning rehabilitation, a baseline for future comparison (ie, outcomes) is established. This information is useful as a patient motivator, a functional link deficiency identifier, and as proof that rehabilitation is "medically necessary." Therefore, there is something for everyone to gain from this information. More specifically, patients gain because their understanding of their problem is enhanced, stimulating rehabilitation compliance and motivation. The HCP benefits through identifying the weak functional link, which leads to the design of an exercise approach that is unique for each individual patient to remedy that weakness as well as to determine endpoints in care. Lastly, the third party payer benefits by better appreciating the "medical necessity" for rehabilitation services and understanding the treatment plan and goals. Therefore, *objective outcomes assessment* can be tracked by using physical performance tests and, when coupled with the subjective paper and pen outcome tools, patient management and data collection are optimized.

WHEN TO INCLUDE PHYSICAL PERFORMANCE TESTS IN PATIENT CARE

When physical performance should be assessed is, of course, case specific; but, in general, it should be as soon as possible. When a physical performance test does not provoke pain, it can be done at the time of the initial examination. For example, hip internal and external rotation can often be performed in a patient with low back pain without reproducing the patient's pain. Similarly, the straight leg raise will quantitatively assess hamstring length often without pain provocation unless acute low back pain is severe and/or nerve tension is present. The bonus of being able to perform physical performance testing on the initial visit is twofold: (1) to identify a baseline measure for future comparison (ie, outcomes assessment); and (2) to identify functional deficiencies and address them immediately to optimize treatment benefit. If hamstring length is, for example, 52 degrees prior to manual release techniques and 68 degrees after stretching, documenting this in the "O" part of the SOAP note provides a "hard" piece of data that supports the "medical necessity" for that visit. Therefore, these tests can also be done periodically during the course of treatment rather than restricting their use to examination time, only.

Once a patient has moved out of the acute stage of a musculoskeletal injury and exercises are being considered, this is an opportune time to assess the patient functionally. **Identification of a specific exercise prescription and baseline measures for outcomes assessment will be determined by the use of physical performance tests that include normative data.** This is the time to assess the patient thoroughly in order to identify as many functional deficiencies as possible and thus allow for identification of weak links, which are sometimes quite removed from the presenting area of complaint. For example, when addressing a patient complaining of headaches, ascending the body during postural and movement analysis often reveals tight hamstrings, weak gluteus maximus, tight iliopsoas, weak quadratus lumborum and lumbosacral erector spinae, tight thoracolumbar erector spinae, weak scapula stabilizers, tight posterior cervicothoracic, and weak anterior scalene muscles. Anterior occiput, shoulder protraction, upper extremity internal rotation, anterior pelvic tilt, leg length imbalance, and ankle pronation may be present as well. The weak kinetic links in this muscular imbalance pattern, common in the layered syndrome (Jull and Janda, 1987), may be far removed from the neck and head in the patient presenting with headache. The qualitative information derived from the postural examination followed by quantifying these functional pathologies by use of physical performance tests "hardens" the documentation and allows for prescriptively useful information and objective outcomes assessment. Timely identification of these findings can result in prompt treatment and enhance patient satisfaction and treatment outcome. Without a complete evaluation of a patient, a short-term improvement with a remitting and exacerbating headache pattern may result.

Therefore, when treatment results fail to procure a successful outcome and rehabilitation of the weak link(s) is clinically indicated, proper identification, quantification, and documentation of the findings are needed. When assessing physical performance as a prerehabilitation examination, grouping together physical performance tests aimed at identifying functional deficits from the upper and lower quarters, as well as the trunk, is appropriate. By doing so, weak links far removed from an area of complaint will not be missed and treatment can address the whole person, not just the area of complaint. **This concept of treating the whole person is the goal of the Quantitative Functional Capacity Evaluation (QFCE)** (Yeomans and Liebenson, 1996a, 1997; Liebenson and Yeomans, 1997), although like all physical performance tests, parts of the QFCE can be done at any time during the course of treatment.

Several researchers have reported opinions as to when physical performance and functional capacity should be evaluated. For example, in order to determine the "weak functional link," Mooney and Matheson (1994) recommend that a functional capacity evaluation (FCE) be considered at 2 weeks postinjury, but indicate this should be mandatory for any patient still suffering pain after 6 to 7 weeks. At 4 weeks, they recommend performing the California Functional Capacity Protocol (Cal-FCP) (Mooney and Matheson, 1994). Triano and Schultz (1994) have reported that 4 weeks of time is an appropriate interval after which to initiate testing. Hart et al (1993) recommend functional testing with the following components:

- Plateau of treatment progress
- Discrepancy between subjective and objective findings
- Difficulty in returning the patient to gainful employment
- Vocational planning, or medical-legal case settlement

TYPES OF PHYSICAL PERFORMANCE TESTS

HEALTH-RELATED FITNESS TEST

Suni et al (1996) reported the reliability of test items included in a health-related fitness (HRF) test battery for adults. In two consecutive studies, the inter-rater reliability, test–retest, and trial-to-trial reproducibility of three balance, two flexibility, and four muscular strength and endurance tests were investigated. These musculoskeletal fitness tests were as follows:

A. One-leg balance (three tests)
   1. Eyes open head straight
   2. Eyes closed
   3. Eyes open, head turning left and right
B. Flexibility (two tests)
   1. Upper body: Shoulder-neck mobility
   2. Trunk: Side-bending
C. Strength and endurance (four tests)
   1. Modified push-up (muscular strength of the upper body)
   2. Isometric sit-up (muscular endurance of the trunk)
   3. Jump and reach test (muscular strength of the legs)
   4. One-leg squat test (muscular strength of the legs)

The first of two studies was made up of 32 volunteers from two work sites and the second group was made up of 510 men and women from a population sample ranging in age from 37 to 57.

The authors indicated that they had two goals for assessing reliability with these tests (Suni et al, 1996). The first goal was to scientifically assess reliability, as identification of objective and reproducible-over-time fitness measures were needed to investigate the interrelationships between physical activity, fitness, and health. The second goal was to design a practical tool that could be used to promote health-enhancing exercise in adult populations. Because fitness evaluators make comparisons between individuals or measure changes in fitness over time, they must be made aware of the errors in their measurements in order to ensure quality of fitness testing and accurate interpretation of the results.

Motor Fitness: Balance

Because there is no single test that can serve as a global measure of balance or posture control, a battery or series of tests are required to assess physical performance (Horak, 1987). Suni et al utilized three methods of one-leg standing assessment previously reported (Bohannon et al, 1984; Stones and Kozma, 1987; Briggs et al, 1989; Johansson and Jarnlo, 1991): (1) eyes open, (2) eyes closed, and (3) head turns to assess different parts of the sensory system, including the visual, vestibular, and proprioceptive (Suni et al, 1996). With the subject wearing sport shoes, the heel of the opposite foot is placed at the level of the opposite knee, on the inner side of the support leg followed by hip external rotation. The arms should hang relaxed at the subject's sides. The subject is instructed to become familiar with the balance position with both legs and then choose the leg that he or she feels would better perform the task. Subjects are advised to stand as long and as relaxed as possible and only use the arms to maintain balance, while being time tested with a stopwatch in seconds for a maximum of 60 seconds for the eyes open test, and 30 seconds for the other two tests (Fig. 16-1). The head is turned in sequence with a metronome set at 50 times per minute to one side. Two trials were recorded with the subject's eyes open, unless the time limit of 60 seconds was achieved in the first trial. Two or three trials with the eyes closed and head turns were performed unless 30 seconds was reached. The authors cautioned that the test should be terminated when any of the following occurs:

- Altered position of the supporting leg
- Loss of knee contact with the heel of the unsupporting leg
- Opening of the eyes when testing eyes closed
- Interruption of the alternating head turns

Prior studies have suggested that one-leg standing tests have validity in relation to falls in the elderly (Gehlsen and Whaley, 1990) and possibly to back pain and injury in middle-aged adults (Videman et al, 1989; Oddsson, 1990; Bly and Sinnot, 1991). Suni et al (1996) reported inter-rater reliability as fair in their first study; this improved to high in the second study (intraclass correlation coefficient [ICC] of .76 vs 1.00, respectively) after standardizing the mensuration methods following the first study. The use of repeated trials to determine if improvement in a subject's performance occurs has been reported (Cohen et al, 1993). A 1-year test–retest correlation of .68 was reported for one leg standing eyes open and .32 for eyes closed (Stones and Kozma, 1987). Similar methods of test performance and forms were used, but Suni et al utilized a different form of statistical analysis. Only the eyes open test proved statistically significant in the first study. However, in the second study, improved mean differences and more narrow 95% confidence intervals indicated small learning effects from trial to trial, and good reproducibility within one rater occurred with trials for eyes closed and head turn tasks.

Bly (1992) reported normative data regarding balance and proprioception, indicating that standardized clinical tests of balance are based on time (Bohannon et al, 1984; Atwater et al, 1990; Chandler et al, 1990; Bly and Sinnot, 1991). Bly derived the following conclusions:

- It is normal for both young and old subjects to balance with both feet together for up to 30 seconds eyes open or closed.
- One-leg balance is much more discriminative.
- In children under 9 years of age, the one-footed balance test revealed good inter-rater reliability but was low on test–retest based on time.

Bly's normative data are summarized in Table 16–1.

Balance skills in athletes have been reported (Crotts et al, 1996; Forkin et al, 1996) as well as balance and proprioception in the elderly population (Heltmann et al, 1989; Frandin et al, 1996; Lord et al, 1996).

Musculoskeletal Fitness: Flexibility of the Upper Body

Mobility restriction of the shoulder joint in older adults often results in activity intolerance and therefore, reduced daily activities. *Shoulder-neck mobility* was scored by the use of a 0-to-3 point ordinal scale, which grades the subject's ability to raise the arms as high as possible overhead while maintaining straight elbows, and keeping the upper arms close to the ears (Suni et al, 1996). The backs of the hands are placed against the wall and the feet are placed 1.5-foot lengths away from the wall with the buttocks, back, and shoulders against the wall (Fig. 16–2). Scoring is as follows:

- 0 = severe restriction of ROM
- 1 = moderate restriction of ROM where only the fingertips reach the wall (Fig. 16–2B)
- 2 = no restriction of ROM; the entire dorsal side of the hand makes wall contact (Fig. 16–2A)

The inter-rater reliability was acceptable using this method, and test repetition within 1 week improved the results. The assessment of change in this test is limited by the use of a 3-point ordinal scale.

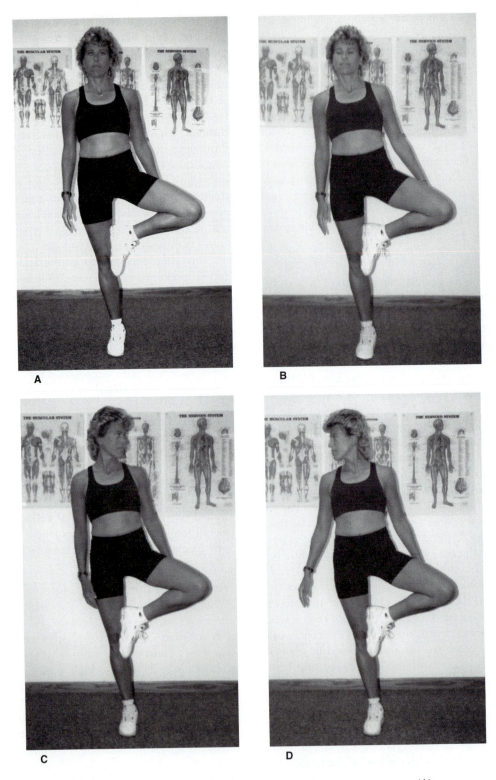

Figure 16–1. *Motor fitness: Balance.* The three methods of one-leg standing assessment are **(A)** eyes open, **(B)** eyes closed, and **(C and D)** head turn. These tests are used to assess different parts of the sensory system, including the visual, vestibular, and proprioceptive systems, respectively.

Table 16-1: Normative Data Regarding One-leg Balance Testing as Derived from Bly et al (1992)

AGE (YRS)	EYES OPEN (SEC)	EYES CLOSED (SEC)
20–59	29–30	21–28.8 (25 ave.)
60–69	22.5 (ave.)	10
70–79	14.2	4.3

Musculoskeletal Fitness: Flexibility of the Trunk (Side Bending)

Spinal mobility restriction has been suggested to be a risk factor for low back trouble (Frymoyer and Cats-Baril, 1987; Burton et al, 1989a; Riihimaki, 1991), but the protective role of mobility against back problems has yet to be proven (Burton et al, 1989b; Battie et al, 1990). *Side bending* was chosen as it is simple to perform and was found to be closely associated with low back pain (Mellin, 1987). Others have reported similar results as well (Frost et al, 1982; Mellin, 1986; Hyytiainen et al, 1991). In this test, the total lateral flexion ROM of the thoracolumbar spine and pelvis is evaluated (Mellin, 1986; Battie et al, 1987; Alaranta et al, 1990; Suni et al, 1996). The feet are placed on two parallel lines marked on the floor spaced 15 cm apart directly in front of a wall, and the subject is instructed to keep the heels on the floor during the movement. The distance between the start and endpoint of lateral flexion is measured with a cloth tape in centimeters, the two sides are added together, and the average for the mean side-bending score is calculated and recorded (Fig. 16–3).

Musculoskeletal Fitness: Muscular Strength of the Upper Body

Muscular endurance capacity of the upper body is measured by the use of a *modified push-up test*, which was revised to improve standardization. The exercise measures the endurance capacity of the upper extremity extensor muscles and the ability to stabilize the trunk. One cycle is completed for practice and the maximum number of push-ups completed in 40 seconds is reported (Fig. 16–4).

Difficulties in differentiating between correct and incorrect performances of conventional push-ups in a straight-leg and bent-leg position for men and women, respectively, has been reported (Invergo et al, 1991). Though acceptable inter-rater reliability and small test–retest variation in the coefficient of variation (CV) measure was found in this study (Suni et al, 1996), a clear learning effect between the first two study days was reported, suggesting some pretest practice may be appropriate. However, the authors warned that undue fatigue may occur from practicing the test before actual testing, especially in those with poor strength.

Musculoskeletal Fitness: Muscular Endurance of the Trunk

The *isometric sit-up test* is used to measure isometric endurance capacity of the trunk flexor muscles as well as the ability to stabilize the trunk following protocols defined by Hyytiainen and colleagues (1991) (Fig. 16–5). The test is performed by having the subject assume a 90-degree knee bent trunk-thigh angle sit-up position, while maintaining a neutral pelvis as lumbar spinal flexion was prohibited. A cardboard model was used to help control the position during the study. The position is maintained as long as possible up to a maximum of 240 seconds, and the subject is told the time every 30 seconds. A 0 (seconds) is reported if the position cannot be assumed or if it cannot be held stable for least 1 second.

Trunk muscle strength has been reported to be the best documented factor of fitness in relation to back health (Biering-Sorenson, 1984; Leino et al, 1987; Holmstrom et al, 1992; Moffet et al, 1993). Although others have reported good reproducibility of the isometric sit-up test (Hyytiainen et al, 1991), Suni et al (1996) reported only fair results with a large standard error of measurement.

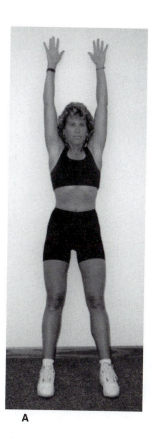 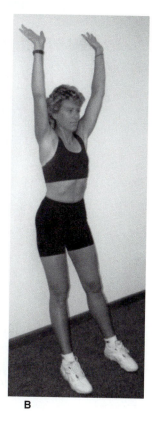

A   **B**

Figure 16–2. *Flexibility, upper body/shoulder-neck mobility.* This test is scored using a 3-point ordinal scale, measured by visual observation. The patient attempts to place the backs of the hands flat on the wall. **A.** The patient is successful in touching the backs of the hands against the wall with elbows placed near the ears (score = 2). **B.** A partially successful attempt where only the fingertips touch (score = 1). A score of 0 is representative of not being able to touch the wall with the fingertips at all.

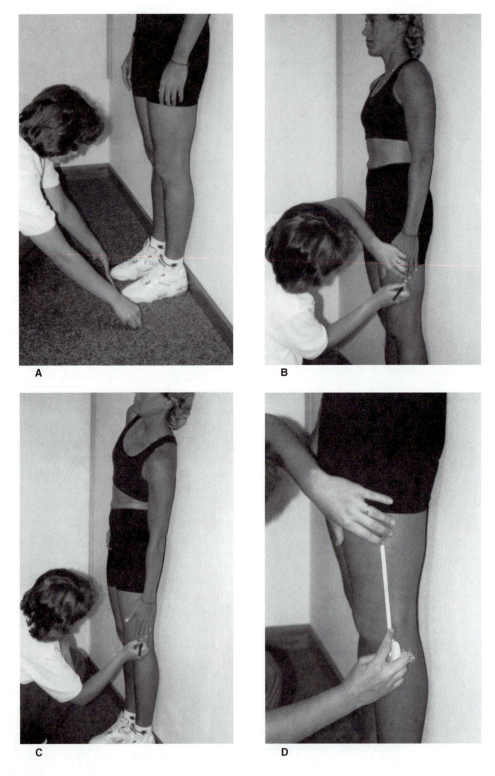

Figure 16–3. *Flexibility, trunk/side-bending test.* **A.** The patient's feet are placed 15 cm apart next to a wall. The scapulae and buttocks are held against the wall to avoid trunk rotation. The arms are held straight at sides with the palms on the lateral thigh. A mark is placed at the tip of the third digit on lateral thigh at neutral **(B)** and at maximum **(C)** lateral flexion. **D.** The distance between the two marks is measured with a cloth tape, and the two readings are averaged.

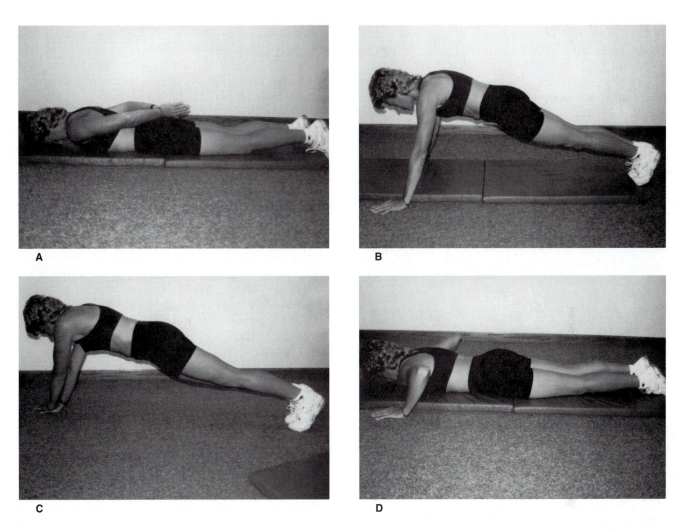

Figure 16–4. *Modified push-up.* The patient is placed prone on a mat. Each cycle begins by clapping hands behind back **(A)** followed by a straight-leg push-up **(B)** to a point of locking the elbows. **C.** The other hand then touches the top of the stabilizing hand, which standardizes the up position of the cycle. **D.** The patient then returns to the prone position to complete the cycle. The maximum number of push-ups completed in 40 seconds is recorded.

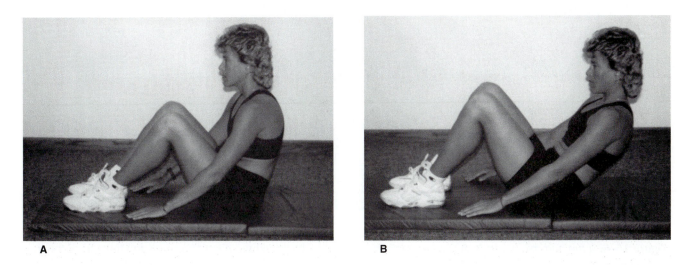

Figure 16–5. *Isometric sit-up test.* **A.** The patient is sitting in the "up" position of a sit-up, with the feet unrestrained on the floor and the knees flexed approximately 90 degrees. **B.** The patient leans straight back, keeping the arms at the side, and fingertips gently touch the mat. No lumbar spine flexion is allowed while the patient leans back to a 90-degree thigh-trunk angle.

A more homogeneous study sample of middle-aged men and/or a different statistical analysis approach are reported to be possible reasons for the difference when comparing other studies to the Suni data. **Standardizing the test position and patient motivation factors are reported as factors that also have a substantial effect on the results (key point).**

Musculoskeletal Fitness: Muscular Strength of the Legs

This category consists of two tests, the jump and reach test and the one-leg squat test (Suni et al, 1996). The *jump and reach test* is used to measure the strength of the leg extensor muscles (Beuker, 1976). The test is performed by having the subject jump as high as possible from a starting position of standing beside the jump and reach board facing forwards. One pretest practice repetition is allowed. A magnesium-powdered third finger then touches the board at the highest point of the jump and at the starting point (taken with the dominant arm reaching as high overhead as possible while keeping the feet/heels on the ground). The distance between the two marks on the board is measured in centimeters and the best of two test trials is recorded (Fig. 16–6).

The jump and reach test was found to be the most reliable of the entire group of tests evaluated as good reproducibility was found (Suni et al, 1996). Suni et al believe that this is due to the natural movement pattern of the performance as the subjects flex the knees, prestretching the leg extensors, and swing their arms during the jump (1996). **This test is the only one that requires speed of movement and, therefore, assesses an important aspect of rehabilitation.**

The *one-leg squat test* assesses functional leg extensor strength, which simulates daily activities such as stair climbing or lifting loads (Suni et al, 1996). The objective is to measure the load limit or maximum strength using up to 30% of the subject's own weight in a successful one-leg squat task, completed bilaterally. The test is preceded by a two-leg squat to a 90-degree knee flexion position followed by the one-leg trials, starting with the subject's own body weight. Next, a 10% increase of body weight is added up to a maximum of 30% of the subject's weight. A weight lifting belt is used to add extra weight. The squat is completed by having the subject take a short step forward and squat down with a straight back in a motion similar to a lunge, until the opposite knee touches the mat. The upright position is then resumed and the test repeated on the opposite side (Fig. 16–7).

Scoring is completed by adding the results of the two sides together and comparing them to a 5-point ordinal scale, which is defined as follows:

- 0 = unable to perform 1 repetition with both legs in the two-leg squat

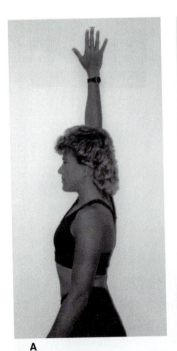 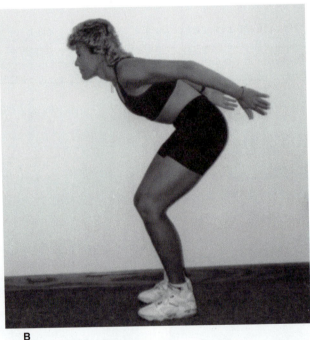 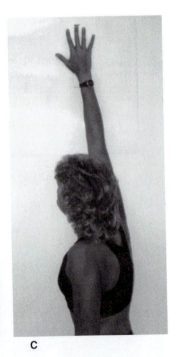

A   B   C

Figure 16–6. *Jump and reach test.* **A.** A starting point is first marked by chalking (magnesium powder) the pad of the third digit and reaching with the dominant arm overhead as high as possible, touching a jump-and-reach board. The test is performed by having the patient jump as high as possible from a starting position of standing beside the board facing forwards. **B.** The knees are allowed to flex but the feet are not allowed to move while preparing for the jump. **C.** The highest point of the jump is marked with a chalked finger. The distance between the starting and the highest mark is then measured.

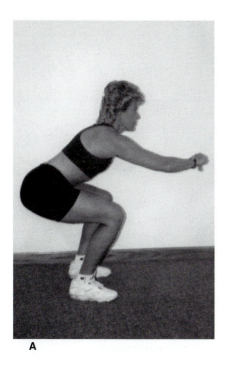
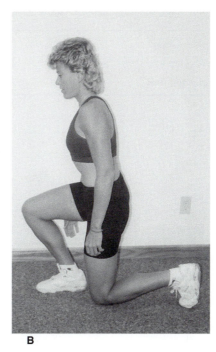
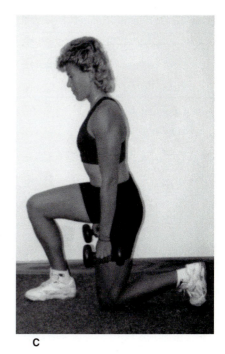

A   **B**   **C**

Figure 16–7. *One-leg squat test.* **A.** The test begins with a two-leg squat to 90 degree knee flexion position. **B.** The patient upon successful completion of the two-leg squat, performs the one-leg squat without weights. See the text for the scoring system. **C.** Weights are gradually added to a 30% maximum body weight amount.

- 1 = able to perform the two-leg squat, only
- 2 = able to perform the one-leg squat with body weight, only
- 3 = able to perform the one-leg squat with 10% extra weight
- 4 = able to perform the one-leg squat with 20% extra weight
- 5 = able to perform the one-leg squat with 30% extra weight

All tests of the fitness test battery (Suni et al, 1996) were completed in a standard sequence:

1. Motor fitness (one-leg standing tests)
2. Flexibility tests (shoulder-neck and side bending tests)
3. Muscular strength tests (modified push-up, isometric sit-up, jump and reach, and one-leg squat tests)

Warm-ups were not used nor were preliminary trials performed of the test unless explicitly instructed to do so. Each subject was tested individually and encouragement by the tester for best performance was done consistently. Reliability was reported with this test.

Table 16–2 includes the HRF tests, and those that met acceptable reliability as methods for field assessment are in bold italic print. Suni et al (1996) emphasize the need for standardization of testing protocols and proper training of those evaluating the patients in order to ensure reliability.

These tests were encouraged to be included in an HRF battery for adults to evaluate baseline information and promote exercises for health. Appendix Form G–1 allows for calculation and summary of scores and provides an excellent method of documenting the results of the HRF for adults.

ABDOMINAL MUSCLE STRENGTH AND ENDURANCE

The abdominal muscle strength and endurance test is also widely accepted as a trunk stabilizer, and strengthening exercises addressing weakness of this muscle group are routinely included in spinal stabilization rehabilitation programs. There are different methods of assessing abdominal strength. One approach is an isometric, one-repetition method to assess abdominal muscle endurance (Janda, 1983; Hyytiainen et al, 1991; Knudson and Johnston, 1995; Ito et al, 1996; Suni et al, 1996; McGill, 1999). Another is a dynamic approach to assess abdominal muscle strength (Ekholm et al, 1979; Hyytiainen et al, 1991; Alaranta et al, 1994). Therefore, the manner and application in which a sit-up is performed has been described in several ways (Table 16–3).

The *traditional straight leg sit-up* has been criticized because the movement involves primarily hip flexors with isometric abdominal muscle activity (Flint, 1964; Nelson, 1964; Soderberg, 1966; Allsop, 1971; Clarke, 1976). This type of sit-up has also been criticized for causing an increased lumbar lordosis and anterior pelvic tilt (Flint,

Table 16–2: Health Related Fitness Tests[a]

BALANCE	MEAN ± SD (N)	ICC	SEM	MEAN DIFFERENCE (95% CI)	CV (%)
Standing on one leg (sec)					
Eyes open	45.6 ± 21.6(40)	.76	13.3	3.7 (−2.2 to 9.6)	5.0
Eyes closed	6.4 ± 5.2(39)	.18	4.6	.6 (−1.6 to 2.8)	10.9
Head turns	8.7 ± 8.9 (39)	.28	7.5	2.6 (−.7 to 5.9)	4.0

FLEXIBILITY	SEVERE RESTRICTION ROM	MODERATE RESTRICTION ROM	NO RESTRICTION ROM	RATIO OF DISCORDANT PAIRS (95% CI)	Kw
Shoulder-neck mobility					
Right	18%	27%	55%	2.3 (.7 to .61)	.61
Left	20%	25%	55%	2.3 (.7 to 7.1)	.62

FLEXIBILITY	MEAN ± SD (N)	ICC	SEM	MEAN DIFFERENCE (95% CI)	CV (%)
Trunk: Side bending (cm)					
Right	21.4 ± 4.9(40)	.90	1.6	−.5 (−1.3 to .3)	4.7
Left	20.8 ± 5.0 (39)	.90	1.7	−.5 (−1.4 to .5)	6.2
Average	21.0 ± 4.8 (39)	.92	1.4	−.5 (−1.3 to .3)	4.7

MUSCULAR STRENGTH AND ENDURANCE	MEAN ± SD (N)	ICC	SEM	MEAN DIFFERENCE (95% CI)	CV (%)
Upper body: *Modified push-up* (reps)	13.6 ± 5.5 (19)	.88	2.6	3.0 (2.1 to 3.9)	.6
Trunk: Isometric sit-up (sec)	41.3 ± 33.4 (20)	.76	20.1	7.9 (− 5.7 to 21.5)	3.7
Legs: *Jump and reach* (cm)	33.1 ± 13.7 (20)	.98	3.0	1.7 (−.2 to 3.6)	2.4
Legs: *One leg squat* (points 0–10)	8.2 ± 2.0 (20)	.86	.9	.1 (−.7 to .5)	12.1

CI, confidence interval; CV, coefficient of variation; ICC, intraclass correlation coefficient; Kw, weighted Kappa coefficient; SD, standard deviation; SEM, standard error of measurement.

[a] Tests that met acceptable reliability as methods for field assessment of Health Related Fitness (HRF) are in bold italic print. The following methods of field assessment of HRF were reported to have acceptable reliability: (1) Standing on one leg with eyes open for balance, (2) side-bending of the trunk for spinal flexibility, (3) modified push-ups for upper body muscular function, and (4) jump and reach.

Reprinted with permission from Suni et al, 1996.

1964; Kendall, 1965; Ito et al, 1996; Mutoh et al, 1983). The *bent knee or "hook-lying"* sit-up has been advocated to reduce iliopsoas muscle activity and, therefore, reduce the lumbar lordosis and anterior pelvic tilt (Institute for Aerobics Research, 1977; Golding et al, 1982; American Alliance for Health, 1988). Most of the tests that describe the bent-knee sit-up recommend stabilizing the feet which tends to, again, increase hip flexor activation and decrease the abdominal muscle activity (Flint, 1965a, 1965b; Gutin and Lipetz, 1971; Godfrey et al, 1977; Mutoh et al, 1983; Andersson et al, 1989; Hall et al, 1990; Carlos et al, 1991).

Trunk curl-ups have been described as the most isolating and safest abdominal muscle strengthening exercise for the majority of people (Soderberg, 1966; Gilliam and Roy, 1976; Vincent and Britten, 1980; Jette et al, 1984; Sharpe et al, 1988; Silvermetz, 1990; Macfarlane, 1993; Ito et al, 1996; Juker et al, 1998). Electromyography (EMG) studies have shown equal or greater abdominal muscle activation and less hip flexor muscle activation compared to the bent-knee sit-up (Bullivant et al, 1986; Robertson et al, 1986; Andersson et al, 1989; Juker et al, 1998). In addition, the limited ROM may favor a reduction in low back strain, and

Table 16–3: Three Common Methods of Sit-up Performance

SIT-UP TYPE	REFERENCE
Least safe:	
Long-lying (other names: supine to long-sitting; straight leg)	Flint, 1964; Nelson, 1964; Kendall, 1965; Soderberg, 1966; Kraus, 1970[a]; Allsop, 1971; Clarke, 1976; Mutoh et al, 1983
Safer but requires feet stabilization:	
Bent-knee (hook lying)	Flint, 1965a, 1965b; Kraus, 1970[a]; Gutin and Lipetz, 1971; Godfrey et al, 1977; Golding et al, 1982; Mutoh et al, 1983; American Alliance for Health, 1988; Andersson et al, 1989; Hall et al, 1990; Carlos et al, 1991.
Safest and most isolating:	
Trunk curl-ups (abdominal crunches)	Walters and Partridge, 1957; Flint, 1965a, 1965b; Soderberg, 1966; Gutin and Lipetz, 1971; Gilliam and Roy, 1976; Ekholm et al, 1979; Vincent and Britten, 1980; Ricci et al, 1981; Jette et al, 1984; Alexander, 1985; Bullivant et al, 1986; Sharpe et al, 1988; Andersson et al, 1989; Silvermetz, 1990; Macfarlane, 1993; Ito et al, 1996.

[a] There are three methods of assessing the flexor strength in the Kraus-Weber test. One involves the long-lying method (for upper abdominal strength); another is the bent-knee approach (lower abdominal strength).

EMG studies indicate that the abdominal muscles are most active in the first 30 to 45 degrees of trunk flexion (Walters and Partridge, 1957; Flint, 1965a, 1965b; Flint and Gudgell, 1965; Gutin and Lipetz, 1971; Borkowitz, 1981; Ricci et al, 1981).

The validity and reliability of a bench truck curl-up test for abdominal muscle endurance has been shown to have good logical validity, weak criterion-referenced validity with isokinetic measures of trunk flexion, and good reliability for college-age persons (Knudson and Johnston, 1995). Data derived from Knutson et al is reported in Table 16–4. The

Table 16–4: Bench Trunk Curl-up Test Data, from Knudson and Johnston[a]

	MALES	FEMALES
Range	30–160	37–163
Mean	87.8	88.1
SD	30.3	28.1
CV (%)	34.5	31.9
Percentiles		
75%	104	100
50%	80	84
25%	68	69

CV, coefficient of variation; SD, standard deviation.

[a] A high degree of reliability is noted for women and men with the bench trunk curl-up test. Bench trunk curl-up test scores in which the number of repetitions are counted in a 2-minute time period for college-aged students in fitness classes are reported.

Reprinted with permission from Knudson and Johnston, 1995.

technique utilized included a supine position, where both the hips and knees are flexed 90 degrees with the lower legs supported on a bench and the posterior thighs and buttocks lying against the bench. The arms are folded on the abdomen, grasping the opposite elbow and the subject performs a curl-up until the forearm approximates the vertically oriented anterior aspect of the thigh (Fig. 16–8A, B).

Recently, McGill reported normative data for the endurance of the low back flexor muscles in a healthy, young (mean age of 23 years) population of 31 men and 44 women (McGill et al, 1999). The subjects were placed on a test bench with the upper body leaning against a 60 degree angled support, arms folded across the chest, and the knees bent so that a 90 degree trunk to leg angle was obtained. The support was then pulled back 10 cm, and the subjects isometrically held the position while being timed in seconds with a stopwatch. The test was concluded when the subjects could no longer hold the position and leaned back into the support. The mean and standard deviation for males was 144 ± 76, and for females 149 ± 99 seconds. The ratio between the low back extensor and flexor endurance was reported at .99 for males and .79 for females.

Ito and colleagues (1996) describe a similar method that is low-tech. In this study, trunk flexor endurance was studied in a normal group and in a chronic low back pain (CLBP) group. A significant difference in endurance was reported. More specifically, subjects included males (n = 37 normals, mean age, 44.3 years; n = 40 CLBP, mean age, 44.9 years; all rated pain < 6/10 and were nonmedicated 1 week prior to testing) and females (n = 53 normals, mean age, 46.8; n = 60 CLBP, mean age, 45.9). The flexor endurance test data ICC when combining the male and female data are .95 and .90 for healthy and CLBP subjects, respectively. The extensor endurance ICC is .97 and .93,

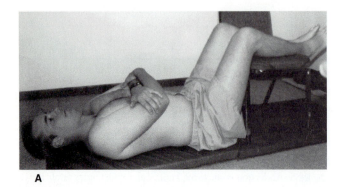
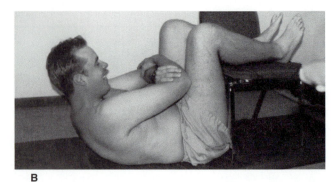

A   **B**

Figure 16–8. The sit-up proposed by Knutson and Johnston (1995) is performed by (**A**) a patient in the supine position with hip and knee flexed 90 degrees, legs resting on a chair seat, and arms folded on the abdomen, grasping the opposite elbows. **B.** The patient sits up, approximating the forearms to the vertical thighs to complete a repetition.

respectively. Table 16–5 lists the endurance strength of both the flexors and the extensor trunk muscles as depicted in Figure 16–9 (A and B, respectively). The authors do not include information about the size of the pillows used in the extensor endurance test. They do, however, emphasize that lumbar lordosis should not be allowed to increase during the test and, hence, the size of the roll must be large enough to allow for extension without an increase in lumbar lordosis.

The authors concluded that these two endurance strength tests have high reliability, reproducibility, and safety. Also, because no expensive equipment is required, they are low in cost compared to high-tech approaches and can be substituted for the latter. Finally, lumbar lordosis was significantly less for flexor endurance testing compared to the Kraus-Weber test ($P < .01$) (Kraus, 1970). More specifically, the radiographic L1 to S1 sagittal angle (2 meter focal film distance) measured 48.3 ± 5.7 and 25.4 ± 2.5 degrees during the Kraus-Weber test and the Ito et al approach, respectively. The Kraus-Weber test consists of three supine trunk flexor strength tests (Kraus, 1970). The

three abdominal strengthening tests include: (1) straight leg sit-up (feet secured); (2) double leg raise 25 degrees off the table; (3) feet flat on table (held down), knee-bent sit-up to 25 degrees (Fig. 16–10).

Before leaving this discussion of abdominal strengthening, it is prudent to discuss the role of psoas muscle function in various positions, especially during sit-up exercises. Juker et al (1998) reported quantitative intramuscular myoelectric activity of lumbar portions of the psoas and abdominal wall musculature during a wide variety of tasks. The psoas major muscle has been reported to be a significant source of spine loading (Bogduk, 1992; Santaguida, 1995) and, therefore, ranking psoas muscle activity during exercises and daily living tasks can give insight to the safest and least-spinal loading exercise approaches. The following conclusions were reported (Juker et al, 1998):

- The psoas muscle does not appear to be involved in lifting and lumbar stabilization; its primary role is to function as a hip flexor.

Table 16–5: Mean Endurance Strength of Flexor and Extensor Trunk Muscles[a]

	HEALTHY		CLBP	
	Males	**Females**	**Males**	**Females**
Flexor endurance	182.6 ± 69.3 sec.	85.1 ± 44.8	107.9 ± 49.6 sec.	57.2 ± 33.2
	$(.95)$[b]	$(.89)$[b]	$(.91)$[b]	$(.85)$[b]
Extensor endurance	208.2 ± 66.2	128.4 ± 53.0	85.1 ± 55.6	70.1 ± 51.8
	$(.97)$[b]	$(.94)$[b]	$(.93)$[b]	$(.95)$[b]

CLBP, chronic low back pain.

[a] The mean endurance strength of the flexor and extensor trunk muscles are reported with the corresponding test–retest correlation (r) values. All test–retest correlations for both groups for the corresponding endurance measurements were significantly high ($P < .01$).

[b] represents the test–retest correlation (r).

Compiled from data in Ito et al, 1996.

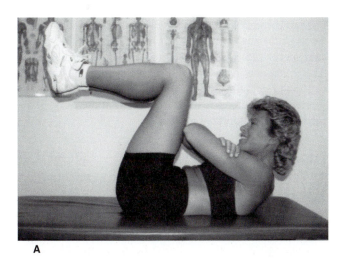
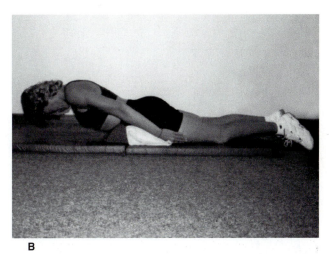

Figure 16–9. Trunk muscle endurance is tested for **(A)** the flexors, and **(B)** the extensors. During both endurance tests, subjects are instructed to attain maximum cervical flexion and pelvic stabilization by contracting the gluteal muscles. A significant difference in strength was found when comparing subjects with and without chronic low back pain.

- The magnetic resonance imaging (MRI) assessed morphology and geometry of the psoas muscle demonstrates that its mechanical advantage gives highest priority to hip flexion.
- The movement generating the maximum psoas activation was produced in the position of standing on one leg and exerting a maximum isometric contraction of hip flexion pushing against the 90-degree flexed hip with both hands (see Table 16–6, no. 11).
- Although it had been popularly hypothesized that the psoas is more active in straight leg versus bent-knee sit-ups, the contrary result was found: psoas activity increased in the bent knee position (see Table 16–6, nos. 4 vs 6).
- Curl-ups always produced psoas activity lower than 10% maximum voluntary contraction (MVC), compared to sit-ups and leg raises, which always resulted in increased levels exceeding 15% MVC.
- The hypothesis of activating the hip extensors by "pressing the heels down" to inhibit the psoas was not supported, as psoas activity increased during this maneuver (Table 16–6, nos. 10 vs 8).
- Substantial loading of the spine occurred during push-ups by psoas activity of 12% to 24% MVC (see Table 16–6, no. 5).
- The side support exercise is the most effective method of stimulating the abdominal obliques with only moderate psoas activity (see Table 16–6, nos. 3 and 7).
- The least spinal loading and most strength and endurance enhancing methods for core strengthening include cross curl-ups, curl-ups, and side support (both isometric and dynamic) (see Table 16–6, nos. 1, 2, 3, and 7).

- All sit-ups are contraindicated to the unstable spine initially after surgical stabilization.
- Both sit-ups and leg raises resulted in high psoas activity and did not significantly challenge the abdominal wall.
- Psoas activity was surprisingly low during lifting of 100-kg (220 lb) loads (<16% MVC).
- Psoas activity was higher during unsupported sitting (both upright and slouched) than during quiet, unloaded upright standing.
- Though the psoas was found to be a stronger external rotator than internal rotator, it is not a prime mover in either of these rotation movements.

HAMSTRING LENGTH

Four methods of measuring the hamstring muscle were evaluated and normative data established (Gajdosik et al, 1993). Utilizing the right lower extremity of 30 men, the following methods of assessing hamstring length were evaluated:

1. Passive straight leg raise (SLR) with the pelvis and opposite thigh stabilized with straps (SLR-SS); norm: 61 ± 6.7 degrees.
2. Passive SLR with the low back flat and, if needed to successfully posterior pelvic tilt, the opposite thigh/knee slightly flexed and supported with a pillow (SLR-LBF); norm: 62 ± 6.2 degrees.
3. Active knee extension with the hip at 90 degrees (AKE); norm: 43 ± 10.2 degrees.
4. Passive knee extension with the hip at 90 degrees (PKE); norm: 31 ± 7.5 degrees.

No significant difference was reported using a dependent t-test comparing methods 1 and 2, but a significant differ-

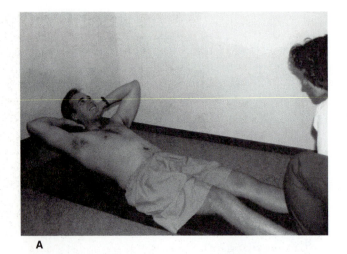

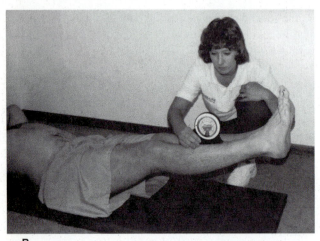

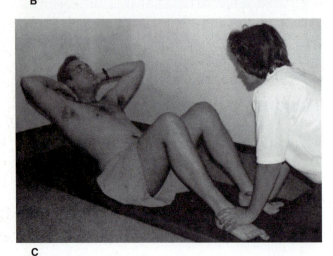

Figure 16–10. Conventional methods for testing trunk/core muscle endurance. **A–C.** Kraus-Weber test for the trunk flexors. **A.** The conventional straight leg sit-up, elevating the trunk to 25 degrees with the feet stabilized. **B.** Double straight leg raise elevating the legs to 25 degrees. **C.** A 90-degree knee flexed, feet fixed on the floor position elevating the trunk to 25 degrees.

ence was noted with methods 3 and 4. The similar angles reported for methods 1 and 2 ($r = .70$, $P < .001$) suggest either method can be used interchangeably (see Chap. 2). The difference in methods 3 and 4 suggests that the AKE test may represent an initial length and the PKE test may represent the maximal length but these should not be interchanged (Gajdosik et al, 1993).

DISCRIMINATIVE PHYSICAL PERFORMANCE TESTS: NIOSH LOW BACK ATLAS TESTS

As introduced in Chapter 14, Moffroid et al (1994) utilized the 25 NIOSH (National Institute of Occupational Safety and Health) tests that were broken down into 53 component items described in the Low Back Atlas (LBA) (Nelson, 1988; Nelson and Nestor, 1988; Moffroid et al, 1992, 1994). Satisfactory reliability was reported with 40 of the 53 tests, while the remaining 13 demonstrated marginal reliability but were felt to be clinically relevant. Twenty-three of the 53 items of the LBA could discriminate between subjects with and without low back pain. Moreover, when taking seven items together, 87% sensitivity for correctly identifying patients with low back pain (true-positives) and 93% specificity for correctly identifying the asymptomatic controls (true-negatives) were calculated. The NIOSH tests for symmetry, strength, passive mobility, and dynamic mobility were addressed by the items listed in Table 16–7. The items printed in bold type make up the seven most reliable tests (Moffroid et al, 1994; Moffroid, personal communication). Appendix Forms G–2 and G–3 represent convenient methods to document the results of the tests.

Moffroid utilized four clustered groups to classify both control subjects and those with low back pain: (1) very fit, (2) flexible, (3) mixed, and (4) unfit and inflexible. Measures that differed by clustered groups included the following:

- *Age:* The "very fit" averaged 25 years of age and the "fit" group, 30 years of age versus the age means of all four subgroups, which varied between 33 and 36 years of age.
- *Davenport Index* (weight/height^2): This was highest in the "very unfit" group (29.9) and the lowest in the "very fit" (22.0). The overall average was 22.5 (Davenport Index, 1978). Other researchers have published findings regarding functional age versus chronological age (Sharkey, 1987).
- *Gender:* The subgroups were equally balanced except the "flexible patient" and "flexible control" subjects were 76% and 92% female, respectively; the "mixed" control group were all female (n = 8); and the "inflexible" patient and control subjects were 65% and 73% male, respectively.
- *Function* (Activities Discomfort Scale [ADS] and Roland-Morris Functional Questionnaire [RMFQ]

Table 16–6: Psoas Muscle Challenges During Various Flexion Exercises Ranked in Chronological Order of Contraction (mean % MVC ± SD)

RANK	EXERCISE	PSOAS 1 (P1)	PSOAS 2 (P2)
1	Cross curl-up	5 ± 3	4 ± 4
2	Curl-up	7 ± 8	10 ± 14
3	Isometric side support	21 ± 18	12 ± 8
4	Straight leg sit-up	15 ± 2	24 ± 7
5	Push-up from feet	24 ± 19	12 ± 5
6	Bent-knee leg raise	24 ± 15	25 ± 8
7	Dynamic side support	26 ± 18	13 ± 5
8	Bent-knee sit-up	17 ± 10	28 ± 7
9	Straight leg raise	35 ± 20	33 ± 8
10	Press heels sit-up	28 ± 23	34 ± 18
11	Isometric hand-to-knee (Right-hand left knee)	56 ± 28	58 ± 18

MVC, maximum voluntary contraction; SD, standard deviation; Pl and P2, test trials 1 and 2.

Compiled from data in Juker et al, 1998.

pertaining to the past week): The "very unfit" group scored significantly higher on the mean number of checked items on the RMFQ (58% vs. 34%, 38%, and 39%, for the other three groups); ADS revealed more difficulty with falling asleep and waking frequently.

- *Psychological measures* (Symptom Check List [SCL90-R]): The "very fit" control subjects were significantly more obsessive/compulsive, and the unfit control and patient subjects were more concerned about overeating (Moffroid et al, 1994).

Measures that were the same among the cluster groups included past history, smoking, handedness, and pain—including nature, duration, and intensity, symptom magnification and outcome (based on working status). The authors stated that others have suggested that physical measures such as those utilized in this study do not have a clear relation to musculoskeletal low back pain. However, they note that when utilized in subclassifications, the physical measures described in this study are able to discriminate, as previously mentioned (Moffroid et al, 1994). Additional study is recommended to further replicate and validate the clustering assignments of patients with musculoskeletal low back pain as described. Also, further study to evaluate the efficacy of specific exercises prescribed by signs and symptoms and, lastly, to study the effect of psychosocial attributes on physical measurements is recommended.

Moffroid and Haugh provide further literature review supporting various approaches for classifying patients by the following categories:

- Physical diagnosis
- Severity
- Length of episode
- Treatment based on specific ROM challenges
- Physical signs
- Self-reported signs
- Disability prediction (Moffroid and Haugh, 1995)

DIAGNOSTIC CLASSIFICATION SYSTEMS

ICD-9 Diagnostic Codes

The 5-digit taxonomy offered by the ICD-9 codes was formulated on the premise that classifications should be true, completely exhaustive, and exclusive (Merskey and Bogduk, 1986). This more detailed classification system recognized that research into low back pain required a more systematic approach, as illustrated by the following example from the taxonomy:

500	low back
30	musculoskeletal
1	single episode
.1	severity indices and times (.1, mild intensity)
.01	cause (.07, unknown origin)

Therefore, the code 531.17 would translate as follows: a single episode of musculoskeletal low back pain of mild intensity lasting less than 6 months and of unknown origin.

Static Back Endurance Test

The static back endurance test measures isometric strength of the back extensor muscles at the point at which the contraction can no longer maintain the patient in the test position. Results are reported in time units (seconds) (see Fig. 16–29, later in this chapter). Since its introduction in 1984, this physical performance test has been included in

Table 16–7: Sensitivity and Reliability of Selected NIOSH Tests[a]

Symmetry	
Pelvic height symmetry (7 tests)	• Iliac crest height: standing (posterior)[a]
	• Iliac crest height: standing (anterior)
	• Iliac crest height sitting (anterior and posterior)
	• **PSIS standing**[a]
	• PSIS sitting
	• ASIS sitting
Hip flexor strength	• Right compared to left
Hip flexor tightness	• Iliopsoas: right compared to left
	• Rectus femoris: right compared to left
Strength	• Upper abdominal muscle strength[a]
	• Lower abdominal strength
	• Dynamic gluteus medius strength (right and left sides)
	• Right hip flexor strength
Passive Mobility	• **Hip rotation (single gravity goniometer) (left and right sides)**[a]
	Internal
	External
	• Single SLR (left and right)
	• Hamstring length (left and right)
	• Gluteus maximus length (left and right)
	• Iliopsoas muscle length (left and right)
	• Rectus femoris muscle length (left and right)
	• Lateral tightness TFL (left and right)
	• Lateral tightness ITT (left and right)
Dynamic Mobility	
Angle difference	• **Forward flexion: Dual inclinometers**[a]
	• **Single straight leg raise**[a]
	• Difference between contour of lumbar spine in erect and slouched sit positions
Lateral bend	• Excursion to the left and right
Presence of *pain* in PPU	• **Whether PPU had any effect**[a]
	• Pain prior to initiation of PPU
	• **Pain at initiation of PPU**
	• Pain at termination of PPU
Characterization of location	(Represents 1 test)
of *pain change* during PPU	• Centralization
	• No change
	• Peripheralization
Presence of *pain after* PPU	• Pain 1 minute after termination of PPU
	• Overall effect of PPU (worse, better, no change in pain)

ASIS, anterior superior iliac spine; ITT: iliotibial tract; PSIS, posterior superior iliac spine; PPU, prone press-up; SLR, straight leg raise; TFL, tensor fascia lata muscle.

[a] Items in bold type make up the 7 NIOSH tests reported to be 87% sensitive and 93% specific for identifying patients verus controls (ie, those with and without low back pain).

Compiled from data in Moffroid et al, 1994.

many studies involving measurement of trunk strength (Biering-Sorensen, 1984; Nicolaisen and Jorgensen, 1985; Jorgensen and Nicolaisen, 1987; Nordin et al, 1987; Mayer and Gatchel, 1988; Hultman et al, 1993; Moffroid et al, 1993; Luoto et al, 1995; Shirado et al, 1995; Ng and Richardson, 1996; Toshikazu et al, 1996; and others). In the original prospective study, this test was reported to have the ability to significantly predict the occurrence of first-time low back pain over a 1-year time period (Biering-Sorensen, 1984). Later, in a cross-sectional study, patients with constant low back pain were found, on average, to have significantly shorter timed endurance compared to healthy controls (Nicolaisen and Jorgensen, 1985). Similarly, those with intermittent low back pain and compared to healthy controls were also found to have weak lumbar extensor endurance (Hultman et al, 1993). Luoto et al (1995) reported that of a total of 126 persons without low back pain at entry, 33 had developed such pain during a 1-year follow-up period. In this group, the static back endurance test was found to be the only physical performance measure associated with first-time low back pain in the follow-up evaluation. Three categories were devised for determining the odds of developing low back pain based on static back endurance performance (Table 16–8).

Concentric and eccentric strength of the trunk flexors and extensors in different test positions was evaluated in 48 subjects with and 50 subjects without low back pain using high-tech equipment (Shirado et al, 1995). Trunk muscle strength was significantly greater in the sitting posture with the feet against the floor ($P < .05$) in both groups. Greater flexor/extensor ratios were found in both the concentric and eccentric contraction modes in patients with chronic low back pain as compared to healthy subjects ($P < .01$), which implies **the extensor muscles weaken more than the flexors in subjects with low back pain.** A significant imbalance between concentric and eccentric strength of LBP patients with low back pain was reported in both the flexors and extensors ($P < .01$). This suggests that the characteristics of trunk muscle strength in patients with chronic low back pain are extremely complicated when being considered in terms of eccentric contraction mode. **Table 16–5 and Figure 16–9 describe an alternative low-tech approach to testing trunk extensor endurance. This approach is reported to be an optional low cost substitute when assessing trunk strength** (Ito et al, 1996).

Because the static back endurance test (Alaranta et al, 1994) **(see Fig. 16–29) and the trunk extensor endurance test** (Ito et al, 1996) **(see Fig. 16–9) are able to differentiate between subjects with and without low back pain, they are important** tests to include in a battery of tests when measuring trunk strength. The section on Quantitative Functional Capacity Evaluation later in this chapter describes the static back endurance procedure (see also Fig. 16–29).

Quebec Task Force Classification

The Quebec Task Force Classification (QTFC) scheme was developed to promote a more uniform diagnostic classification that could "help in making a clinical decision, establishing a prognosis, evaluating the quality of care, and conducting scientific research" (Spitzer et al, 1987) (Table 16–9). A group of 516 patients with sciatica and/or spinal stenosis, who were also part of the Maine Lumbar Spine Study (MLSS) were followed from August 1990 to June 1992 to assess the usefulness of the QTFC scheme (Atlas et al, 1996). ICD-9 categories 5 (fracture), 8 and 9 (postsurgical status), 10 (chronic pain), and 11 (other diagnoses) were omitted in order to standardize the patient population for this study (see Table 16–9). Outcomes were assessed at 1 year for patients treated surgically and nonsurgically utilizing the QTFC scheme. Study results revealed that the **QTFC category did not correlate with resolution of symptoms in postsurgically treated patients with sciatica but did correlate for the nonsurgically treated group of patients.** In addition, spinal stenosis patients were less likely to become asymptomatic as compared to patients with sciatica ($P<.005$, Cochran-Mantel-Haenszel test controlling for treatment received). Similarly, the duration of symptoms at baseline was only significant for the patient group treated nonsurgically. The following percentages of asymptomatic patients were reported:

- Symptoms of less than 6 weeks' duration—56% became asymptomatic
- Symptoms lasting 6 weeks to 3 months—50% became asymptomatic
- Symptoms lasting more than 3 months ($P = .008$, test of trend)—31% became asymptomatic

Patients whose scores were at baseline were also more likely to be asymptomatic at 1 year regardless of whether they were treated surgically or nonsurgically. In the surgical

Table 16–8: Performance Results Utilizing the Static Back Endurance Tests[a]

	NO. OF SUBJECTS	INCIDENCE OF LOW BACK PAIN	ODDS RATIO	MEN (TIME/SEC)	WOMEN (TIME/SEC)
Good performance	43	7	1.0	104–240	110–240
Medium performance	40	9	1.4	58–104	58–110
Poor performance (at risk)	43	17	3.4	<58	<58

[a] The odds of developing low back pain in a 1-year time period were found to be 3.4 times greater when comparing those with poor static back endurance performance to those with good performance.

Reprinted with permission from Luoto et al, 1995.

Table 16–9: Quebec Task Force Classification (modified for the Maine Lumbar Spine Study)[a]

1. **Pain without radiation**
   Duration of pain
   <1 week
   1–6 weeks
   >6 weeks
   Working status
   Working
   Idle

2. **Pain with proximal extremity radiation**
   Duration of pain
   <1 week
   1–6 weeks
   >6 weeks
   Working status
   Working
   Idle

3. **Pain with distal extremity radiation**
   Duration of pain
   <1 week
   1–6 weeks
   >6 weeks

Working status
Working
Idle

4. **Pain with radiation and neurological finding**
   Duration of pain
   <1 week
   1–6 weeks
   >6 weeks
   Working status
   Working
   Idle

6. **Spinal nerve root compression**
   Duration of pain
   <1 week
   1–6 weeks
   >6 weeks
   Working status
   Working
   Idle

7. **Spinal stenosis**

[a] The QTFC scheme has been modified omitting categories 5 (fracture), 8 and 9 (post-surgical), 10 (chronic pain), and 11 (other diagnoses).

Compiled from data in Spitzer et al, 1987.

group, 80% of working versus 55% of idle subjects were asymptomatic ($P<.05$). In the nonsurgical group, 52% of working versus 32% of idle subjects were asymptomatic ($P<.05$).

The severity of baseline symptoms, including frequency and intensity, increased across QTFC categories 2 through 6, whereas baseline functional status, age, gender, education, and disability compensation did not. The percentage of patients who required surgical intervention increased proportionally from 7% in QTFC 1 (low back pain only) to 84% in QTFC 6 (nerve root compression). Similar percentages of patients treated surgically and nonsurgically were noted in QTFC categories 2 through 4 (45% to 56% received surgical treatment), suggesting greater variability and ambiguity regarding treatment decisions for patients in these categories. Surprisingly, in the nonsurgical group, the authors noted that improvement in functional status and symptoms was associated with increasing QTFC category from 2 to 6. In other words, **the more severe the neurological and imaging abnormalities, the *better* the nonsurgical outcome.** Atlas et al (1996) state that this was not a result of later surgical treatment for patients initially treated nonsurgically. Additional long-term analyses were recommended and underway. Spitzer et al (1987) indicated that

only validity, not reliability, was assessed in their study and stressed the need for future reliability studies (Spitzer et al, 1987).

This study supports the following prognostic indicators (Atlas et al, 1996):

- Work status at baseline should be established in all categories, as those not working had worse outcomes.
- Duration of symptoms was significant in the nonsurgical group, only.
- The QTFC scheme was useful in showing improvement in the nonsurgical group, only.
- The QTFC scheme differentiated surgical from nonsurgical patients well in categories 1 and 6, but not in categories 2 through 4.
- The presence of nerve root compression led to a paradoxical improved outcome in the nonsurgically treated group in this study.

Treatment Group Classifications Based on Range of Motion

Delitto, Erhard, and Cibulka published a series of articles between 1988 and 1994 describing the use of McKenzie tests to classify patients with low back pain into various treatment groups (Cibulka et al, 1988; Delitto et al, 1992, 1993; Erhard et al, 1994). By utilizing these tests, they were able to describe "prescriptive validity" for arranging patients into distinct treatment groups (Delitto et al, 1993). For example, a classification category called "extension-biased" included patients whose symptoms improved with at least two extension movements and worsened with at least one flexion movement. Reliability was reported with respect to these tests (Delitto et al, 1992).

In 1993, Delitto et al described four sacroiliac (SI) tests that were performed on their patient population. These tests included (see Appendix Form G–4):

1. Altered posterior superior iliac spine (PSIS) heights in a sitting position
2. Standing flexion PSIS test—a change in the PSIS heights when testing standing versus in forward flexion
3. Supine to long-sitting test—a change in leg length measured at the medial malleolli when comparing supine to a sit-up ("long-sitting") position (similar to a straight leg sit-up)
4. Prone knee flexion test—a leg length change when comparing straight knee versus flexed knee positions.

When three of the four sacroiliac tests are positive, the patient is considered to have a sacroiliac lesion. A percentage of agreement beyond chance of identifying the three or four tests was previously reported (kappa = .88) (Cibulka et al, 1988).

In their 1994 study, Erhard et al, showed that manipulation was a crucial component of the group treated with the exercise program. More specifically, the group treated with exercise alone compared poorly to the combined exercise and manipulation treatment group to a level of statistical significance ($P<.05$). In this study, 24 patients were randomly assigned to either an extension exercise–only group or a manipulation and extension exercise group by the toss of a coin. The "extension-bias" group was treated by an extension-oriented approach proposed by McKenzie (1989). This approach included such exercises as prone press-ups, the use of a lumbar roll, and postural instruction. The second group was treated with manipulation, which was performed with the patient supine and the pelvis held flat to the table while the shoulders were rotated toward the therapist (Fig. 16–11).

The second group was instructed in an exercise referred to as the hand-heel rock (Fig. 16–12). This exercise combines nonweight-bearing repetitions of flexion, followed by extension, prone press-ups. **I have found the hand-heel rock exercise to be very effective in re-establishing spinal functional ROM in both flexion- and extension-biased patients (after the radicular component remains centralized).**

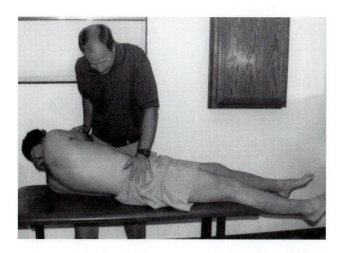

Figure 16–11. The manipulation approach utilized is designed to affect the sacroiliac joint. This is accomplished by stabilizing the supine patient's pelvis by maintaining downward pressure on the contralateral anterior superior iliac spine (ASIS) and applying torque to the trunk toward the ipsilateral side, using the lower elbow for leverage.

Test outcomes were measured by the Oswestry Low Back Pain Disability scores (see Chap. 6) administered initially, midway, at discharge, and at 1 month after discharge. An Oswestry score below 11 was used as the cutoff for discharge or preparation for return to work (RTW), which was determined case specifically. Results favored the manipulation group, as discharge criteria at 1 week post-treatment were met by 9 of 12 manipulation/extension subjects compared to only 2 of the 12 extension group subjects. The initial, 3-day, and 5 day Oswestry scores for the extension group were 40, 32, and 25, and for the manipulation group, 47, 19, and 6, respectively. At 1 month post-discharge, only 6 of 12 subjects from each group (total of 12) responded to a mailed Oswestry questionnaire. The average scores of those who responded were 22.16 and .66 for the exercise and manipulation/exercise groups, respectively. Also, only 2 of the 6 subjects from the exercise only group met the < 11 score discharge or RTW cutoff defined by Erhard, while all 6 subjects met the criteria (5 of the 6 subjects scored 0 and 1 subject scored 4). Physical examination forms for various McKenzie tests can be found in the Appendix (Forms G–2, G–3, G–4, and G–8).

More recently, Cibulka et al (1998) reported that, in patients with low back pain, without evidence of SI dysfunction, hip external rotation was greater than internal rotation bilaterally. However, in patients with SI dysfunction, hip external rotation was significantly greater unilaterally on the side of posterior innominant. The authors utilized the four SI tests previously described (see Appendix Form G–4) and concluded that **the presence of unilaterally greater hip external rotation in patients with low back pain may help identify those with SI dysfunction.**

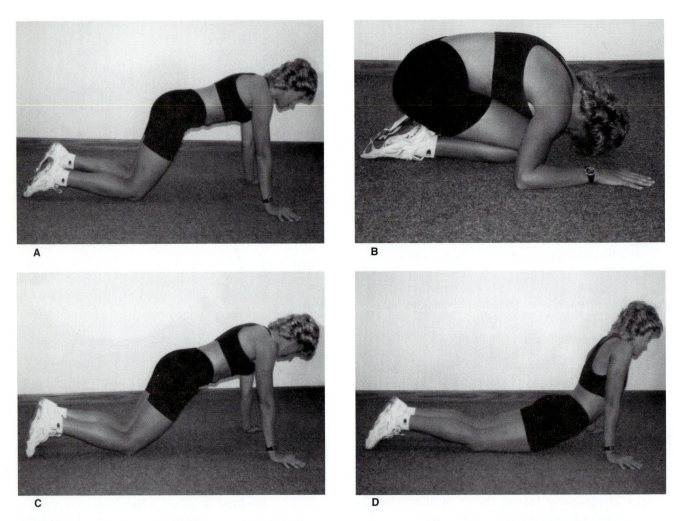

Figure 16–12. The hand-heel rock exercise begins in **(A)** the hands-knee position with the elbows straight. **B.** The patient rocks back approximating the buttock to the heels, curling up in a maximum flexed position. **C.** Next, the patient rocks forward, keeping the elbows straight and allowing the hips and pelvis to sag downward into **(D)** a prone press-up position. The patient then returns to the hands-on-knees position with the elbows straight. The exercise is repeated 6 to 8 times or to patient tolerance, with the patient trying to painlessly reach the extremes of forward and backward rocking. The maneuver is modified according to the patient's symptoms.

CERVICAL SPINE PHYSICAL PERFORMANCE TESTS

CERVICAL SPINE STRENGTH

Thus far, the majority of the discussion has focused on the trunk and low back. Silverman et al (1991) discussed the use of a hand-held dynamometer (MicroFET with three integrated strain gauges) used to test cervical spine strength. Two techniques were used: (1) an isometric approach, and (2) a technique in which the muscle group being tested was overpowered until the isometric force was broken. The subject's head was tested in two different planes of motion: sagittal (flexion, extension), and transverse (right and left

rotation). Chin retraction was used to flatten the cervical lordosis and the neck was flexed. The dynamometer was placed over the forehead and resistance was applied. In rotation, the supine patient rotated the head followed by the chin tuck, limited to the pain-free range. The dynamometer was positioned just above the ear (to avoid auricular nerve compression). The isometric test was applied in a manner so as to maintain a constant head position as the subject initiated the head lift. The break test included a full flexion starting position, and resistance was applied until the muscles "gave way." The contractions were held for 3 to 5 seconds and, a 30- to 60-second resting time factor was allowed between trials. The average of three trials of each technique in each plane of motion was reported initially in pounds and then converted to Newtons (reported force relative to body weight, N-kg⁻¹). Only the break technique was used to compare strength in the neck pain population. Similar to the findings of Vernon et al (1992), results revealed that **subjects with neck pain had significantly weaker anterior cervical flexor muscle strength compared to the control group.** In addition, strength was greater in both planes of movement compared to the control group (*P*<.05). The neck pain group consisted of 11 subjects who were involved in motor vehicle accidents; 13 who had insidious onset; 4 who were injured in falls; and 2 whose etiologies were unknown. Myofascial trigger points or tender points were located in 73% of the neck pain group versus 7% of the pain-free control group. Weakness of the flexors was postulated to be caused by an injury that resulted in reflex inhibition of the flexor muscles via the muscle spindle system. Over time, this causes the anterior neck muscles to weaken and atrophy, leading to postural alteration and increased susceptibility to injury (Silverman et al, 1991). Refer to Figure 16–32 and the associated text, later in this chapter, for a modification of this described technique.

CERVICAL RANGE OF MOTION, SAGITTAL MUSCLE STRENGTH, FLEXION RELAXATION PHENOMENON

Bussieres (1994) measured the reliability, validity, and usefulness of three outcome measures, including cervical ROMs, sagittal neck muscle strength, and the presence or absence of **flexion relaxation phenomenon (FRP)** in the neck. After reviewing 59 articles and 2 textbooks, normative data for cervical range of motion (CROM) was cited, based on the results segregated by age and gender (Foust et al, 1973; Lind et al, 1989; Youdas et al, 1992) (see Chapter 14 for more information). Muscle strength revealed a flexor/extensor ratio of 1:1.1 to 1:75 (average, 1.43) in normal subjects, suggesting the extensors are, on average, 43% stronger than the flexors (Foust et al, 1973). Others have reported similar findings (Moroney et al, 1988). Flexion relaxation refers to relaxation of the extensor muscles at full flexion. More specifically, **the antagonistic role the extensor muscles play during flexion is replaced at full flexion by passive support offered by the ligamentous and articular structures in normal subjects** (Gracovetsky et al, 1990). Loss of this phenomenon is indicative of an abnormal condition and has been demonstrated in the cervical (Harms-Ringdahl and Ekholm, 1987; Schuldt and Harms-Ringdahl, 1988) and lumbar spine (Triano and Schultz, 1987; Ahern et al, 1990).

RAPIDITY OF ARM MOTION IN PREDICTING NECK PAIN

The speed of repetitive arm motion and its ability to predict neck pain was studied in a population of 486, 35- to 54-year-old subjects in Finland (Lauren et al, 1997). Because psychomotor factors have been theorized to play a role in the cause of spinal disorders, the hypothesis was made that motor skills, as demonstrated by arm motion speed, can provide protection against neck pain. Outcomes were followed by the use of a questionnaire regarding neck pain and several tests including arm motion speed as well as upper extremity static and dynamic strength. Of the 124 subjects that reported no neck pain in the prior year, 23 (19%) reported neck pain on re-examination. Neck pain incidence was significantly greater in both the least and the most rapid quintiles of arm motion speed compared to the medium quintiles. This finding did not take into account factors such as age, sex, smoking, physical activity at work or leisure, psychological distress score, or strength measures of the upper extremities, although these factors were significant covariates of the arm motion speed at the baseline assessment. When adjusted for these factors, the odds ratio of having neck pain in the most and least rapid quintiles of arm motion speed were 8.68 (confidence interval [CI], 1.85 to 40.75), and 9.57 (CI, 2.21 to 41.52), respectively. Arm speed was measured by counting the time taken to move the dominant hand from one testboard to the other as rapidly as possible. The speed at which neck pain was more prevalent was less than 14.9 seconds and greater than 23.8 seconds, and the incidence of neck pain was 8 and 9, respectively, compared to 6, total, in the middle three groups collectively (arm speed, 14.9 to 3.7). This means that people with either very slow or rapid arm motion speeds are significantly at higher risk of developing neck pain versus those ranked in the medium categories. Factors associated with high risk include the following:

Predicted Slowness

- Gender (females—odds ratio [OR], 1.48)
- Static arm endurance (OR .98)
- Physical activity at work or leisure (OR—light/work, 1.00; light to moderate/leisure, 1.00)

Predicted Rapidity

- Gender (males—OR, 1.00)
- Physical activity at work or leisure (OR—heavy/leisure, .69)
- Dynamic hand strength (OR—.87)
- Finger dexterity (Purdue Pegboard) (OR, 1.09)

The authors speculate that rapidity in arm motion might be related to repetitive overloading to proximal upper extremities due to high peak forces and subsequent high inertial forces (Lauren et al, 1997). Also, minor trauma may be more prevalent with high-speed activities. On the other hand, slowness in arm movement may support early degenerative signs resulting in psychomotor slowness as a reaction to pain production. The findings of this study suggest that psychomotor or motor control tests such as this may be worthwhile additions to future studies focusing on risk factors for neck pain.

TEST FOR CERVICAL
SPINE PROPRIOCEPTION

Altered proprioception from the articular capsules of the facet joints and other mechanoreceptors of the surrounding soft tissues of the spine have been implicated with spinal injury (Bly and Sinnot, 1991; Bullock-Saxton et al, 1993; Fitz-Ritson, 1995).

Anatomy and Pathogenesis
of the Proprioception System

Before discussing the test associated with cervical spine proprioceptive function, a short discussion of the anatomy and pathogenesis of the proprioception system will heighten the reader's appreciation of this topic. Four types of neural receptors have been identified either in or near joints. Three have been classified as mechanoreceptors and one as a nociceptor, or pain receptor (Wyke, 1967). The mechanoreceptors have been considered to be important participants in the proprioceptive system (Newton, 1982; Fitz-Ritson, 1991). The receptors located in the deep intervertebral muscles are thought to participate significantly in proprioceptive input as there is a greater concentration of mechanoreceptors in deep versus superficial muscles (Richmond and Bakker, 1982). It is these deep muscles of the paraspinal region that are thought to play an important role in the ability to position the head and are important during head and neck movement in general. The functional significance of this point was demonstrated in 1951 when McCouch et al showed that the cat's tonic neck reflex was lost only after the deeper nerves close to the intervertebral joints were severed as opposed to those nerves supplying the superficial, prime moving muscles. Similarly, a change in the vestibulo-ocular reflex occurred only after deep cervical spine muscle stimulation, not after stimulation of the larger, less proprioceptive superficial muscles (Hikosaka and Maeda, 1973). In addition, results of returning proprioceptive function for patients with chronic neck pain (greater than 4 months) were obtained by cervical manipulation significantly more often than with muscle stretching only (Rogers, 1997). This latter study helps to differentiate the role of the joint proprioceptors compared to the mechanoreceptors of the paraspinal musculature, and results suggest **the mechanoreceptors of the joint play the more important role in proprioception.** When comparing balance and body sway in healthy middle-aged adults versus those with low back pain (Bly and Sinnot, 1991), as well as the kinesthetic dysfunction in patients with cervical pain (Revel et al, 1991), the concept of treating spinal dysfunction for balance and dizziness disturbance appears to make good sense.

These data—in addition to the studies discussing altered proprioceptive sensory input following ankle, knee, and other joint related injuries—strongly support the **importance of articular function in the treatment of proprioceptive disorders** (Bosien et al, 1955; Freeman et al, 1965; Hocherman et al, 1984; Reid et al, 1987; Slosberg, 1988; Barrack et al, 1989; Bullock-Saxon et al, 1993; Hall

et al, 1995; Murphy, 1995; Rogers, 1997). Further detailed information on this subject can be found in *Conservative Management of Cervical Spine Syndromes,* by Donald R. Murphy, DC, DACAN (in press, 1999).

QUANTITATIVE FUNCTIONAL
CAPACITY EVALUATION

The Quantitative Functional Capacity Evaluation (QFCE) was developed in 1995 with the objective of creating a low-cost, time-efficient, valid and reliable method of evaluating the functional capacity of a patient (Yeomans and Liebenson, 1996). The QFCE provides objective baselines of physical performance. These baselines can track outcomes in an active care rehabilitation program when repeated during the course of active care and/or at the conclusion of the program. **The QFCE provides an outcome assessment instrument that can be used both as an objective barometer for measuring change in function over time ("descriptive"), and as an aid in determining weak functional links to be addressed specifically in the rehabilitation program ("prescriptive").** The functional tests measure factors such as flexibility, strength, coordination, endurance, aerobic capacity, posture, and balance. There is a common thread that connects the subjective outcome assessment instrument(s) and the objective QFCE: both instruments enable the HCP to document changes in symptoms and function over time. Therefore, as an outcome tool, the QFCE serves as a method that the HCP can use when making clinical decisions such as changes in treatment approach, referral, and discharge with or without permanent residuals. The QFCE is designed not to replace but, rather, to compliment other qualitative, less "objective," tests such as motion or end-feel palpation, postural and gait analysis, and observation of altered movement patterns. These tests are well described elsewhere (Liebenson, 1996).

Another goal—to incorporate the QFCE into a computerized format in order to prepare a database for clinical research objectives—has been accomplished. More specifically, the CareTrak program will calculate the percent difference from the published normative data and the patient's results as well as the percent change from exam 1 to exam 2 dates. When both the QFCE data and the subjective tool data (such as Oswestry Low Back Pain Disability Questionnaire) are entered into CareTrak, the information can be used to generate reports by patient, diagnostic classification, age/gender, and other categories on a weekly, monthly, quarterly, or other basis. These options allow the HCP to offer his or her personal outcomes data in such practical situations as when negotiating for an insurance contract or applying for a position in a learning facility, or in the many other applications where quality control measures are useful. **Having the capability to establish quality control measures in the current health care marketplace offers distinct advantages by placing the HCP well ahead of the competition who may not offer this type of infor-**

CLINICAL TIP 16–2
Obtaining the CareTrak Program

The CareTrak program can be obtained by contacting: The Gym Ball Store, 16776 Bernardo Center Dr., Suite 101, San Diego, CA 92128-2558, or by phone at (800) 393-7255. Try out CareTrak at www.caretrak-outcomes.com

---

mation. Whether or not the data derived from the QFCE is utilized in a computerized or noncomputerized format, it can be used to generate reports to document "medical necessity." This, in turn, will enhance patient education, as well as communication with insurance companies to support the need for further care or special testing needs, and with other co-treating physicians and therapists to facilitate the process of establishing maximum therapeutic benefit and, thus, support case closure or treatment change. Therefore, the value of the information derived from objective outcomes assessment using the QFCE has many applications and can help guide the HCP in clinical decision making, especially at a time in care when provocative testing is often not very helpful.

In the following pages, each test of the QFCE is fully explained and the appropriate reference given. If the original reference was not clear, I contacted the principal author of the article in which the specific test was described, and the additional information that I gathered has been incorporated into the text. Because low-tech functional testing is gaining such interest in the research community, it is probable that the QFCE will be updated from time to time to stay current as well as to utilize new valid and reliable approaches that measure function.

TEST COMPONENTS OF THE QFCE

When performing the tests included in the QFCE, it is important to follow the instructions of each test as precisely as possible. One example of the benefit of performing the tests correctly was noted in Ekstrand et al's (1982) study. After using the tests for 2 months and making subsequent refinements, the authors observed an improvement in the CV from 7.5 ± 2.9 to 1.9 ± .7. This was accomplished by paying attention to the following details (Ekstrand et al, 1982):

- Standardizing inclinometer placement and making sure the pendulum of the gravity type swings freely
- Stiffening up the examination table (plywood with Velcro bands)
- Identifying bony anatomical landmarks (placing marks on skin)
- Standardizing the examination bench height for each visit

Each test of the QFCE is described in the following pages in the order in which it should be performed.

Pain Rating Test
Test 1. Visual Analogue Scale
This test evaluates the patient's perception of his or her pain level on a 0–10 pain scale and is completed at the beginning and conclusion of the QFCE. For a more in-depth description of outcome tools for pain assessment, refer to Chapter 6. The approach utilized is the Visual Analogue Scale (VAS), a 10-cm line containing two pain descriptors at each end ("no pain" or "0" and "unbearable pain" or "10"). Specific instructions are given to the patient to answer each question as to the pain level that is perceived "right now." Overlaying a transparent 10-cm ruler on the line and recording the centimeter and millimeter markings completes scoring. For example, a 0–10 scale is used where 1 cm = 1/10 pain, 5.5 cm = 5.5/10 pain, and so on. The VAS is completed both before and after the QFCE (see Appendix Form G–5). (For further information, see the following sources: Reading, 1979; Melzack, 1987; Dworkin et al, 1990; Von Korff et al, 1992, 1993).

Standing Tests
Test 2. Repetitive Squat
The repetitive squatting test assesses joint mobility of the hip, knee, ankle, and foot as well as the strength, endurance, and coordination of the hip and knee extensors. The patient is instructed to stand with the feet 15 cm apart and squat downward to a point where the thighs are parallel to the floor, and then return to the upright position. Each repetition is completed in a 2- to 3-second period, and the test is repeated until a maximum number of repetitions are achieved or the number 50 is reached, whichever occurs first. Both the quality of movement and the number of repetitions are observed; the information derived from the quality of movement gives rise to treatment and exercise prescription, while recording the number of repetitions tracks outcomes (Fig. 16–13). If the patient is having a difficult time and compensating significantly to complete a squat, it may be safest to end the test and record the maximum number of repetitions to the point of quality of movement failure. **Therefore, the quantitative information assesses outcomes while the qualitative data drives treatment goals.** The normative data is age-, gender-, and occupational-specific as depicted in Table 16–10 (Alaranta et al, 1994). (For further information, see the following sources: Alaranta et al, 1994; Rissanen et al, 1994.)

Test 3. Range of Motion: Lumbar Spine
Lumbar ROMs assess both the articular structures as well as the muscular components of the spine (Fig. 16–14). For a complete description of the proper procedure for using inclinometers, refer to Chapter 14. In general, for sagittal plane assessment (flexion/extension), the center of one inclinometer is placed at the T12 spinous process and a second inclinometer over the sacrum, with the center placed at a line connecting the posterior superior iliac spines, or at S2. Placing the base of the inclinometer horizontally at the same bony landmarks so that the needle hangs freely assesses frontal plane motion (lateral flexion). The true lum-

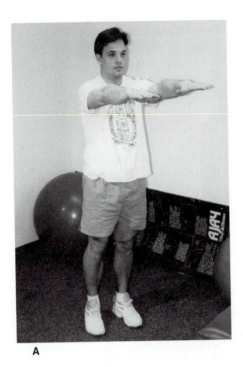 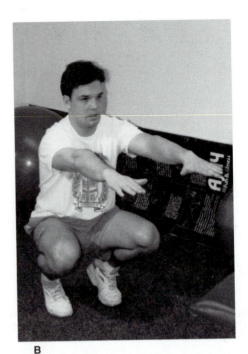

A   B

Figure 16–13. *Repetitive squatting test.* This test is performed by squatting to a thigh-horizontal position, returning upright, and repeating each repetition in a 2- to 3-second cadence. The score is reported by counting the number of repetitions (maximum 50) that the patient completes.

bar ROM is calculated by taking the difference between the two inclinometers at the endpoint of movement using the equation, T12 − S2 = x degrees. The average of three consecutive readings is calculated and if the three individual readings fall within 5 degrees or 10% of the average, the highest of the three readings is recorded. This may be repeated a maximum of six times in an attempt to achieve three consecutive readings within the 5-degree/10% validity rule (American Medical Association, 1993). Table 16–11 includes normative data for the lumbar spine

(Mayer et al, 1984, 1994). Refer to Chapter 14 for a discussion of age- and gender-adjusted normative data. (For further information, see the following sources: Mayer et al, 1984; Hyytiainen et al, 1991; American Medical Association, 1993; Mayer et al, 1994).

Waddell Nonorganic Low Back Pain Signs

The Waddell nonorganic low back pain (LBP) signs are objective measures for evaluating abnormal psychosocial issues. These tests are performed by purposely *not* attempting

Table 16–10: Normative Data for Repetitive Squatting Test[a]

	MALES (N = 242)						FEMALES (N = 233)					
	Blue Collar		White Collar		All		Blue Collar		White Collar		All	
AGE	X	SD	x	SD	x	SD	x	SD	x	SD	x	SD
35–39	39	13	46	8	42	12	24	11	27	12	26	12
40–44	34	14	45	9	38	13	22	13	18	8	20	12
45–49	30	12	40	11	33	13	19	12	26	13	22	13
50–54	28	14	41	11	33	14	13	10	18	14	14	11
35–54	33	14	43	10	37	13	20	12	23	12	21	12

[a] Data are broken down by age (left column), gender (males, left half; females, right half), and occupation (blue collar, white collar, and the average [all]). The average or mean number of repetitions is found in the column labeled "x" and the standard deviation (SD) is in the adjacent column. The last row is the average of all subjects tested (34 to 54 years old). A maximum of 50 repetitions is allowed.

Reprinted with permission from Alaranta et al, 1994.

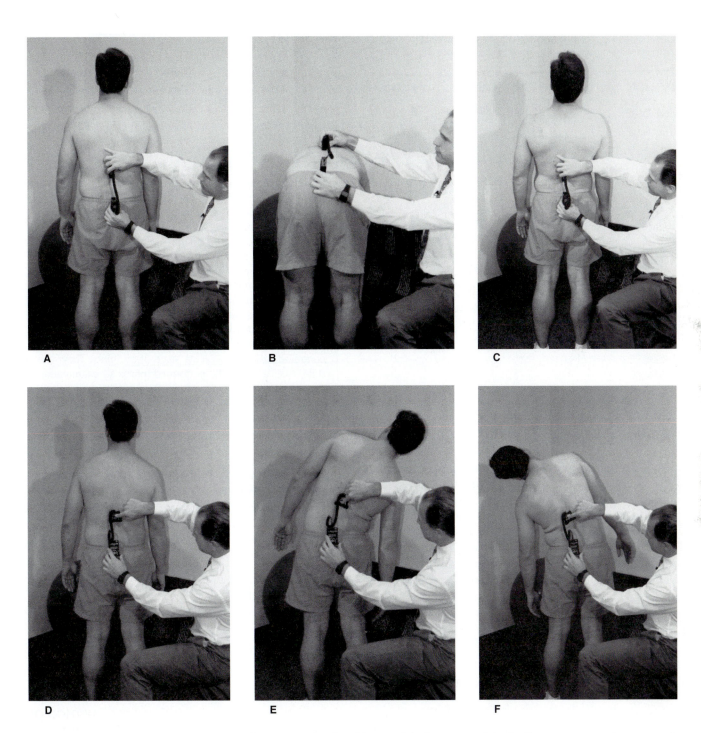

Figure 16–14. *Lumbar ranges of motion.* This test is completed by careful placement of the inclinometers over the appropriate bony landmarks as described in the text. **A.** Neutral standing. **B.** Flexion. **C.** Extension. **D.** Lateral flexion neutral. **E.** Right lateral flexion. **F.** Left lateral flexion.

to provoke pain, which is in direct opposition to the typical provocative orthopedic test in which pain reproduction is the goal. The result of the nonorganic test is reported as "positive" or "negative." It is important to determine if a physiological or organic explanation for the test response exists and repeat the test as many times as needed in order to assure evaluator reliability. Hence, these tests must be performed carefully, as it is easy to apply the test too vigor-

ously, which may result in a false positive test result. There are a total of eight tests that make up the five Waddell signs because three of the five signs include two separate tests (Table 16–12). If one of the two tests in a sign is positive, the sign is considered positive. In other words, **when a sign consists of two tests, it is not necessary for both tests to be positive to result in a positive sign.** The final score is documented as the total number of positive signs

Table 16–11: Normal Lumbar Ranges of Motion

MOTION	MEAN AND SD[a]	% OF NORMAL[b]
True flexion	58° +/– 9.6°	89.2 (65°)
True extension	22° +/– 9.7°	72.7 (30°)
Pelvic flexion	60° +/– 13.8°	109.1 (55°)
Straight leg raise		
Right	77° +/– 12.5°	102.9 (75°)
Left	77° +/– 12.0°	102.9 (75°)
Right lateral flexion	24° +/– 7.4°	96.9 (25°)
Left lateral flexion	25° +/– 8.2°	100.6 (25°)

[a] The normal lumbar ROMs of the railroad workers studied by Mayer et al (1994), including the mean and standard deviation, are found in the middle column.
[b] The percent of normal is located in the right hand column, and the normal ROMs are in parentheses. For 160 male railroad workers, average age, 35 years (+/– 8); height, 70 in (+/– 3); weight, 187 lbs (+/– 29).

Compiled from data in Mayer et al, 1994.

over five (eg, 2/5). When three or more of the five signs are positive (3/5, 4/5, or 5/5), nonorganic LBP must be considered and the psychosocial issues clinically addressed.

Test 4. Nonorganic Low Back Pain—Sign 1: Tenderness
The first of the Waddell signs is called *tenderness,* which consists of two tests for superficial and deep tenderness. **Superficial tenderness** is tested by applying a light touch over the lumbar skin in a manner that should *not* normally provoke pain (Fig. 16–15). The tenderness associated with a localized band of tissue (a trigger point) can be ignored as pain can normally occur due to the innervation supplied by the posterior primary rami when nerve irritation is present. A nonorganic pain response is a disproportionate or exag-

<table>
<tr><td colspan="1">CLINICAL TIP 16–3
Organic and Nonorganic Application
of Orthopedic Provocative Tests</td></tr>
<tr><td>

I have observed that any orthopedic provocative test can be performed in an organic and a nonorganic manner. More specifically, the test can first be performed in a nonorganic manner or in a manner that should not physiologically create a pain response. For example, a Kemp's test is performed first with only slight lateral flexion, extension, and rotation of the lumbar spine. If a pain response occurs, the patient should be quite acute in presentation; or the response can be interpreted as a nonorganic pain response. Of course, only the Waddell signs have been validated and time-tested; therefore, **caution must be exercised when using the many published provocative tests in a nonorganic manner. Furthermore, any non-Waddell test that is positive for nonorganic pain should not be included in the 0–5 Waddell scoring scheme.** Waddell et al point out in the original 1980 article that these signs are contraindicated in the acute stage of an injury. They also state that a carefully performed physical examination should yield the same conclusion or results, which supports my own observations regarding application of provocative tests in a nonprovocative manner.

</td></tr>
</table>

gerated reaction to a non-noxious stimulus resulting in inappropriate pain behavior such as a "jump-sign" or withdrawal response. **Deep tenderness** is characterized by a nonanatomical, wide area of pain, not localized to one structure or anatomical region. (For more information, see Waddell et al, 1980.)

Test 5. Nonorganic Low Back Pain—Sign 2: Simulation
The second of the Waddell signs, **simulation,** is also comprised of two tests: axial compression and trunk rotation.

Table 16–12: Tests that Comprise Waddell's Low Back Pain Signs

SIGNS	EXAMINATION METHOD	METHOD OF REPORTING
1. Tenderness		+ or –
a. Superficial	Light pressure to skin	
b. Deep	Non-anatomical, widespread pain	
2. Simulation		+ or –
a. Axial compression	Light downward pressure on calvarium	
b. Trunk rotation	Minimal twisting of the pelvis without excess shoulder rotation	
3. Distraction	Sitting (distracted) SLR is nonpainful versus nondistracted supine SLR	+ or –
4. Regional neurology		+ or –
a. Motor	Nonanatomical or inconsistent findings during a routine neurological	
b. Sensory	examination	
5. Exaggeration	Noted at any time during the physical examination	+ or –

SLR, straight leg raise.

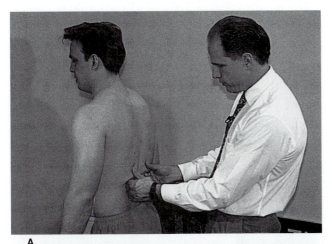

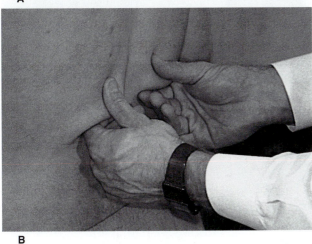

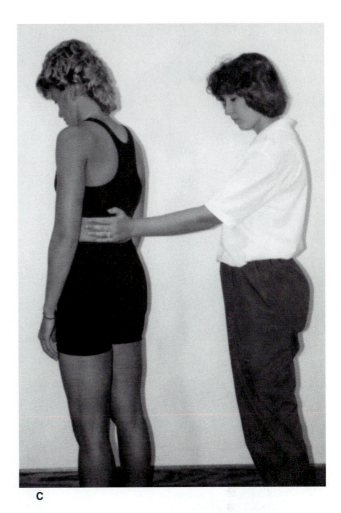

Figure 16–15. *Tenderness* (Waddell sign 1). The test was originally described as lightly pinching the skin over the paraspinal lumbar area as depicted in **(A)** and **(B).** However, false-positive results can occur, especially in those with little subcutaneous adipose tissue. **C.** A modification of this test is recommended by lightly touching the patient's low back in a manner that should not provoke pain. When a pain response is reported, this sign is considered positive.

With the patient standing, the **axial compression** test is performed by placing light pressure on the occiput in the direction of the floor, similar to a cervical compression test but performed in a manner that should *not* provoke a pain response (Fig. 16–16A). A positive test for nonorganic low back pain is documented if an exaggerated low back pain response is observed. Neck pain may occur with axial loading and, hence, this test may be contraindicated as described in the original article (Waddell et al, 1980). If this occurs, a modification of the test should be performed in which downward pressure is employed on the shoulders (Fig. 16–16B).

The second of the two tests that make up the **simulation sign** is that of **trunk rotation.** The HCP stands behind the weight-bearing patient and, while grasping the patient's wrists and pressing them against the hips, the pelvis and trunk are manually rotated in a manner that should *not* normally provoke a pain response (Fig. 16–16C through E). This procedure will ensure that the patient will not rotate the shoulders beyond the move-

ment that is occurring at the pelvis. A positive test for nonorganic low back pain is documented if an exaggerated pain response is observed. Note that if lumbar nerve root pain is present, the test may be contraindicated as a false-positive pain response may occur. Therefore, the decision as to whether or not to perform this test should be made by correlating other tests, including a straight leg raise for nerve tension assessment and neurological examination findings. (For more information, see Waddell et al, 1980.)

Test 6. Gastrocnemius/Ankle Dorsiflexion Test
The function assessed by the gastrocnemius and soleus dorsiflexion tests are important in the QFCE evaluation because of the vital role the ankle joint plays in maintaining balance and coordination and its important relationship to the **"kinetic chain."** The kinetic chain refers to the human structure, in which the first link is in contact with the floor and last link represents the head. Each "link" of the chain represents a kinetic body part that, when dysfunctional, al-

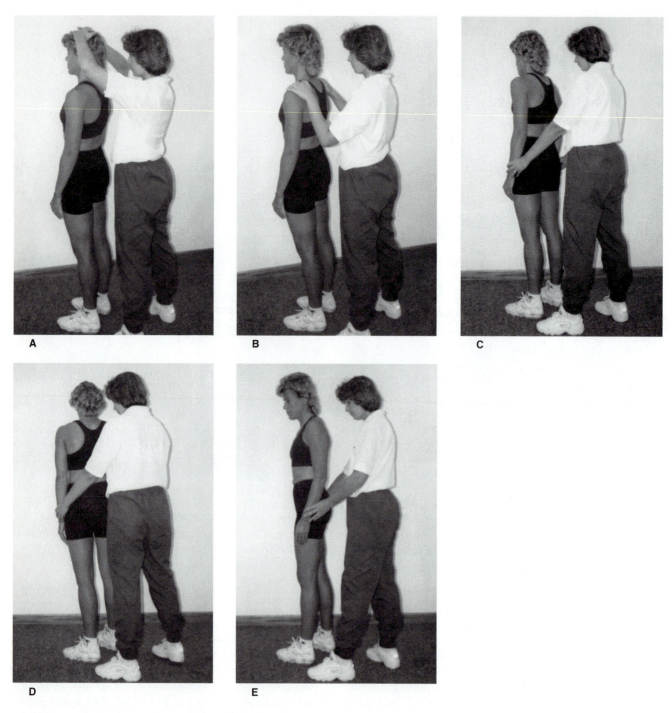

Figure 16–16. *Simulation* (Waddell sign 2). This test is made up of two tests: axial compression (**A** and **B**) and trunk rotation (**C–E**). **A.** Axial compression is performed by applying a light downward pressure on the patient's occiput in a manner that should not provoke low back pain. **B.** If cervical spine problems exist, a modification of applying downward pressure at the shoulders is suggested. **C–E.** Trunk rotation is performed by mildly rotating the patient, grasping their wrists in the neutral position (**C**). Grasping the patient by the wrists and pressing the arms against the hips will minimize the chance for excessive trunk rotation. The patient is then rotated *slightly* to the right (**D**) and left (**E**). Provocation of pain is indicative of a positive sign.

ters biomechanics results. For example, the stability of the subtalar joint is highly dependent on the flexibility of the ankle and must be intact for proper proprioceptive function and kinetic integration with locomotion.

Patient position is upright, standing with the feet par-

allel and knees straight (Ekstrand et al, 1982). The muscle length of the gastrocnemius is measured at maximum knee extension and ankle dorsiflexion and, hence, evaluates the tension of the gastrocnemius muscle as well as the integrity of the ankle joint (Fig. 16–17). The inclinometer is posi-

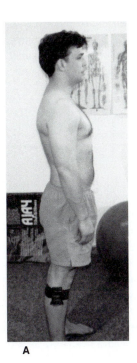
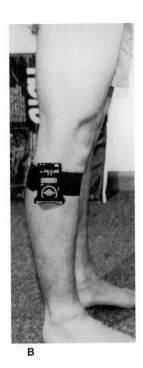
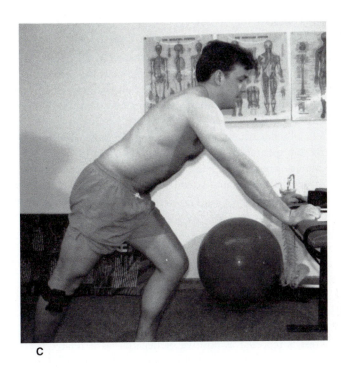

A   **B**   **C**

Figure 16–17. *Gastrocnemius/ankle dorsiflexion test.* **A** and **B.** With the knee extended, an inclinometer is "zeroed out" in the neutral standing position. **C.** Keeping the knee locked in extension, the patient steps forward with opposite leg and may lean on a wall or table to maintain balance. After the heel lifts up slightly and is then returned to the floor, the measurement is read and the degrees of ankle dorsiflexion range of motion is recorded.

tioned above the lateral malleolus and "zeroed" in the upright standing neutral position. The angle of the lower leg is then measured at maximum ankle dorsiflexion while keeping the heel down. To facilitate this process, the patient may place the hands on a wall while leaning forward to a point just as the heel raises off the floor. The patient then rocks back slightly so that the heel comes in contact with the floor at which point the angle is measured. The normative data reveals 22.5 degrees, standard deviation (SD) .7; intra-assay CV 2.2%, and inter-assay CV 2.5% (Ekstrand et al, 1982). (For more information, see Ekstrand et al, 1982.)

Test 7. Soleus/Ankle Dorsiflexion Test (Knee Flexed)
This test is similar to the gastrocnemius dorsiflexion test except the measurement is taken with knee flexion, which essentially removes the tension of the gastrocnemius muscle. At this point, the length of the soleus muscle as well as the integrity of the ankle joint articulation can be assessed (Fig. 16–18). The patient's position in this test is standing with one leg on the floor and the ankle being tested placed on a bench (Ekstrand et al, 1982). The knee is flexed and the ankle is dorsiflexed to a maximum angle while maintaining heel-to-bench contact. The normative data reveals 24.9 degrees, SD .8; intra-assay CV 2.2%; and inter-assay CV 2.6% (Ekstrand et al, 1982). (For more information see the following sources: Ekstrand et al, 1982; Wang et al, 1993.)

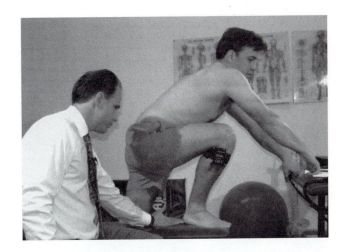

Figure 16–18. *Soleus/Ankle dorsiflexion test.* The same procedure is followed as described in Figure 16–17A and B. The foot is placed on a flat bench allowing the knee to flex and the ankle to dorsiflex. The measurement is taken after the slightly raised heel is returned down to the table top. Eliminating or reducing the table top padding is suggested to minimize the error in assessment when the heel is returned down to the position in which the measurement is taken.

Sitting Tests

Test 8. Nonorganic Low Back Pain—Sign 3:
Distraction (Sitting versus Supine Straight Leg Raise)
This test evaluates for abnormal psychosocial issues. The patient position is seated. The HCP performs a sitting SLR test, mentally distracting the patient and focusing his or her attention away from the low back by performing a plantar superficial reflex, then rapidly extending the knee. Another distraction technique is for the HCP to say "I'm now going to evaluate the range of motion of your knee joint" and then repeatedly flex and extend the knee from the seated patient position (Fig. 16–19). A positive test is present when little to no pain is noted in the distracted sitting SLR position and a disproportionately high level of pain is observed during the nondistracted supine SLR test. This is often referred to as a positive "flip" sign. Note that, if true sciatic nerve tension signs exist, this test is contraindicated as sharp pain can occur. Also, be cautious as to the speed at which the sitting SLR is performed if nerve tension is suspected. As with the other Waddell nonorganic LBP signs, this test is reported as positive or negative as it relates to nonorganic low back pain, rather than a number (see Table 16–12). (For more information, see Waddell et al, 1980.)

Test 9. Nonorganic Low Back Pain—Sign 4: Regional Neurology
This Waddell sign consists of two tests, which are essentially inconsistent and/or nonanatomical **motor** and/or **sensory** examination findings. This test is performed by completing a standard neurological physical examination that includes deep tendon reflexes, muscle strength, and sensory perception. A positive test is present when the neurological examination findings do not follow an expected anatomical pattern and/or are highly inconsistent.

These findings can include altered motor functions where many muscle groups representing several myotomes are weak. The presence of "breakaway" weakness, whereby the patient suddenly relaxes during muscle testing, indicates one of three possibilities:

1. Pain induced weakness (physiological)
2. A poor voluntary effort (nonorganic)
3. A myopathy (physiological)

The altered sensory findings are of a nondermatomal variety, often with hyperpathia (heightened sensory perception) with or without dysesthesia. **Dysesthesia** is defined as an unpleasant abnormal sensation, whether spontaneous or evoked (Merskey, 1986; Merskey and Bogduk, 1994) (Fig. 16–20). The differential diagnosis of sclerotomal pain must also be considered. **Sclerotomal pain** can arise from any structure derived from the embryological layer of the somite called the sclerotome. The pain origin commonly includes the posterior third of the disc and the articular capsule and joint structure. Symptoms are usually described as a deep ache that is nonspecific with a rather global distribution, sometimes described "bone pain," which does not follow any obvious anatomical pathway. Consider these possible origins of pain and expect multiple signs of nonorganic low back pain before feeling secure about this assessment. This test is reported as positive or negative as it relates to nonorganic low back pain (Table 16–9). (For more information, see Waddell et al, 1980.)

Test 10. Nonorganic Low Back Pain—
Sign 5: Exaggeration/Overreaction
This sign does not consist of a specific test, but rather is applicable to the entire physical examination—whenever ex-

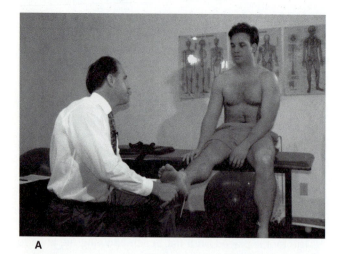

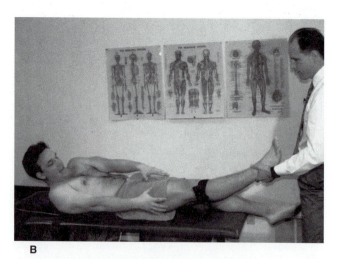

Figure 16–19. *Distraction* (Waddell sign 3). This test includes a nonpainful expression response when a sitting straight leg raising (SLR) test is performed while distracting the patient into thinking about something other than his or her low back pain. **A.** As the knee is extended, the patient is told that the reflex on the bottom of the foot is going to be tested. The second half of the test is a nondistracted supine SLR. **B.** During the supine SLR test without distraction, a positive Waddell sign is reported when an exaggerated expression of pain is observed and no pain behavior was observed during the sitting SLR.

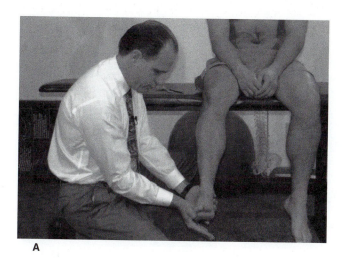
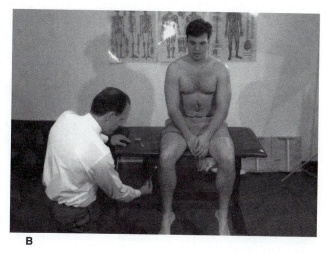

A   **B**

Figure 16–20. *Regional neurology* (Waddell sign 4). This sign of nonorganic pain behavior includes two tests; the motor and sensory components comprising a good neurological examination. **A.** The peroneus longus and brevis muscle is tested bilaterally when assessing the S1 nerve root function in the seated patient. **B.** The sensibility of the skin over the lateral calf is tested and compared bilaterally for symmetry in sensibility perception. When inconsistent and/or nonanatomical findings are encountered with either the motor or sensory test, a positive sign is reported.

aggeration, overreaction, or a disproportionate response such as a tremor, outcry, or collapse occurs. Overreaction may be noted at any time during the consultation or examination. For example, if performing an orthopedic test (such as Kemp's test) results in an verbal outburst response of pain that occurs early into the maneuver, before an end-feel of tissue tension is palpated, a positive test for exaggeration is reported (Fig. 16–21). This test is reported as positive or negative as it relates to nonorganic low back pain (Table 16–12).

When a score of 3 or more Waddell's signs is noted, nonorganic behavior has been demonstrated. This is typi-cally reported as "3/5," communicating to those who re-view the file that the assessment has resulted in a score of 3 out of 5 Waddell signs. It has been my experience that of-ten, only one test is reported as positive, yet nonorganic pain is concluded. Documentation of the Waddell signs can be handwritten, dictated, or completed on a preprinted form (see Appendix Form J–5D). (For more information, see Waddell et al, 1980.)

Test 11. Range of Motion: Cervical Spine
Cervical ROM assessment evaluates both the articular structures and the muscular components of the spine (Fig. 16–22). For a complete description of the proper procedure for using inclinometers, refer to Chapter 14. In general, for sagittal plane assessment (flexion/extension), the center of an inclinometer is placed at the vertex of the calvarium and the other over the T1 spinous process. Frontal plane motion (lateral flexion) is assessed by placing the base of the inclinometer horizontal at the same bony landmarks so that the needle hangs freely. The true cervical ROM is cal-culated by taking the difference between the two incli-nometers at the endpoint of movement, using the equa-tion, $Occip - T1 = x$ degrees. The average of three consecutive readings is calculated, and if the three readings fall within 5 degrees or 10% of the average, the highest of the three readings is recorded. This may be repeated a maximum of six times in an attempt to achieve three con-secutive readings within the 5 degree/10% validity rule (American Medical Association, 1993). Table 16–13 in-cludes normative data for the cervical spine (Mayer et al, 1994). Refer to Chapter 14 regarding a discussion of age- and gender-adjusted normative data. (For more informa-tion, see the following sources: Loebl, 1967; American Medical Association, 1993; Mayer et al, 1994.)

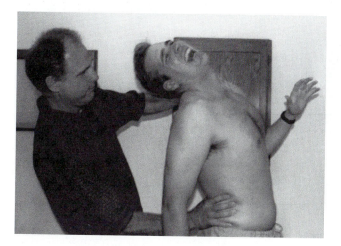

Figure 16–21. *Exaggeration* (Waddell sign 5). Any occur-rence of exaggeration during the physical examination constitutes a positive sign. The photograph shows an exag-gerated response to a Kemp's orthopedic test.

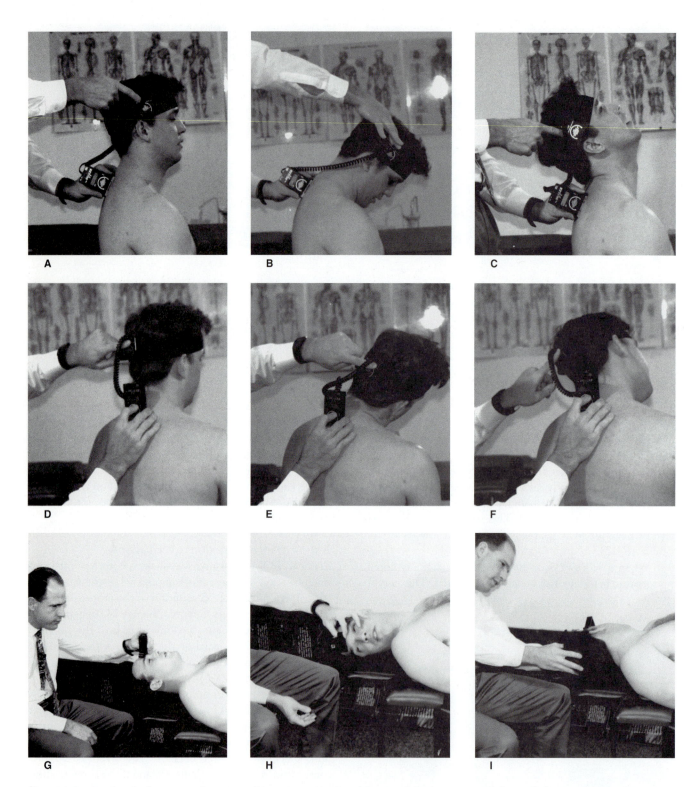

Figure 16–22. *Cervical ranges of motion.* This test is completed by careful placement of the inclinometers over the appropriate bony landmarks, as described in the text. **A.** Neutral sitting. **B.** Flexion. **C.** Extension. **D.** Lateral flexion neutral. **E.** Right lateral flexion. **F.** Left lateral flexion. **G.** Neutral rotation. **H.** Right rotation. **I.** Left rotation

Supine Tests

Test 12. Modified Thomas Test/Hip Extension Test
The modified Thomas test evaluates ROM of the hip and the length or tension of the iliopsoas muscle (Fig. 16–23).

After following the steps outlined in Figure 16–23, record the angle at which tested leg is fully relaxed, hip is extended, and lumbar lordosis is removed.

The normative data is 83.5 degrees, SD 1.1; intrassay

Table 16–13: Normative Data for Cervical Spine Range of Motion

MOTION	MEAN AND SD[a]	% OF NORMAL[b]
Flexion	53° +/– 12.1°	105.6 (50°)
Extension	71° +/– 14.1°	112.6 (63°)
Right lateral flexion	49° +/– 7.2°	109.6 (45°)
Left lateral flexion	50° +/– 7.8°	112.0 (45°)
Right rotation	88° +/– 10.6°	103.3 (85°)
Left rotation	90° +/– 9.6°	105.5 (85°)

[a] The normal cervical ROM of the railroad workers studied by Mayer et al (1994), including the mean and standard deviation, are found in the middle column.

[b] The percent of normal is located in the right-hand column and the normal lumbar ROMs are found in parentheses. For 160 male railroad workers, average age 35 years (+/– 7.5); height 64.9 in. (+/– 2.6); weight 187 lbs (+/– 28.6).

Compiled from data in Mayer et al, 1994.

CV .7%; and interassay CV 1.2% (Ekstrand et al, 1982). (For more information, see Ekstrand et al, 1982; Wang et al, 1993.)

Test 13. Sitting and Supine Straight Leg Raise

Test 13 contains two tests: (a) the sitting/distracted straight leg raise (SLR), which is the second half of test 8 (the Waddell Distraction test, previously described); and (b) the supine SLR, measuring for hamstring length and/or hip ROM. For test 13a, refer to test 8, Figure 16–19, and Table 16–11. The supine SLR is needed to complete Waddell's nonorganic low back pain sign 3 (Waddell et al, 1980).

Test 13b is the SLR or hamstring flexibility test. The SLR hamstring flexibility test evaluates the integrity of the hip joint and the length or tension of the hamstring muscle group (Fig. 16–24). The examiner supports the patient's lower extremity (with the crook of the elbow) and passively raises the straight leg while holding a "zeroed-out" inclinometer on the mid-tibia or on a strap of Velcro to the lateral thigh (5 cm above patella), with the indifferent hand stabilizing the pelvis. The leg is raised to a point of knee flexion (of the leg being tested) or until the pelvis begins to rock and/or the opposite knee flexes. Record the hip flexion angle. Normative data is 70 to 90 degrees (average, 80 degrees) (Ekstrand et al, 1982). (For more information, see Ekstrand et al, 1982.)

Test 14. Repetitive Sit-up

The repetitive sit-up test evaluates the strength and endurance of the rectus abdominus muscle, particularly, the upper portion. The patient is positioned supine with the knees flexed 90 degrees and the ankles secured. The patient performs a sit-up and approximates the thenar pads of the hands to the superior pole of the patella, then curls back down fully to the supine position (Fig. 16–25). The number of repetitions is counted to a maximum of 50, each repetition should take 2 to 3 seconds. The normative data is age-, gender-, and occupation-specific (for blue vs white collar workers) (Table 16–14) (Alaranta et al, 1994). (For more information, see Alaranta et al, 1994.)

Prone Tests

Test 15. Knee Flexion Test/Nachlas

The knee flexion test measures the length or tension of the quadraceps femoris muscle group. The patient is placed in the prone position with the knees straight. The inclinometer is placed on the lower leg and with the knee fully extended (the feet may hang over the edge of the table to ensure the proper position). The inclinometer is reset to "0." The pelvis is strapped down and the knee is passively flexed so that the heel is brought toward the buttocks. The moment hip flexion or hip-hiking occurs, the angle is recorded (Fig. 16–26). The normal angle is 147.9 degrees, SD 1.6; intra-assay CV .5%; and inter-assay CV 1.1 (Ekstrand et al, 1982). (For more information, see Ekstrand et al, 1982.)

Test 16. Repetitive Arch-up Test

The repetitive arch-up test evaluates the strength and endurance of the back extension muscle group. The patient is placed prone supporting the weight of the upper body on a chair with the elbows while the ankles and thighs are strapped down. The anterior superior iliac spines lie just on the table, while the trunk from the waist to the head extend off the table. The patient raises the trunk to the horizontal position, lowers down to a 45-degree angle, and then returns to the horizontal position to complete one cycle (Fig. 16–27). This is repeated for a maximum total of 50 repetitions and is performed at a rate of 2 to 3 seconds per repetition. The number of repetitions is counted and compared to the normative data calculating the percent change using Table 16–15, which is age-, gender-, and occupation-specific (Alaranta et al, 1994). (For more information, see Alaranta et al, 1994.)

Test 17. Hip Range of Motion—Internal and External Rotation

The hip ROM tests measure the physical capacity of the hip in rotation in the prone position. The inclinometer is fixed to the anterior distal third of lower leg with the knee flexed 90 degrees. The pelvis is stabilized with a strap to prevent pelvic rotation, and internal and external rotation of the hip is performed to a point of firm end-feel. The angle is recorded at maximum internal rotation (IR) and external rotation (ER) of the hip, and the test is performed bilaterally (Fig. 16–28). The normative data established by Chesworth et al (1994) are 41 to 45 degrees (mean, 43 degrees) for internal rotation and 41 to 43 degrees (mean, 42 degrees) for external rotation. (For more information, see the following sources: Ellison et al, 1990; American Medical Association, 1993; Chesworth et al, 1994.)

Test 18. Static Back Endurance Test

The static back endurance test measures the endurance of the back extensor muscle group. The starting position is

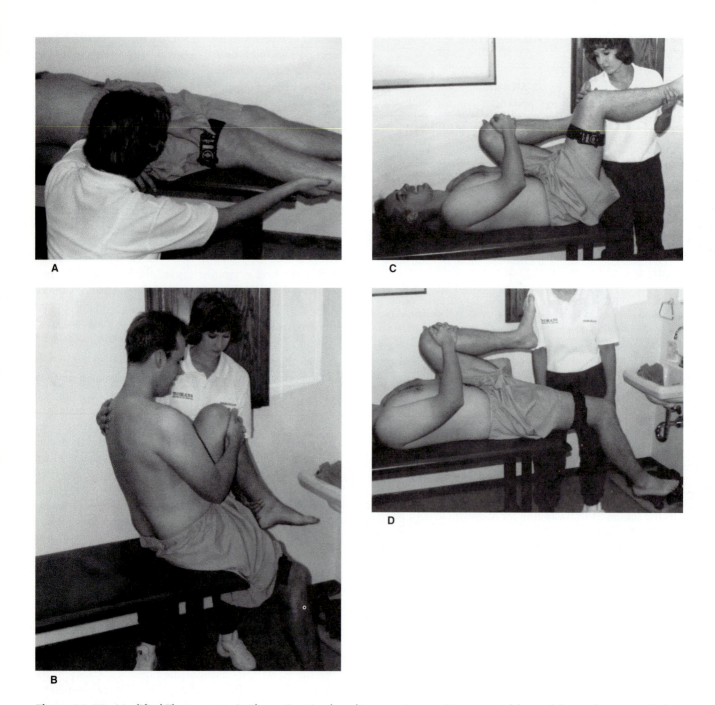

Figure 16–23. *Modified Thomas test.* **A.** The patient is placed in a supine position on a table, and the inclinometer is "ze-roed out." **B.** The patient is carefully repositioned to the end of the table so that the ischii approximate the table's edge and the nontested knee is held to the chest. **C.** The patient is rocked back into a supine position keeping the knee held tight to the chest by both the patient's arms and the examiner's hip by leaning into the foot while the leg being tested is brought to 90 degrees (as read on the inclinometer). **D.** The inclinometer is reset to "0" and the tested leg is brought down to hang freely off the end of the table; the measurement is then recorded.

the same as that for the repetitive arch-up test, earlier: the patient is prone with the anterior superior iliac spines on the end of the table; arms at the sides; and ankles, thighs, and buttocks strapped (Fig. 16–29). The static neutral, horizontal position is held for as long as possible, or 240 seconds, whichever occurs first. The normative data is age-, gender-, and occupation-specific as depicted in Table

16–16 (Alaranta et al, 1994). More recently, McGill reported normative data for the endurance of the low back extensor muscles in a healthy, young (mean age of 23 years) population of 31 men and 44 women (McGill et al, 1999). The mean and standard deviation for males was 146 ± 51, and for females 189 ± 60 seconds. When comparing this to the normative data reported by Alaranta in healthy

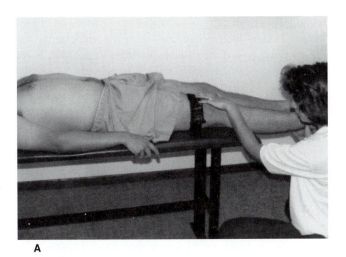

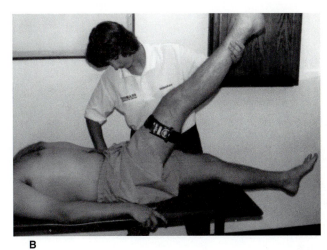

A   **B**

Figure 16–24. *Straight leg raise (SLR).* The "zeroed-out" inclinometer is placed on the patient's distal lateral thigh **(A)** while the lower extremity is passively raised **(B)** until pelvic rotation, opposite knee flexion, and/or homolateral knee flexion occurs.

35- to 54-year-old male and female white-collar workers, the greatest endurance strength was found in the 45- to 49-year-old population reported at 131 ± 64 and 122 ± 73, males and females, respectively (Alaranta, 1994). In this population, males were found to have greater extensor endurance compared to females, opposite of that reported by McGill. (For more information, see Biering-Sorenson, 1984; Hyytiainen et al, 1991; Alaranta et al, 1994; and Rissanen et al, 1994.)

Test 19. Grip Strength Dynamometry
Grip strength dynamometry tests for upper extremity grip strength and can also facilitate the evaluation of psychosocial issues such as patient effort and fear-avoidant behavior. The patient position may be sitting or standing, and the test arm is held at a 90 degree elbow-flexed position (Fig. 16–30). **It is my opinion that the most important concept when performing this test is to locate a pain-free arm position in order to avoid a "false-positive" test due to pain-induced weakness.** Because the normative data tables were derived from grip testing performed on a Jamar hand dynamometer (Swanson et al, 1970), the use of any other brand of dynamometer may not accurately match the data in the tables. Therefore, it is necessary to compare and calibrate a non-Jamar brand dynamometer with a calibrated Jamar. There are five handle settings on a Jamar grip dynamometer, of which the second (4 cm) or third position (6 cm) is most often utilized, depending on hand size. The average of three readings is calculated and documented. The three tests may be taken at different times during the examination to assess reliability, as when there is greater than 20% variation in the three readings, a differential diagnosis between full effort versus psychosocial issues is necessary (Swanson et al, 1970). Pain-induced weakness must also be clinically considered when greater than 20% variation in the three readings occurs. Usually, there is no reason to use the normative data tables unless a bilateral prob-

lem exists, as the normal side is compared to the abnormal side (Table 16–17) (Swanson et al, 1970). (For more information, see the following sources: Swanson et al, 1970; American Medical Association, 1993.)

Test 20. Subjective Outcome Assessment Instrumentation
The self-administered, subjective outcome assessment instruments are included here to prompt the HCP to readminister these questionnaires as a part of the QFCE assessment. This allows for comparison of a baseline and/or follow-up evaluation of activity intolerance, as reported subjectively, to the functional losses determined objectively in the QFCE. The two should jibe or agree with each other; if not, some other issues, such as psychosocial variables, may need to be addressed. Valuable, reliable information regarding the patient's perception of the condition specific problems, general health issues, patient satisfaction, and psychometrics (eg, depression) are also assessed. In addition, subjective questionnaires serve as valuable and sensitive ways to assess clinical outcomes; an area in which functional tests, in general, fall short in terms of sensitivity and specificity (see Chaps. 4 through 7). Finally, much has been written regarding the utility and practicality of subjective instruments, and they compliment the functional assessment the same way that the history compliments the physical examination. Because there are so many different types of questionnaires to choose from, **it is important to utilize the same instrument(s) as initially completed.** Changing to a different instrument at a later point in the case management process will preclude comparisons and, hence, outcomes assessment.

Test 21. The Post-QFCE Visual Analogue Scale
(See also test 1, earlier, for a description of this test.) The post-test VAS is necessary to properly identify a patient who has been perhaps aggravated by the test so that proper

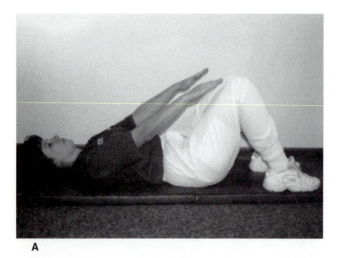

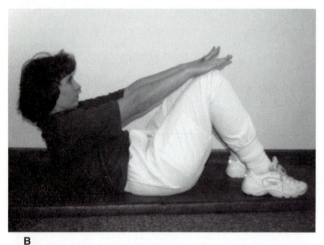

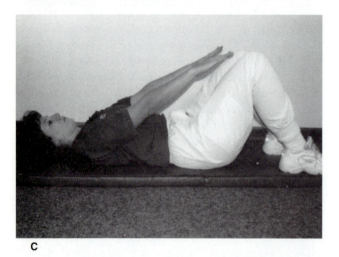

Figure 16–25. *Repetitive sit-up.* **A.** The supine patient is positioned with knees flexed and feet fixed. The patient reaches forward with the arms, elbows locked into extension. **B.** When the thenar pad approximates the superior pole of the patella, the patient returns to the full supine position using a 2- to 3-second per repetition cadence. **C.** The patient then returns to a neutral position so that the head touches the mat prior to performing the next repetition. A maximum of 50 repetitions is allowed before the test is terminated.

home instructions such as ice, walking, or avoidance of prolonged flexion such as counter-top work, etc can be discussed. **The most difficult tests included in the QFCE are those that assess strength and endurance: the repetitive squat (test 2), sit-up (test 14), arch-up (test 16) and static back endurance (test 18).** Alaranta et al (1994) noted no significant trouble in their patient sample with respect to back injuries associated with these tests and in general, this is consistent with my own observations and experience. Rather, these tests serve as practical tools to screen for fear-avoidance behavior, which becomes quite apparent when the patient lacks the courage to try the tests. There may, indeed, be times when it is not safe to perform some of these tests, and this should be carefully considered on a case-by-case basis. It has been observed that some patients who refuse to perform a test on the initial evaluation will later allow the test to be done after 2 to 4 weeks of rehabilitation. This is probably a result of reduced fear-avoidance behavior, the patients having "proven" to themselves during this period that they are capable of doing many of the exercises they were afraid of initially. This is, of course, a sign that the patients are succeeding in their rehabilitation process, as it has been shown that depression, anxiety, and fear-avoidance improve as the functional deficiencies and condition improve (Cherkin et al, 1996). (For more information, see the following sources: Reading, 1979; Dworkin et al, 1990; Chapman-Smith, 1992; Von Korff et al, 1992, 1993.)

NEW ADDITIONS TO THE QFCE

Three additional tests were recently added to the QFCE: the one-leg balance test, the double leg lowering test, and cervical spine muscle strength assessment test (see also Table 16–20).

One-Leg Balance Test

The **one-leg balance test** is performed with the patient standing and assesses proprioceptive awareness, a function that is commonly lost following a traumatic event to both the extremities and the spine (Inamura, 1983; Videman et al, 1989; Oddsson, 1990; Bly and Sinnot, 1991). This test is performed by having the patient stand on one foot at a time while assessing by time the position is maintained and by quality of balance. The test is first performed with eyes open followed by eyes closed (see Fig. 16–1A and B). If the subject can successfully maintain balance for 30 seconds, the test is terminated. This test has been validated, is safe, has good utility, and is reliable and practical (Bohannon et al, 1984; Stones and Kozma, 1987; Briggs et al, 1989; Johansson and Jarnlo, 1991). In addition, normative data have been published, allowing a baseline comparison with the subject's results and a percentage of normal to be calculated. When a functional problem, which is defined as less than 85% of normal is identified, specific proprioceptive exercises addressing this problem can be prescribed in the active care rehabilitation program. This test, like the others of the QFCE, serves as an outcome assessment tool

Table 16–14: Normative Data for Repetitive Sit-up Test[a]

| | MALES (N = 242) | | | | | | FEMALES (N = 233) | | | | | |
| | Blue Collar | | White Collar | | All | | Blue Collar | | White Collar | | All | |
AGE	*x*	*SD*	*x*	*SD*	*x*	*SD*	*x*	*SD*	*x*	*SD*	*x*	*SD*
35–39	29	13	35	13	32	13	24	12	30	16	27	14
40–44	22	11	34	12	27	13	18	12	19	13	19	12
45–49	19	11	33	15	24	14	17	14	22	15	19	14
50–54	17	13	36	16	23	16	9	10	20	13	11	11
35–54	23	13	35	13	27	14	17	13	24	15	19	14

[a] Data are broken down by age (left column), gender (males, left half; females, right half), and occupation (blue collar, white collar, and the average [all]). The average number of repetitions is found in the column labeled "x" and the standard deviation (SD) is adjacent. The last row is the average of all subjects tested (35 to 54 years old). A maximum of 50 repetitions is allowed.

Reprinted with permission from Alaranta et al, 1994.

when the test is repeated later in a re-examination. Balance dysfunction also correlates with the subjective paper and pen Dizziness Handicap Inventory (see Chap. 7) (Jacobson et al, 1991). Table 16–1, earlier in this chapter, includes the normative data for different age groups (Bly and Sinnot, 1991). Figure 16–1 is similar to the test described by Bly; however, in Bly's test head rotation is not necessary, and the foot does not need to be maintained against the medial knee.

Double Leg Lowering Test

The **double leg lowering test** evaluates the strength of the lower abdominal muscles (Basmajian and Nyberg, 1993; Moffroid, personal communication 1997, 1998). The patient is placed in the supine position with the hips flexed approximately 70 to 90 degrees, and the soles of the feet resting on the table. The inclinometer can be strapped to the lateral thigh with Velcro or held on the mid-shaft of the tibia and "zeroed out" with the knees fully extended (Fig. 16–31). The examiner stands at the side of the patient and places his or her cephalic hand palm up under the patient's mid-lumbar spinous processes to monitor the posterior pelvic tilt. The examiner assists the patient in raising the legs to a starting position of 70 to 90 degrees of hip flexion and continues to monitor the posterior pelvic tilt as the patient voluntarily contracts the abdominal muscles while lowering the legs, but with assistance. This is repeated up to two times, and the third time, the patient completes the maneuver on his or her own without assistance. The angle of the legs to the table or horizontal is measured with an inclinometer at the point at which the posterior pelvic tilt is lost by releasing the hand monitoring the lumbar spine and supporting the legs at the endpoint of the test. The angle that is recorded may be compared to an initial reading taken previously or to a future

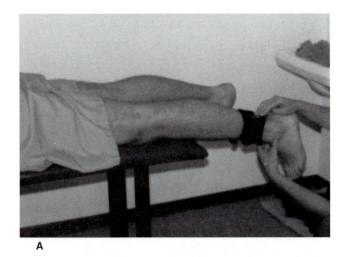
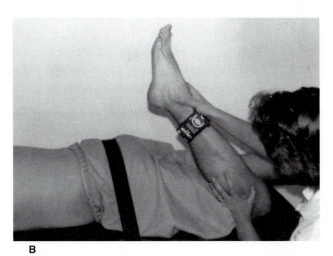

A   B

Figure 16–26. *Knee flexion test.* **A.** The inclinometer is placed on the prone patient's distal lateral lower leg and "zeroed out." **B.** The lower extremity is then flexed approximating the heel to the buttock until hip hiking or pelvic rotation is noted and the degrees are recorded. The test is then repeated on the opposite side.

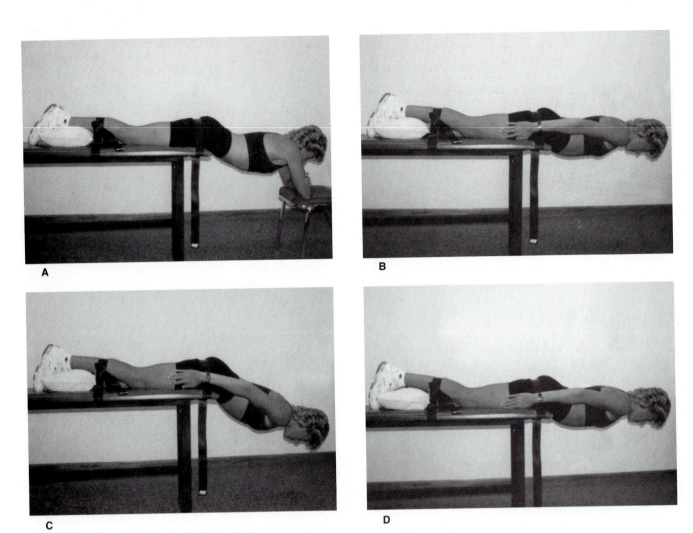

Figure 16–27. *Repetitive arch-up test.* **A.** The prone patient is strapped so that the upper half of the body is suspended off the edge of the table, supporting his or her weight by leaning on a chair while straps are applied to the pelvis and lower leg. **B.** The chair is then pulled out and the patient suspends outward. **C.** The trunk flexes downward to approximately 45 degrees and returns to the neutral position **(D).** Each repetition should be completed in 2 to 3 seconds.

Table 16–15: Normative Data for Repetitive Arch-up Test[a]

| | MALES (N = 242) | | | | | | FEMALES (N = 233) | | | | | |
| | Blue Collar | | White Collar | | All | | Blue Collar | | White Collar | | All | |
AGE	x	SD	x	SD	x	SD	x	SD	x	SD	x	SD
35–39	26	11	34	14	29	13	28	13	27	11	27	12
40–44	23	12	36	14	28	14	25	14	20	11	23	13
45–49	24	13	34	16	28	15	25	15	31	16	27	15
50–54	21	11	35	17	26	15	18	14	26	14	19	14
35–54	24	12	35	15	28	14	24	14	26	13	24	14

[a] Data for the repetitive arch-up test are broken down by age (left column), gender (males, left half; females, right half), and occupation (blue collar, white collar, and the average [all]). The average number of repetitions is found in the column labeled "x" and the standard deviation (SD) is adjacent. The last row is the average of all subjects tested (35 to 54 years old). A maximum of 50 repetitions is allowed.

Reprinted with permission from Alaranta et al, 1994.

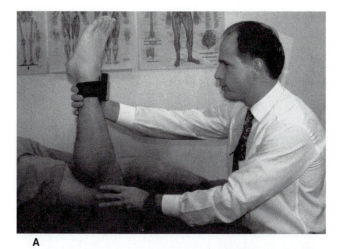

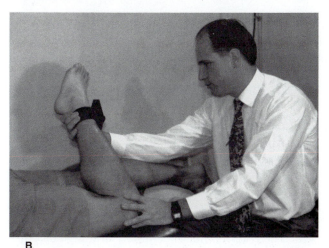

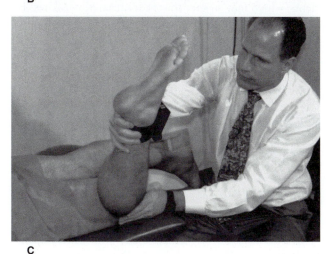

Figure 16–28. *Hip rotation test.* **A.** The patient is placed in a prone position with the pelvis strapped down. The patient flexes the knee 90 degrees while maintaining a neutral hip rotation position. **B.** External hip rotation is accomplished by moving the lower leg medially. **C.** Internal hip rotation occurs when the lower leg is moved laterally.

reading for outcomes assessment of lower abdominal muscle strength. This test is considered normal if the horizontal-to-leg angle is 60 degrees or less.

Cervical Spine Muscle Strength Assessment Test

The third new test is a **cervical spine muscle strength assessment test.** This test was originally described using a modified sphygmomanometer dynamometer (MSD) [no longer available] (Magnatec Co. Ltd., Concord, Ontario, Canada) with reported reliability (Vernon et al, 1992). Vernon et al performed paired trials on 40 normal subjects (average age 25 ± 2 years) and 24 symptomatic subjects (39 ± 7 years). The latter trials were made up of 8 patients with "whiplash"-type injuries (average duration 22.5 weeks) and 16 patients with nontraumatic chronic neck pain (average duration 110 weeks). The isometric pressure levels produced by the subjects were measured in millimeters of mercury (mm Hg) by the MSD and converted to kilopascals (kPa). The first part of the study included repeated paired trials using a standardized weight of 20 lbs, which produced a coefficient of variation of .84% with virtually no difference between the means of the two trials. When testing subjects, the test–retest correlation coefficients were high (.79 to .97) for all ROMs and right to left asymmetries in rotation and lateral flexion were within 6% to 8%. The ratio between flexion and extension was reported at .57:1, indicating that flexion was approximately 40% lower than extension in normal subjects. The differences in paired trials were analyzed by intraclass coefficients, which ranged from 4% to 10.4% (average 7%), supporting the presence of a high degree of intraclass correlation. The symptomatic subjects fell well below the normal cutoff values, and the flexion/extension ratio for whiplash subjects was .25:1.00, which is about half of that reported for the normal subjects. The MSD was found to be reliable and normative data and flexion/extension ratios were reported. **The authors concluded that the MSD was "very promising" in evaluating neck-injured patients** (Vernon, 1992).

Subject positioning was standardized by placing the patient in a standing position with the feet placed on markers directly under the testing device and the head maintained in a starting position within 10 degrees of neutral. A preload pressure of 15 to 35 mm Hg was allowed on the testing device, which was described as an insignificant amount compared to the range of subsequent values. In flexion, the pressure is placed just above the subject's eyebrows. A test interval time of 5 seconds was used, of which the last 3 seconds of sustained maximal effort was recorded. A second trial was completed following a 5-second rest interval. Verbal cues such as "keep pushing" or "push as hard as you can" were used during the time in which resistance was measured. Table 16–18 includes data derived from the study and a conversion from KPa to mm Hg is included so that comparisons can be made when instruments are used that measure in mm Hg.

As noted in Table 16–18, the strength difference between the flexors and the extensors is significant and is

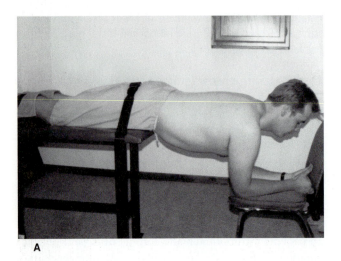
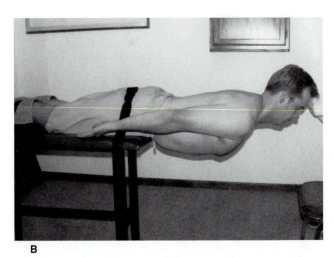

A

B

Figure 16–29. *Static back endurance test.* The patient's position is identical to that of the repetitive arch-up test. The prone patient is strapped at the lower leg and pelvis so that the trunk extends off the end of the table. This position is maintained for a maximum time of 240 seconds, and the total time completed prior to trunk flexion and loss of the static neutral position is recorded.

consistent with findings reported regarding trunk strength (Triano and Schultz, 1987). This may be caused by lordosis of both spinal regions. In whiplash patients, all cervical ROM strength values were decreased compared to the normative data, with the most significant loss being that of flexor strength. More specifically, the losses were as follows:

- Flexion strength loss: 75%
- Extensor strength loss: 41%
- Lateral flexion strength loss: 40%
- Rotation strength loss: 64%

In addition, the flexor/extensor ratio decrease of the normal (.57) versus the whiplash group (.25) supports the finding that the most significant functional deficiency in

acute cervical spine injuries from motor vehicle accidents occurs to the anterior cervical musculature (the flexors). There was, however, no mention in this study of the mechanism of injury such as rear-end collisions versus front-end impacts. Interestingly, the flexor/extensor ratio of patients with chronic pain was .62, which is slightly greater than the .57 flexor/extensor ratio reported for the normal subjects. There was no traumatic history in this group of patients, which may suggest that flexor strength weakness is a unique finding in acute traumatic cervical spine injuries. Or, it may simply mean that sufficient time had passed for the previously weak flexor muscle group to gradually regain its strength. Unfortunately, the chronic pain group is only segregated out in the data reporting the flexor/extensor ratios, as the remaining data was grouped together with the whiplash cases. As a total symptomatic group (chronic

Table 16–16: Normative Data for Static Back Endurance Test[a]

| | MALES (N = 242) | | | | | | FEMALES (N = 233) | | | | | |
| | Blue Collar | | White Collar | | All | | Blue Collar | | White Collar | | All | |
AGE	x	SD	x	SD	x	SD	x	SD	x	SD	x	SD
35–39	87	38	113	47	97	43	91	61	95	48	93	55
40–44	83	51	129	57	101	57	89	57	67	51	80	55
45–49	81	45	131	64	99	58	90	55	122	73	102	64
50–54	73	47	121	56	89	55	62	55	99	78	69	60
35–54	82	45	123	55	97	53	82	58	94	62	87	59

[a] Data are broken down by age (left column), gender (males, left half; females, right half), and occupation (blue collar, white collar, and the average [all]). The average amount of time (sec) is found in the column labeled "x" and the standard deviation (SD) is adjacent. The last row is the average of all subjects tested (35 to 54 years old). A maximum amount of time allowed is 240 seconds.

Reprinted with permission from Alaranta et al, 1994.

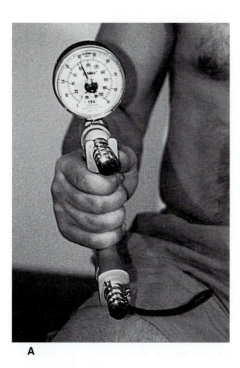
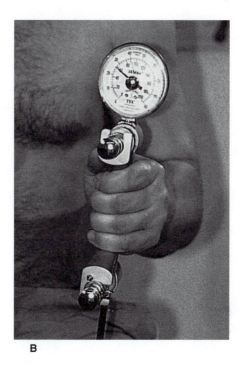

A   **B**

Figure 16–30. *Grip strength test.* Right **(A)** and left **(B)** grip strength is recorded by averaging three readings, which must be within 20% of each other to be valid.

neck pain and whiplash subjects combined), significant weakness compared to normative data is reported in all ranges, and as a result, the flexor/extensor ratio of the chronic group was nearly equal to the normative data. This suggests that a fairly uniform loss of both flexor and extensor strength resulted.

After establishing dialogue with the main author (Vernon et al, 1992), the company that produced the MSD has discontinued production of the unit. This author has utilized a modified Nexus Ball dynamometer, which works quite well (Nexerciser, PO Box 516, Bedford, NH 03102). The dynamometer was modified by exchanging the LED light indicator for strength, with the bulb and gauge of a sphygmomanometer, allowing pressure to be read in mm Hg rather than with a four-light indicator. The Nexus ball is inflated to 20 mm Hg, the hose is clamped to prevent air leakage, and the remaining protocol, similar to that previously described for the MSD is utilized. The ball is placed between the subject's head and the wall in a close to neutral position and strength measurements are taken in the frontal and sagittal planes (flexion, extension, and right and left lateral flexion). Similar results are often obtained, especially the flexion/extension ratio as reported by Vernon et al (1992). The purpose of converting the kPa to mm Hg in Table 16–18 is to offer an opportunity for results to be compared to previously established normative data published by Vernon and colleagues when using a modified Nexus dynamometer. However, it should be clear that until the va-

lidity and reliability are properly evaluated, the modified Nexus dynamometer approach should be used with the understanding that the normative data may be less reliable with this unit. The importance of its inclusion in the QFCE is, however, to follow outcomes at the point of re-examination as the ratios between tests, especially the flexion/extension ratio, can be followed to assess improvement in flexion strength loss through rehabilitative approaches. **Since cervical spinal muscle strength is such an important clinical aspect in cases involving trauma, having the ability to quantify strength in a fairly low-tech manner strengthens the utility of the QFCE significantly.** This test is depicted in Figure 16–32.

Another low-tech option for assessing cervical spine flexor muscle strength that has great practicality and utility as an outcome assessment test is a modified chin-flexion test. This test was originally described as a qualitative test to assess for weakness of the anterior neck flexor muscles and is described as the "Head/Neck Endur/Coord" test in the Appendix Form F–8, test 16. A modification can be applied by measuring the time (in seconds) with a stopwatch to the point of chin poking or head drop, which allows for quantification and, hence, outcomes assessment. This test can be further modified by placing a modified Nexus ball dynamometer behind the head so the test could be terminated when a decrease **or** an increase in pressure occurs (Fig. 16–33). A partially inflated sphygmomanometer may be used in place of the modified Nexus ball dynamometer.

Table 16–17: Normative Data for Grip Strength and Pinch Strength[a]

| | GRIP STRENGTH (KG) | | | |
| | MALES | | FEMALES | |
	Major Hand	Minor Hand	Major Hand	Minor Hand
Occupation				
Skilled	47.0	45.4	26.8	24.4
Sedentary	47.2	44.1	23.1	21.1
Manual	48.5	44.6	24.2	22.0
Average	47.6	45.0	24.6	22.4
Age Group				
<20	45.2	42.6	23.8	22.8
20–29	48.5	46.2	24.6	22.7
30–39	49.2	44.5	30.8	28.0
40–49	49.0	47.3	23.4	21.5
50–59	45.9	43.5	22.3	18.2

| | PINCH STRENGTH (KG) | | | |
| | MALES | | FEMALES | |
	Major Hand	Minor Hand	Major Hand	Minor Hand
Occupation				
Skilled	6.6	6.4	4.4	4.3
Sedentary	6.3	6.1	4.1	3.9
Manual	8.5	7.7	6.0	5.5
Average	7.5	7.1	4.9	4.7

Data for dominant ("major hand") and nondominant ("minor hand") grip or pinch strength (in kilograms) are broken down by occupation (left-hand column) and gender.

Reprinted with permission from Swanson AB, Matev IB, de Groot Swanson G. The strength of the hand. In: American Medical Association. Guides to the Evaluation of Permanent Impairment. 4th ed. Chicago, Ill: AMA; 1993: pp. 64–65, Tables 31–33.

APPLICATIONS OF THE QUANTITATIVE FUNCTIONAL CAPACITY EVALUATION

FUNCTIONAL REHABILITATION OUTCOMES TOOL

The original intent of the QFCE was to track outcomes in a rehabilitation setting. By performing a battery of tests that meet the criteria of a good test (see Chap. 2) and include normative data, reliable baseline measures are established. When these baseline measures are repeated at an interim or concluding/discharge examination, the benefits as well as the failures of the rehabilitation program can be assessed and additional recommendations can appropriately follow. Without this form of objective guidance, the HCP can only base clinical decisions on subjective infor-

mation. Moreover, **the objective outcomes assessment approach of the QFCE is important, as it allows the HCP to promptly identify weak areas of physical performance, which can then be addressed through customization of the patient's rehabilitation program.**

One of the motivating factors that prompted the formation of the QFCE was the number of rehabilitation services that did not use any kind of low-tech assessment process that could be implemented in a rehabilitation center to track functional outcomes. For example, before developing the QFCE, this author interviewed staff at approximately 50 rehabilitation centers throughout Wisconsin and inquired about current outcome assessment approaches that were being used at the time, and was surprised to find that most rehabilitation centers did not use *any* type of outcome tool, including subjective paper-driven questionnaires. However, among those who indicated that such a device was important, all felt strongly that a need existed for the development of such an assess-

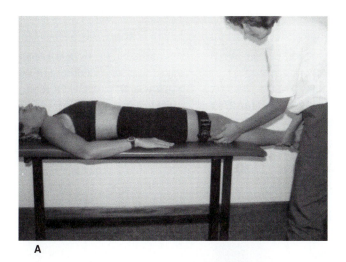

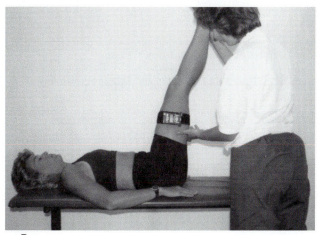

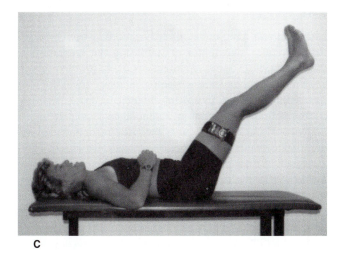

Figure 16–31. *Double leg lowering test.* **A.** The patient is placed in a supine position and the inclinometer is "zeroed out" on the lower leg while the legs are extended at rest. The knees are then flexed and brought to the chest. **B.** The knees are then extended with the legs pointing upwards toward the ceiling. **C.** The legs are then actively lowered while maintaining a posterior pelvic tilt. A measurement is taken when the lumbar spine raises off the table (the posterior pelvic tilt is lost). A hand under the lumbar spine helps to monitor the point of lordosis failure (not pictured).

ment approach. Many also indicated that they would like to implement a practical functional outcomes assessment approach, "if one existed." After an extensive literature search and development of the QFCE, instruction of this approach has been made available in the postgraduate rehabilitation diplomate program sponsored, since 1995, by the Los Angeles College of Chiropractic postgraduate division and the feedback from those who have adopted its use has been tremendous. A videotape of the tests and a manual were designed to help guide the HCP through the process of performing a QFCE. After two or three examinations, the evaluation becomes progressively easier to perform. The average time for an experienced examiner to complete the QFCE is 35 minutes (excluding data analysis). With respect to "warnings" or cautions that may apply to the QFCE, the same concerns previously discussed regarding all FCE or WCE approaches should be exercised.

I have not noted significant problems of exacerbation occurring as a result of performing the QFCE, particularly, the strength and endurance tests. Alaranta et al (1994) published similar success with the strength and endurance tests cited above. However, at times patients have refused to perform the repetitive arch-up, static back endurance, and/or repetitive sit-up tests. This was often due to fear-avoidant behavior and upon subsequent re-examination, they did not exhibit the same fear-avoidant characteristics. **In some cases of lumbar instability, herniated disc, or other cases that are clinically sensitive to movement intolerance, especially in the sagittal plane, it may be safest to avoid some of these strength and endurance tests.** As always, clinical decisions such as these must be made on a case-by-case basis.

EXERCISE PRESCRIPTION: THE QFCE AND OTHER IMPORTANT TESTS

Another important application of the QFCE is in prescribing specific exercises through identification of weak links in the kinetic chain of the locomotor system. The "kinetic chain" refers to the body as a whole divided into links that make up the chain. A popular concept in rehabilitation is to assess all the functional links of the kinetic chain as, sometimes, the key functional pathology may be well separated from the presenting complaint. Therefore, assessment of the entire "chain" may be necessary to obtain the desired affects of patient treatment. **Once a functional "link" is disrupted, "chain reactions" in the locomotor system can further alter other functions.** For instance, joint capsule tightening may result in loss of articular ROM and subsequent accelerated cartilage degeneration; or, joint hypermobility and resultant instability may lead to other functional impairments. Because of neurophysiological responses such as reciprocal inhibition, whereby an overactive antagonist results in inhibition of an agonist muscle, each key link of the kinetic chain that is altered must be restored if long-term success is to be achieved with treatment (Bullock-Saxton, 1994). For example, the exer-

Table 16–18: Normative Data for Cervical Spine Strength[a]

	NORMAL ± SD (KPa)	NORM ± SD (mm Hg) (KPa × .0075)	CV (%)	LOWER CUTOFF (MEAN – 1) (KPa/mm Hg)	RELIABILITY COEFFICIENT	AVERAGE % DIFFERENCE, TRIAL 1 VS 2	INTRACLASS CORRELATION COEFFICIENT, TRIAL 1 VS TRIAL 2
Flexion	4615 ± 1317	34.61 ± 9.88	28	3300/.93	.93	10.4	.98
Extension	7927 ± 2128	59.45 ± 15.96	27	5800/.97	.97	7.0	.95
Right Lateral Flexion	7930 ± 1995	59.48 ± 14.96	25	6200/46.5	.87	6.4	.99
Left Lateral Flexion	8512 ± 2261	63.84 ± 16-95	27	6200/46.5	.95	NA	NA
Right Rotation	7315 ± 1862	54.86 ± 13.97	26	5200/39.0	.79	4.0	.98
Left Rotation	6783 ± 1859	46.37 ± 13.94	28	5200/39.0	.79	NA	NA
Total	NA	NA	NA	NA	NA	7.0	.98

CV, coefficient of variation; KPa, kilopascals; mm Hg, millimeters of mercury; NA, not available; SD, standard deviation.

[a] Data and standard deviations are converted from KPa to mm Hg by multiplying the KPa by a factor of .0075 (columns 2 and 3). The lower cutoff was computed by subtracting 1 SD from the mean. The reliability coefficient values reveal that moderate to high reliability was obtained by this testing approach.

Modified with permission from Vernon et al, 1992.

cise/rehabilitation program for a patient whose hamstring muscle measures short must include methods of resolving this impairment if functional restoration of the whole person is to occur. Specific hamstring stretching maneuvers can be prescribed for home use. In-office manual release techniques may include neuromuscular reeducation such as contract-hold, post-isometric relaxation, reciprocal inhibition, and eccentric stretching under a submaximal load (Liebenson, 1996). These techniques can be applied directly to the hamstrings, and/or an overactive synergist such as the gastrocnemius/soleus muscle, an under-active antagonist such as a weak abdominal muscle, or an inhibited agonist such as the gluteus maximus muscle may require strengthening. Similarly, an overactive antagonist such as the iliopsoas muscle may have to be inhibited prior to achieving significant benefit. Health care providers with a clear understanding and appreciation of the various links in the "kinetic chain" and the chain reactions involving muscle imbalances, along with a strong commitment to learning the information found in Table 16–19, will greatly enhance their ability to prescribe rehabilitation on an individual basis.

Specific rehabilitation/exercise protocols that can be utilized for each corresponding failed QFCE test (< 85% of normal) are presented in Table 16–20. The appropriate method(s) of exercise and other rehabilitation approaches are well described elsewhere (Liebenson, 1996) and should be reviewed concurrently with this section. **It should be emphasized that once the rehabilitation principles are established, adapting the various exercises to the individual patient will typically yield the best outcome rather than forcing the individual patient into a "pre-canned" pro-** **gram that cannot be individually tailored.** Appendix Forms G–6 and G–7 function as tools to facilitate documentation.

OTHER TESTS THAT COMPLEMENT THE QFCE

The quadratus lumborum muscle has recently been reported to be a major contributor to stabilizing the lumbar spine (McGill, 1998). Spinal stabilization exercises have classically included "core" strengthening exercises, including various approaches to the sit-up maneuver, back extensor strengthening, and combinations/modifications of these maneuvers. These exercises have included recommended abdominal strengthening exercises, as well as extensor exercises such as lying prone and raising both the upper half and lower half of the body, sometimes referred to as a "superman." McGill recommends avoidance of this exercise as facet and annulus loading and high spine compressive loads of 4000 to 6000 Newtons (N) were recorded (McGill, 1998). McGill also reports that when compression is applied to the spine in an upright position without bending, the muscular activity of the quadratus lumborum increases as much as any other muscle. Though the psoas muscle has frequently been cited as a lumbar spine stabilizer, this function has been questioned based on EMG findings that revealed the quadratus lumborum to play a much more significant role in the upright, nonbending posture (Juker et al, 1998; McGill et al, 1996). A less common exercise, the horizontal side support, appears to challenge the lateral oblique muscles without inducing high lumbar compressive loading (Fig. 16–34). More specifically, high levels of activ-

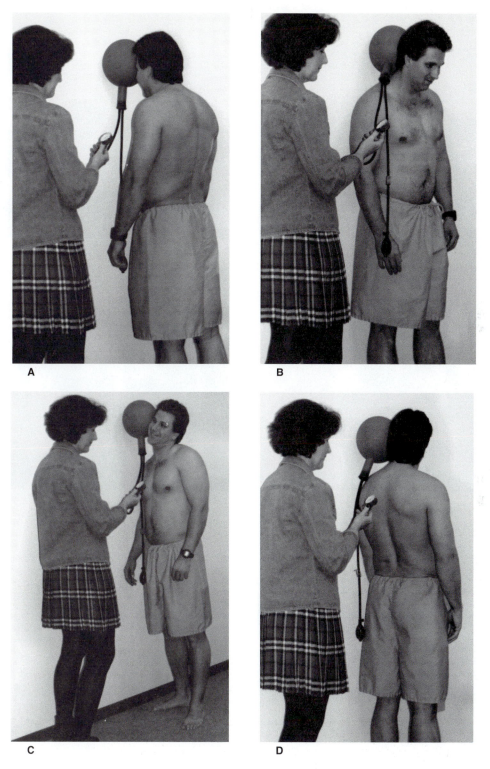

Figure 16–32. Assessment of cervical spine strength can be accomplished by the use of modified Nexus ball dynamometer. The LED light indicator can be replaced with a sphygmomanometer bulb and gauge so that quantification of a more sensitive variety can be accomplished. Though no specific normative data exists for this particular unit, the ratio between flexors and extensors can be calculated and the quantity of strength in the sagittal and frontal planes (**A, B** and **C, D,** respectively) can be used as an outcome tool later at re-examination.

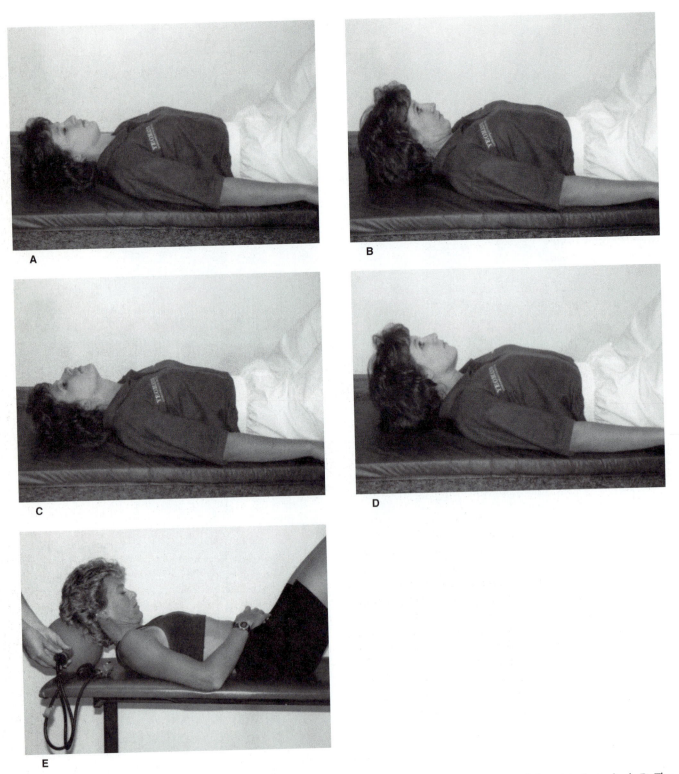

Figure 16–33. *Modified head-flexion test.* **A.** The patient is placed in the supine position and the chin is tucked. **B.** The head is raised one inch off the table, maintaining the chin-flexed posture. The examiner records (in seconds) the length of time the patient can statically hold the position, ending the test when **(C)** the head falls back to the table and/or **(D)** the chin-tuck is lost. **E.** A partially inflated blood pressure cuff or a modified Nexus ball dynamometer can be added and the test terminated when an increase or decrease in pressure on the cuff or ball occurs.

CLINICAL TIP 16–4
Using the QFCE with Subjective Tools

The QFCE should be coupled with the subjective tools, which help the HCP to gather information pertaining to disability, psychosocial issues, quality of life, and pain intensity. This information, in turn, assists the HCP in identifying those patients most likely to fail to respond to treatment (regardless of what is done). Furthermore, by the use of these tools, identification of these patients can be accomplished on day 1 rather than 2 or 3 months into care. By identifying such patients early on, specific treatment objectives addressing chronic pain behavior and disability can be established, which may include the initiation of psychosocial support. **This approach allows the HCP to treat the whole person, not just the functional impairments identified through the QFCE.**

---

ity in the quadratus lumborum muscle were recorded (54 ± 28% MVC) as no other exercise stimulated quadratus lumborum activity above a 12% MVC, over four times less stimulation compared to the bent-knee leg raise (12 ± 6) and bent-knee sit-up (12 ± 7). This is important, as the quadratus lumborum was found to be one of the most important stabilizers of the spine (McGill, 1998). Recently, McGill reported normative data of the side bridge (see Figure 16–34) using a healthy, young (mean age of 23 years) population of 31 men and 44 women (McGill et al, 1999).

The subjects were instructed to maintain the side bridge position as long as possible while the time in seconds was monitored using a stopwatch. The mean and standard deviation for males were reported as follows: right 94 ± 34, left 97 ± 35; and for females: right 72 ± 31, left 77 ± 35. The ratio between the side bridge to low back extensor endurance as determined by the static back endurance test (Figure 16–29) was .65 for males and .39 for females. In early stage rehabilitation for abdominal strengthening and endurance, McGill recommends the following considerations:

- Use of several variations of curl-ups to strengthen the rectus abdominus muscle
- Isometric horizontal side support, initially from the knees and later, from the feet, by supporting the upper body with one elbow on the floor
- Avoidance of most back extensor exercises using resistance from either free weights or resistance machines, because of the high spinal loads produced during such exercises

Muscular *endurance* (high repetitions and/or long holds at low loads/force) are, in McGill's view, more advantageous than *strength* (low repetitions and/or short holds at high loads/force) (McGill, 1998). Hence, an isometric hold of 5 to 10 seconds per repetition to a point of fatigue makes sense for determining the dose of this exercise. Owing to the popularity of back extensor muscle strengthening exercises, their respective spinal loads during six back extensor exercises are reviewed in Table 16–21.

Table 16–19: Chain Reactions in the Locomotor System

SKILL	MOVEMENT PATTERN	TIGHT OR OVERACTIVE MUSCLE	WEAK OR INHIBITED MUSCLE	STIFF JOINTS	HYPERMOBILE JOINTS
Gait/toe off, lifting, standing posture	Hip extension	Psoas, hamstring, erector spinae	Gluteus maximus	Hip joint	Lumbar
Gait/stance	Hip abduction	TFL, QL, adductors, piriformis	Gluteus medius	Hip joint	SI joint and LS joint
Lifting and trunk stabilization	Trunk flexion	Psoas, erector spinae	Rectus abdominus	Lumbar flexion	Lumbar extension
Prehension, reaching grasping	Shoulder abduction	Upper trapezius, levator scapulae	Lower and middle trapezius	C/T junction, S/C joint	C5-6, G/H joint
Pushing/pulling	Trunk lowering from a push-up	Pectoralis major/minor, subscapular	Serratus anterior	C/T junction, mid-upper thoracic	G/H joint
Mastication, sitting posture	Head/neck flexion	SCM, Suboccipitals	Deep neck flexors	C/T junction in flexion, TMJ	C5-6
Respiration	Respiration	Scalenes	Diaphragm	Rib cage, lower cervical spine	NA

C, cervical; C/T, cervicothoracic; G/H, glenohumeral; LS, lumbosacral; NA, not applicable; QL, quadratus lumborum; S/C, sternoclavicular; SCM, sternocleidomastoid; TFL, tensor fascia lata; TMJ, temporomandibular joint.

Reprinted with permission from Rehabilitation of the Spine: A Practitioner's Manual. *C. Liebenson, ed. Williams & Wilkins, 1996, p. 359.*

Table 16–20: Rehabilitation Options Related to Specific Components of the QFCE

TEST	REHABILITATION OPTIONS: SCORE < 85% OF NORMAL
1. Visual analogue scale	NA: note if pain > 6/10, consider safety in QFCE, catastrophization/chronic pain
2. Repetitive squat	Lunges; wall squats; quad sets; muscle stretch of hamstrings, iliopsoas, gastrocnemius/soleus; proprioception exercises ball, one-leg stand, rocker and wobble boards, balance sandals
3. ROM: Lumbar spine	Exercises:
Flexion	*Nerve tension*—McKenzie (promote centralization)
	Mechanical—*Williams*. Stretch: hamstrings, adductors, gastrocnemius/soleus; lumbar erector spinae. *Pelvic stabilization (floor and gym ball):* pelvic tilt, 4-point, lunges, dead-bug, swimmers, bridges, curl-ups. *Proprioceptive retraining:* ball, one-leg stand, rocker and wobble boards, balance sandals
Extension	Same—emphasize Mckenzie within safe pain limits; stretch iliopsoas
Lateral Flexion	Same—emphasize lateral flexion within safe pain limits
4. Waddell—sign 1: Tenderness	When 3 of 5 positive signs—psychometrics: promote active care/minimize passive care, emphasize work return; consider comanagement if off work > 4 weeks; identify early!
5. Waddell—sign 2: Simulation	Same as 4
6. Gastrocnemius/Ankle dorsiflexion	Stretch gastrocnemius/soleus muscles: calf-wall stretch, heels off step-ankle DF/PF stretch, rocker and wobble board with appropriate balance challenges
7. Soleus/Ankle dorsiflexion	Same as 6
7a. One-leg standing test	Proprioception exercises: ball, one-leg stand, rocker and wobble boards, balance sandals; playing catch during trunk curl
7b. Cervical spine strength	Use slightly deflated beach ball with isometric resistance in frontal and sagittal planes; PIR, self-stretches, self-strengthening exercises
8. Waddell—sign 3: Distraction (part I, with no. 13)	Same as 4
9. Waddell—sign 4: Regional neurology	Same as 4
10. Waddell—sign 5: Exaggeration	Same as 4
11. ROM: Cervical Spine	Exercises
Flexion	Stretch extensors, strengthen flexors, promote chin retraction posture correction
Extension	Stretch flexors, strengthen extensors, promote chin retraction posture correction
Lateral Flexion	Stretch contralateral LF, strengthen homolateral LF, promote chin retraction posture correction
Rotation	Circumduction, stretch and strengthen appropriate muscles (based on examination findings)
11a. Double leg lowering	Lower abdominal strengthening; sit-up track
12. Modified Thomas/Hip extension	Stretch iliopsoas, stretch erector spinae (L and T/L spine), strengthen GMax; posture/coordination retraining
13a. Waddell—sign 3: Distraction (part II with no. 8)	Same as 4
13b. Straight leg raise	Stretch hamstrings, adductors, TFL, iliopsoas, MRTs
14. Repetitive sit-up	Strengthen: abdominals (obliques > rectus) curl-ups, GMax; QL. Stretch: iliopsoas, L-erector spinae; side-bridge (see Fig. 16–34)
15. Knee flexion/Nachlas	Quadraceps stretch and strengthening (emphasize last 5 degrees of extension—VMO); stretch Hamstrings
16. Repetitive arch-up	Strengthen: Lumbar extensors—see pelvic stabilization; reverse sit-ups; side-bridge
17. Hip ROM: Rotation	
Internal rotation ROM	Stretch tight external rotators (pirirormis, GMed), hip capsule stretch
External rotation ROM	Stretch tight internal rotators, hip capsule stretch
18. Static back endurance	Strengthen lumbar extensors—see pelvic stabilization: superman, see-saw; lumbar extensions; repetitions of arch-ups, or from floor, reverse sit-up, side-bridge

Table 16–20: *(continued)*

TEST	REHABILITATION OPTIONS: SCORE < 85% OF NORMAL
19. Grip strength	Stretch flexor antebrachial musculature (wall wrist DF with thumb extension); grip strengthening devices; theratube wrist curls; squeeze putty
20. Subjective outcome Instrument(s)	Include the subjective tools such as Neck Disability Index, Oswestry LBDQ, SF-36
21. Post-test Visual Analogue Scale	Compare to initial score, give home instructions of appropriate item such as ice, rest

DF, dorsiflexion; GMax, gluteus maximus; GMed, gluteus medius; L, lumbar; LBDQ, low back disability questionnaire; LF, lateral flexors; MRTs, manual release techniques; NA, not applicable; PF, plantar flexion (ankle); PIR, post-isometric relaxation; QFCE, quantitative functional capacity evaluation; QL, quadratus lumborum; SF-36, Short Form-36; TFL, tensor fascia latae; T/L, thoracolumbar; VMO, vastus medialis oblique.

There are many different ways to assess functional losses. The QFCE offers one method that has the added benefit of having established normative data available; therefore, it can be used quantitatively to track outcomes. However, more qualitative tests such as posture/gait analysis, movement pattern assessment, and McKenzie protocols offer important information that can provide specific treatment prescriptions; hence, such tests should be included in the assessment process as well (see Table 13–8 for a description of each test). This is especially true when regional losses are not well addressed quantitatively by the QFCE or some other validated/reliable physical performance test with normative data. An example previously described is cervical strength assessment by the chin flexion test, which assesses weak or *inhibited* cervical flexor musculature. Though no normative data has yet been established, the *quantitative* information gathered can be used to track outcomes when repeated later, after rehabilitation protocols have addressed the weakness. Many other qualitative tests can be quantified and made practical for outcomes measurement in a similar manner even though no normative data exist for an initial baseline comparison. A partial list of some examples follows.

- **McKenzie tests**—*measure* with dual inclinometry the ROM when peripheralization occurs. As the condition improves, a greater ROM of flexion is expected prior to pain radiation.

- **Chin flexion test**—count the *time* to test failure of chin poking, head dropping, or pain intolerance
- **Shoulder abduction test**—*measure* with an inclinometer the point at which the upper trapezius muscle contracts with shoulder abduction (should not contract <30 degrees)
- **Hip abduction test**—*measure* abduction with an inclinometer and report the point at which the pelvis rocks and the hip deviates from the frontal plane (compensatory motion occurs); *time* the point the leg drops from the abducted position (endurance test)
- **Hip extension test**—quantify as mild, moderate, or severe the altered muscular contraction of the erector spinae muscles compared to the gluteus maximus. For instance, mild represents an abnormal contraction pattern of homolateral quadratus lumborum toward the end range of hip extension, as compared to severe, which represents premature contraction of both contralateral and homolateral quadratus lumborum and lumbar erectors prior to the gluteus maximus early into the hip extension test. An endurance test, by actively maintaining hip extension and timing the held position to the point when the patient returns the leg back to the table, can also be performed.
- **Adductor length**—*measure* hip abduction with a goniometer and compare to contralateral side for comparison retest poststretch for change.

Quantification of tests can be achieved by the following methods:

- Measuring time (in seconds) to the point of fatigue or test failure
- Measuring the range of motion at which a positive provocative response occurs (ie, "early," "midrange," "toward endpoint")
- Measuring in degrees (inclinometer, goniometer) the point of test failure

Once quantified, an outcome can be objectively assessed. When designing various methods of quantifying softer (qualitative) tests, it is necessary to measure the placement of the inclinometer (such as 10 cm above superior pole of

Table 16–21: Spinal Loads in Various Exercises[a]

EXERCISE/TEST	SPINAL COMPRESSION (KN)
Right leg extension	2.3 ± .9
Left leg extension	2.0 ± .2
Right leg/left arm elevation	3.2 ± 1.0
Left leg/right arm elevation	2.9 ± 1.2
Superman	4.3 ± 1.1
Static back endurance	4.3 ± 1.2

[a] Data suggest single leg extension from the kneeling/all fours position is the safest exercise and may, therefore, be a wise choice for instituting an early postinjury thoracolumbar extension strengthening exercise program.

Compiled from data in McGill, 1998.

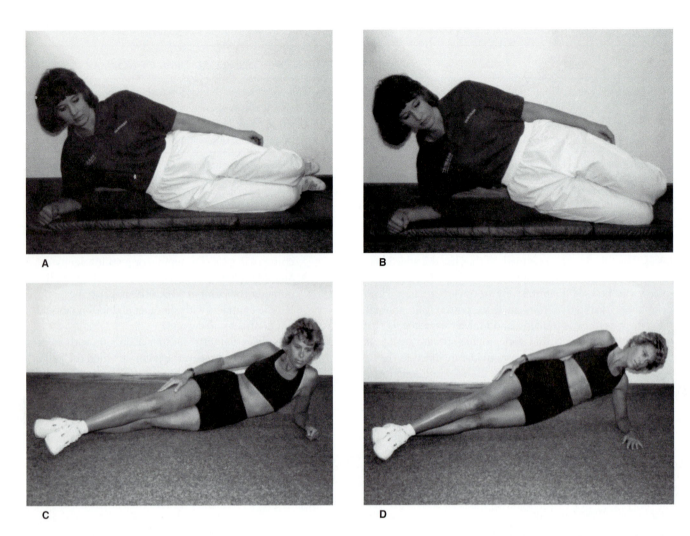

Figure 16–34. The horizontal side bridge (HSB) is the most effective way to stimulate the quadratus lumborum and, at the same time, minimize spinal loading. An exercise patterned after this test should be included early in the rehabilitation of trunk endurance, initially performed from the knees (**A** and **B**). As strength and endurance improve, it can be performed from the feet (**C**). As a test, the patient is instructed to hold the HSB as long as possible, which is timed in seconds with a stopwatch (**D**).

the patella) as well as establish the criteria to terminate the test. This will allow for duplication of the protocols at the time of the follow-up examination. Failure to do so will jeopardize the validity and reliability of the testing method, negating the practicality and meaningfulness of the test. Therefore, it is ideal to utilize those tests that include established valid and reliable protocols and normative data (ie, QFCE tests) whenever possible. Table 16–22 offers a summary of many softer, objective, qualitative tests, as well as treatment prescription options. An examination form and test description is offered in Appendix Form G–8 for documentation of the various tests described in Table 16–22.

As stated previously, treatment prescription can be obtained from multiple sources including in part, the QFCE, movement patterns, McKenzie protocols, and posture/gait assessment. Integration of all these methods minimizes the risk of missing a key functional pathology or "link" of the

kinetic chain. Table 16–23 includes functional pathologies and the associated clinical findings when assessing patients using posture and gait analysis. Appendix Form G–9 facilitates documentation.

RETURN-TO-WORK ISSUES: THE RELATIONSHIP BETWEEN THE DOT AND QFCE

The issue of returning the worker to a safe work environment prior to completion of healing has long plagued both HCP and employer. Very often, the worker returns to work and is reinjured owing to an overestimation of function by the HCP or to poor job selection by the employer. Patient motivation, psychological stressors both inside (internal factors) and outside (external factors) the workplace, and employer/patient compliance with carrying out the job restrictions further complicate the return-to-work process.

Table 16–22: Summary of Selected Qualitative Tests[a]

TEST	REHABILITATION OPTIONS
Pre-test visual analogue scale	Perform carefully if pain level is < 6/10
1. **Repetitive squat** (feet 15 cm apart)	Lunges; wall squats; quad sets; muscle stretch including hamstrings, iliopsoas, gastrocnemius/soleus; proprioception exercises ball, one-leg stand, rocker and wobble boards, balance sandals
2. **Lunge-kneel**	Same as 1
3. **Extension in standing (EIS)**	If pain centralizes: McKenzie exercises or prone press-up, standing extension, and avoidance of flexion exercises
	If pain worsens: avoid extension exercises and promote exercises into the pain-free direction
4. **Flexion in standing (FIS)**	If pain peripheralizes: McKenzie exercises or prone press-up, standing extension, and avoidance of flexion exercises
	If pain lessens: promote flexion exercises (William's) within a pain-free ROM
5. **Standing flexion test** (Delitto et al, 1993: SIJ test no. 1)	This test is one of four that was used to help categorize patients into an extension exercise/spinal manipulation treatment group; three of the four tests are required (see tests 7, 13, 26); refer to text discussion (Delitto et al, 1993).
6. **Side-gliding** (McKenzie no. 1)	This test is used to classify patients into a McKenzie classification syndrome; it is applied to antalgic patients, often due to nerve root irritation and, hence, the derangement syndrome
7. **PSIS sitting (PSISSI)** (Delitto et al, 1993: SIJ test no. 2)	This test is one of four that was used to help categorize patients into an extension exercise/spinal manipulation treatment group; three of the four tests are required (see tests 4, 13, 26); refer to text discussion (Delitto et al, 1993).
8. **ASIS sitting (ASISSI)**	Facilitates assessment of sacroiliac lesions; prescription extension exercise and manipulative therapy
9. **PSIS FL in sitting (PSISSI)**	Facilitates assessment of sacroiliac lesions; prescription extension exercise and manipulative therapy
10. **T/L rotation** (goniometer)	Manipulation of T/L fixation, ROM spinal exercises, especially extension
11. **Shoulder abduction, coordination, and endurance**	MRTs of the shoulder girdle/upper quarter; scapulohumeral mobilization; facilitate lower and middle trapezius; inhibit upper trapezius and levator scapulae muscles; SMT: C/T junction, glenohumeral joint, sternoclavicular joint.
12. **Hip adductors**	Stretch hamstrings, adductors, homolateral TFL
13. **Supine to long sitting** (SIJ no. 3)	This test is one of four that was used to help categorize patients into an extension exercise/spinal manipulation treatment group; three of the four tests are required (see tests 4, 7, 26); refer to text discussion (Delitto et al, 1993).
14. **Pelvic tilt coordination** (supine hook lying)	*Pelvic stabilization (floor and gym ball):* pelvic tilt, 4-point, lunges, dead-bug, swimmers, bridges, curl-ups; side-bridge
	Proprioceptive retraining: ball, one-leg stand, rocker and wobble boards, balance sandals
15. **Trunk flexion, coordination/ endurance**	Strengthen: abdominals (obliques>rectus) curl-ups, GMax; QL
Janda Coordination	Stretch: iliopsoas, L-erector spinae
16. **Head/Neck endurance/ coordination**	Use slightly deflated beach ball with isometric resistance in frontal and sagittal planes; PIR, self-stretches, self-strengthening exercises
	SMT: occiput, cervical, thoracic spinal regions
17. **Flexion supine** (McKenzie no. 4) Repeat 1 repetition	See 15
18. **Flexion supine** (McKenzie no. 5) Repeat 10 repetitions	See 15
19. **Flexion supine** (McKenzie no. 6) Sustain last repetition 10 seconds	See 15
20. **Respiratory synkinesis**	Stretch scalenes; facilitate/strengthen diaphragm
	SMT: lower C upper T, ribs
21. **Hip abduction coordination**	Stretch tight QL, TFL, hamstrings, adductors, piriformis; facilitate weak gluteus medius
	SMT: hip joint, fixation patterns in lower lumbar, SIJ, hip capsule stretch

Table 16–22: Summary of Selected Qualitative Tests[a] *(continued)*

TEST	REHABILITATION OPTIONS
22. **Hip extension coordination** Hamstrings Gluteus maximus Contralateral erector spinae Ipsilateral erector spinae Contralateral shoulder/neck	*Record the order in which each muscle contracts* Stretch: hamstrings, adductors *Pelvic stabilization (floor and gym ball):* pelvic tilt, 4-point, lunges, dead-bug, swimmers, bridges, curl-ups *Proprioceptive retraining:* ball, one-leg stand, rocker and wobble boards, balance sandals Lumbar erector spinae Lumbar erector spinae Self-strengthening exercise SMT: occiput, cervical, thoracic spinal regions
23. **Single extension in lying (SEL)** (McKenzie no. 7)	If pain centralizes: McKenzie exercises or prone press-up, standing extension, and avoidance of flexion exercises If pain worsens: avoid extension exercises and promote exercises into the pain-free direction
24. **Repeated extension in lying (REIS)** (McKenzie no. 8) (a) pain; (b) syndrome; (c) lateral shift	Same as 23
25. **Sustained extension in standing (SusEIS)** (McKenzie no. 9) (a) pain; (b) syndrome; (c) lateral shift	Same as 23
26. **Prone knee flexion test** (SIJ no. 4)	This test is one of four that was used to help categorize patients into an extension exercise/spinal manipulation treatment group; three of the four tests are required (see tests 4, 7, 13); refer to text discussion (Delitto et al, 1993).
27. **Push-up** Janda: Scapular Winging Maximum reps	Stretch pectoralis major/minor, subscapularis muscle; strengthen serratus anterior SMT: C/T junction, mid-upper thoracic
28. **Sit-to-stand test**	Lunges; wall squats; quad sets; muscle stretch of hamstrings, iliopsoas, gastrocnemius/ soleus; proprioception exercises ball, one-leg stand, rocker and wobble boards, balance sandals
Post-test visual analogue scale	Compare to initial score; give home instructions of appropriate item such as ice, rest (especially if pain >6/10)

C/T, cervicothoracic; GMax, gluteus maximus; L, lumbar; PIR, post-isometric relaxation; QL, quadratus lumborum; ROM, range of motion; SIJ, sacroiliac joint; SMT, spinal manipulative therapy; TFL, tensor fascia latae; T/L, thoracolumbar.
[a] There are several ways in which muscle imbalances can be assessed, including posture and gait analysis, and movement pattern assessment. Usually, only small subgroups of these tests are performed at one time. However, if a prerehabilitation screen to assess prescription needs is the application, performing the QFCE in total is recommended.

The goal of the work capacity evaluation (WCE) is to help bridge the communication gap between HCP and employer so that repeated failures in returning the injured patient to work can be avoided. For this process to succeed, the HCPs must determine the patient's functional capacities, while the employer must provide the "demand minimum functional capacity" of the job site to the HCP. If the minimum demands of a job site are not established or appreciated by the HCP, there will be no baseline against which to compare the patient's current functional or work capacities. In this situation, reinjury may more readily occur. Therefore, success at returning the patient to work without exacerbation of the injury is dependent on matching the worker's limitations, as determined by a WCE, to the minimum demands of a job site. Perhaps of even more importance to a successful return to work is that the limitations set forth by the HCP be taken seriously by both the worker and the employer. Often a worker is embarrassed to tell the foreman he or she is worse or needs a lighter duty task. Similarly, a foreman may feel that the worker is simply trying to get out of performing his or her regular duties and, as a result, may not take the worker's concerns seriously.

Unfortunately, attempts to reproduce the workplace environment, especially the psychosocial issues and interpersonal relationship stressors between fellow workers and/or management, fall well short of ideal, as replicating this environment and all its associated stressors cannot be

Table 16–23: Functional Pathologies and Associated Clinical Findings When Assessing Patients Using Posture and Gait Analysis[a]

GAIT ANALYSIS	
SIGN	**FUNCTIONAL PATHOLOGY**
1. Hyperpronation during swing phase	1. Forefoot/subtalar instability
2. Hip hiking during gait	2. QL overactivity, gluteus medius weakness or inhibition

CHECKLIST FOR POSTURE	
Sign: *Anterior to Posterior*	**Functional Pathology**
1. Hypertrophied SCM	1. Overactive SCM
2. Gothic shoulders	2. Shortened upper trapezius
3. UE internal rotation/round shoulders	3. Shortened pectorals
4. Prominence of the iliotibial tract	4. Shortened TFL and ITB
5. Lateral deviation of the patellae	5. Shortened TFL or ITB and/or lengthened vastus medialis
Sign: *Posterior to Anterior*	6. Weak Glutei
6. Flattening superior/lateral buttock quadrant	7. Overactive T/L erector spinae muscle
7. Hypertrophied T/L erector spinae	8. Lengthened serratus anterior
8. Scapula winging	9. Shortened upper trapezius or levator scapulae and/or lengthened lower and middle trapezius
9. Medial rotated scapula	
Sign: *Lateral*	
10. Protruding abdomen	10. Lengthened rectus abdominus
11. Forward head carriage	11. Lengthened deep neck flexors and/or shortened suboccipitals

ITB, iliotibial band; QL, quadratus lumborum; SCM, sternocleidomastoid; TFL, tensor fascia latae; T/L, thoracolumbar; UE, upper extremity.
[a] The posture and gait portion of the examination can yield clinically useful information when assessing outcomes.

accurately accomplished outside the workplace. In addition, cumulative trauma effects cannot be properly assessed in a nonwork environment in a short time duration. More specifically, many occupational injuries are caused by a series of events that occur over time (ie, **cumulative trauma disorders**). Hence, no laboratory, clinic, or job simulator can reproduce the type of environment in which a gradual onset of a symptom over days, weeks, or months results in an injury. **In such cases, an evaluation of the patient at their work station may be of equal or even greater benefit as a WCE, especially when a high percentage of workers are injured in a particular job site.** In general, it has been

reported that is easier to change a work site than to change the worker (Putz-Anderson, 1988). It is necessary to acknowledge these weaknesses or pitfalls of WCE in order to benefit from the strengths of functional assessments. For more information concerning WCEs, refer to Chapter 17.

The term "functional capacity evaluation" or FCE is used in several contexts in the literature and, as a result, can be quite confusing. Functional tests such as those included in the QFCE measure physical or functional performance. These tests assess individual functional kinetic links such as hamstring length, iliopsoas length, and spinal ROM. The term "functional capacity," however, has also been used when assessing whole body or "real-world" movements, which are commonly assessed in a WCE. Examples of whole body functional tests include reaching, climbing, bending, stooping, crouching, and so forth. The Dictionary of Occupational Titles (DOT) has defined these movements, and the correlation between the QFCE and the DOT is described in Table 16–24. A lift and carry assessment is considered an important part of a WCE (Mayer et al, 1988; Matheson, 1991). This evaluation can be accomplished by adding weights to a crate, which are typically masked or unknown to the patient. The crate is then moved from floor to waist, waist to shoulder, and shoulder to overhead position. The test is typically terminated when poor body mechanics are observed and/or pain occurs and the patient elects to stop the test.

The WCE has traditionally been performed by occupational therapists (OTs). The duration of the test can range

---

CLINICAL TIP 16–5
Finding a Functional Pathological Link

Some of my difficult-to-manage patients who presented with chronic headaches have responded best to treatment only after treatment that addressed a distant key functional pathological link. One example of such a distant pathological link is ankle pronation and resulting muscle imbalances in the lower extremity, pelvis, and lumbar spine. The inclusion of corrective prescription foot orthotics, followed by facilitation of the weak muscles and stretching of overactive muscles higher in the kinetic chain, brought about the most satisfying results for these patients.

Table 16–24: Comparison of QFCE with DOT Basic Job Traits[a]

TEST	DESCRIPTION
Standing	Postural muscles allow for maintenance of an upright standing posture; these muscles tend to be short and tight as they must remain tonic or active in order to keep us vertical
	The QFCE tests that assess the postural/tonic muscle groups include: gastrocnemius and soleus, modified Thomas test/hip extension (iliopsoas), knee flexion test (quadriceps femoris, particularly if contracture is present), repetitive squat, and static back endurance
Walking	This function is a dynamic, multi-muscular functional task, the same tests described above, for "Standing," would apply, in addition to hamstring length (SLR test) and hip ROM
Sitting	Trunk stabilization, which includes the static back endurance, repetitive arch-up, and repetitive sit-up, are utilized
	The hip must also be flexible in the sagittal plane (flexion, extension) in order to sit; hence, the modified Thomas, SLR, and hip rotation are important tests in assessing osteoarthritis of the hip
	The act of changing positions from sitting to standing or vice versa incorporates the action of almost all the tests, with exception of CROM and grip strength
Lifting	In a WCE, lifting is measured by floor to waist, waist to shoulder, and floor to shoulder lift tasks; these tests incorporate combinations of bending, squatting, and stooping
	All of the QFCE tests are needed in order to test these three functions except for CROM and repetitive sit-up, although the latter (abdominal muscles) are needed for trunk stabilization, which is required in lifting
Carrying	The same muscle groups as noted in "Walking" are needed, in addition to grip strength test
Pushing	All QFCE tests with the exception of CROM and grip strength are needed
Pulling	All QFCE tests are required with exception of CROM and LROM
Climbing	Requires repetitive squat, gastroc/soleus, modified Thomas/hip extension, SLR, knee flexion, and hip ROM tests
	It is also important to assess the one-leg standing test for balance
Balancing	The one-leg standing test for balance and trunk stabilization, which includes all functions that are tested by the QFCE are required with the exception of grip strength
	Because of the deep tonic neck reflexes, CROM and strength tests are important
Stooping	This complex movement requires function measured by all of the QFCE tests with exception of CROM and grip strength
Kneeling	Repetitive squat, gastroc/soleus, modified Thomas/hip extension, SLR, knee flexion, and hip ROM
Crouching	Repetitive squat, LROM, CROM, modified Thomas, SLR, hip ROM, and static back endurance
Crawling	Modified Thomas, SLR, knee flexion, and hip ROM
Reaching	The qualitative test of shoulder abduction testing will facilitate shoulder function assessment; this could be modified by the use of an inclinometer or goniometer and recording the abduction ROM at the point of upper trapezius contraction
Handling	Grip strength
Fingering	Grip and pinch strength

CROM, cervical range of motion; LROM, lumbar range of motion; QFCE, quantitative functional capacity evaluation; ROM, range of motion; SLR, straight leg raise.

[a] The items included in the Dictionary of Occupational Titles (DOT) are listed and cross-references to the QFCE discussed. The 20 DOT items test global motion, whereas the QFCE tests for physical performance of smaller functioning units. Although the two methods overlap somewhat, the global movement tends to be less sensitive at detecting deficiency in the kinetic chain but more practical in assessing return-to-work issues.

from 4 hours to up to 2 days. The WCE is usually ordered when prior attempts to return a patient back to work with restrictions have either failed or resulted in exacerbations of the condition and, often, a return to regular duties cannot be achieved. Therefore, it is primarily used in the small percentage of patients who consume a large portion of health care dollars—patients who are often chronically injured, difficult to treat, and unable to work. The WCE is used to place the patient into a specific physical demand characteristic (PDC) level, which includes sedentary, light, medium, heavy, and very heavy lift and carry categories (Table 16–25).

Because the WCE is usually reserved for the difficult-to-manage patient population, and the evaluation is quite time intensive, it lacks utility and practicality for the primary care provider. Also, many patients do not require a full 4-hour (or more) WCE when initially being returned to work. Therefore, an intermediate type of examination or something less than the full WCE may play a significant role in filling this void to help the patient with a less-complicated treatment plan safely return to work. This type of examination should include physical performance testing, such as the QFCE, as these tests have been reported to be

Table 16–25: Physical Demands Characteristics[a]

ABBREVIATION	TERM	MAXIMUM LIFTING (LBS)	MAXIMUM CARRYING (LBS)
S	Sedentary	10	5
L	Light	20	10
M	Medium	50	25
H	Heavy	100	50
V	Very Heavy	over 100	over 50

[a] The Dictionary of Occupational Titles (DOT) maximum lift (third column) and maximum carry (fourth column) definitions.

Reprinted with permission from Yeomans and Liebenson, 1996b.

sensitive, specific, reliable, and valid and give functional clues to whole-body movement failure(s) or activity limitations (see Table 16–24). However, physical performance tests are not a substitute for the WCE or whole-body, real-world tests, which are needed in order to identify specific occupational/DOT activity intolerance (Kishino et al, 1985; Curtis et al, 1994). Mooney and Matheson (1994) designed the California Functional Capacity Protocol (Cal-FCP), which incorporates an assessment of the DOT items. Included in the Cal-FCP is the **Performance Assessment and Capacity Testing (PACT) Spinal Function Sort (SFS),** which is completed by having the patient review pictures of various tasks of daily living that include work-related items as well as domestic activities covering the 20 items of the DOT (Fig. 16–35) (Matheson et al, 1993). The patient completes a worksheet, scoring his or her perceived tolerance to the activity pictured on a 1 to 5 scale (where 1 = able, 5 = unable) (Fig. 16–36).

Several important items are derived from this evaluation, as follows:

- The score, of Rating of Perceived Capacity (RPC) categorizes the patient into one of the five PDC work levels (from sedentary to heavy)
- A perceived maximum lift/carry load is identified.
- Internal reliability is checked by comparing similar tasks.
- The RPC score is compared to normative data collected on both working and disabled males and females.
- The PDC level into which the RPC score places the patient is compared to a Jobs Demands Questionnaire (which describes the demands of the patient's current job). The ability of the patient to perform the current job is then determined.
- Work-related duties are circled so that tolerance to specific work activities can be appreciated and separated from nonoccupational duties. This can also be used to institute work-specific exercise protocols or work simulation.

When all 50 items are completed, the total RPC score is calculated. This information can be used to guide the HCP

in issuing return-to-work restrictions for the patient (see Fig. 16–37). It takes approximately 5 to 7 minutes for the patient to complete the SFS, and approximately 10 to 15 minutes for the HCP to calculate the score, interpret the results of maximum lift/carry, and compare it to the patient's current work demands (Job Demands Questionnaire) and the normative data (Table 16–26).

The patient's ability to perform and maintain static positions is assessed in the functional ROM tests or **Static Position Tolerance Tests (SPTTs).** These tests use the patient's own stature as a frame of reference. This anthropometric ROM assessment assesses five static positions, which include:

CLINICAL TIP 16–6
Results of Comparison Between SFS and WCE

When comparing over 75 SFSs to the full WCE, the results are usually strikingly similar. Less frequently, when the SFS and the WCE do not agree with each other, it has been my experience that significant psychosocial issues often exist, such as fear-avoidant behavior, marital distress, economic difficulties, anxiety, depression, catastrophization, job dissatisfaction, poor self-rated health, and/or others. Utilizing the questionnaire provided in Appendix 4 can help the HCP to identify "yellow flags" such as these and may help predict patients whose recovery will be prolonged. Keeping in perspective the practicality of the SFS, SPTT, and QFCE (approximately 45 minutes are required to complete all three tests) as compared to the WCE (4 hours or more to complete), a balanced way of assessing return-to-work limitations objectively without the time or expense of the full WCE can be appreciated. I recommend this more practical approach when returning the worker to light duty after a short period of **total temporary disability (TTD)** or when graduating the worker from light to regular duties. However, the full WCE is recommended if the patient has repeatedly failed to return safely to light duty from TTD or repeated failures to successfully graduate the patient from light to regular duties have occurred.

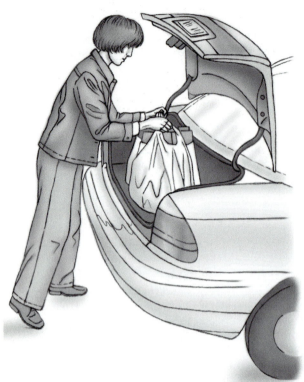

A. Unload two 10-pound grocery bags from the trunk of an automobile.

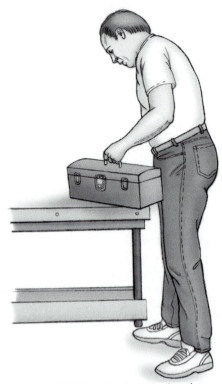

B. Lift a 20-pound tool box from the floor to a bench.

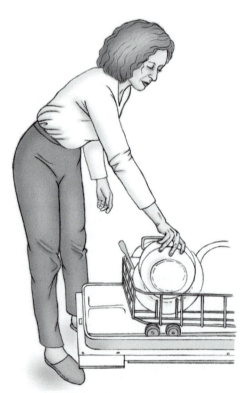

C. Load or unload a dishwasher.

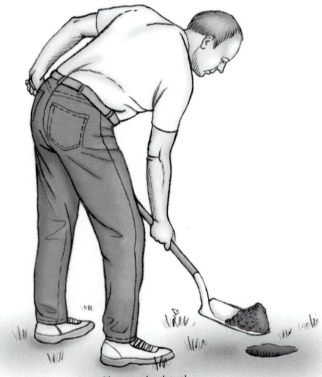

D. Dig in a garden with a spade-shovel.

Figure 16–35. The Spinal Function Sort consists of pictures representing activities of daily living, both domestic and occupational, which are reviewed by the patient and scored on a 1-to-5 (1 = able, 5 = unable) ordinal scale.
Reprinted with permission granted by Matheson LN. *PACT Spinal Function Sort Examiner's Manual.* Employment Potential Improvement Corporation, 1451 Ridgetree Trails Drive, Wildwood, MO 63021, and Matheson LN et al, 1993.

P.A.C.T. SPINAL FUNCTION SORT

© Copyright 1993 Performance Assessment and Capacity Testing

Section 2 (right half)

	Able	Restricted	Unable ?	
2 Retrieve/Tool/Floor	① 2 3 4		5 ?
4 Push/Pull Shopping Cart	① 2 3 4		5 ?
6 Place or Retrieve 5# Waist to Overhead	① 2 3 4		5 ?
8 Lower10# Crate Bench to Floor	1 2 ③ 4		5 ?
10 Lift 10# Crate Floor to Bench	1 2 ③ 4		5 ?
12 Lower 20# Crate Eye-Level to Floor	1 2 ③ 4		5 ?
14 Lift 20# Crate Floor to Eye-Level	1 2 ③ 4		5 ?
16 Lift 20# Box Floor to Bench	① 2 3 4		5 ?
18 Hammer Nails	1 2 3 4		5 ⑦
20 Trim Shrubs	1 2 3 4		5 ⑦
22 Install Face-Plate	1 2 ③ 4		5 ?
24 Pull Nail	1 2 3 4		5 ⑦
26 Move Barrel with Dolly	1 2 ③ 4		5 ?
28 Dig with Shovel	1 2 3 ④		5 ?
30 Get into Driver's Seat	1 ② 3 4		5 ?
32 Get out of Driver's Seat	1 ② 3 ④		5 ?
34 Carry 30# Bucket	① 2 3 4		5 ?
36 Carry 10# Groceries x 2	① 2 3 4		5 ?
38 Carry 20# Bucket Up Step-Ladder	1 2 3 ④		5 ?
40 Sweep Kitchen Broom	1 2 3 4		5 ?
42 Lower 50# Crate Bench to Floor	1 2 3 4		⑤ ?
44 Lift 50# Tool Box Floor to Bench	1 2 3 4		⑤ ?
46 Lower 100# Crate Bench to Floor	1 2 3 4		⑤ ?
48 Lift 100# Crate Floor to Bench	1 2 3 4		⑤ ?
50 Place or Retrieve 5#	① 2 3 4		5 ?

Section 2 totals: Able 6 (4x) 24, 2 (3x) 6, Restricted 6 (2x) 12, 3 (1x) 3 — **Section 2 Total RPC 45 / 02** %tile 25–50%

Name: **Ken Esthetic** Date: **12-16-99** ER: _____

PDC Sedentary	PDC Light	PDC Medium	PDC Heavy	PDC Very Heavy
100–110	125–135	165–175	180–190	196+

Section 1 (left half)

	Able	Restricted	Unable ?
1 Place/Bottle/Floor	① 2 3 4		5 ?
3 Push/Pull/Vacuum	1 2 ③ 4		5 ?
5 Place or Retrieve 5# Waist to Eye-Level	① 2 3 4		5 ?
7 Lower10# Eye-Level to Floor	1 2 ③ 4		5 ?
9 Lift 10# Floor to Eye-Level	1 2 ③ 4		5 ?
11 Load 20# Trunk of Auto	1 2 ③ 4		5 ?
13 Unload 20# Trunk of Auto	1 2 ③ 4		5 ?
15 Unload 2 x 10# Trunk of Auto	1 ② 3 4		5 ?
17 Paint Brush Eye-Level	① 2 3 4		5 ?
19 Wash Dishes Sink	1 2 ③ 4		5 ?
21 Light Bulb Overhead	① 2 3 4		5 ?
23 Cut Lumber	1 2 3 4		5 ⑦
25 Pour Soap	1 2 ③ 4		5 ?
27 Load/Unload Dishwasher	1 2 3 ④		5 ?
29 Push Heavy Door	① 2 3 4		5 ?
31 Pull Heavy Door	① 2 3 4		5 ?
33 Carry 10# Stool	1 2 ③ 4		5 ?
35 Carry 20# Groceries	1 2 ③ 4		5 ?
37 Climb Step-Ladder	① 2 3 4		5 ?
39 Sweep Push Broom	① 2 3 4		5 ?
41 Lower 50# Crate Eye-Level to Floor	1 2 3 4		⑤ ?
43 Lift 50# Crate Floor to Eye-Level	1 2 3 4		⑤ ?
45 Lower 100# Crate Eye-Level to Floor	1 2 3 4		⑤ ?
47 Lift 100# Crate Floor to Eye-Level	1 2 3 4		⑤ ?
49 Paint Brush Eye-Level	1 ② 3 4		5 ?

Section 1 totals: Able 8 (4x) 32, 2 (3x) 6, Restricted 9 (2x) 18, 1 (1x) 1 — **Section 1 Total 57**

FCE at: _____ RPC Score: _____

Dis	DK	Int
0–2	0–3	1
0–2	4+	②
3–4	na	3
5+	na	4

Figure 16–36. Sample Spinal Function Sort evaluation. The patient's Rating of Perceived Capacity (RPC) is calculated and compared to normative data and the physical demands characteristics chart.

Reprinted with permission granted by Matheson LN. *PACT Spinal Function Sort Examiner's Manual.* Employment Potential Improvement Corporation, 1451 Ridgetree Trails Drive, Wildwood, MO 63021 and, Matheson LN et al, 1993.

ATTENDING PHYSICIAN'S RETURN TO WORK RECOMMENDATIONS

Employer: _____ XYZ Corp _____

Employee Name: _____ Ken Esthetic _____

TO BE COMPLETED BY ATTENDING PHYSICIAN:

Diagnosis: _____ Lumbar sprain/strain (847.2) _____

Injury or Illness: _____ Injury _____ Work or Non-work related? _____ Work _____

I saw and treated this employee on (date) _____ 12-16-99 _____ and:

1. _____ Recommended his/her return to work with no limitations on (date) _____

2. _X_ He/She may return to work capable of performing the degree of work checked below with the following limitations.

DEGREE	LIMITATIONS
_____ **Sedentary Work**. Lifting 10 pounds maximum and occasionally lift and/or carrying such articles as dockets, ledgers and small tools. Although a sedentary job is defined as one which involves sitting, a certain amount of walking and standing is often necessary in carrying out job duties. Jobs are sedentary if walking and standing are required only occasionally and other sedentary criteria are met.	1. In a 10 hour work day patient may: a. Stand/Walk ___ None ___ 4–6 Hours _X_ 1–4 Hours ___ 6–10 Hours b. Sit ___ 1–3 Hours _X_ 3–5 Hours ___ 5–10 Hours

2. Patient may use hands for repetitive actions such as:

	Simple Grasping	Firm Grasping	Fine Manipulating
Right:	___ Yes ___ No	___ Yes ___ No	___ Yes ___ No
Left:	___ Yes ___ No	___ Yes ___ No	___ Yes ___ No

_X_ **Light Work**. Lifting 20 pounds maximum with frequent lifting and/or carrying of objects weighing up to 10 pounds. Even though the weight lifted may be only a negligible amount, a job is in this category when it requires walking or standing to a significant degree or when it involves sitting most of the time with a degree of pushing and pulling of arm and/or leg controls.

3. Patient may use feet for repetitive movement as in operating foot controls: ___ Yes ___ No

4. During work day, patient is able to:

	67–100%	34–66%	1–33%	0%
a. Bend	___	___	X	___
b. Squat	___	X	___	___
c. Climb	___	X	___	___
d. Twist Body	___	X	___	___
e. Push	___	X	___	___
f. Pull	___	___	X	___
g. Balance	X	___	___	___
h. Kneel	___	___	___	___
i. Crawl	___	X	___	___
j. Grasp	X	___	___	___
k. Reach	___	X	___	___

_____ **Medium Light Work**. Lifting 35 pounds maximum with frequent lifting and/or carrying of objects weighing up to 30 pounds.

_____ **Medium Work**. Lifting 50 pounds maximum with frequent lifting and/or carrying of objects weighing up to 35 pounds.

_____ **Heavy Work**. Lifting 75 pounds maximum with frequent lifting and/or carrying of objects weighing up to 50 pounds.

_____ **Very Heavy Work**. Lifting objects in excess of 100 pounds with frequent lifting and/or carrying of objects weighing 75 pounds or more.

Other restrictions and/or limitations: Please allow him a sit/stand option to avoid prolonged static positions. Please rotate him to a different task if pain increases and cannot be controlled.

3. These restrictions are in effect until (date) _____ 12-30-99 _____ or until employee is re-evaluated on (date) _____

4. He/She is totally incapacitated at this time. Employee will be re-evaluated on (date) _____

PHYSICIAN'S SIGNATURE: _____ Dr. Frank Lee Concerned MD, DC, RPT _____ DATE: _____ 12-16-99 _____
(No rubber stamp, please)

Figure 16–37. Return-to-work form. The Rating of Perceived Capacity (RPC) score and the individual answers obtained from the patient can be applied directly to a standard return-to-work form. This process is a logical step before returning a patient to work after a period of total temporary disability. A full Work Capacity Evaluation (WCE) is recommended if there have been prior attempts to return the patient to light duty work or back to regular duty.

Table 16–26: Spinal Function Sort Male and Female Rating of Perceived Capacity Scores Derived from Normative Data from Both Healthy and Disabled Subjects

	MALES		FEMALES	
PERCENTILE	**Employed** Healthy (n = 62)	**Unemployed** Disabled (n = 161)	**Employed** Healthy (n = 116)	**Unemployed** Disabled (n = 66)
90th	200	159	186	146
75th	195	140	178	115
50th	191	113	161	94
25th	155	76	147	66
10th	144	50	129	48

Compiled from data in Matheson and Matheson ML, 1991.

1. Standing and reaching to shoulder level
2. Standing and reaching to eye level
3. Stooping and reaching to knee level
4. Crouching and reaching to knee level
5. Kneeling and reaching to knee level

Each posture is held for 15 seconds during a countdown from 15 backwards, as the HCP observes the patient's quality of posture. The following scoring method is utilized:

- 1 = able to perform without restrictions
- 2 = slightly restricted; the patient can maintain the position for the full 15 seconds with only minimal complaints
- 3 = moderately restricted; the patient cannot maintain the position for 15 seconds but can maintain for more than 5 seconds
- 4 = very restricted; this score is assigned to patients who cannot hold the position for 5 seconds.

- 5 = unable; the patient cannot assume the position at all

It takes about 5 minutes to perform the SPTTs and no additional calculation or interpretation time is required. (Refer to Appendix Form G–10.)

The patient's SPTT and SFS make up the whole-body, "real-world" movement assessment. When this information is combined with the QFCE, the functional limitations derived from the QFCE describe the **impairment,** while the SPTT and SFS describe the **disability.** This low-tech approach is appropriate initially when returning a patient to work. If the patient cannot perform the limited duties as recommended by the results of this approach, or if there is a history of poor work tolerance, a prior history of poor return to work success, and/or a significant number of psychosocial barriers to recovery, then a full WCE is recommended.

Conclusion

The utilization of physical performance tests such as those included in the QFCE are very practical, as they fulfill the following objectives:

- Weak links in the kinetic chain that can lead to functional losses are identified, often at a time when traditional provocative testing is of little to no value. This qualifies as an "objective" reason to support ongoing patient complaints (a common third-party payer expectation to support "medical necessity" of care).
- The inclusion of normative data allows for a direct comparison to be made and, therefore, the QFCE tests serve as objective outcome measures to assess progress following antecedent therapeutic intervention.

- Exercise prescription and rehabilitation approaches can be derived from the tests that fall below the 85% cutoff and repeating the test following rehabilitation allows for objective outcomes assessment.
- Comparing the QFCE tests with other tests, such as the spinal function sort, static position tolerance tests and the DOT facilitates returning the injured worker back to work safely.
- When documentation includes subjective questionnaire outcome data and objective outcome data from the QFCE, the HCP can make timely and rational clinical decisions that are supported both subjectively and objectively.

Conclusion (*continued*)

Many tests that can be utilized have been reviewed in this chapter. The strength of the physical performance tests lies in their ability to assess functional deficiencies and, therefore, they drive treatment and exercise prescriptions. When normative data exists, the test results can be compared to the norms on the initial examination data and a percentage of normal calculated. This will allow for identification of weak kinetic links, quantitative outcomes assessment, as well as treatment prescription.

These tests should be performed when the patient continues to complain symptomatically, often at a time when objective provocative testing fails to substantiate a problem. All too often when this occurs, the patient is viewed as behaving inappropriately or as having a hidden agenda such as secondary gain. Although the latter may sometimes be accurate, it is well established that functional losses continue to exist after healing is complete (Kishino et al, 1985; Curtis et al, 1994). Failure to address these deficiencies can result in a higher probability of failure, leading to chronicity. It is well accepted that rehabilitation following an injury or after any prolonged time period of inactivity is standard care in today's health care market (Mooney, 1994). Informed patients are also beginning to request these services if they are not first offered by the HCP. The utilization of physical performance testing allows a program to be specifically designed for the individual patient, tailoring the rehabilitation protocols most precisely for that person.

Combinations of different types of tests were discussed to allow for rational decision making in various scenarios including:

- Rehabilitation prescription
- Returning the patient to work
- Assessing outcomes

The real strength of applying these tests clinically becomes evident when they are repeated a second time and outcomes arising from a functional restoration program can be objectively determined and compared to the subjective tools to assess for consistency between the subjective complaints and the objective findings. Moreover, this link seems to be more popular as a prerequisite for reimbursement from third-party payers, for review organizations, and for quality determination of managed care groups striving for national accreditation. The standard in health care regarding the musculoskeletal system is becoming rehabilitation oriented. Similarly, outcomes-based practice is also becoming expected. Utilization of these tests will help fulfill the outcomes requirements objectively, while use of the administration of questionnaires will do the same subjectively. Regardless of the model HCPs are forced into following, utilization of these approaches will fulfill the most important reason to make this paradigm change: to provide the best service possible to the patient for the best value.

REFERENCES

Ahern DK, Hannon DJ, Goreczny J, Follick MF, Parziale JR. Correlation of chronic low-back pain behavior and muscle function examination of the flexion-relaxation response. *Spine* 1990;15:92–95.

Alaranta H, Hurri H, Heliovaara M et al. Non-dynamometric trunk performance tests: Reliability and normative data. *Scand J Rehabil Med* 1994;26:211–215.

Alaranta H, Soukka A, Harju R, Heliovaara M. Selan ja niskahartiaseudun suoritustestisto tyoterveyshuollon terveystarkastuksiin. *Tyosuojelurahaston Julkaisuja C21*. Helsinki, Finland: Invalidisaatio; 1990.

Alexander MJL. Biomechanics of sit-up exercises. *CAHPER J* 1985;51:36–38.

Allsop KG. Potential hazards of abdominal exercises. *JOHPER* 1971;42:89–90.

American Alliance for Health, Physical Education, Recreation and Dance. *Physical Best*. Reston, Va: AAHPERD; 1988.

American Medical Association. *Guides to the Evaluation of Permanent Impairment*, 4th ed. Chicago, Ill: AMA; 1993:78.

Andersson E, Ma Z, Nilsson J, Thostensson A. Abdominal and hip flexor muscle involvement in various training exercises. In: Gregor RJ, Zernicke RF, Whiting WC, eds. *Proceedings of the XXI International Congress of Biomechanics*. Los Angeles, Calif: UCLA; 1989:no.245.

Atlas SJ, Deyo RA, Patrick DL, et al. The Quebec Task Force Classification for Spinal Disorders and the severity, treatment, and outcomes of sciatica and lumbar spinal stenosis. *Spine* 1996;21:2885–2892.

Atwater SW, Crowe TR, Deitz JC, et al. Interrater and test retest reliability of two pediatric balance tests. *Phys Ther* 1990;20:79–87.

Barrack RL, Skinner HB, Buckley SL. Proprioception in the anterior cruciate deficient knee. *Am J Sports Med* 1989;17:1–6.

Basmajian JV, Nyberg R. *Rational Manual Therapies*. Balitimore, Md: Williams & Wilkins; 1993:47.

Battie MC, Bigos SJ, Fisher LD, et al. The role of spinal flexibility in back pain complaints within industry. *Spine* 1990;15:768–773.

Battie MC, Bigos SJ, Sheehy A, Wortley M. Spinal flexibility and individual factors that influence it. *Phys Ther* 1987;67:653–658.

Beuker F. *Leistungsprüfungen im Freizeit und Erholungssport*. Leipzig, Germany: 1976.

Biering-Sorenson F. Physical measurement as risk indicators for low back trouble over a one-year period. *Spine* 1984;9:143–148.

Bigos S, Bowyer O, Braen G et al. Acute low back problems in adults. *Clinical Practice Guideline No. 14*. Rockville, Md: Agency for Health Care Policy and Research, Public Health Service, US Department of Health and Human Services; 1994. AHCPR Publication No. 95-0642.

Bly N. Spatial orientation to gravity and implication for balance training. *Orthop Phys Ther Clin North Am* 1992;1(2):207–236.

Bly N, Sinnot PL. Variations in balance and body sway in middle-aged adults: subjects with healthy backs compared with subjects with low-back dysfunction. *Spine* 1991;16:325–330.

Bogduk N, Pearcy M, Hadfield G. Anatomy and biomechanics of psoas major. *Clin Biomech* 1992;7:109–115.

Bohannon RW, Larkin PA, Cook AC, Gear J, Singer J. Decrease in timed balance test scores with aging. *Phys Ther* 1984;64:1067–1070.

Borkowicz R. Sit-ups: With and without resistance. *Athletic J* 1981;62:42–44.

Bosien WR, Staples OS, Russell SW. Residual disability following acute ankle sprains. *J Bone Joint Surg [Am]* 1955;37:1237.

Brady S, Mayer T, Gatchel RJ. Physical progress and residual impairment quantification after functional restoration. Part II: Isokinetic trunk strength. *Spine* 1994;19:395–400.

Briggs RC, Gossman MR, Birch R, Drews J, Shaddeau S. Balance performance among noninstitutionalized elderly women. *Phys Ther* 1989;69:748–756.

Bullivant AM, Burchell C, Chamberlain J, Miller EK, Wareham MP. An electromyographic and biomechanical investigation of a variety of sit-up techniques. *Br J Phys Ed* 1986;17:38–39.

Bullock-Saxton J. Local sensation changes and altered hip muscle function following severe ankle sprain. *Phys Ther* 1994;74:17–34.

Bullock-Saxton JE, Janda V, Bullock MI. Reflex activation of gluteal muscles in walking: An approach to restoration of muscle function for patients with low back pain. *Spine* 1993;18:704–708.

Burton AK, Tillotson KM, Troup JDG. Prediction of low-back trouble frequency in a working population. *Spine* 1989a;14:939–946.

Burton AK, Tillotson KM, Troup JDG. Variation in lumbar sagittal mobility with low-back trouble. *Spine* 1989b;14:584–590.

Bussieres A. A review of functional outcome measures for cervical spine disorders: Literature review. *JCCA* 1994;38:32–40.

Carlos A, Guimaraes S, Aurelia B, Ines M, DeCampos A, Marantes R. The contribution of the rectus abdominis and rectus femoris in twelve selected abdominal exercises. *J Sports Med Phys Fitn* 1991;31:222–230.

Chandler JM, Duncan PW, Studenski SA. Balance performance on the postural stress test: Comparison of young adults, healthy elderly and fallers. *Phys Ther* 1990;70:410–415.

Chapman-Smith D. Measuring results—the new importance of patient questionnaires. *Chiro Report* 1992;7(1):1–6.

Cherkin DC, Deyo RA, Street JH, Barlow W. Predicting poor outcomes for back pain seen in primary care using patients' own criteria. *Spine* 1996;21:2900–2907.

Chesworth BM, Padfield BJ, Helewa A, Stitt LW. A comparison of hip mobility in patients with low back pain and matched healthy subjects. *Physio Can* 1994;46:267–274.

Cibulka MT, Delitto A, Koldehoff R. Changes in innominate tilt after manipulation of the sacroiliac joint in patients with low back pain: An experimental study. *Phys Ther* 1988;68:1359–1363.

Cibulka MT, Sinacore DR, Cromer GS, Delitto A. Unilateral hip rotation range of motion asymmetry in patients with sacroiliac joint regional pain. *Spine* 1998;23:1009–1015.

Clarke HH. Exercise and the abdominal muscles. *Phys Fitn Res Dig* 1976;6:1–21.

Cohen H, Blatchly CA, Gombash LL. A study of the clinical test of sensory interaction and balance. *Phys Ther* 1993;73:346–354.

Crotts D, Thompson B, Nahom M, Ryan S, Newton RA. Balance abilities of professional dancers on select balance tests. *J Orthop Sports Phys Ther* 1996;23:12–17

Curtis L, Mayer T, Gatchel R. Physical progress and residual impairment quantification after functional restoration, part III: Isokinetic and isoinertial lifting capacity. *Spine* 1994;19:401–405.

Delitto A, Cibulka MT, Erhard RE, et al. Evidence for use of an extension-mobilization category in acute low back syndrome: A prescriptive validation pilot study. *Phys Ther* 1993;73:216–228.

Delitto A, Shulman AD, Rose SL, et al. Reliability of a clinical examination to classify patients with low back syndrome. *Phys Ther Prac* 1992;1:1–9.

Dworkin SF, Von Korff M, Whitney WC, et al. Measurement of characteristic pain intensity in field research. *Pain Suppl* 1990;5:S290.

Ekholm J, Arborelius UP, Fahkrantz A, Larsson AM, Mattson G. Activation of abdominal muscles during some physiotherapeutic exercises. *Scand J Rehabil Med* 1979;11:75–84.

Ekstrand J, Wiktorsson M, Oberg B, Gillquist J. Lower extremity goniometric measurements: A study to determine their reliability. *Arch Phys Med Rehabil* 1982;63:171–175.

Ellison JB, Rose SJ, Sahrmann SA. Patterns of hip rotation range of motion: A comparison between healthy subjects and patients with low back pain. *Phys Ther* 1990;70:537–541.

Erhard RE, Delitto A, Cibulka MT. Relative effectiveness of an extension program and a combined program of manipulation and flexion and extension exercises in patients with acute low back syndrome. *Phys Ther* 1994;74:1093–1100.

Fitz-Ritson D. Assessment of cervicogenic vertigo. *J Manipulative Physiol Ther* 1991;14:193–198.

Fitz-Ritson D. Phasic exercises for cervical rehabilitation after "whiplash" trauma. *J Manipulative Physiol Ther* 1995;18:21–4.

Flint M. Effect of increasing back and abdominal muscle strength on low back pain. *Res Q Exer Sport* 1955;29:160–171.

Flint MM. Selected exercises. *JOHPER* 1964;35:19–23.

Flint MM. Abdominal muscle involvement during the performance of various forms of sit-up exercises. *Am J Phys Med* 1965;44:224–234.

Flint MM. An electromyographic comparison of the function of the iliacus and the rectus abdominis muscles. *J Am Phys Ther Assoc* 1965;45:248–253.

Flint MM, Gudgell J. Electromyographic study of abdominal muscular activity during exercise. *Res Q Exer Sport* 1965;36:29–37.

Forkin DM, Koczur C, Battle R, Newton RA. Evaluation of kinesthetic deficits indicative of balance control in gymnasts with unilateral chronic ankle sprains. *J Orthop Sports Phys Ther* 1996;23:245–250.

Foust DR, Chaffin BC, Snyder RG, Baum JK. Cervical range of motion and dynamic response and strength of cervical muscles. *SAE Transaction* 1973;82:3222–3234.

Frandin K, Sonn U, Svantesson U, Grimby G. Functional balance tests in 76-year-olds in relation to performance, activities of daily living and platform tests. *Scand J Rehabil Med* 1996;77:37–43.

Freeman MAR, Dean MRE, Hanham IWF. The etiology and prevention of functional instability of the foot. *J Bone Joint Surg [Br]* 1965;47:678–685.

Frost M, Stuckey S, Smalley L, Darman G. Reliability of measuring trunk motions in centimetres. *Phys Ther* 1982;62:1431–1437.

Frymoyer JW, Cats-Baril W. Predictors of low back pain disability. *Clin Orthop* 1987;221:89–98.

Gajdosik RL, Rieck MA, Sullivan DK, Wightman SE. Comparison of four clinical tests for assessing hamstring muscle length. *J Orthop Sports Phys Ther* 1993;18:614–618.

Gehlsen BM, Whaley MH. Falls in the elderly: Part II, balance, strength, and flexibility. *Arch Phys Med Rehabil* 1990;71:739–741.

Gilliam TB, Roy RR. "Abdominal" exercises: More harm than good? *J Phys Ed Rec* 1976;47:46, 67.

Godfrey KE, Kinding LE, Windell EJ. Electromyographic study of duration of muscle activity in sit-up variations. *Arch Phys Med Rehabil* 1977;58:132–135.

Golding LA, Myers CR, Sinning WE. *The Y's Way to Physical Fitness*. rev ed. Chicago, Ill: National Board of the YMCA; 1982.

Gracovetsky S, Kary DJ, Ben Said R, Pitceh I, Helie J. Analysis of spinal and muscular activity during flexion/extension and free lifts. *Spine* 1990;15:1333–1339.

Gutin B, Lipetz S. An electromyographic investigation of the rectus abdominis in abdominal exercises. *Res Q Exer Sport* 1971;42:256–263.

Hall MG, Ferrell WR, Sturrock RD, Hamblen DL, Baxendale RH. The effect of the hypermobility syndrome on knee joint proprioception. *Br J Rheumatol* 1995;34:121–125.

Hall SJ, Lee J, Wood TM. Evaluation of selected sit-up variations for the individual with low back pain. *J Appl Sport Sci Res* 1990;4:42–46.

Harms-Ringdahl K, Ekholm J. Influence of arm position on neck muscular activity levels during flexion-extension movements of the cervical spine. In: Jonsson B, ed. *Biomechanics X-A*. Champaign, Ill: Human Kinetics; 1987:249–254.

Hart DL, Isernhagen SJ, Matheson LN. Guidelines for functional capacity evaluation of people with medical conditions. *J Orthop Sports Phys Ther* 1993;18:682–686.

Heltmann DK, Gossman MR, Shaddeau, Jackson JR. Balance performance and step width in noninstitutionalized, elderly, female fallers and nonfallers. *Phys Ther* 1989;69:923–931.

Hikosaka O, Maeda M. Cervical effects on abducens motoneurons and their interaction with vestibulo-ocular reflex. *Exp Brain Res* 1973;18:512–530.

Hocherman S, Dickstein R, Pillar T. PlatForm training and postural stability in hemiplegia. *Arch Phys Med Rehabil* 1984;65:588–592.

Holmstrom E, Moritz U, Andersson M. Trunk muscle strength and back muscle endurance in construction workers with and without low back disorders. *Scand J Rehabil Med* 1992;24:3–10.

Horak FB. Clinical measurement of postural control in adults. *Phys Ther* 1987;67:1881–1885.

Hultman G, Nordin M, Saraste H, Ohlsen H. Body composition, endurance, strength, cross-sectional area, and density of MM erector spinae in men with and without low back pain. *J Spinal Disord* 1993;6:114–123.

Hyytiainen K, Salminen J, Suvitie S, Wickstrom G, Pentti J. Reproducibility of nine tests to measure spinal mobility and trunk muscle strength. *Scand J Rehabil Med* 1991;23:3–10.

Inamura K. Re-assessment of the method of analysis of electrogravitiograph and the one foot test. *Aggressologie* 1983;24:107–108.

Institute for Aerobics Research. *FITNESSGRAM User's Manual*. Dallas, Tex: IAR; 1977.

Ito T, Shirado O, Suzuki H, et al. Lumbar trunk muscle endurance testing: An inexpensive alternative to a machine for evaluation. *Arch Phys Med Rehabil* 1996;77:75–79.

Invergo JJ, Ball TE, Looney M. Relationship of push-ups and absolute muscular endurance to bench press strength. *J Appl Sport Sci Res* 1991;5:121–125.

Jacobson GP, Newman CW, Hunter L, Balzer GK. Balance function test correlates of the dizziness handicap inventory. *J Am Acad Audiol* 1991;2:253–260.

Janda V. *Muscle Function Testing*. London, England: Butterworths; 1983.

Jette M, Sidney K, Cicutti N. A critical analysis of sit-ups: A case for the partial curl-up as a test of abdominal muscular endurance. *CAHPER J* 1984;50:4–9.

Johansson G, Jarnlo G-B. Balance training in 70-year-old women. *Physiother Theor Pract* 1991;7:121–125.

Jorgensen K, Nicolaisen T. Back muscle strength and body weight as limiting factors for work in the standing slightly-stooped position. *Scand J Rehabil Med* 1970;2:259.

Juker D, McGill SM, Kropf P, Steffen T. Quantitative intramuscular myoelectric activity of lumbar portions of psoas and the abdominal wall during a wide variety of tasks. *Med Sci Sports Exerc* 1998;30:301–310.

Jull G, Janda V. Muscles and motor control in low back pain. In: Twomey LT, Taylor JR, eds. *Physical Therapy for the Low Back; Clinics in Physical Therapy*. New York, NY: Churchill Livingstone; 1987.

Kendall FP. A criticism of current tests and exercises for physical fitness. *J Am Phys Ther Assoc* 1965;45:187–197.

Kishino N, Mayer T, Gatchel R, et al. Quantification of lumbar function. Part 4: Isometric and isokinetic lifting simulation in normal subjects and low back dysfunction patients. *Spine* 1985;10:921–927.

Knudson D, Johnston D. Validity and reliability of a bench truck-curl test of abdominal endurance. *J Strength Cond Res* 1995;9:165–169.

Kondraske G. Towards a standard clinical measure of postural stability. In: Kondraske G, Robinson C, eds. *Proceedings of the 8th Annual Conference of the IEEE Engineering in Medicine and Biology Society* 1986;3:1579–1582.

Kraus H. *Clinical Treatment of Back and Neck Pain*. New York, NY: McGraw-Hill; 1970:28–56.

Lauren H, Luoto S, Alaranta H, et al. Arm motion speed and risk of neck pain: A preliminary communication. *Spine* 1997;22:2094–2099.

Leino P, Aro S, Hasan J. Trunk muscle function and low-back disorders: A ten-year follow-up study. *J Chronic Dis* 1987;40:289–296.

Lewit K. *Manipulative Therapy in Rehabilitation of the Motor System*. 2nd ed. London, England: Butterworths; 1991.

Liebenson C, ed. *Rehabilitation of the Spine: A Practitioner's Manual*. Baltimore, Md: Williams & Wilkins; 1996.

Liebenson C, Yeomans, S. Outcomes assessment in musculoskeletal medicine. *Man Ther* 1997;2:67–74.

Lind B, Sihlbom H, Norwall A, Malchau H. Normal range of motion of the cervical spine. *Arch Phys Med Rehabil* 1989;70:692–695.

Loebl W. Measurements of spinal posture and range in spinal movements. *Ann Phys Med* 1967;9:103–110.

Lord SR, Ward JA, Williams P. Exercise effect on dynamic stability in older women: A randomized controlled trial. *Arch Phys Med Rehabil* 1996;77:232–236.

Luoto S, Heliovaara M, Hurri H, Alaranta H. Static back endurance and the risk of low-back pain. *Clin Biomech* 1995;10:323–324.

Macfarlane PA. Out with the sit-up, in with the curl-up! *JOPERD* 1993;64:62–66.

Matheson L. An introduction to lift capacity testing as a component of functional capacity evaluation. IRG, Summer 1991.

Matheson LN, Matheson ML. *Examiner's Manual for the Spinal Function Sort*. Trabuco Canyon, Ca: Performance Assessment and Capacity Testing; 1991.

Matheson L, Matheson M, Grant J. Development of a measure of perceived functional ability. *J Occup Rehabil* 1993;3:15–30.

Mayer L, Greenberg B. Measurements of the strength of trunk muscles. *J Bone Joint Surg* 1942;24:842–856.

Mayer T, Barnes D, and Kishino N, et al. Progressive isoinertial lifting evaluation. I. A standardized protocol and normative database. *Spine* 1988;13:993–997.

Mayer TG, Gatchel RJ. Functional restoration for spinal disorders: The sports medicine approach. Philadelphia, Pa: Lea & Febiger; 1988.

Mayer TG, Gatchel RJ, Keeley J, Mayer H, Richling D. A male incumbent worker industrial database. *Spine* 1994;19:762–764.

Mayer TG, Tencer A, Kristoferson S, Mooney V. Use of noninvasive techniques for quantification of spinal range-of-motion in normal subjects and chronic low-back dysfunction patients. *Spine* 1984;9:588–595.

McCouch GP, Deering ID, Ling TH. Location of receptors for tonic neck reflexes. *J Neurophysiol* 1951;14:191–195.

McGill SM. Low back exercises: Evidence for improving exercise regimens. *Phys Ther* 1998;78:754–765.

McGill SM, Juker D, Kropf P. Quantitative intramuscular myoelectric activity of quadratus lumborum during a wide variety of tasks. *Clin Biomech* 1996;11:170–172.

McGill SM, Childs A, Liebenson C. Endurance times for low back stabilization exercises: Clinical targets for testing and training from a normal database. *Arch Phys Med Rehabil* 1999;80.

McKenzie RA. *The Lumbar Spine: Mechanical Diagnosis and Therapy*. Upper Hutt, New Zealand: Spinal Publications/Wright & Carman; 1989 (reprinted).

Mellin G. Accuracy of measuring lateral flexion of the spine with a tape. *Clin Biomech* 1986;1:85–9.

Mellin G. Correlations of spinal mobility with degree of chronic low-back pain after correction for age and anthropometric factors. *Spine* 1987;12:464–468.

Melzack R. The short-form McGill Pain Questionnaire. *Pain* 1987;30:191–197.

Merskey H. Classification of chronic pain. Descriptions of chronic pain syndromes and definitions of terms. In: International Association for Study of Pain, Subcommittee on Taxonomy. *Pain* 1986;24(suppl 3):S1–S222.

Merskey H, Bogduk N. In: Task Force on Taxonomy, eds. *Classification of Chronic Pain: Descriptions of Chronic Pain Syndromes and Definitions of Pain Terms*. 2nd ed. International Association for the Study of Pain. IASP Press; 1994:207.

Moffet JAK, Hughes GI, Griffiths P. A longitudinal study of low back pain in student nurses. *Int J Nurs Stud* 1993;30:197–212.

Moffroid MT, Haugh LD. Classification schema for acute and subacute low back pain. Part I: Managing acute low back pain in the new health care environment. *Orthop Phys Ther Clin North Am*, 1995;4(2):179–191.

Moffroid MT, Haugh LD, Haig AJ, Henry SM, Pope MD. Endurance training of trunk extensor muscle. *Phys Ther* 1993;73:3–10.

Moffroid MT, Haugh LD, Henry SM, Short B. Distinguishable groups of musculoskeletal low back pain patients and asymptomatic control subjects based on physical measures of the NIOSH low back atlas. *Spine* 1994;19:1350–1358.

Moffroid MT, Haugh LD, Hodous T. Sensitivity and specificity of the NIOSH low back atlas. NIOSH Final Report RFP 200-89-2917; May 1992.

Mooney V. The place of active care in disability prevention. In: Liebenson CL, ed. *Rehabilitation of the Spine: A Practitioner's Manual*. Baltimore, Md: Williams & Wilkins; 1994.

Mooney V, Matheson LN. Objective measurement of soft tissue injury: Feasibility study. *Examiner's Manual*. October 1994:4.

Moroney SS, Schultz AB, Miller JAA. Analysis and measurements of neck loads. *J Orthop Res* 1988;6:713–720.

Murphy DJ. Soft tissue research-pain and proprioception. *Clin Chiro* 1995;3:8.

Murphy DR. *Conservative Management of Cervical Spine Syndromes*. Stamford, Conn: Appleton & Lange; 1999.

Mutoh Y, Mori T, Nakamura Y, Miyashita M. The relation between sit-up exercises and the occurrence of low back pain. In: Matsui H, Kobayashi K, eds. *Biomechanics VII-A*. Champaign, Ill: Human Kinetics, 1983:180–185.

Nachemson A. Work for all. *Clin Orthop Rel Res* 1983;179–82.

Nelson DO. Focus on two fitness exercises. *JOHPER* 1964;35:22–23.

Nelson RM. NIOSH low back atlas of standardized tests/measures. US Department of Health and Human Services, National Institute for Occupational Safety and Health; December 1988.

Nelson RM, Nestor DE. Standardized assessment of industrial low-back injuries: Development of NIOSH low-back atlas. *Top Trauma Acute Care Rehabil* 1988;2:16–30.

Newton RA. Joint receptor contributions to reflexive and kinesthetic responses. *Phys Ther* 1982;62:22–29.

Ng JK-F, Richardson CA. Reliability of electromyographic power spectral analysis of back muscle endurance in healthy subjects. *Arch Phys Med Rehabil* 1996;77:259–264.

Nicolaisen T, Jorgensen K. Trunk strength, back muscle endurance and low-back trouble. *Scand J Rehabil Med* 1985;17:121–127.

Nordin M, Kahanovitz N, Verderame R, et al. Normal trunk muscle strength and endurance in women and the effect of exercises and electrical stimulation. *Spine* 1987;12:105.

Oddsson LI. Control of voluntary trunk movements in man: Mechanism for postural equilibrium during standing. *Acta Physiol Scand* 1990;140(suppl):595.

Pederson O, Peresen R, Staffeldt E. Back pain and isometric back muscle strength of workers in a Danish factory. *Scan J Rehabil Med* 1975;7:125–128.

Pederson O, Staffeldt E. The relationship between four tests of back muscle strength in untrained subjects. *Scan J Rehabil Med* 1972;4:175–181.

Putz-Anderson V, ed. *Cumulative Trauma Disorders. A Manual for Musculoskeletal Diseases of the Upper Limbs*. Philadelphia, Pa: Taylor and Francis; 1988:7.

Reading AE. A comparison of pain rating scales. *J Psychosom Res* 1979;24:119–124.

Reid DC, Burnham RS, Saboe LA, Kushner SF. Lower extremity flexibility patterns in classical ballet dancers and their correlation to lateral hip and knee injuries. *Am J Sports Med* 1987;15:347–352.

Revel M, Andre-Deshays C, Minguet M. Cervicocephalic kinesthetic sensibility in patients with cervical pain. *Arch Phys Med Rehabil* 1991;72:288–291.

Ricci B, Marchetti M, Figura F. Biomechanics of sit-up exercises. *Med Sci Sports Exerc* 1981;13:54–59.

Richmond FJR, Bakker DA. Anatomical organization and sensory receptor content of soft tissues surrounding upper cervical vertebrae in the cat. *J Neurophysiol* 1982;48:49–61.

Riihimaki H. Low-back pain, its origin and risk indicators. *Scand J Work Environ Health* 1991;17:81–90.

Rissanen A, Allaranta H, Sainio P, Harkonen H. Isokinetic and non-dynamometric tests in low back pain patients related to pain and disability index. *Spine* 1994;19:1963–1967.

Robertson LD, Darville D, Magnusdottir H. Abdominal fitness testing—A new approach. In: Reilly T, Watkins J, Borms J, eds. *Proceedings of the VIII Commonwealth and International Conference on Sport, Physical Education, Dance, Recreation, Health, and Kinanthropometry II*. London, England: Spon, 1986:227–232.

Rogers RG. The effects of spinal manipulation on cervical kinesthesia in patients with chronic neck pain: A pilot study. *J Manipulative Physiol Ther* 1997;20:80–85.

Santaguida PL, McGill SM. The psoas major muscle: A three-dimensional geometric study. *J Biomech* 1995;28:339–345.

Schuldt K, Harms-Ringdahl K. Cervical spine position versus EMG activity in the neck muscles during maximum isometric neck extension. *Clin Biomech* 1988;3:129–136.

Sharkey BJ. Functional vs chronologic age. *Med Sci Sports Exerc* 1987;19:174–178.

Sharpe GL, Liemohn WP, Snodgrass LB. Exercises prescription and the low back—Kinesiological factors. *JOPERD* 1988;59:74–78.

Shirado O, Toshikazu I, Kaneda K, Straz TE. Concentric and eccentric strength of trunk muscles: Influence of test postures on strength and characteristics of patients with chronic low-back pain. *Arch Phys Med Rehabil* 1995;76:604–611.

Silverman JL, Rodriquez AA, Agre JC. Quantitative cervical flexor strength in healthy subjects and in subjects with mechanical neck pain. *Arch Phys Med Rehabil* 1991;72:679–681.

Silvermetz MA, Pathokinesiology of supine double leg lifts as an abdominal strengthener and suggested alternative exercises. *Athl Training* 1990;25:17–22.

Slosberg M. Effects of altered afferent articular input on sensation, proprioception, muscle tone and sympathetic reflex responses. *J Manipulative Physiol Ther* 1988;11:400–408.

Soderberg GL. Exercise for the abdominal muscles. *JOHPER* 1966;37:67–70.

Spitzer WO, LeBlanc FE, Dupuis M, et al. Scientific approach to the assessment and management of activity-related spinal disorders. *Spine* 1987;12:7S.

Stones M, Kozma A. Balance and age in the sighted and blind. *Arch Phys Med Rehabil* 1987;68:85–89.

Suni JH, Oja P, Laukkanen RT, et al. Health-related fitness test battery for adults: Aspects of reliability. *Arch Phys Med Rehabil* 1996;77:399–405.

Swanson AB, Matev IB, de Groot Swanson G. The strength of the hand. *Bull Prosthet Res*, Fall 1970;145–53.

Toshikazu I, Shirado O, Suzuki H, et al. Lumbar trunk muscle endurance testing: An inexpensive alternative to a machine for evaluation. *Arch Phys Med Rehabil* 1996;77:75–79.

Triano JJ, Schultz AB. Correlation of objective measures of trunk motion and muscle function with low back disability ratings. *Spine* 1987;12:561–565.

Tropp H, Ekstrand J, Gillquist J. Stabilometry in functional instability of the ankle and its value in predicting injury. *Med Sci Sports Exerc* 1984;16:54–66.

Vernon HT, Aker P, Aramenko M, et al. Evaluation of neck muscle strength with a modified sphygmomanometer dynamometer: Reliability and validity. *J Manipulative Physiol Ther* 1992;15:343–349.

Videman T, Rauhala H, Asp S, et al. Patient-handling skill, back injuries and back pain: An intervention study in nursing. *Spine* 1989;14:148–156.

Vincent WJ, Britten SD. Evaluation of the curl up—A substitute for the bent knee sit up. *JOPER* 1980;51:74–75.

Von Korff M, Deyo RA, Cherkin D, Barlow SF. Back pain in primary care: Outcomes at 1 year. *Spine* 1993;18:855–862.

Von Korff M, Ormel J, Keefe F, Dworkin SF. Grading the severity of chronic pain. *Pain* 1992;50:133–149.

Waddell G, McCulloch JA, Kummel E, Venner RM. Nonorganic physical signs in low-back pain. *Spine* 1980;5:117–125.

Walters CE, Partridge MJ. Electromyographic study of the differential action of the abdominal muscles during exercise. *Am J Phys Med* 1957;36:259–268.

Wang S, Whitney SL, Burdett RG, et al. Lower extremity muscular flexibility in long distance runners. *J Orthop Sports Phys Ther* 1993;2:102–107.

Wiktorsson M, Oberg B, Gillquist J. Lower extremity goniometric measurements: A study to determine their reliability. *Arch Phys Med Rehabil* 1982;63:171–175.

Wyke BD. The neurology of joints. *Ann R Coll Surg Engl* 1967;25:50.

Yeomans S, Liebenson C. Quantitative functional capacity evaluation: The missing link to outcomes assessment. *Top Clin Chiro* 1996;3(1):32–43.

Yeomans S, Liebenson C. Functional capacity evaluation and chiropractic case management. *Top Clin Chiro* 1996;3(3):15–25.

Yeomans S, Liebenson C. Applying outcomes management to clinical practice. *J Neuromusculoskel System* 1997;5(1):1–15.

Youdas JW, Garret TR, Suman VJ, et al. Normal range of motion of the cervical spine: An initial goniometer study. *Phys Ther* 1992;72:16–26

CHAPTER 17

Functional Capacity Assessments and Low Back Pain

BRUCE HOFFMANN & JEFF GULLICKSON

INTRODUCTION

Low back injuries are of increasing concern and cost in the U.S. workplace. Incidence, cost, and disability are continuing to rise (Frymoyer and Cats-Baril, 1991). The injury incidence rate from lifting has been associated with low back injuries up to 65% of the time (Mayer et al, 1988b). Furthermore, injury rates up to eight times higher have been reported for individuals required to lift heavy objects regularly (Keyserling et al, 1980). These statistics led to the development of lifting tests for use as a preventative tool. These tests were used to compare a job applicant's physical ability to the physical requirements of the job and sometimes to a normative database. Later, these testing methods were used to assess an injured worker's capacity to return to work. This use has led to a rise in testing methodologies, manufacturing of specialized instrumentation, and facilities for performing functional capacity assessments (FCEs).

This chapter reviews the purpose, importance, proper methods, and applications of functional capacity assessments. Special attention is given to lift assessment methods. Issues regarding FCEs, return-to-work outcomes, and cost-effectiveness are also discussed.

OVERVIEW OF FUNCTIONAL CAPACITY EVALUATIONS

PURPOSE OF THE FUNCTIONAL CAPACITY EVALUATION

Definitions of FCEs have been presented by numerous authors with a fair amount of consistency. Tramposh (1991) describes FCE as a systematic, comprehensive, objective measurement of individuals' maximum work ability. Matheson (1989) defines it as a systematic process of measuring and developing an individual's capacity to dependably sustain performance in response to broadly defined work demands. Isernhagen (1988) describes the process through its basic makeup:

- Function—purposeful activity that by its result can be measured
- Capacity—maximum ability
- Evaluation—an outcome statement that is explanatory and objective in measurement of activity

From these definitions, there appears to some consensus regarding what an FCE is and its purpose, but this is where the similarities end. **The specific evaluation protocols can differ greatly from provider to provider and from clinic to clinic.** It is not the purpose of this chapter to discuss and compare each FCE system or approach; rather, the chapter seeks to provide guidelines for proper test selection, implementation, and data interpretation.

On the most fundamental level, functional testing helps substantiate a finding of impairment, disability, and—when compared with job demands—a job handicap. These comparisons to job demands may demonstrate an ability to return to work fully, or suggest that placement on restricted duty is appropriate. On the other hand, it may be suggested that return to work is inappropriate, and work hardening or work conditioning may be necessary. In these situations, the FCE may serve as an objective functional database to guide specific rehabilitation goals and objectively monitor functional gains or lack thereof. This is a critical element and tool in the functional rehabilitation of patients with low back pain (Mayer and Gatchel, 1988). In summary, reasons for performing an FCE may include:

- Substantiate impairment
- Determine level of disability
- Determine specific job handicap
- Establish return-to-work recommendations
- Establish work restrictions
- Demonstrate indications for rehabilitation with specific goals
- Objectively monitor physical capacity improvement, or lack thereof
- Litigation
- Social security

COMPONENTS OF A FUNCTIONAL CAPACITY EVALUATION

When asked to determine an individual's capacity to work, some health care providers (HCPs) continue to rely on personal experience and opinion, or solely on the patient's report of ability. This approach continues even though new technologies and advancements in human performance measures have evolved with both high- and low-tech methodologies. On the other hand, many new technologies lack credibility and are based on unsubstantiated manufacturer claims. **It is the HCP's responsibility to choose appropriate methods for testing.**

When evaluating functional abilities, one must understand that many facets affect human performance and, thus, no "gold standard" is available. **Instead, a functional capacity test needs to consist of a battery of tests to evaluate all the necessary or applicable aspects of functional abilities with an emphasis that is patient and job-demand specific.** As Waddell (1987) points out, low back pain and the associated disability is an intertwining of physical impairment, psychological reactions, and illness behavior. Therefore, the test battery may evaluate common physical measures, such as range of motion, various strength and functional values, and cardiovascular fitness, as well as psychosocial and psychophysical values.

A template for performing FCEs is founded in the hierarchical view of disease, impairment, disability, and handicap (Menard and Hoens, 1994). *Disease* refers to disruption of normal health, whether physical or psychological in nature. *Impairment* is defined as the change in function caused by the disease. If an impairment prevents a person from performing at a given level or functional task, then a disability is present. It is possible to have an impairment yet not demonstrate a disability. As stated in the *Guide to Evaluation of Permanent Impairment*, **impairment gives rise to disability only when the condition limits the individual's capacity to meet demands that pertain to activities** (AMA, 1988). And, finally, a handicap is present when disabilities are severe enough to alter social role performance.

This hierarchical view gives rise to an evaluation system that first identifies pathology, typically during an examination, and records the presence of any impairment of function that arises from the presence of this pathology. The effect of any impairment on functional activities is assessed during the testing portion of the FCE. If an individual's impairment has caused difficulty or inability to perform a given task, the impairment is now defined as a disability. This hierarchical view puts the evaluation findings into a simple context, as follows: an individual is unable to lift a 5-lb bundle of towels out of the tub due to decreased lumbar flexion from a previous lumbar fusion. In this example, we have listed the disability in relation to the impairment and pathology. In another example, an individual is unable to lift more than 15 lbs from floor to waist at a frequent rate due to decreased strength and cardiovascular fitness, measured by lumbar strength dynamometry and submaximal VO_2 bicycle ergometry.

A common problem that confronts HCPs using this ideology is seen in the case of an individual who presents with no remarkable objective findings yet is functionally impaired. This presentation is common and supports the literature's assertion that much of occupational disability is rooted in psychosocial issues. **This fact underscores the importance of including a psychosocial assessment as part of the test battery.** Does a subjective report of pain alone substantiate an impairment or disability?

Although this model presents a systematic template of evaluating and presenting data that will reflect human performance, there are no reported standard test components, or common functional components described in the literature at this time. Fishbain et al (1994) have reported on their use of a standardization of testing components based on the *Dictionary of Occupational Titles*. These components are listed in Table 17–1. This approach provides an excellent baseline, yet should be defined by each patient and must be job specific, if possible. A second review presented in the literature compared results from a variety of functional testing techniques and concluded that a concurrent validity exists between the methods reviewed (Dusik et al, 1993).

Although many tasks commonly need to be evaluated, traditionally an emphasis is placed on lifting capacity. This is due to the prevalence of low back injuries and faulty lifting mechanics.

GUIDELINES FOR TEST SELECTION

Proper test selection and execution is critical in providing objective values for the HCP. Standardized criteria are made available for which testing methods should be judged. This pursuit of objectivity may be the most important aspect of testing. This is especially true when applying test results in medical-legal arenas or when making return-to-work recommendations that ultimately can affect an individual's earning capacity. Keyserling et al (1980) suggest the several criteria that are necessary for human performance measurements, including:

- Safety—risk of injury should be of primary concern
- Relationship to job requirements—recent laws make such requirements mandatory (Americans with Disabilities Act)
- Reliability—the repeatability of a test to measure its designated outcome over time on subsequent tests
- Predictive ability—whether the test provides the HCP with information that is consistent with what is expected.

For individuals with medical conditions, Hart et al (1993) suggests the following criteria:

- Safety—the procedure should not be expected to cause injury

Table 17–1: FCE Testing Components Based on the Dictionary of Occupational Titles

Standing
Walking
Sitting
Lifting
Carrying
Pushing
Pulling
Climbing
Balance
Stooping
Kneeling
Crouching
Crawling
Reaching
Handling
Fingering
Feeling

- Reliability—the data produced should be dependable across evaluators, the evaluee, and the date or time performed
- Validity—the data and its interpretation should be able to predict or reflect the evaluee's performance
- Practicality—the evaluation of cost, time, and usefulness of the information gained
- Utility—the usefulness to the assessment in terms of meeting the needs of the parties involved

If our goal is to provide objective data for our given purpose of performing the FCE, then the above criteria act as an additional guide for test selection. A more comprehensive list of standards for such tests and physical measurements is available, and provides an excellent resource for protocol establishment (Task Force on Standards for Measurement in Physical Therapy, 1991).

LIFT ASSESSMENT METHODS

The methods for lift assessment can be broken down primarily into two categories: static and dynamic. Dynamic testing includes isokinetic and isoinertial/psychophysical methods; these methods are described in the following sections.

ISOKINETIC TESTING (DYNAMIC LIFTING)

Isokinetic testing consists of an external variable force designed or programmed to maintain a constant and predetermined speed. This technique of performance measure was popularized initially in the sports medicine arena and had primarily been utilized for extremity strength measures. Later, trunk testing and lifting assessment protocols followed. High cost factors have resulted in decreased accessibility, acceptance, and usage of isokinetic methods.

Mayer and Gatchel had popularized the use of isokinetic dynamometry with lumbar flexion/extension and rotational machines (Mayer et al, 1985, 1989). These tools were used to evaluate strength at varying speeds, with comparisons made to a normative database. They found this to be an excellent tool in their multidisciplinary program for making pre- and postprogram comparisons and monitoring improvement. Beyond this, there is minimal support for the use of single plain testing in determining, limiting, or predicting functional performance (Newton and Waddell, 1993). Such tests do, however, allow the HCP to evaluate for a specific weak link when lifting or functional deficits are present. Furthermore, functional status has been shown to improve when isolated strength deficits are addressed (Brady and Mayer, 1994).

Isokinetic lifting was introduced as one type of dynamic assessment because it was thought to more closely reflect actual lifting activities. Theoretically and biomechanically, this is somewhat true, yet one must recall that isokinetic testing is performed at a constant velocity. A review of biomechanical data on lifting assessment demonstrates that lifting velocity changes between lifts as well as within a single lift. Isokinetic lifting techniques eliminate these variables of acceleration and deceleration and, thus, do not fully reduplicate actual lifting. In terms of safety, very little has been reported on injuries that have occurred while performing isokinetic lift testing.

Newton and Waddell (1993) performed a lengthy review of the literature on isokinetic methods. They concluded that isokinetic methods typically provide reliable measures of torque and force production. There is a strong learning affect and two separate testing sessions may be warranted. In terms of normative data, the lift task provides sufficient normative data for comparisons. More important, there is little data that currently supports its ability to predict workplace performance.

ISOINERTIAL/PSYCHOPHYSICAL LIFTING TESTS

Another form of dynamic lifting commonly utilized includes those tests categorized as psychophysical lifting. Typically, this type of test encompasses lifting a box through a predetermined range, with self-adjustment of weight.

Snook and co-workers popularized this concept in determining safe manual material handling limits (Snook and Ciriello, 1991). The protocol is based on psychophysical principles for which an individual's perception of fatigue, pain, and/or exertion is used as an endpoint as well as heart rate monitoring and examiner observation of control and postural safety. This technique is built on the premise that the individual is best suited to interpret physiological re-

sponses to different loading situations and determine the extremes.

The initial use of this branch of psychology was in the prevention of industrial lifting injuries. Snook published large databases utilizing psychophysical lifting protocols. They included many variables such as lifting posture, frequency of lift, and box size. Snook concluded that 75% of the male or female population performing jobs requiring physical exertion greater than that acceptable through psychophysical testing were at a three-fold increased risk of injury (Snook, 1978). The science of psychophysical estimation gained further support by reports demonstrating a higher injury rate in workers who believed their jobs to be more physically demanding (Snook, 1985).

Instructions for psychophysical testing are fairly consistent between studies, with only slight variation. An article by Ciriello et al (1993) provides a good reference for standard instructions. Generally, a candidate is asked to lift a box at a given frequency. Weight adjustments are made throughout the test period to achieve a weight that could be handled for an 8-hour day without straining oneself or becoming unusually tired, weakened, overheated, or out of breath. Typically, the amount of weight is concealed from the individual, forcing him or her to self-monitor physiological indicators while avoiding any preconceived or self-determined arbitrary limits. Common test postures include floor-to-knuckle, knuckle-to-shoulder, shoulder-to-overhead, carry, and push/pull maneuvers.

Psychophysical tests offer a moderate advantage over other tests. First, this branch of testing allows for an extremely high ability to recreate specific job requirements and their many variables. The importance of such job specific modifications is made more apparent when reviewing the new NIOSH equation for the design and evaluation of manual lifting tasks (Waters et al, 1993). Specifically, it was found necessary to account for deviations in horizontal distance of the load from the body, any asymmetry of the load, and frequency of performance. All these variables are found to change an individual's lift ability and, if not accounted for, may greatly overestimate the individual's capacity for that given situation. Second, this method is quite cost-effective as equipment costs are minimal. Third, safety is rarely an issue unless one is presented with an overachiever or if a poor candidate selection process is utilized.

No other form of lift assessment has undergone as many clinical investigations and trials, or been reported on as often in the literature, as psychophysical lifting. Studies have reported on utility and reliability in uninjured and injured patient populations, along with comparisons to other lift assessment techniques.

Snook and Campanelli (1978) best demonstrated the utility of psychophysical lifting. They found that lifting injuries were three times more likely to occur when work requirements were above acceptable levels for 75% of the population as determined by psychophysical testing. If one accepts the basic premise that the individual is best suited to judge his or her physical limitations, then this is an excellent source. **No other testing methods come as close to reduplicating true lifting as it occurs in the workplace.**

The reliability issue concerning the psychophysical protocol lies in the test's inherent subjectivity; the test is primarily based on the patient's subjective report of pain or exertion. Can a motivated individual discriminate a safe endpoint and, if so, can it be performed repeatedly? Can the same be said when applied to an injured population?

In a study by Legg and Myles (1985), repeated testing over 5 days on a healthy population found that maximum acceptable lift did not vary greatly over repeated efforts. Furthermore, there was no subjective, cardiovascular, or physiological evidence of fatigue when the selected weights were lifted for an 8-hour day. Subjects were tested and worked at a frequency of five lifts every 2 minutes. This study sample was found to be working at 21% VO_2 max, which is well below the NIOSH recommended upper limit of 33% VO_2 max. Differences were also reported between experienced and nonexperienced material handlers. Experienced material handlers chose higher maximal acceptable lifts when compared to inexperienced material handlers and showed less variability on test–retest scores. This occurred even though both groups had similar isometric strengths.

Alpert et al (1991) reported on a variation of this psychophysical technique for determining safe occasional lifts. These authors used healthy individuals for their study. On single test–retest series, for which the retest was performed an average of 8 days later, good reliability was found.

In a similar study, Mital (1983) had shown a 35% decrease in psychophysically determined values for high frequency lifts performed for 8 hours as estimated by a 25-minute psychophysical testing session. Fernandez et al (1991) showed a similar change with an average decrease of 15% for high-frequency lifts performed for 8 hours (lift frequency ranged from two to eight lifts per minute). In this same study, a second group was not allowed to alter their chosen weights for the 8-hour shift. Nine of the twelve subjects withdrew because of soreness. The authors concluded that psychophysical lifting estimates are valid for low- or medium-frequency lifts, but tend to overestimate high-frequency lifts greater than eight per minute.

Other investigators have evaluated and compared psychophysical reports of stress with estimates of stress through biomechanical models. Walker et al (1991) found an inverse relationship between the two. Subjectively, more stress was reported in the low back with the above-waist lifts, as compared to below-waist lifts. On the other hand, biomechanical estimates demonstrated more stress to the low back with the below-waist lifts than the above-waist lifts. This study points out the importance of subjective report and perception, yet also raises questions regarding the ability of an individual to interpret these physiological signals in an unbiased fashion. This is particularly significant if the person being tested has been injured recently or is recovering from an injury.

ISOMETRIC LIFT ASSESSMENT (STATIC LIFTING)

Isometric strength testing was popularized in part by the work of Chaffin and co-workers as well as from its inclusion in NIOSH publications (Chaffin and Park, 1973; Chaffin, 1974; Chaffin et al, 1978).

The early use of isometric testing was in the area of prevention of material handling injuries by matching workers to jobs based on strength. Keyserling et al (1990) found that individuals with work requirements greater than their static strength had an injury occurrence nearly three times higher than those whose strength was greater than their job requirements. This finding was further supported by Chaffin et al (1978) in an evaluation of 500 individuals. They found that when workers' job requirements exceeded their isometric lifting strength, injury rates increased significantly. Based on this information, **protocols were developed in which safe lifting limits for occasional, frequent, and constant rates were extrapolated as a percentage of the maximal isometric strength.**

The early benefits offered by this form of testing included standardized posturing and setup, and objectification of force production. Variance of force production over repeated efforts allows for more objective estimations of effort. It was also felt that in the lifting sequence, the most stressful aspect occurred at the initiation of the lift, when force is needed to overcome inertia. This is ultimately a static contraction. Furthermore, lifting is considered most stressful at the postural end-ranges; this is the basis for the NIOSH standardized postures.

Test–retest reliability of isometric testing is very high (Sapega, 1990). Issues of safety have arisen, particularly when using the NIOSH torso lift, although no reports of the injury incidence rate are available in the literature (Kishino et al, 1985). Biomechanically, this posture would seem to lend itself to producing moderate loading of the lumbar spine. We have personally chosen to eliminate this from our battery of test postures, yet this safety factor could seemingly be better addressed if psychophysical protocols were used instead of maximum contraction instructions.

Some caution must be used when making safe lifting recommendations from static strength values. As pointed out by Chaffin and Anderson (1984), assumptions are made that lifting is smooth and unrestrictive, objects are only of moderate width, and ideal environmental factors are present such as handles, flooring, lighting, and temperature.

The use of static lifting assessments has come under much scrutiny, primarily because of the many variables involved in dynamic lifting that are not accounted for in static testing. Numerous reports have documented the discrepancy between dynamic and static testing results in similar populations (Pytel and Kamon, 1981; Kumar et al, 1988; Kumar and Garand, 1992).

COMPARISONS BETWEEN STATIC AND DYNAMIC LIFTING

Much has been made of the debate regarding static and dynamic lifting evaluations. Much of the difficulty in evaluating the literature for which comparisons have been made lies in the diverse methodologies employed and instructions used.

Khalil et al (1987b) confirmed a poor correlation between lifting results from psychophysical protocols and maximal contraction isometric protocols. A much closer correlation was found between static and dynamic testing when both used psychophysical protocols of maximum acceptable lift. Similar reports and confirmations were given by Foreman et al (1984), Khalil et al (1987b), and Matheson et al (1993).

In a comprehensive review of the literature concerning muscular strength and its evaluation, Sapega (1990) reported that isometric lift assessment bears a stronger relationship to human functional capacity than was previously believed.

TESTING IN AN INJURED POPULATION

Although much of the standardization and validation of the various tests were performed on a healthy population, one must question the validity of these tests when applied to an injured population. **This concern arises primarily because of the psychological differences between healthy and injured populations. In particular, fear-avoidant behavior is common in injured populations, especially those with chronic injury sequelae** (Christ et al, 1993).

DYNAMIC TESTING IN AN INJURED POPULATION

In terms of dynamic testing with injured populations, very little has been published in the literature. Griffin et al (1984) found that individuals who reported back injuries selected much lower weights than those who had no injury and, more importantly, findings on psychophysical lifting assessment were less reproducible on repeated efforts. Troup et al (1987), in a subsequent report, stated that the experience of low back pain may lead to an exaggerated perception of pain or discomfort and may affect performance on psychophysically based assessments. Mayer et al (1988a, 1988b) popularized the Progressive Iso-inertial Lifting Evaluation (PILE) technique, which is similarly based on a psychophysical approach. They found this technique useful for monitoring improvement in a population with chronic low back pain participating in a functional restoration program.

Kishino et al (1985) reported on the use of both static and dynamic/isokinetic lift assessment for an injured and uninjured population. Both techniques demonstrated the ability to discriminate between injured and uninjured persons, and both were able to document improvement in performance after participation in a functional restoration program.

STATIC TESTING IN AN INJURED POPULATION

The use of static lift assessment in an injured population is also not often reported in the literature. Khailil et al (1987a) have shown static lift assessment using psychophysical instructions for back pain patients to be highly reliable with a good test–retest reliability. Furthermore, they found this to be an excellent tool to evaluate functional changes from treatment in a quantitative manner in patients with chronic low back pain. Harber and SooHoo (1984) supported this finding in their report. They found a good coefficient of variation on repeated exertions in an injured population using a psychophysical approach to static strength measurements.

MAINTAINING TEST–RETEST AND INTER-TESTER RELIABILITY

INFLUENCE OF TESTER INSTRUCTION ON SUBJECT PERFORMANCE

A key component in maintaining test–retest and inter-tester reliability is standardization of instructions. Instruction sets have been shown to greatly affect effort and force production.

The choice of instructions is critical in achieving maximal voluntary effort. Voluntary muscular control is achieved through an integration of a variety of bodily systems, and any inhibition placed on these coordinated events, whether it be physiological, neural, or behavioral, will affect performance. For example, it has been specifically cited that fear of injury may act as an inhibitory mechanism (Christ et al, 1993). This same study evaluated the effect of simple instructions such as "contract as hard as you can," or "contract as fast as you can," compared to more complex instructions such as "contract as fast and as hard as you can." **Each instruction group produced different results in terms of the magnitude and force-time recordings.** The authors concluded that substantial consideration must be given to instruction sets, especially when accurate values are required for comparison between muscle groups, against normative data, and/or during retesting at a later date for outcomes assessment.

Matheson et al (1992) evaluated the effect on two different sets of instructions on isokinetic lifting and strength. They compared a high demand set of instructions ("put forth high effort") with another set of instructions ("put forth a consistent effort") and found that different instructions greatly affect the reliability, variability, and magnitude of results from these isokinetic measures. In general, **high demand instructions were more effective.**

Caldwell et al (1974) similarly reported on the effect of instructional sets on values recorded during isometric testing. They concluded that instructions must be explicit to prevent subjects from developing their own strategies, based on their diverse interpretation of the task. Gamerale (1988) also reported on a reduction of reliable data when inconsistent instructions were given during psychophysical lifting evaluations.

THE EFFORT VALIDATION PROCESS

Validity of effort is the cornerstone of an objective FCE, yet detecting submaximal effort has, to this point been challenging. The terms *force* and *effort* are sometimes used interchangeably, and the use of these terms needs to be clarified as they are both involved in evaluation procedures. *Force* is the amount of resistance given by the individual being tested. *Effort* is the amount of force given as a percentage of the individual's maximum ability for the given task. One must ask, is force or effort being measured during a given task?

COEFFICIENT OF VARIATION

A common method for quantifying effort in lifting assessment is through the statistical outcome of coefficient of variation. It has been estimated that repeated trials of force production that show minimal variation are consistent with maximal effort. This measurement of consistency is defined as a coefficient of variation and is typically recorded as a percentage. Most values that are below 15% are considered valid. This value does not universally signify maximal effort, but it is more indicative of a valid maximal acceptable effort (Mayer et al, 1988a). This finding can differ greatly from maximal physical capacity, and more research will help in clarify the relationship of these two measures.

POSTURAL CHANGES

Other authors have suggested that observation of the individual while looking for postural changes or cues can help in indicating maximal effort. Smith (1994) has shown that inter-tester evaluations using preset safety endpoint definitions to judge safe lifting endpoints has good agreement. The basis for this methodology is that as an individual approaches or exceeds a safe maximal lift, body mechanics will deteriorate and reflect a biomechanical endpoint. This change was also noted in uninjured individuals while performing psychophysical lift assessment in a study outlined by Alpert et al (1991). **Postural changes were noted as in-**

dividuals approached their maximum lifting capacity. These changes include shifting from a leg lift (using the legs with maintenance of lordosis) to a back lift (knee extension preceding back extension). It was also noted that individuals began rising onto the toes and/or shrugging their shoulders as they approached their maximums for above-the-shoulder lifts. Although the basis of this method is posturally and biomechanically oriented, there is currently no well-accepted ideal lifting posture.

Hazard and co-workers have provided an in-depth look at verification of patient effort during lifting assessments. In one report, they evaluated the test–retest variation of several commonly used indices that reflect patient effort (1993). This study used an uninjured, supposedly well-motivated population. The authors concluded that heart rate was a poor indicator of effort during isometric testing but was better for isoinertial or isokinetic tests. In a second study, Hazard et al (1992) studied several indices of effort in an uninjured and well-motivated population. Of special interest was the finding that peak force variance may not be as good an indicator of maximal effort in isokinetic or isometric testing. The authors suggest that **a trained observer is better able to distinguish maximal from submaximal efforts than the most accurate physiological indicators.**

OTHER METHODS OF EFFORT VALIDATION

When evaluating patient effort, one must consider the many facets of human function and complicating factors that affect its production. Hirsch et al (1991) have described these as nonorganic causes of poor motor performance. They include:

- Misunderstanding of instructions to perform maximal effort
- Test anxiety
- Depression
- Nociception
- Fear of pain
- Unconscious symptom magnification

The influence of such factors becomes even more evident when the findings of Menard, Cook, and Hirsch are reviewed. Menard et al (1994) evaluated a large patient population that differed only in Waddell disability scores. Those with higher Waddell scores performed statistically significantly, and consistently as a group, lower on dynamometry tests (Menard et al, 1994). Similarly, Cooke et al (1992) performed lumbar dynamometry on patients with chronic low back pain before and after a rehabilitation program. Once again, patients were classified according to Waddell scores. Patients with higher Waddell scores produced significantly lower strength values than controls or those with low Waddell scores. A retest performed after completion of a work conditioning program demonstrated

CASE STUDY 17–1
LEFT-SIDED LOW BACK AND LEG PAIN

HISTORY

A 32-year-old male experienced a work-related injury $3^{1}/_{2}$ months ago. Initially he experienced left-sided low back and leg pain, with pain extending to the left foot. The patient received conservative care which included spinal manipulative therapy as the primary intervention, and he also recently completed a work conditioning program. Currently, he experiences left-sided low back pain with a mild amount of pain radiating into the left gluteal region. He is employed as a driver for a freight company and is required to lift/carry between 75 and 150 lbs. He is required to make deliveries to rural areas; functionally, this requires prolonged sitting/driving, lifting, carrying, and repetitive bending and squatting. He has been unable to work for 2 months and has been under work restrictions for the past month. He is currently working 3 days a week, and is limited to 4-hour work shifts each day. He is under a restriction to lifting no more than 25 lbs.

This patient was referred for an FCE to help determine his safe candidacy for increasing work related demands.

PHYSICAL EXAMINATION

Lumbar range of motion revealed flexion of 90 degrees, extension of 20 degrees, left lateral flexion of 35 degrees, and right lateral flexion of 25 degrees with mild pain. Palpable tenderness was generalized throughout the lumbosacral spine. Hamstring flexibility was 70 degrees on the left and 60 degrees on the right. Nerve tension signs were unremarkable. Prone lumbar extension was mildly limited, by pain centrally.

The patient ranked his pain at a 3/10, on a scale of 0 to 10, with 10 being unbearable (Visual Analogue Scale). He scored a 10/50 on an Oswestry questionnaire, which places him at a 20% disability level for perceived activity intolerance.

Computed tomography of the lumbar spine revealed multilevel degenerative disc disease of the lumbar spine with a small partially calcified, right-sided disc herniation at the L5–S1 level, moderate bony lateral spinal stenosis with mild impingement on the left L5 nerve root, and a small, broad-based central bulging of the L4–5 disc annulus with mild subarticular impingement of the transversing left L5 nerve root.

FUNCTIONAL CAPACITY EVALUATION

A series of lift tasks were presented to the patient to assess safe occasional lifting recommendations. The patient was oriented to the goal and purpose of the FCE. He was encouraged to perform at maximum ability on each test. He was also instructed that each test could be terminated at any point. This procedure typically consists of six trials of lifts, with the weight increased with each trial of lifts.

- *Preferred floor-to-knuckle lift* (Fig. 17–1). The patient performed six trials, and terminated the test on the sixth trial, stating that the weight was too much. In addition, postural changes were noted during the final series of lifts. The patient was able to consistently lift 85 lbs; above 85 lbs, the patient stated that he had reached his maximum. The physician also observed postural changes.
- *Knuckle-to-shoulder lift* (Fig. 17–2). The patient performed five trials of lifts, with the final trial being terminated by the physician due to poor lifting mechanics. It would have been unsafe for the patient to continue the test. The patient was able to effectively lift 77.5 lbs.
- *Shoulder-to-overhead lift* (Fig. 17–3). The patient self terminated the testing procedure during the fifth trial, subjectively reporting that he had reached his maxi-

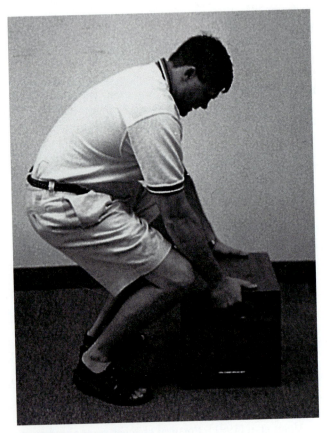

Figure 17–1. A preferred floor-to-knuckle lift.

CASE STUDY 17–1 *(continued)*
LEFT-SIDED LOW BACK AND LEG PAIN

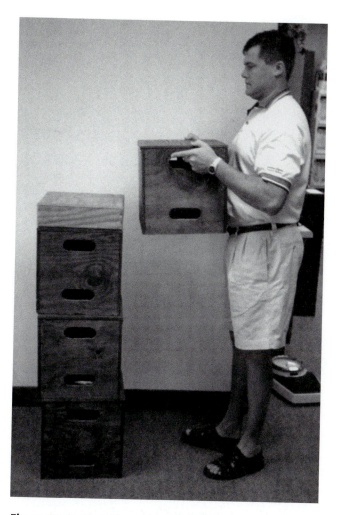

Figure 17–2. Knuckle-to-shoulder lift.

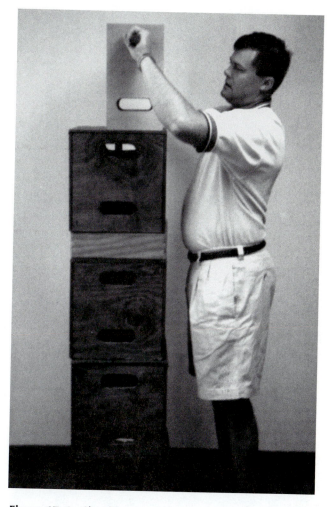

Figure 17–3. Shoulder-to-overhead lift.

mum. The physician also noted postural changes during the fifth lifting series. The patient was able to lift 64 lbs consistently.

- *Carry 8.5-m test* (Fig. 17–4). This test was terminated by the physician after four trials of carries, due to postural changes of increased lordosis, shortened stride, and carrying the weight on the thighs. The patient was able to carry 70 lbs without discomfort.

The patient was tested with a series of repetitive flexion bending to a 12 inch height, and instructed to touch his palms on top of a box. The patient was able bend 25 times without discomfort. Additionally, the patient was asked to repetitively squat to a 12-inch height, and touch his palms to the top of a box; he was able to perform this task without discomfort.

VALIDITY OF EFFORT

Several areas of this FCE demonstrate the validity of effort from this patient. No gross pain behaviors or psychosocial indicators were noted. The patient demonstrated excellent effort on the lifting tasks; in addition, postural cues suggest excellent effort.

RESULTS

This patient demonstrated the ability to perform the following tasks on an occasional basis:

- Floor lift: 85 lbs
- Knuckle-to-shoulder lift: 77.5 lbs
- Shoulder-to-overhead lift: 64 lbs
- Carry: 70 lbs

CASE STUDY 17–1 *(continued)*
LEFT-SIDED LOW BACK AND LEG PAIN

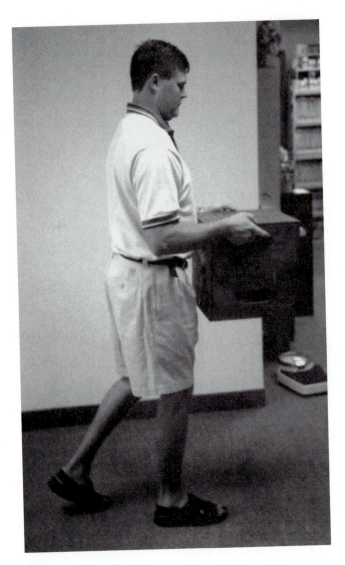

Figure 17–4. Carry test.

Other tasks critical to this patient's job include bending and squatting. He demonstrated good ability to tolerate repetitive bending and squatting.

CONCLUSIONS

This patient demonstrated the capacity to increase his work ability from the previous weight of a 25-lb restriction to the weight listed above. He should be able to continue

to increase his work ability as his condition improves. The patient has demonstrated excellent effort in performing the tests and has not shown any pain behaviors, supporting the validity of the results.

QUESTIONS

1. Is this patient a good candidate for an FCE? Why?

   Yes, this patient is a good candidate for an FCE for several reasons; to determine current work restrictions, because the patient has been off of work for over 3 months, and because he has heavy occupational work demands. As previously discussed in the text of the chapter, the longer an individual is away from work, the worse the outcome for return to work in the same capacity.

2. Why was a dynamic lifting assessment performed?

   A dynamic lift assessment was utilized based upon the patient's job demands as driver for a freight company. These job demands include lifting from a variety of positions, along with repetitive bending and squatting. A dynamic lift assessment will present a variety of lifting postures and can closely duplicate the job requirements.

3. Why would a lift trial be terminated if the patient showed postural cues of increased lordosis, shortened stride, and carrying a weight on the thighs?

   This trial should be terminated by the physician because the patient has shown that he has reached his near maximal lifting capacity. To allow the patient to continue would put the patient at risk of injuring himself.

4. Would an isokinetic lift assessment provide sufficient information to determine workplace performance, as compared to the dynamic lift assessment performed in this situation?

   No, as mentioned previously in this chapter, there is little evidence to support the premise that isokinetic testing can determine workplace performance.

5. Is further testing appropriate for this patient?

   This patient has continued to show improvement with care and his lifting ability has increased; however, his work requirements require him to lift between 75 and 150 lbs. As his improvement progresses, it may be necessary to retest him to remove the work restrictions.

CASE STUDY 17–2
LOW BACK PAIN

HISTORY

A 34-year-old, right-handed male experienced a work-related accident 7 months ago. He continues to experience considerable low back pain. He works as a baggage handler at a local airport. He has been returned to work on several occasions with work restrictions. On each of these occasions he has experienced flare-ups and has had requested to be off duty. He has not been able to return to work for the past 2 months. He reports that he does not do many activities because of increased low back pain.

He reports that he feels a lot of anger towards his employer and the insurance company for returning him to work before he felt physically capable of doing so.

PHYSICAL EXAMINATION

The patient's movements were slow and guarded. Lumbar range of motion is limited and painful; with flexion of 50 degrees, extension of 5 degrees, left lateral flexion of 20 degrees, and right lateral flexion of 25 degrees. Increased pain was felt in all ranges. Palpable tenderness was severe and generalized throughout the entire lumbar spine. Palpation revealed mild muscle hypertonicity of the lumbar paraspinal muscles. Cervical compression increased low back pain, as did straight leg raise, sitting root, and Kemp tests. Waddell's tests of axial compression, trunk rotation, and superficial tenderness were positive, for a score of 3/5. The patient scored 37/50 on his Oswestry questionnaire, and ranked his pain at 8/10. He states that his pain will get worse with activity but rarely ever is better than 8/10. A pain diagram showed multiple pain descriptors (ie, descriptive words to describe the pain quality, arrows to the area of pain, and so on).

Because of the possibility that psychosocial issues might be involved, as revealed in the patient's history and pain questionnaires, grip testing was performed to look for testing inconsistencies. This test utilized a Jamar dynamometer to measure grip strength in a variety of grip positions, repetitive grip trials in position 2, and grip test in the five positions from position 1 through position 5. In the grip test, position 2 test for the right hand was scored as 45, 40, and 42 lbs, respectively. Five-position testing for the right hand revealed values of 20, 30, 40, 40, and 45 for positions 1 through 5.

FUNCTIONAL CAPACITY EVALUATION

Initially the patient was orientated to the goal and purpose of the FCE. He was encouraged to perform at a maximum ability on each test. He was informed that any test could be terminated at any point if there was too much pain, if maximum effort was reached, or at the physician's discretion.

He appeared to understand the instructions and the purpose of the FCE.

The patient was tested initially on a static strength machine, during a series of isometric lifts (three repetitions). A Promatron 3000 Lift Task Evaluation System was utilized for this procedure. This device was used to document static strength and record the coefficient of variation to document effort of the subject. The resulting coefficient of variation greater than 15% suggests that the subject may not have understood the directions, did not produce maximal effort, or is limited by pain.

- *High far lift* (Fig. 17–5). The patient lifted an average of 46 lbs with a coefficient of variation of 2.2%.

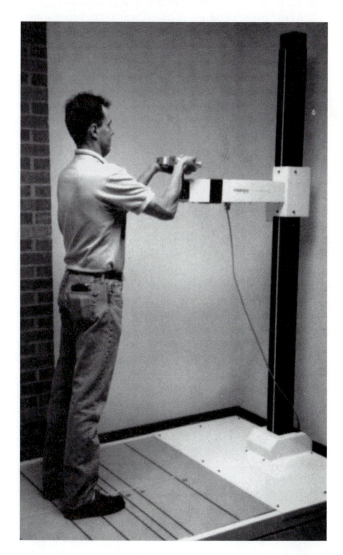

Figure 17–5. High far lift performed on a Promatron 3000.

CASE STUDY 17–2 *(continued)*
LOW BACK PAIN

- *High near lift* (Fig. 17–6). The patient lifted an average of 59 lbs with a coefficient of variation of 1.0%.
- *Arm lift* (Fig. 17–7). The patient lifted an average of 49 lbs with a coefficient of variation of 1.2%.
- *Leg lift* (Fig. 17–8). The patient lifted an average of 35 lbs with a coefficient of variation of 30.1%.
- *Floor lift* (Fig. 17–9). The patient lifted an average of 29 lbs with a coefficient of variation of 18.2%.

The patient was asked to perform a series of repetitive flexion bending from the waist to a height of 12 inches from the floor, and to place palms on top of a box 12 inches high. This required the patient to utilize 90 degrees of lumbar flexion. He was able to perform six repetitions before self-terminating the test, reporting increased pain.

In the dynamic lifting segment, a series of lifts was presented to the patient to assess safe occasional lifting recom-

mendations. He was instructed that each test could be terminated at any point. This procedure typically consists of six trials of lifts, with the weight increased with each lift trial.

- Floor-to-knuckle lift (see Fig. 17–1). The test was terminated at 25 lbs due to increased pain after the patient performed 3 repetitions.
- Knuckle-to-shoulder lift (see Fig. 17–2). The patient was able to lift 25 lbs and terminated the test due to increased pain.
- Shoulder-to-overhead lift (see Fig. 17–3). The patient was able to lift 25 lbs and terminated the test due to increased pain.
- Carry (see Fig. 17–4). The patient was able to carry 45 lbs and stated that he had reached his maximum effort. No postural observations were noted to suggest that the patient was near his physical maximal effort.

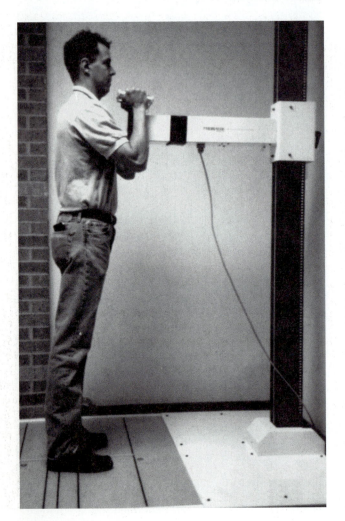

Figure 17–6. High near lift.

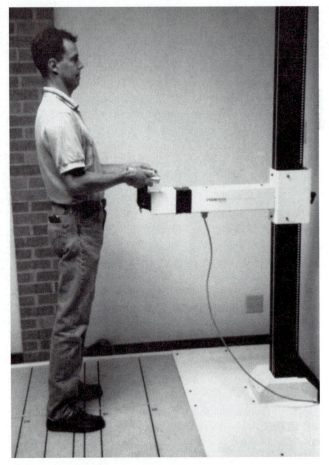

Figure 17–7. Arm lift.

CASE STUDY 17–2 *(continued)*
LOW BACK PAIN

VALIDITY OF EFFORT

Several areas of the history, physical examination, and FCE reveal the possibility of psychosocial issues in this patient's case. These include the patient's positive Waddell's findings, positive orthopedic tests, grip strength tests, pain questionnaire, rating, and diagram results.

His static strength results also revealed discrepancies in his effort, with coefficient of variation scores being greater than 15%. A coefficient of variation greater than 15% is considered invalid; this can result from not understanding the directions, failure to produce maximal effort, or being limited by pain.

The dynamic lifting tests were terminated by the patient due to increased low back pain, there were no postural suggestions that the patient was near his maximal effort.

Comparing scores from the static and the dynamic lifting tests reveals the patient's scores were not consistent with comparable lifts.

Grip strength testing for the five-position test is considered valid when the scores follow a bell-shaped curve, when plotted.

CONCLUSIONS

This patient has demonstrated numerous inconsistencies in his FCE. In addition, he has demonstrated the likelihood of psychosocial issues being involved in his injury. The presence of these issues does not rule out the presence of an organic injury. However, the psychosocial issues need to be addressed by an appropriate referral.

QUESTIONS

1. Is this patient a good candidate for an FCE? Why?

   Yes, this patient is a good candidate for an FCE due to the length of time missed from work, occupational demands, and the possibility of psychosocial issues.

2. Why would a grip strength test be performed on a patient with a low back complaint?

   A grip strength test was performed to look for testing inconsistencies that would suggest the presence of other issues being involved with his low back injury.

3. What would be considered as multiple descriptors on a pain diagram?

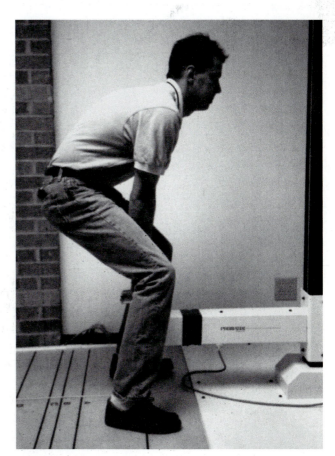

Figure 17–8. Leg lift.

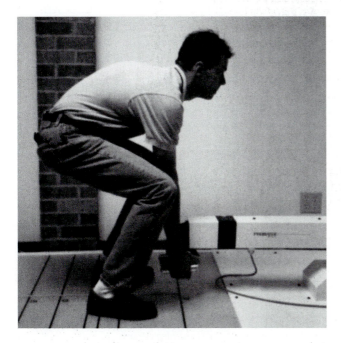

Figure 17–9. Floor lift.

CASE STUDY 17–2 *(continued)*
LOW BACK PAIN

These descriptors can include descriptive words, arrows drawn to the area of injury, or other forms to make sure that you are aware of the patient's injured areas (ie, stars, multiple circles, bold drawings).

4. Does the presence of psychosocial issues suggest that there is not an injury?

No, the patient may have an injury; however, other issues have now affected the outcome. These issues can arise from

a variety of sources, such as animosity toward the employer, presence of litigation, or a lack of job satisfaction.

5. What are some of the options available for HCPs managing a case of this nature?

A trial period of active care would be warranted in this case. If the active care did not produce satisfactory results, a referral to a pain behavior specialist would be appropriate.

---

an increase in performance greater than that expected from any therapeutic or physiological intervention on the group with high Waddell scores. The authors concluded that dynamometry and performance testing, alone, do not reflect true musculoskeletal impairment, nor can they be assumed to reflect true maximal physical capacity in patients who complain of low back pain (Cooke et al, 1992). Hirsch et al (1991), finding similar outcomes, concluded that **dynamometry and functional testing for patients with low back pain should be considered a psychophysical test,** and underscored the many facets affecting human performance in the population.

There is inherent subjectivity in many of the testing methods utilized during functional assessment. One key to improving the quality of this type of evaluation lies in better objectifying protocols that will accurately and more reliably measure patient effort.

CLINICAL APPLICATIONS

In the chapter thus far, we have discussed the various principles of FCEs, including purpose, testing methodologies, and guidelines. The accompanying case studies present two scenarios that apply the principles of FCE to specific clinical situations.

Conclusion

The FCE can serve as an excellent tool for outcomes and clinical management of patients with low back and neck pain. The cornerstone of the FCE is its objectivity, which can be greatly affected by the particular lift test selected and the methods by which it is applied. Choosing a proper candidate for the FCE, along with the specific tests that will best help the HCP monitor and evaluate the patient's ability to work, while maintaining objectivity of the FCE. Finally, evaluating a patient's level of effort while considering the variety of factors that may affect this level, and understanding its effects on the data collected, will greatly enhance the interpretation of the results reported, clinical management, and return-to-work plans.

REFERENCES

Alpert J, et al. The reliability and validity of two new tests of maximum lifting capacity. *J Occ Rehabil* 1991;1:13–29.

American Medical Association. *Guides for the Evaluation of Permanent Impairment*, 3rd ed. Chicago, Ill: AMA; 1988.

Brady S, Mayer T. Physical progress and residual impairment quantification after functional restoration: Part III isokinetic trunk strength. *Spine* 1994;19:395–400.

Caldwell L, et al. A proposed standard procedure for static muscle strength testing. *Am Ind Hyg Assoc* 1974;35:201–206.

Chaffin D. Human strength capability and low back pain. *JOM* 1974;16:248–254.

Chaffin D, Anderson G. *Occupational Biomechanics*. New York, NY: Wiley; 1984.

Chaffin D, Park K. A longitudinal study of low back pain as associated with occupational weight lifting factors. *Am Ind Hyg Ass J* 1973;34:513–525.

Chaffin D, et al. Pre-employment strength testing: An updated position. *J Occup Med* 1978;20:403–408.

Christ C, et al. The effect of test protocol instructions on the measurement of muscle function in adult women. *J Orthop Sports Phys Ther* 1993;18:502–510.

Ciriello V, et al. Further studies of psychophysically determined maximum acceptable weights and forces. *Ergonomics* 1993;35:175–186.

Cooke C, et al. Serial lumbar dynamometry in low back pain. *Spine* 1992;17:653–662.

Dusik L, et al. Concurrent validity of the ERGOS work simulator versus conventional functional capacity evaluation techniques in a workers compensation population. *JOM* 1993;35:759–767.

Fernandez J, et al. Psychophysical lifting capacity over extended periods. *Ergonomics* 1991;34:23–32.

Fishbain D, et al. Measuring residual functional capacity in chronic low back pain patients based on the dictionary of occupational titles. *Spine* 1994;19:872–880.

Foreman T, et al. Ratings of acceptable load and maximal isometric lifting strengths: The effect of repetition. *Ergonomics* 1984;27:1283–1288.

Frymoyer J, Cats-Baril W. An overview of the incidence and cost of low back pain. *Orthop Clin* 1991:22;263–271.

Gamerale F. Maximum acceptable work loads for repetitive lift tasks. *Scand J Work Envir Health* 1988;14:85–87.

Griffin A, et al. Tests of lifting and handling capacity, their repeatability and relationship to back symptoms. *Ergonomics* 1984;27:305–320.

Harber P, SooHoo K. Static ergonomic strength testing in evaluating occupational back pain. *JOM* 1984;26:877–884.

Hart D, et al. Guidelines for functional capacity evaluation of people with medical conditions. *J Orthop Sports Phys Ther* 1993;18:682–686.

Hazard R, et al. Test–retest variation in lifting capacity and indices of subject effort. *Clin Biomech* 1993;8:20–24.

Hazard R, et al. Lifting capacity, indices of subject effort. *Spine* 1992;17:1065–1070.

Hirsch G, et al. Relationship between performance on lumbar dynamometry and Waddell score in a population with low back pain. *Spine* 1991;16:1039–1043.

Isernhagen S. *Work Injury: Management and Prevention*. Gaithersburg, Md: Aspen; 1988.

Keyserling M, et al. Isometric strength testing as a means of controlling medical incidents on strenuous jobs. *JOM* 1980;22:332–336.

Khalil T, et al. Acceptable maximum effort. A psychophysical measure of strength in back pain patients. *Spine* 1987a;12:372–376.

Khalil T, et al. Determination of lifting abilities: A comparison study of four techniques. *Am Ind Hyg Assoc J* 1987b;48:951–956.

Kishino N, et al. Quantification of lumbar function: Part 4, isometric and isokinetic lifting simulation in normal subjects and low back dysfunction patients. *Spine* 1985;10:921–927.

Kumar S, et al. Isometric and isokinetic back and arm lifting strengths: Device and measurement. *J Biomech* 1988;21:35–44.

Kumar S, Garand D. Static and dynamic lifting strength at different reach distances in symmetrical and asymmetrical planes. *Ergonomics* 1992;35:861–880.

Legg S, Myles W. Metabolic and cardiovascular cost, and perceived effort over an 8 hour day when lifting loads selected by the psychophysical method. *Ergonomics* 1985;28:337–343.

Matheson L. Work hardening. In: Tollison D, Kriegel M, eds. *Interdisciplinary Rehabiliation of Low Back Pain*. Baltimore Md: Williams & Wilkins;1989:325–342.

Matheson L, et al. Effect of computerized instructions on measurement of lift capacity: Safety, reliability, validity. *J Occup Rehabil* 1993;3:65–81.

Matheson L, et al. Effect of instructions on isokinetic trunk strength testing variability, reliability, absolute value, and predictive value. *Spine* 1992;17:914–921.

Mayer T, et al. Progressive isoinertial lifting evaluation. A standardized protocol and normative data. *Spine* 1988a;13:993–997.

Mayer T, et al. Progressive isoinertial lifting evaluation. Comparison with isokinetic lifting in a disabled chronic low back pain industrial population. *Spine* 1988a;13:998–1002.

Mayer T, Gatchel R. *Functional restoration of spinal disorders: The sports medicine approach*. Philadelphia, Pa: Lea and Febiger; 1988.

Mayer R, et al. Objective assessment of spine function following industrial injury. *Spine* 1985;10:482–493.

Mayer R, et al. Quantifying postoperative deficits of physical function following spinal surgery. *Clin Orthop* 1989;224:147–157.

Menard M, et al. Pattern of performance in workers with low back pain during a comprehensive motor performance evaluation. *Spine* 1994;19:1359–1366.

Menard M, Hoens A. Objective evaluation of functional capacity: Medical, occupational, and legal settings. *J Orthop Sports Phys Ther* 1994;19:249–260.

Mital A. The psychophysical approach in manual lifting: A verification study. *Hum Factors* 1983;25:485–491.

Newton M, Waddell G. Trunk strength testing with iso-machines. *Spine* 1993;18:801–811.

Pytel J, Kamon, E. Dynamic strength test as a predictor for maximal and acceptable lifting. *Ergonomics* 1981;24:663–672.

Sapega A. Muscle performance evaluation in orthopedic practice. *J Bone Joint Surg* 1990;72-A:1562–1574.

Smith R. Therapists' ability to identify safe maximum lifting in low back pain patients during functional capacity evaluation. *J Orthop Sports Phys Ther* 1994;19:277–281.

Snook S. The design of manual handling tasks. *Ergonomics* 1978;21:963–985.

Snook S. Psychophysical acceptability as a constraint in manual working capacity. *Ergonomics* 1985;28:331–335.

Snook S, Campanelli R. A study of three preventative approaches to low back injury. *JOM* 1978;20:478–481.

Snook S, Ciriello V. The design of manual handling tasks: revised tables of maximum acceptable weights and forces. *Ergonomics* 1991;34:1197–1213.

Task Force on Standards for Measurement in Physical Therapy. Standards for tests and measurements in physical therapy practice. *Phys Ther* 1991;71:589–622.

Tramposh A. The functional capacity evaluation: Measuring maximal work abilities. *Spine* 1991;5:437–448.

Troup J, et al. The perception of back pain and the role of psychophysical test of lifting capacity. *Spine* 1987;12:645–657.

Waddell G. A new clinical model for the treatment of low back pain. *Spine* 1987:10;632–644.

Walker A, et al. Evaluating lifting tasks using subjective and biomechanical estimates of stress at the lower back. *Ergonomics* 1991;34:33–47.

Waters T, et al. Revised NIOSH equation for the design and evaluation of manual lifting tasks. *Ergonomics* 1993;36:749–776.

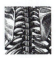

CHAPTER 18

Cardiovascular Fitness Testing

WILLIAM D. DEFOYD

INTRODUCTION

A safe and effective exercise program will often include the testing of cardiovascular fitness. It is performed prior to beginning an exercise program, at specified intervals during a physical training regimen, and upon completion of an exercise program. The information gathered by testing cardiovascular fitness serves many purposes, including:

- Screening for cardiovascular risk factors prior to beginning an exercise program
- Determining the need for further medical evaluation, including medically monitored exercise testing (ie, "stress testing" with a trained physician evaluating electrocardiogram and blood pressure)
- Establishing a baseline cardiovascular fitness level
- Documenting progress
- Selecting an appropriate training program
- Providing motivation for exercise participants

This chapter is intended to provide the rehabilitation-oriented health care provider (HCP) with the necessary tools to safely and effectively perform cardiovascular fitness testing. **The emphasis is on a relatively "low-tech" approach utilizing minimal equipment.** Much of the information presented here is from two primary sources: the American College of Sports Medicine (Kenney et al, 1995) and the YMCA (Golding et al, 1989). The testing protocols and normative data from these two sources are widely used as part of physical fitness evaluations across the United States, and apply well to the musculoskeletal rehabilitation setting.

Other information that can be found in this chapter includes:

- Clinical examples of situations in which cardiovascular fitness testing can be helpful
- An informed consent form for exercise testing
- The process and worksheets for performing cardiovascular risk factor screening
- The protocol and worksheets for measuring cardiovascular fitness using cycle ergometer (stationary bicycle) testing, the 3-minute bench step test, and treadmill testing

EFFECTIVENESS OF CARDIOVASCULAR EXERCISE

While an in-depth review of the benefits of regular sustained cardiovascular activities or exercise is beyond the scope of this chapter, these benefits are generally widely known and well accepted. Adherence to a regular cardiovascular exercise program has been shown to decrease the risk for the most common chronic diseases, including coronary artery disease, hypertension, obesity, stroke, adult-onset diabetes, peripheral vascular disease, several types of cancer, anxiety and depression (Golding et al, 1989).

There is also some evidence to support the use of regular cardiovascular or aerobic exercise in the treatment of certain musculoskeletal conditions, including low back pain. The Agency for Health Care Policy and Research's (AHCPR) *Acute Low Back Problems in Adults* practice guideline recommends aerobic exercise within the first 2 weeks of onset of symptoms to speed recovery and to promote activity tolerance (Bigos et al, 1994). This practice guideline further states that exercise quotas that are gradually increased result in better outcomes than recommending that patients stop exercising if pain occurs (Bigos et al, 1994). Patients (particularly sedentary people) who are given advice to exercise and "to let your pain be your guide" will often respond with "my pain tells me to do nothing." It is becoming more widely accepted that **early return to activity promotes recovery** from an acute onset of back or neck pain. These patients should be given specific recommendations to begin low-stress aerobic activities such as walking or swimming, with modifications if necessary, within the first few days or weeks of onset of the acute episode.

It is important that the HCP consider the patient's health status, motivation, and access to private or community facilities when prescribing cardiovascular exercise. For these reasons, the HCP may determine that it is appropriate to assess an individual's cardiovascular fitness level, as described in this chapter, before initiating an exercise program.

POTENTIAL ROLES FOR CARDIOVASCULAR FITNESS TESTING

Examples of the role of cardiovascular fitness testing in the outpatient musculoskeletal clinical setting include:

- Performing cardiovascular risk factor screening prior to prescribing cardiovascular exercise for the majority of patients seen in this type of environment
- Performing cardiovascular fitness testing as part of a functional capacity evaluation, which is often done to more accurately assess an individual's physical capacity to return to work or continue working
- Performing cardiovascular fitness testing prior to beginning, during, and upon completion of a physical rehabilitative exercise program to measure and document progress in the management of a variety of conditions including coronary artery disease, hypertension, obesity, stroke, adult onset diabetes, peripheral vascular disease, several types of cancer, anxiety, and depression

! CLINICAL ALERT 18–1

Cardiovascular Risk Factor Screening

Before beginning an exercise program, patients should be screened for cardiovascular risk factors, as well as signs and symptoms suggestive of cardiorespiratory disease.

CARDIOVASCULAR RISK FACTOR SCREENING

An assessment of an individual's cardiovascular risk factors can be obtained using a set of worksheets, as depicted in Tables 18–1 through 18–4, which are adapted from ACSM's *Guidelines for Exercise Testing and Prescription* (Kenney et al, 1995). This will indicate if, prior to beginning a moderate or a vigorous exercise program, the patient needs to undergo a medical examination and exercise testing supervised by an HCP trained and equipped to manage an emergent cardiac or other life-threatening event.

Some patients will not require the use of cardiovascular fitness capacity testing prior to beginning an exercise program based on their **risk profile;** however, you may want to test them for other reasons as discussed earlier (establishing a baseline for goal setting, functional capacity evaluation, documenting outcomes, etc). Individuals with lower cardiorespiratory risk will require testing only if engaged in vigorous exercise, whereas others will require testing before beginning even moderate levels of exercise. Some individuals with "increased risk" or "known disease," as depicted in Table 18–4, will require exercise testing under the supervision of an HCP prepared to deal with a potential cardiac or other emergency.

CASE STUDY 18–1
PRESCRIBING CARDIOVASCULAR EXERCISE
FOR A PATIENT WITH MECHANICAL LOW BACK PAIN

Maurice is a 56-year-old executive who has had right sided lower back pain and "stiffness" for 8 weeks after playing golf. In the past, he has been able to minimize the frequency of lower back pain by following an exercise program 3 to 4 days per week consisting of walking at a brisk pace for at least 30 minutes, followed by stretching for 10 to 15 minutes. However, he saw an HCP a few days after the episode 8 weeks ago who, among other things, prescribed rest and the avoidance of exercise and physical activity "as long as it hurts." His back pain and stiffness have persisted and, as a result, Maurice has been hesitant to resume his normal physical activities including his walking and stretching program.

TREATMENT RECOMMENDATIONS

- Performance of cardiovascular risk factor screening to determine if cautions should be given regarding exercise intensity or if Maurice needs further evaluation or testing prior to exercising (this process is described in the section of the chapter entitled "Cardiovascular Risk Factor Screening"). Maurice has two risk factors (age > 45 and sedentary lifestyle) and, as a result, is in the "increased risk" category. However, he has no cardiorespiratory signs or symptoms, and is told to exercise at a moderate intensity level (one that he could comfortably sustain for a prolonged time such as 60 minutes—this approximates 40% to 60% of his heart rate reserve [HRR]).
- Maurice is encouraged to resume his walking program, initially for 10 minutes, twice per day, at a moderate intensity as discussed earlier.
- Modifications are made to his stretching program. He is also encouraged to take "mini stretch breaks" throughout the day and to get up from his chair at work and home to walk around as frequently as possible.
- He is advised to delay resumption of his golf game for 2 weeks, and then to begin slowly, initially by going to the driving range for two occasions the first week, then, by playing 9 holes the following week (walking as much as possible), then proceeding to 18 holes as tolerated, again with as much walking as possible.

FOLLOW-UP

Maurice reports substantial improvement within a week, with less pain, more mobility, and a sense of having some control of his back pain. Outcome assessment tools used included the Oswestry Low Back Pain Disability Questionnaire, which improved from an initial score of 38% to 12%. Similarly, the visual analogue pain scale measuring pain levels "right now," on average ("usual"), and in the "range from best to worst" improved from 7/10, 5/10, and 3–9/10 to 3/10, 2/10, and 0–4/10, respectively.

Table 18–1 reproduces the cardiovascular risk factor analysis worksheet (CRFAW), which should be completed by the patient. In some circumstances, additional evaluation and completion by an HCP may be required (eg, questions about terminology; values for blood pressure, serum glucose, and serum cholesterol). The CRFAW should be reviewed and scored by the HCP. Note that positive risk factors each have a value of +1 and negative risk factors, such as a high-density lipoprotein (HDL) cholesterol level of 60 mg/dl, values of −1.

Table 18–2, signs and symptoms suggestive of cardiopulmonary disease, should be completed by the HCP. Each category of sign or symptom—such as angina, shortness of breath at rest or with mild exertion, dizziness, or syncope—is given a score of 1 if present and 0 if absent. The total score should be calculated, and the need for additional evaluation and the potential risks of exercise determined.

Table 18–3, the cardiovascular risk factor summary, should also be completed by the HCP. The scores from Tables 18–1 and 18–2 should be reviewed to determine whether the patient is in the category "apparently healthy," "increased risk," or "known disease," as described in Table 18–3.

Table 18–4 is a worksheet designed to determine the type of cardiovascular exercise testing needed before beginning exercise. Again, it should be completed and analyzed by the HCP, who should determine if the patient requires a medical examination and/or a clinical cardiovascular exercise test prior to beginning a moderate or a vigorous exercise program. The HCP should also determine whether the exercise test needs to be supervised by a physician trained and equipped to manage an emergent cardiac or other life-threatening event. As shown in Table 18–4, "moderate" exercise is performed at an intensity level that could be comfortably sustained for a prolonged time (60 minutes or longer), which corresponds to 40% to 60% of an individual's maximal cardiovascular or aerobic capacity. "Vigorous" exercise means exercising at an intensity that represents substantial cardiorespiratory challenge or produces fatigue within 20 minutes (Kenney et al, 1995).

Table 18–1: Cardiovascular Risk Factor Analysis Worksheet

To Be Completed by the Patient

Patient Name _____

Date _____

Please circle any of the following which apply

Category	Positive Risk Factors		Score (The maximum score for each category = 1)
Age	Male >45 years	Female >55 or 55 or less with early menopause without estrogen replacement therapy	0 or 1
Family History	Heart attack in father or brother before age 55	Heart attack in mother or sister before age 65	0 or 1
Cigarette Smoking	Current cigarette smoker		0 or 1
Blood Pressure	Blood Pressure ≥140/90 on two separate occasions	Taking high blood pressure medication	0 or 1
Cholesterol	Total serum cholesterol >200 mg/dl	HDL cholesterol <35 mg/dl	0 or 1
Diabetes Mellitus	Age >30 with IDDM or IDDM for 15 >years	Age >35 with NIDDM	0 or 1
Sedentary Lifestyle	Sedentary job and no regular exercise or regular active physical recreational activities		0 or 1
		Subtotal	_____
Negative Risk Factors			
High serum HDL Cholesterol	HDL >60 mg/dl	(Subtract 1 if you have this high level of "good" HDL cholesterol)	0 or −1
		Total Score	_____

HDL, high-density lipoprotein; IDDM, insulin-dependent diabetes; NIDDM, noninsulin-dependent diabetes.

Adapted with permission from Kenney et al, 1995.

Table 18–2: Signs and Symptoms Suggestive of Cardiopulmonary Disease

To Be Completed by the Health Care Provider

Patient Name _____

Date _____

	Yes = 1	No = 0
1. Pain, discomfort (or other anginal equivalent) in the chest, neck, jaw, arm, or other areas that may be ischemic in nature		
2. Shortness of breath at rest or with mild exertion		
3. Dizziness or syncope		
4. Orthopnea or paroxysmal nocturnal dyspnea		
5. Ankle edema		
6. Palpitations or tachycardia		
7. Intermittent claudication		
8. Known heart murmur		
9. Unusual fatigue or shortness of breath with usual activities		
Total Score	_____	

Adapted with permission from Kenney et al, 1995.

Table 18–3: Cardiovascular Risk Factor Summary

To Be Completed by the Health Care Provider

Apparently Healthy	Increased Risk	Known Disease
If the score from Table 18–1 <2 (less than 2 major CV risk factors); *and* the score from Table 18–2 = 0 (asymptomatic)	If the score from Table 18–1 ≥2 (2 or more major CV risk factors); *and/or* the score from Table 18–2 ≥1 (Any signs or symptoms suggestive of cardiopulmonary disease)	Individuals with known cardiac, pulmonary, or metabolic disease

CV, cardiovascular.

Adapted with permission from Kenney et al, 1995.

❗ CLINICAL ALERT 18–2

Special Considerations for Cardiovascular Fitness Testing

Caution should be used when testing patients with acute musculoskeletal conditions. In general, cardiovascular fitness capacity testing should be postponed and performed later at a time when patients' condition and activity tolerance have improved. Patients with weight-bearing intolerance in the lower extremities may not be able to perform a step test or even, in some rarer cases, a cycle or treadmill test. Patients with poor balance or lower extremity weakness may also find the step test too difficult.

the metronome at 50 bpm if the patient will count the cadence of only one leg; the setting should be at 100 bpm if each leg (right and left) will be counted. A **cadence meter** attached to the bicycle may be easier than the amplified or recorded metronome system and these are available at most bike stores.

The test procedure is explained in Figure 18–2. The initial workload is set at 150 kgm/min and this is maintained for at least 3 minutes. The heart rate is recorded at the beginning of the second and third minutes. A heart rate monitor can make this easier than counting using a stethoscope and watch. The difference in the heart rates between the second and third minutes should be 5 bpm or less. If

---

Table 18–4: Determining the Type of Cardiovascular Exercise Testing Needed Prior to Beginning Exercise

To Be Completed by the Health Care Provider

Medical Exam and Exercise Testing Recommended Prior to Beginning Exercise

	Apparently Healthy		Increased Risk		Known Disease
Exercise Intensity	*Men ≤40; Women ≤50*	*Men >40; Women >50*	*No Symptoms*	*Symptoms*	
Moderate (40%–60% Vo₂ max or a level that is comfortably sustained for 60 minutes)	Not necessary	Not necessary	Not necessary	Recommended	Recommended
Vigorous (>60% Vo₂ max or level of substantial CV challenge or fatigue within 20 minutes)	Not necessary	Recommended	Recommended	Recommended	Recommended

Physician Supervision Recommended During Exercise Test

	Apparently Healthy		Increased Risk		Known Disease
Type of Testing	*Men ≤40; Women ≤50*	*Men >40; Women >50*	*No Symptoms*	*Symptoms*	
Submaximal testing	Not necessary	Not necessary	Not necessary	Recommended	Recommended
Maximal testing	Not necessary	Recommended	Recommended	Recommended	Recommended

CV, cardiovascular.

Adapted with permission from Kenney et al, 1995.

CASE STUDY 18–4
CARDIOVASCULAR RISK FACTOR SCREENING

Mike is a 46-year-old computer software engineer who would like to begin an exercise program to lose weight and increase his cardiovascular fitness level, upper and lower body strength, endurance, and flexibility.

He recently had his annual physical examination, including a blood serum chemistry profile. His total cholesterol value was 187 mg/dl, with HDL level of 52 mg/dl. Mike's father died following a heart attack at age 62. He does not smoke cigarettes. His blood pressure is 135/82 and he is not diabetic. He exercises occasionally on the weekends, but otherwise is relatively sedentary. Using Table 18–1, these findings indicate that he has two cardiovascular risk factors.

Mike does not have any signs or symptoms of cardiopulmonary disease, as described in Table 18–2. Therefore, he is in the "increased risk" category of Table 18–3, given that he has two cardiovascular risk factors from Table 18–1 and no cardiopulmonary signs or symptoms from Table 18–2.

According to Table 18–4, a medical examination and a clinical cardiorespiratory exercise test are not necessary if Mike exercises at a moderate level. However, a medical examination and clinical exercise test are recommended if Mike wants to exercise at an increased ("vigorous") intensity level. Physician supervision of the exercise test is not necessary for submaximal testing as long as Mike does not experience cardiorespiratory symptoms.

TREATMENT RECOMMENDATIONS

- Mike is advised to begin a cardiovascular exercise program of moderate intensity, for at least 20 to 30 min-

utes, at a frequency of at least 3 days per week. Moderate intensity is exercise that could be comfortably sustained for 60 minutes, and that requires approximately 70% of his full effort level of exertion.
- Mike receives instruction in the use of isotonic weight machines, again at an approximate 70% effort level, performing two to three sets of exercises on 10 to 12 different pieces of equipment. He is told that these exercises should be performed at least two to four times per week.
- Mike receives instruction in an individualized self-stretching exercise program, performing 8 to 10 stretching exercises slowly, holding each for at least 30 seconds and repeating these three to four times per session. He is told that he can stretch on a daily basis, and that his flexibility will be greater if he does these exercises in the afternoon or evening (not first thing in the morning upon awakening).

FOLLOW-UP

Mike joins a local health facility and begins exercising 3 to 4 days per week for an hour or so. After 12 weeks, he has lost 8 pounds, notices his clothes fit differently, has more energy, and that he sleeps more soundly. His blood pressure has dropped to 118/72 and his cholesterol is 180 mg/dl with HDL level of 58 mg/dl.

---

it exceeds 5 bpm, extend the first workload for another minute, or even 2 minutes, checking the heart rate at the end of each minute. A steady state heart rate should be achieved. **The second workload should not be started until this steady state heart rate is maintained.**

The second workload intensity is based on the heart rate at the end of the first workload. If the heart rate at the end of the first workload is:

- <80 bpm, the second workload = 750 kgm
- 80–89 bpm, the second workload = 600 kgm
- 90–100 bpm, the second workload = 450 kgm
- >100 bpm, the second workload = 300 kgm

The heart rate is recorded at the second and third minutes of the second workload. Again, **the workload should be**

maintained until a steady state heart rate is reached. The third and fourth workloads are determined using the values listed in Figure 18–2. Record the data on Figure 18–3, as described earlier. The values from the heart rate in the final minute of each workload or stage are plotted on Figure 18–3 against work rate and in relationship to the age predicted maximal heart rate (220 minus age). A corresponding maximal cardiovascular fitness/aerobic capacity level (VO_2 max) can be determined using Figure 18–4.

Figures 18–6 and 18–7 show age and gender rankings for cardiovascular fitness and estimated VO_2 max from the cycle ergometer test. The corresponding values for the bike test are found in the "PWC max (kgm)" column. The rankings allow for comparison of cardiovascular fitness levels to others in the same age and gender categories.

Informed Consent for Exercise Test

You will perform a step exercise test, an exercise test on a stationary bike or a treadmill exercise test. We may stop the test at any time because of signs of fatigue or changes in your heart rate or blood pressure. It is important for you to realize that you also may choose to stop the test at any time if you become fatigued or experience any discomfort.

There exists the possibility of certain changes occurring during the test. They include abnormal blood pressure; fainting; irregular, fast, or slow heart rhythm; and, in rare instances, heart attack, stroke, or death. Every effort will be made to minimize these risks by evaluation of preliminary information relating to your health and fitness and by observations during testing. Trained personnel are available to deal with any unusual situations that may arise.

Information you possess about your health status or previous experiences of unusual feelings with physical effort may affect the safety and value of your exercise test. Your prompt reporting of feelings with effort during the exercise test itself is also of great importance. You are responsible for fully disclosing such information when requested by the testing staff.

The results of this test will assist in evaluating if you may safely begin an exercise program and at what level of activity you should start.

Any questions about the procedures used in the exercise test or the results of your test are encouraged. If you have any concerns or questions, please ask us for further explanations.

Your permission to perform this exercise test is voluntary. You are free to stop the test at any point, if you so desire.

I have read this form and I understand the test procedures that I will perform and the attendant risks and discomforts. Knowing these risks and discomforts, and having had an opportunity to ask questions that have been answered to my satisfaction, I consent to participate in this test.

_____   _____
Date   Signature of patient

_____   _____
Date   Signature of witness

_____   _____
Date   Signature of physician

Figure 18–1. Informed Consent for Exercise Test form.

(Reprinted with permission of Aspen Publishing, Gaithersburg, MD. In Mootz, RD, ed. Informed Consent for Exercise Test. *Top Clin Chiro* 1997;2:69.)

YMCA 3-MINUTE BENCH STEP TEST

The 3-minute bench step test, as described by the YMCA (Golding et al, 1989), is the least expensive method of car-

diovascular testing presented in this chapter, and it is easy to perform in many different environments. The patient continuously steps up and down on a 12-inch bench at a rate of 24 steps per minute for 3 minutes (Fig. 18–8). At the end of 3 minutes of stepping, the patient immediately sits down and the recovery heart rate is counted for a full minute (Fig. 18–9). **It is important that the recovery heart rate be counted within 5 seconds of ending the 3 minutes of exercise.**

The following equipment is required for this test:

- A stable sturdy 12-inch bench
- A metronome set at 96 bpm (24 steps/minute— each click of the metronome equals a step with each leg—"up, up, down, down")
- A timer or watch for timing the 3 minutes of stepping and the 1-minute recovery
- A stethoscope for counting the recovery heart rate (the number of beats for the full minute following 3 minutes of stepping are counted—therefore, a heart

---

CLINICAL TIP 18–3
Benefits of Tracking Patient Progress

The ability to show change over time offers the patient, the HCP, and the third-party payer information about progress. This information can lead to better clinical decision making, such as modification of the aerobic exercise program, discontinuation/discharge, or the need for further testing. In addition, the information obtained from testing will often provide patient motivation and allow the HCP to determine whether or not the goals of the rehabilitation program are being met.

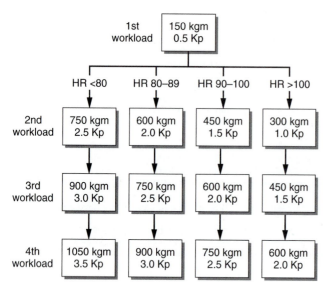

Directions:

1. Set the first workload at 150 kgm/min (0.5 Kp).
2. If the HR in the third min is
   • less than (<) 80, set the second load at 750 kgm (2.5 Kp);
   • 80 to 89, set the second load at 600 kgm (2.0 Kp);
   • 90 to 100, set the second load at 450 kgm (1.5 Kp);
   • greater than (>) 100, set the second load at 300 kgm (1.0 Kp).
3. Set the third and fourth (if required) loads according to the loads in the columns below the second loads.

Figure 18–2. Guide to setting workloads on bicycle ergometer.

(Reprinted from *Y's Way to Physical Fitness* with permission of the YMCA of the USA, 101 N. Wacker Drive, Chicago, IL 60606.)

rate monitor should *not* be used as it measures the heart rate at any given moment)
• The Aerobic Capacity tables shown in Figures 18–6 and 18–7

The test should be explained to the patient, and the stepping in time to the metronome should be demonstrated. The participant should step up with one foot on the first beat, up with the second foot on the second beat, down with the first foot on the third beat and down with the second foot on the fourth beat. The cadence is "up, up, down, down" repeatedly. It is helpful to count this out for the patient, especially if the metronome is difficult to hear. Let the patient try this until he or she can do this successfully prior to beginning the test. **Find the patient's heart rate before beginning the test, and make sure he or she understands the instruction to sit down on the bench or a chair next to the bench immediately following the test.** Always remember to assure the patient that the test will be stopped at any time if he or she experiences any unusual symptoms.

It is important to remember that **the recovery heart rate is counted for the *full minute* starting within 5 seconds immediately following the 3 minutes of stepping.**

Once you have determined this value, refer to Figures 18–6 and 18–7 to assess the patient's relative cardiorespiratory fitness level estimated VO_2 max from the 3-minute step test. The corresponding values for the bike test are found in the "3-min step test" column. The rankings allow for comparison of cardiovascular fitness levels to others in the same age and gender categories.

TREADMILL TESTS

Although cycle ergometry is the most popular form of cardiovascular fitness testing, treadmill testing is tolerated well by many patients as it involves walking or running, activities to which most of us are accustomed. However, treadmills are more expensive than either a cycle ergometer or a 12-inch bench for a step test. Also, walking on a motorized treadmill belt requires different skills than walking on land, and **most individuals will benefit from some time spent practicing this activity before testing.**

PERFORMING TREADMILL TESTS

Before beginning, the patient should receive instructions describing the test. Walking or running shoes should be worn. The treadmill should have rails for the patient to use if needed (especially at first) and there should be an emergency stop button or switch mechanism. The patient should initially straddle the belt and start "pawing" or "pedaling" the belt using one foot as it begins to move. Patients will often look down at the belt, walk with a very short stride, and drift to the rear of the belt at first. They should be encouraged to look forward, walk with a more lengthened normal stride, and walk in the center of the belt.

The patient's heart rate will need to be measured while exercising. Relatively inexpensive accurate heart rate monitors made by companies such as Polar are recommended. (Polar can be reached at 1-800-227-1314 or on their web site at http://www.polar.fi/sampola/.)

TREADMILL PROTOCOL TESTS

There are several submaximal treadmill protocols, including the **Balke protocol** (Kenney et al, 1995). These often involve having the individual exercise until he or she attains a predetermined intensity level, which is often a percentage of his or her predicted maximal cardiorespiratory or aerobic capacity (Fig. 18–10). The Balke treadmill protocol uses increasing speed and/or incline until the patient reaches 85% of his or her **maximal heart rate reserve.** The maximal heart rate reserve is calculated as follows:

Maximal heart rate (HR max) = 220 − age
Resting heart rate (HR rest) = heart rate at rest
[(HR max − HR rest) × .85] + HR rest =
85% of maximal heart rate reserve

(*Text continues on p. 389.*)

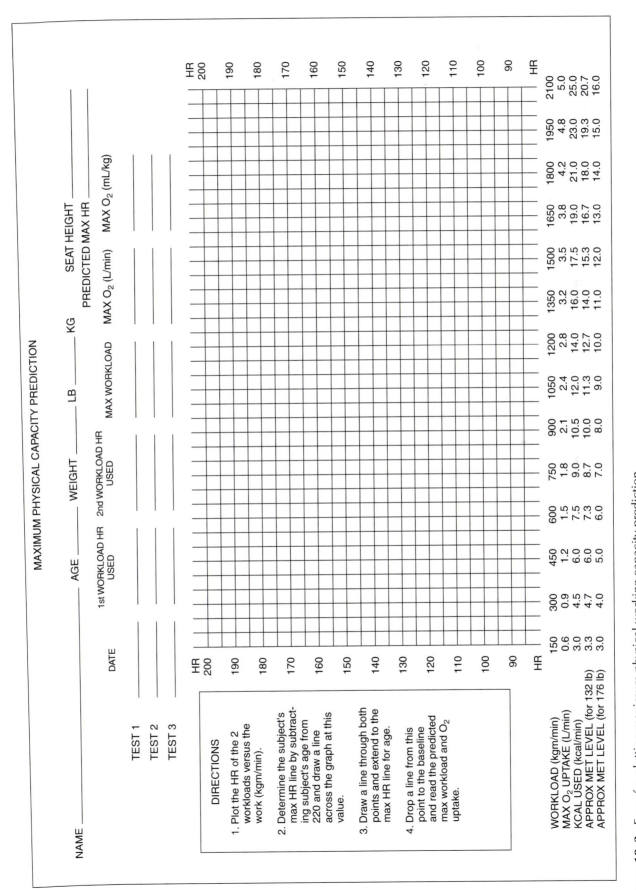

Figure 18–3. Form for plotting maximum physical working capacity prediction.
(Reprinted from *Y's Way to Physical Fitness* with permission of the YMCA of the USA, 101 N. Wacker Drive, Chicago, IL 60606.)

Rating	% ranking	Women Age 18–25 3-min step test	PWC max (kgm)	$\dot{V}O_2$ max (mL/kg)	Women Age 26–35 3-min step test	PWC max (kgm)	$\dot{V}O_2$ max (mL/kg)	Women Age 36–45 3-min step test	PWC max (kgm)	$\dot{V}O_2$ max (mL/kg)
Excellent	100	72	1830	71	72	1800	69	74	1780	66
	95	79	1640	67	80	1440	59	80	1360	53
	90	83	1440	58	86	1330	54	87	1215	46
Good	85	88	1320	54	91	1245	51	93	1135	44
	80	93	1235	50	93	1180	48	97	1085	41
	75	97	1175	48	97	1115	46	101	1035	39
Above average	70	100	1120	46	103	1065	43	104	980	37
	65	103	1075	43	106	1020	42	106	925	36
	60	106	1030	42	110	985	40	109	880	34
Average	55	110	990	41	112	955	38	111	835	33
	50	112	950	40	116	925	37	114	800	32
	45	116	915	39	118	885	35	117	765	31
Below average	40	118	880	37	121	840	34	120	745	30
	35	122	845	35	124	805	33	122	720	29
	30	124	810	34	127	765	31	127	695	28
Poor	25	128	775	32	129	730	30	130	670	26
	20	133	740	31	131	695	28	135	625	25
	15	137	705	29	135	655	26	138	575	23
Very poor	10	142	640	26	141	600	25	143	530	21
	5	149	555	22	148	530	22	146	490	19
	0	155	500	18	154	490	20	152	470	18

Rating	% ranking	Women Age 46–55 3-min step test	PWC max (kgm)	$\dot{V}O_2$ max (mL/kg)	Women Age 56–65 3-min step test	PWC max (kgm)	$\dot{V}O_2$ max (mL/kg)	Women Age Over 65 3-min step test	PWC max (kgm)	$\dot{V}O_2$ max (mL/kg)
Excellent	100	76	1700	64	74	1650	57	73	1190	51
	95	88	1245	48	83	1165	43	83	860	39
	90	93	1130	42	92	1015	38	86	820	33
Good	85	96	1045	39	97	970	36	93	725	31
	80	100	980	36	99	895	34	97	665	30
	75	102	930	35	103	840	32	100	640	28
Above average	70	106	885	33	106	790	31	104	610	27
	65	111	850	32	109	750	30	108	585	26
	60	113	815	31	111	720	28	114	560	25
Average	55	117	790	30	113	690	27	117	540	24
	50	118	760	29	116	660	26	120	525	23
	45	120	730	28	117	635	25	121	510	22
Below average	40	121	700	27	119	605	24	123	495	22
	35	124	670	26	123	575	23	126	480	21
	30	126	640	25	127	550	22	127	470	20
Poor	25	127	610	24	129	530	21	129	460	18
	20	131	585	23	132	510	20	132	425	17
	15	133	545	21	136	475	19	134	395	17
Very poor	10	138	495	19	142	420	17	135	370	16
	5	147	430	18	148	355	15	149	340	15
	0	152	400	16	151	340	14	151	320	14

Figure 18–7. Aerobic capacity values and rankings for 3-minute step test and YMCA cycle ergometer test for women. (Adapted from *Y's Way to Physical Fitness* with permission of the YMCA of the USA, 101 N. Wacker Drive, Chicago, IL 60606.)

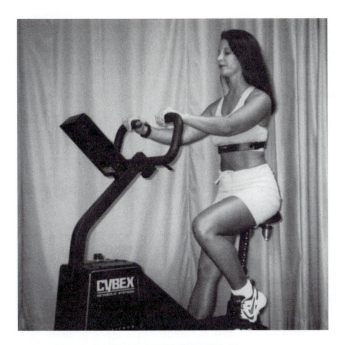

Figure 18–5. Patient performing cycle ergometer test.

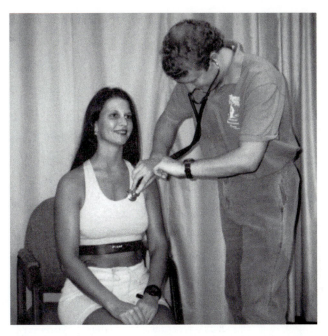

Figure 18–9. Measurement of recovery heart rate after 3-minute step test.

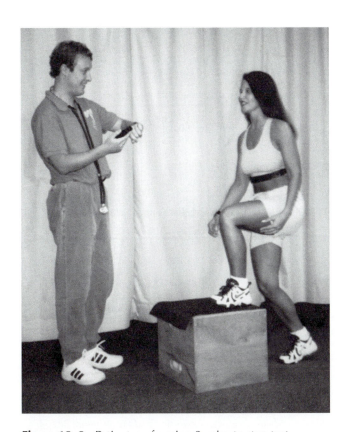

Figure 18–8. Patient performing 3-minute step test.

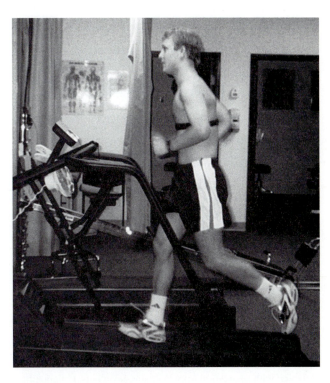

Figure 18–10. Patient performing treadmill test.

		Age 20–29		Age 30–39		Age 40–49		Age 50–59		Age 60+	
%		Balke treadmill (time)	$\dot{V}O_2$ max (mL/kg/min)	Balke treadmill (time)	$\dot{V}O_2$ max (mL/kg/min)	Balke treadmill (time)	$\dot{V}O_2$ max (mL/kg/min)	Balke treadmill (time)	$\dot{V}O_2$ max (mL/kg/min)	Balke treadmill (time)	$\dot{V}O_2$ max (mL/kg/min)
99		30:20	58.79	29:00	58.86	28:00	55.42	26:00	52.53	24:29	50.39
95	S	27:00	53.97	26:00	52.53	24:30	50.36	22:15	47.11	20:56	45.21
90		25:11	51.35	24:30	50.36	23:00	48.20	21:00	45.31	19:00	42.46
85		24:00	49.64	23:00	48.20	21:00	45.31	19:00	42.42	17:00	39.53
80	E	23:00	48.20	22:00	46.75	20:10	44.11	18:00	40.98	16:00	38.09
75		22:10	46.99	21:00	45.31	20:00	43.89	17:00	39.53	15:00	36.65
70		22:00	46.75	20:30	44.59	18:32	41.75	16:15	38.45	14:04	35.30
65		21:00	45.31	20:00	43.87	18:00	40.98	15:40	37.61	13:22	39.29
60	G	20:15	44.23	19:00	42.42	17:15	39.89	15:00	36.65	12:53	33.59
55		20:00	43.87	18:25	41.58	17:00	39.53	14:30	36.10	12:03	32.39
50		19:03	42.49	18:00	40.98	16:00	38.09	14:00	35.20	11:40	31.83
45		19:00	42.42	17:00	39.53	15:30	37.37	13:15	34.12	11:00	30.87
40	F	18:00	40.98	16:32	38.86	15:00	36.69	13:00	33.76	10:30	30.15
35		17:30	40.26	16:00	38.09	14:15	35.56	12:07	32.48	10:00	29.43
30		17:00	39.53	15:30	37.37	13:57	35.13	12:00	32.31	9:30	28.70
25		16:00	38.09	15:00	36.65	13:00	33.76	11:08	31.06	8:54	27.89
20	P	15:20	37.13	14:06	35.35	12:30	33.04	10:30	30.15	8:00	26.54
15		15:00	36.65	13:10	34.00	12:00	32.31	10:00	29.43	7:00	25.09
10		13:30	34.48	12:09	32.53	10:59	30.85	9:00	27.98	5:35	23.05
5	VP	11:30	31.57	11:00	30.87	6:21	28.29	7:00	25.09	4:00	20.76
1		8:23	27.09	8:00	26.54	6:21	24.15	4:54	22.06	2:17	18.28
		N = 1675		N = 7094		N = 6837		N = 3808		N = 1005	

Figure 18–11. Aerobic power tests (men).

(Adapted with permission from Williams & Wilkins, Philadelphia, PA. *ACSM—Guidelines for Exercise Testing and Prescription,* 5th ed, 1995.)

		Age 20–29		Age 30–39		Age 40–49		Age 50–59		Age 60+	
%		Balke treadmill (time)	$\dot{V}O_2$ max (mL/kg/min)	Balke treadmill (time)	$\dot{V}O_2$ max (mL/kg/min)	Balke treadmill (time)	$\dot{V}O_2$ max (mL/kg/min)	Balke treadmill (time)	$\dot{V}O_2$ max (mL/kg/min)	Balke treadmill (time)	$\dot{V}O_2$ max (mL/kg/min)
99		26:21	53.03	23:22	48.73	22:00	46.75	18:44	42.04	20:25	44.47
95	S	22:00	46.75	20:00	43.87	18:00	40.98	15:07	36.81	15:34	37.46
90		20:12	44.15	18:00	40.98	17:00	39.53	14:00	35.20	14:00	35.20
85		19:00	42.42	17:30	40.26	15:35	37.49	12:53	33.59	12:00	32.31
80	E	18:00	40.98	16:20	38.57	14:45	36.28	12:00	32.31	11:15	31.23
75		17:00	39.53	15:30	37.37	13:56	35.11	11:43	39.90	11:00	30.87
70		16:00	38.09	15:00	36.65	13:00	33.76	11:00	30.87	10:00	29.43
65		15:30	37.37	14:10	35.44	12:30	33.04	10:14	29.76	9:00	27.98
60	G	15:00	36.65	13:35	34.60	12:00	32.31	10:00	29.43	8:28	27.21
55		14:39	36.14	13:10	33.85	11:30	31.59	9:30	28.70	8:00	26.54
50		14:00	35.20	13:00	33.76	11:00	30.87	9:10	28.22	7:30	25.82
45		13:30	34.48	12:10	32.41	10:48	30.58	9:00	27.98	7:00	25.09
40	F	13:00	33.76	12:00	32.31	10:01	29.45	8:13	26.85	6:35	24.49
35		12:17	32.72	11:09	31.09	10:00	29.43	7:43	26.13	6:16	24.03
30		12:00	32.31	10:45	30.51	9:11	28.25	7:16	25.48	6:08	23.80
25		11:03	30.94	10:00	29.93	9:00	27.98	7:00	25.09	6:00	23.65
20	P	10:50	30.63	9:30	28.70	8:00	26.54	6:25	24.25	5:24	22.78
15		10:00	29.43	9:00	27.98	7:20	25.57	6:00	23.65	5:00	22.21
10		9:17	28.39	8:00	26.54	7:00	25.09	5:05	22.33	4:00	20.76
5	VP	7:33	25.89	7:00	25.09	5:55	23.53	4:14	21.10	3:15	19.68
1		5:15	22.57	5:12	22.49	4:00	20.76	2:36	18.74	2:00	17.87
		N = 764		N = 2049		N = 1630		N = 878		N = 202	

Figure 18–12. Aerobic power tests (women).

(Adapted with permission from Williams & Wilkins, Philadelphia, PA. *ACSM—Guidelines for Exercise Testing and Prescription,* 5th ed, 1995.)

For example, the maximal heart rate reserve of a 30-year-old patient with a resting heart rate of 70 would be calculated as follows:

$$[(190 - 70) \times .85] + 70 = 172 \text{ beats/minute}$$

In this example, the patient would exercise until reaching 172 beats/minute, at which point the test should be stopped.

The Balke protocol works well in the outpatient rehabilitation setting. It uses small incremental increases in workload and is gradual and, therefore, is generally tolerated reasonably well by individuals in poor physical condition. It does, however, require a treadmill that elevates up to a 25% grade incline, especially for more physically fit patients who require more workload to achieve their 85% maximal heart rate reserve level.

This test requires the following equipment:

- A treadmill with variable speed and incline with a top speed of in excess of 3.3 mph and an elevation of 25 degrees or greater
- A heart rate monitor or other device(s) to record heart rate at the 85% maximal heart rate reserve level.

The Balke protocol begins with a constant speed of 3.3 mph with the treadmill grade set at 0% for the first minute. At the end of the first minute the grade should be increased to 2%. The incline should thereafter be increased at 1% per minute, and the speed remain constant at 3.3 mph. If the patient has not reached 85% of his or her maximal heart rate reserve by the time a 25% incline is reached, then the incline should be maintained at 25% and the speed increased .2 mph/min, until the 85% maximal heart rate reserve level is reached.

The patient's heart rate should be monitored and the test stopped when the 85% maximal heart rate reserve level is attained. The number of 1-minute stages performed should be recorded. This value corresponds to a predicted level of aerobic fitness for similarly aged men or women. Percentile ranking and cardiovascular fitness/aerobic capacity (VO_2 max) values are provided in Figures 18–11 and 18–12.

Conclusion

The information gained through cardiovascular fitness risk factor screening and testing can help the rehabilitation-oriented HCP ascertain if additional testing is indicated before an individual should begin an exercise program, and what intensity of exercise is recommended for that individual.

Cardiovascular fitness testing can be valuable if performed prior to beginning, during, and upon completion of a physical rehabilitative exercise program to measure and document progress in the management of a variety of conditions. A partial list of conditions includes many musculoskeletal conditions, coronary artery disease, hypertension, obesity, stroke, adult-onset diabetes, peripheral vascular disease, anxiety, depression, and several types of cancer.

Three methods for assessing cardiovascular fitness testing are discussed in this chapter: the YMCA cycle ergometer test, the YMCA 3-minute bench step test, and the Balke treadmill test. All are relatively safe, inexpensive, and easy to perform in an outpatient musculoskeletal rehabilitation setting. Each method has its benefits, and the reader is urged to consider which of these methods best fit an individual set of circumstances.

Retesting at specified intervals to show change over time offers the patient, the HCP, and the third-party payer information about progress. This information can often increase patient motivation, allow the practitioner to determine whether or not the goals of the rehabilitation program are being met, and lead to better clinical decision making, such as modification of the exercise program, discontinuation/discharge, or the need for further testing.

REFERENCES

Bigos SJ, Bowyer O, Braen G, et al. *Acute Low Back Problems in Adults*. Washington, DC: US Department of Health and Human Services, Agency for Health Care Policy and Research; 1994. Clinical Practice Guideline No. 14.

Golding LA, Myers CR, Sinning WE, eds. *Y's Way to Physical Fitness*. 3rd ed. Champaign, Ill: Human Kinetics; 1989.

Kenney WL, Humphrey RH, Bryant CX, eds. ACSM—*Guidelines for Exercise Testing and Prescription*. 5th ed. Baltimore, Md: Williams & Wilkins; 1995.

Mootz RD, ed. Informed consent for exercise test. *Top Clin Chiro* 1997;2:69.

SECTION

IV

Application of Outcomes Assessment to Clinical Practice

The objective of this section is to bring together methodologies of implementing the various outcome tools that are the subject of Sections II and III into the clinical setting. Chapter 19 offers a timeline for data collection through the various stages of care. Chapter 20 addresses the integration of outcomes assessment and the documentation process. This section closes with Chapter 21, which addresses factors that are useful in the identification of patients who are at risk for a prolonged recovery. This domain is of significant value as it helps the health care provider identify, on the first visit, patients who are not likely to succeed with passive treatment intervention.

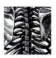

CHAPTER 19

Case Management in an Evidence-based Practice

STEVEN G. YEOMANS

INTRODUCTION

As we move further into the era of accountability, the use of an evidence-based, outcomes-oriented practice style is gaining popularity. As mentioned in previous chapters, health care providers (HCPs) who decide to make this "paradigm shift" to becoming outcomes based will be in an advantageous position with respect to negotiating for group privileges and managed care contracts, reducing insurance dispute losses, and most importantly, will sharpen their case management skills to optimize case management/patient care. These issues are more thoroughly presented in Chapter 24.

GOALS OF OUTCOMES MANAGEMENT

The following outline summarizes information that is discussed in this section of the chapter.

A. Acute, Subacute, and Chronic Stages of Healing
B. Steps to Follow in Case Management
  1. Perform Diagnostic Triage
    a. Identifying Red Flags
      (1) Cauda Equina Syndrome
      (2) Tumor/Cancer
      (3) Infection
      (4) Fracture
      (5) Referred Pain from Viscera
    b. Identifying Nerve Root Lesions
    c. Identifying Yellow Flags
      (1) What Are Psychosocial Yellow Flags?
      (2) Why Is There a Need to Identify Psychosocial Yellow Flags?
      (3) Who Is at Risk?
  2. Provide Reassurance and Advice
  3. Provide Symptomatic Relief
  4. Utilize Outcomes Management
  5. Promote Functional Restoration
  6. Determine Endpoints of Care

ACUTE, SUBACUTE, AND CHRONIC STAGES OF HEALING

In the acute stage of healing, the primary goals of care are providing symptomatic relief of pain, protecting against reinjury, and reassuring the patient to reduce unnecessary anxieties and perhaps unnecessary or premature costly emergent evaluations or tests. In the subacute to chronic stage, however, identification and prevention of disability must be primary considerations. To achieve the goal of disability prevention, the HCPs primary focus must be on promoting a return of function to minimize activity limitations. The use of outcomes management can help the HCP determine whether these goals are being met, allowing for prompt identification of patients who fail to respond to care and implementation of alternative care options.

Two patients who present with identical signs, symptoms, and diagnoses can respond in ways that are completely opposite to each other. It is thus necessary to identify the differences between such seemingly identical cases. For example, in an "uncomplicated case," there are usually few, if any, **"yellow flags"** or risk factors that interfere with the natural historical resolution of the presenting complaint (see Case Study 1). However, in a complicated case where many risk factors exist, a poor outcome may result (see Case Study 2). Unless these risk factors are being captured, poor management and promotion of chronicity may occur.

In complicated cases such as that depicted in Case Study 2, especially those patients who present with chronic conditions in which multiple risk factors exist, a successful outcome is often dependent upon identifying the risk factors that may be interfering with recovery. The care one renders to the complicated case may necessitate treatment/referral for management of psychosocial issues such as job dissatisfaction, prior childhood abuse, anxiety and/or depression, and a host of other possibilites. Also, an ergonomic evaluation for those in a high-risk occupation with modifications in the workstation may be required if control of a chronic condition is to be achieved. **These barriers to recovery may be more important to address than the actual physical impairment the patient presents with because often, disability is significantly greater than impairment.** Therefore, in a primary care setting, proper case management necessitates obtaining a complete current and past history (including medical, family, occupational, social, and habits history), performing a complete examination, and reviewing past patient records. The HCP must then weigh the information obtained to determine treatment goals and direct care where it is most needed.

STEPS TO FOLLOW IN CASE MANAGEMENT

To simplify this process, the steps to follow in case management to achieve quality care are presented in Table 19–1.

By following these steps, the HCP can remain focused on the patient's specific treatment goals and address important issues as they arise.

PERFORM DIAGNOSTIC TRIAGE

In diagnostic triage, there are three primary tasks: (1) identifying red flags, (2) identifying nerve root lesions, and (3) identifying risk factors of chronicity (yellow flags).

Identifying Red Flags

The importance of identifying a red flag is obvious, since an emergent referral for proper management is necessary (McCarthy, 1994). The AHCPR has identified the following red flags (Bigos et al, 1994): cauda equina syndrome, tumor/cancer, infection, and fracture. McCarthy (1994) has also discussed an additional "red flag," referred pain from viscera.

Cauda Equina Syndrome

The occurrence of cauda equina syndrome is rare; when present, however, emergent surgical referral is considered appropriate (Floman et al, 1980). From a historical and physical examination perspective, urinary retention was reported to be the most consistent finding with a sensitivity of .90, specificity of .95, and negative predictive factor of .99 (Deyo et al, 1992). Loss of anal sphincter tone, sciatic leg pain, motor and sensory deficits, nerve tension signs (positive straight leg raise [SLR]), and saddle anesthesia were reported as other important distinguishing features.

Tumor/Cancer

Cancer is quite rare affecting less than 1% of patients presenting with low back pain (Deyo and Diehl, 1988). Primary cancer, such as multiple myeloma, accounts for <10% whereas metastatic cancer accounts for 80% of those patients over 50 years in age. It has been shown that history is more discriminating than physical examination in unveiling the tumor/cancer patient (Deyo, 1991). More specifically, in a group of known cancer patients, Deyo found at least one of the first five historical finding items listed in Table 19–2 to be present, while routine physical examination findings were essentially negative. This illustrates quite pointedly the importance of the clinical history, which is usually reported to be subjective and, therefore, less important than the objective physical examination (McCowin et al, 1991) (see Chap. 3).

Infection

The occurrence of a spinal infection is uncommon. Historical findings, again, play an important role in identifying low back pain patients who may be presenting with a spinal infection. These important historical findings include:

- Urinary tract infection history
- Skin infection
- Respiratory tract infection (Waldvogel and Vasey, 1980)
- Intravenous drug users
- Elderly or the debilitated patient at any age

CASE STUDY 19–1
CASE 1: NONRADICULAR LOW BACK PAIN PATIENT

SUBJECTIVE

Bob is a 28-year-old male of mesomorphic stature who presented with his first episode of nonradicular low back pain of a 5-day duration. He has missed 2 days of work due to the complaint; this is not a worker's compensation issue as the mechanism of injury was lifting a 5-gallon can of gas out of his trunk. The *past history* is uneventful and there are no yellow (see table p. 389) or red flags identified using the classification checklist (see Appendix Forms H–1 and H–2), the SF–12, and the three depression screening questions (Appendix Form A–4), and the Severity Index (Appendix Form I–1). The Oswestry Low Back Pain Disability Questionnaire reveals 33% disability score (Appendix Form C–2). The pain drawing is physiologically consistent with the presenting history. The Quadruple Visual Analogue Scale (VAS) scores 83% (see Appendix Form B–1). Refer to the Outcomes Assessment (OA) summary form, later in this presentation for OA results.

OBJECTIVE

Vital signs: BP 128/76; pulse 68; respiration 16; height 5'11"; weight 205 lbs. *Observation:* Elevated left occiput, shoulder, and hemipelvis with suspected right leg length deficiency. Minor's sign was present and rising from sitting was painful unless completed very slowly. Normal gait assessment was noted except the left foot toed inwards. *Palpation:* Reveals muscle hypertrophy of the erector spinae musculature and tenderness in the lumbosacral region (L3-S1, symmetrical). Vertebral fixation was noted in the lumbosacral junction, right L5, and bilateral SI joints. Lumbar *range of motion* (LROM) reveals: flexion of 50 degrees with endpoint pulling pain graded at 0/4, without radiation, but 2/4 when rising back to neutral; extension of 10 degrees with sharp endpoint pain localized at the lumbosacral junction, grade 4/4. Extension LROM reveals more pain/dysfunction versus flexion, which was pain relieving. Extension-related *provocative orthopedic tests* were pain provocative localizing pain in the lumbosacral region, which include Kemp's and Yeoman's tests bilaterally; nerve tension signs were negative at straight leg raises (SLRs) were hamstring-restricted, only. No motor or sensory L2-S2 neurological losses were noted. *Physical performance tests* revealed SLRs at 52 degrees/58 degrees (left/right, respectively) (normal: 80 degrees); hip internal rotation at 32 degrees/36 degrees (normal: 42 degrees); hip external rotation 38 degrees/40 degrees (43 degrees); hip extension/psoas 68 degrees/74 degrees (normal: 82 degrees).

ASSESSMENT

Reveals an uncomplicated, flexion-biased, mechanical low back injury consistent with a lumbar sprain/strain.

Short-term goals include:

1. Reassure patient.
2. Reduce pain 50% by week 2.
3. Restore range of motion (ROM) and activities of daily living (ADL) losses by week 4.
4. Maintain employment by limiting duties as needed.

Long-term goals include:

1. Educate about proper body mechanics with bend, lift, pull, push, and occupational-specific movements.
2. Implement active care: Williams' exercises, self-stretch—contract and hold hamstrings against wall; eccentric stretch hip internal rotation (IR) and external rotation (ER), abdominal strengthening, and pelvic stabilization emphasizing strengthening of the lumbar extensors, especially the quadratus lumborum (QL) by use of the side bridge (see Chap. 16 for assessment of functional losses and rehabilitation prescriptions).

PLAN

The treatment plan includes:

Week 1: Three treatments on week 1, including spinal manipulative treatment (SMT), manual release techniques (MRTs), Interferential Current (IFC), initiation of Williams' exercises, and ADL modifications eliminating over stressing the low back at work and home.

Week 2: Two treatments (SMT) for second week, adding side bridges to tolerance (have patient record hold times in seconds at home for outcomes data and comparison); a walking program will be initiated, starting with 5 to 10 minutes followed by a gradual increase in time and pace/speed. Initiate regular duties if able.

Week 3: One treatment (SMT); pelvic stabilization exercises; increased pace/distance in walking; patient may use aerobic exercise machine (bicycle, stepper, treadmill); resume ADLs without restrictions.

Week 4: Re-evaluation of subjective tools and discharge with full resolution. One treatment (SMT)

(continued)

CASE STUDY 19–1 *(continued)*
CASE 1: NONRADICULAR LOW BACK PAIN PATIENT

Outcomes Assessment Record (extracted from Appendix Form H–4)

DATE	PAIN			FUNCTION			
	VAS (miscell.) a. Now b. Ave. c. Range CC *LBP*	Pain Drawing/ Severity Index	Options: 1. UE 2. CTS 3. Shoulder 4. Knee	Options: 1. Headache 2. Dizziness 3. SCL-90R 4. _____	VAS and Neck Disability (NDI)	VAS and LB Disability: • *Oswestry* • Roland- Morris	Patient Satisfaction
Baseline							
2/24/99	a. 9/10 b. 6/10 c. 5–10/10 QVAS = 83%	Physiological **1. Yes** 2. No SI:108 (mild)				Osw. 33%	
Progress							
3/31/99	a. 1/10 b. 0/10 c. 0–1/10 QVAS = 7%	Physiological **1. Yes** 2. No SI: 0 (none)				Osw. 4%	98

HSQ-12 (from Appendix Form A–3)

SCALE	HSQ-12 MEAN[a]	INITIAL BASELINE 2-24-99	FIRST RE-EXAM 3-31-99
1. Health perception	72	85	100
2. Physical function	84	50	100
3. Role—physical	81	25	100
4. Role—emotional	81	65	100
5. Social functioning	83	75	100
6. Bodily pain	75	0	100
7. Mental health	75	80	93
8. Energy fatigue	61	60	80
9. Major depression	yes/no	yes/**no**	yes/**no**
10. Dysthemia	yes/no	yes/**no**	yes/**no**
11. Both 9 and 10	yes/no	yes/**no**	yes/**no**
[a] Not yet established (1996); the mean scores are those derived from the HSQ 2.0 (36-item questionnaire).			

CASE STUDY 19–1 *(continued)*
CASE 1: NONRADICULAR LOW BACK PAIN PATIENT

		QUESTION	SCORE		
			Baseline	2nd	3rd
1.	1.	Pain location (×2/region)	2	0	NA
2.		Duration of the **current** episode (×2 for score indicated)	2		
3.		Number of prior episodes (×2 for score indicated)	0		
4.		Prior surgery or hospitalizations (yes = 10; no = 0)	0		
5.	2.	Usual level of pain (0–10) this week (score is no. circled)	9	0	NA
6.		Frequency of pain 0–10 (score is no. circled)	10		
7.	3.	Frequency of radiating pain (0–10) (score is no. circled)	0	0	NA
8.	4.	Frequency of medication use (0–10) (score is no. circled)	5	0	NA
9.	5.	Patient satisfaction if no change (0–10) (score is no. circled)	7	0	NA
10.	6.	How anxious the past week (0–10) (score is no. circled)	3	0	NA
11.	7.	Ability to control/cope (0–10) (score is no. circled)	2	0	NA
12.	8.	How depressed the past week (0–10) (score is no. circled)	3	0	NA
13.		General health rating (0–10) (score is no. circled)	0		
14.		Smoking? (yes = 10; no = 0)	0		
15.	9.	Pain = stop activity (0–10) (score is no. circled)	5	0	NA
16.	10.	Physical activity = worse pain (0–10) (score is no. circled)	7	0	NA
17.	11.	Light work tolerant for 1 hour (0–10) (score is no. circled)	4	0	NA
18.	12.	Can sleep at night (0–10) (score is no. circled)	6	0	NA
19.		Physical demanding (0–10) (score is 10 − no. circled)	9		
20.		Any disability in last 12 months? (yes = 10; no = 0)	0		
21.	13.	Should not do normal duty? (0–10) (score is 10 − no. circled)	8	0	NA
22.		Do you like work? (yes = 0; no = 10)	10		
23.	14.	Ability to sit/stand 6 wks from now? (0–10) (score is no. circled)	8	0	NA
24.	15.	Ability to work 6 mo. from now (0–10) (score is no. circled)	8	0	NA
25.		**Total**	108	0	NA

Note: the re-examination form has only 15 questions versus the 24 of the standard form.

(continued)

CASE STUDY 19–1 *(continued)*
CASE 1: NONRADICULAR LOW BACK PAIN PATIENT

INTERPRETATION

Standard Form (Score = 108)		
None	Scores < 82	= no risk of a prolonged recovery
Mild:	**Scores ≥ 82 to 114**	**= mild risk of a prolonged recovery**
Moderate:	Scores ≥ 115 to 143	= moderate risk of a prolonged recovery
Severe:	Scores ≥ 144 +	= severe risk of a prolonged recovery (initial exam)
Re-exam Form (Score = 0)		
None	**Scores < 51**	**= no risk of a prolonged recovery**
Mild:	Scores ≥ 51 to 71	= mild risk of a prolonged recovery
Moderate:	Scores ≥ 72 to 89	= moderate risk of a prolonged recovery (2nd re-exam)
Severe:	Scores ≥ 90 +	= severe risk of a prolonged recovery (1st re-exam)

YELLOW FLAGS SUMMARY CHART

☐ A past history of prior episodes	☐ Depression	☐ Duration of symptoms before the 1st visit (>1 wk)
☒ Severe pain intensity (>6/10)	☐ Sciatica	☐ Multiple sites of pain
☐ Duration of symptoms (>1 mo.)	☐ Catastrophizing	☐ Tolerance for light work
☐ Anxiety	☐ Job dissatisfaction	☐ Physical activity makes pain worse
☒ Sleep is affected by pain	☒ Activity intolerance	☐ Belief that shouldn't work with current pain

OTHER RISK FACTORS SUMMARY CHART

☐ Abnormal illness behavior	☐ Weak back extensor musculature
☐ Heavy job classification	☐ Smokes 1 pack or greater/day
☐ Pre-existing structural pathology/skeletal anomaly	☐ Poor self-rated health

Total: 3 yellow flags and other risk factors.

(Table extracted from Appendix Form G–6)

Duration of care (in weeks): 5 weeks	Duration of disability: 2 days total temporary disability (TTD), 5 days partial temporary disability (PTD)
Total no. of visits: 7	Patient satisfaction score: 98%
Total treatment cost: $525 (figured at $75/tx)	Pre-Oswestry: 33%
	Post-Oswestry: 4%

CASE SUMMARY

Given the uncomplicated presentation of this patient, resolution occurred as expected, within a "natural history" of 4 to 6 weeks for a lumbar sprain/strain. The tables in Case 1 indicate the patient's response and value of the care, leading to a successful conclusion with both long- and short-term goals being met.

CASE STUDY 19–2
CASE 2: NONRADICULAR LOW BACK PAIN PATIENT WITH PROLONGED RECOVERY

In a presenting patient with similar history and physical examination findings as the subject of case 1, one would expect similar results if all things were indeed equal. However, when a significant number of yellow flags and other risk factors of chronicity exist, the risk of a prolonged recovery is probable. The following table includes outcome assessment results and other risk factors extracted from Appendix Form H–4. This case exemplifies a patient who experienced a delay in recovery in spite of a diagnosis of a lumbar sprain/strain.

OUTCOMES ASSESSMENT RECORD

DATE	PAIN			FUNCTION			
	VAS (miscell.) a. Now b. Ave. c. Range CC *LBP*	Pain Drawing/ Severity Index	Options: 1. UE 2. CTS 3. Shoulder 4. Knee	Options: 1. Headache 2. Dizziness 3. SCL-90R 4. _____	VAS and Neck Disability (NDI)	VAS and LB Disability: • *Oswestry* • Roland-Morris	Patient Satisfaction
Baseline							
2/12/99	a. 9/10 b. 8/10 c. 7–10/10 QVAS = 90%	Physiological 1. Yes **2. No** SI: 197 (Severe)				Osw. 79%	
Progress							
3/15/99	a. 6/10 b. 5/10 c. 4–7/10 QVAS = 60%	Physiological 1. Yes **2. No** SI: 93 (Severe)				Osw. 52%	92
4/16/99	a. 4/10 b. 4/10 c. 3–5/10 QVAS = 43%	Physiological 1. Yes **2. No** SI: 78 (Moderate)				Osw. 40%	96

SCALE	HSQ-12 MEAN[a]	INITIAL BASELINE 2-12-99	FIRST RE-EXAM 3-15-99	SECOND RE-EXAM 4-16-99
1. Health perception	72	25	25	60
2. Physical function	84	0	17	33
3. Role—physical	81	0	10	25
4. Role—emotional	81	20	20	45
5. Social functioning	83	25	25	50
6. Bodily pain	75	0	25	45
7. Mental health	75	0	7	27
8. Energy fatigue	61	20	20	40
9. Major depression	yes/no	**yes**/no	**yes**/no	**yes**/no
10. Dysthemia	yes/no	**yes**/no	**yes**/no	**yes**/no
11. Both 9 and 10	yes/no	**yes**/no	**yes**/no	**yes**/no

[a] Not yet established (1996); the mean scores are those derived from the HSQ 2.0 (36-item questionnaire).

CASE STUDY 19–2 (*continued*)
CASE 2: NONRADICULAR LOW BACK PAIN PATIENT WITH PROLONGED RECOVERY

Appendix Form I–1 has been completed for this patient, as follows:

		QUESTION	SCORE		
			Baseline	2nd	3rd
1.	1.	Pain location (×2/region)	2	2	2
2.		Duration of the *current* episode (×2 for score indicated)	10	0	0
3.		Number of prior episodes (×2 for score indicated)	10	0	0
4.		Prior surgery or hospitalizations (yes = 10; no = 0)	0	0	0
5.	2.	Usual level of pain (0–10) this week (score is no. circled)	9	6	5
6.		Frequency of pain 0–10 (score is no. circled)	10	0	0
7.	3.	Frequency of radiating pain (0–10) (score is no. circled)	5	4	4
8.	4.	Frequency of medication use (0–10) (score is no. circled)	9	7	5
9.	5.	Patient satisfaction if no change (0–10) (score is no. circled)	10	9	8
10.	6.	How anxious the past week (0–10) (score is no. circled)	8	5	6
11.	7.	Ability to control/cope (0–10) (score is no. circled)	8	6	6
12.	8.	How depressed the past week (0–10) (score is no. circled)	9	7	6
13.		General health rating (0–10) (score is no. circled)	8	0	0
14.		Smoking? (yes = 10; no = 0)	10	0	0
15.	9.	Pain = stop activity (0–10) (score is no. circled)	8	7	5
16.	10.	Physical activity = worse pain (0–10) (score is 10 – no. circled)	8	6	5
17.	11.	Light work tolerant for 1 hour (0–10) (score is 10 – no. circled)	9	8	6
18.	12.	Can sleep at night (0–10) (score is no. circled)	9	6	4
19.		Physical demanding (0–10) (score is 10 – no. circled)	9	0	0
20.		Any disability in last 12 months? (yes = 10; no = 0)	10	0	0
21.	13.	Should not do normal duty? (0–10) (score is 10 – no. circled)	10	8	6
22.		Do you like work? (yes = 0; no = 10)	10	0	0
23.	14.	Ability to sit/stand 6 wks. from now? (0–10) (score is no. circled)	8	6	5
24.	15.	Ability to work 6 mo. from now (0–10) (score is no. circled)	8	6	5
		Total	197	93	78

Note: the re-examination form has only 15 questions versus the 24 of standard form.

CASE STUDY 19–2 (*continued*)
CASE 2: NONRADICULAR LOW BACK PAIN PATIENT WITH PROLONGED RECOVERY

Score Interpretation

Standard Form		
Mild:	Scores ≥ 82 to 114	= mild risk of a prolonged recovery
Moderate:	Scores ≥ 115 to 143	= moderate risk of a prolonged recovery
Severe:	**Scores ≥ 144+**	= **severe risk of a prolonged recovery (initial exam)**
Re-exam Form		
Mild:	Scores ≥ 51 to 71	= mild risk of a prolonged recovery
Moderate:	**Scores ≥ 72 to 89**	= **moderate risk of a prolonged recovery (2nd re-exam)**
Severe:	**Scores ≥ 90+**	= **severe risk of a prolonged recovery (1st re-exam)**

YELLOW FLAGS SUMMARY CHART

☒ A past history of prior episodes	☒ Depression	☐ Duration of symptoms before the 1st visit (>1 wk)
☒ Severe pain intensity (>6/10)	☐ Sciatica	☐ Multiple sites of pain
☒ Duration of symptoms (>1 mo.)	☒ Catastrophizing	☒ Tolerance for light work
☒ Anxiety	☒ Job dissatisfaction	☒ Physical activity makes pain worse
☒ Sleep is affected by pain	☒ Activity intolerance	☒ Belief that shouldn't work with current pain

OTHER RISK FACTORS SUMMARY CHART

☒ Abnormal illness behavior	☐ Weak back extensor musculature
☐ Heavy job classification	☒ Smokes 1 pack or greater/day
☐ Pre-existing structural pathological/skeletal anomaly	☒ Poor self-rated health

Total: 15 yellow flags and other risk factors.

VALUE

Duration of care (in weeks): 8.5 weeks	Duration of disability: 4 weeks TTD, 4.5 weeks PTD
Total no. of visits: 23	Patient satisfaction score: 96
Total treatment cost: $1725 (figured at $75/tx)	Oswestry scores: Pre-79; Intermediate 52; Final 40%

CASE SUMMARY

Given the same treatment plan as outlined for case 1, less than optimal outcomes are noted due to the significant number of psychosocial variables that are present in this second case. In this example of a lumbar sprain/strain, the clinical data suggest this to be a complicated case as many risk factors are present and the outcomes assessment data support slowly responding activity intolerance and pain levels. Even though the same diagnosis exists in this and the first case, the prognosis in this case is much more bleak.

Table 19–1: A Case Management Approach to Care Rendered for Musculoskeletal Low Back Pain

Steps to Follow in Case Management

1. Perform diagnostic triage (rule out red flags)
2. Identify yellow flags and attend to those that are manageable
3. Provide reassurance/advice
4. Provide symptomatic relief
5. Utilize outcomes management
6. Promote functional restoration
7. Determine endpoints of care

Laboratory/objective findings typically found with infections include a temperature greater than 100°F, an elevated erythrocyte sedimentation rate (ESR), and a positive blood culture. X-ray evidence is often delayed for up to 2 months after laboratory changes occur. In order of highest sensitivity, bone scan is followed by x-ray and computed tomography (CT) scan, respectively, which also assist in making the diagnosis (McCowin et al, 1991). Physical examination includes percussion, for which an 86% sensitivity is reported for a bacterial infection, although specificity is quite poor (Deyo et al, 1992).

Fracture

A patient who presents with low back pain and a history of osteoporosis must be suspected of having a compression fracture until proven otherwise. Other historical information yielding suspicion of a compression fracture includes recent *mild* trauma in patients over the age of 50, which carries a sensitivity and specificity of 84% and 61%, respectively. Low back pain in a patient presenting over the age of 70 without trauma has a 22% sensitivity and 96% specificity rate. The history of *significant* trauma at any age carries 30% sensitivity and 85% specificity. Also, the pro-

Table 19–2: Historical Findings Suggestive of Spinal Cancer[a]

1. > 50 years old
2. + Past history of cancer: 98% specificity (Deyo et al, 1992)
3. Unexplained weight loss
4. Pain > 1 month
5. No improvement with conservative treatment
6. Low back pain
7. Positive neurological losses (Weinstein and McLain, 1987)
8. X-ray: 99% were identified on initial x-ray
9. No improvement with bed rest ($\uparrow$ sensitivity, $\downarrow$ specificity)

[a] Deyo reported that at least one of the first five items listed were present in a group of known cancer patients, while physical examination findings were essentially normal.

longed use of a corticosteroid has a very low sensitivity rate of 6% but a very high specificity rate of 99.5%.

In ruling out red flags, x-ray is described as not being necessary in the first month unless the criteria previously described for fracture, infection, cauda equina, or tumor/cancer is suspect. Magnetic resonance imaging (MRI) and electromyography (EMG) should be postponed until conservative therapy has failed to manage the patient to his or her satisfaction and/or a surgical consult is indicated and desired. No nerve root signs of improvement after 1 month; severe, disabling, and progressive low back pain; a positive neurological examination; and/or progressive neurological losses are indicators of the need to obtain a surgical opinion.

Referred Pain from Viscera

Referred pain to the low back can result from the viscera; examples include low back pain arising from genitourinary, gastrointestinal, or a vascular disease (Souza, 1994). Clinically, the quality of pain is sharp and well localized, with reflex muscle contraction and hyperalgesia (Table 19–3) (McCowin et al, 1991).

It appears that the patient's history plays a significant role in the diagnostic process when ruling out red flags. **Moreover, as illustrated by the Deyo study** (Deyo, 1991; Deyo et al, 1992), **physical examination findings may be completely benign in patients presenting with cancer but at least one of five historical pieces of information were present in all cases.** The history appears to carry sensitivity and specificity that often exceed the best of the orthopedic tests, which are considered objective. Table 19–4 illustrates the historical findings for several red flags and, when available, the sensitivity and specificity of the historical item is included.

It is essential to reduce the chances of missing a red flag as much as possible because of the obvious prognostic and medico-legal implications. A survey of the patient presenting with low back pain can be easily completed in less than 3 minutes by use of forms designed to minimize the risk of missing a red flag and to assist in the process of diagnostic triage (see Appendix Forms H–1, H–2, and H–3). This form may prove to be one of the most important inclusions in the patient's file. More specifically, if use of this checklist helps identify even one patient with a red flag, the value of such a form may have far reaching effects, both from the patient's viewpoint (morbidity/mortality) and from a medico-legal standpoint.

Identifying Nerve Root Lesions

Diagnostic triage next must differentiate patients with mechanical back pain from those presenting with nerve root–oriented pain. This is due to the potential for surgery in the nerve root group of patients (Selim et al, 1998). Nerve root symptoms and signs include:

- Leg symptoms below the knee (BK)
- Positive nerve root tension signs
- Positive neurological examination

Table 19–3: Differential Diagnosis of Low Back Pain: "Ruling Out Red Flags"

CONDITION	CAUDA EQUINA	CANCER/TUMOR	INFECTION	VISCERAL REFERRED PAIN
Unisciatic	X			
Bisciatic	X			
Saddle anesthesia	X			
Bowel/bladder incontinence	X			
	.95 sensitivity			
	.90 specificity			
	.99-pre.fac			
Straight leg raise	X			
Unexplained weight loss		X		
+Past history cancer		X		
No improvement with conservative care		X		
>50 yrs old		X		
+Erythrocyte sedimentation rate			X	
Reflex muscle spasm and hyperalgesia			X	X

ESR, erythrocyte sedimentation rate.

Nonspecific mechanical low back pain represents 85% of all LBP cases. Symptoms include:

- Pain change with movement
- Pain localized (usually) to the lower back, buttock, or thigh; that is, above the knee (AK)
- Negative neurological findings

Care must be taken to avoid an inaccurate diagnosis of a nerve root lesion based on a history of leg pain alone. More specifically, referred pain of a sclerotomal origin such as a facet capsule, sacroiliac joint, or a contained disc lesion in the posterior third of the disc (e.g., an annular tear) can refer pain into an extremity and, therefore, is commonly mistaken for a nerve root lesion. The main differentiating factors are the following:

- The location of the radiating pain of sclerotomal origin is described as deep, global, and not anatomically specific to a dermatome
- The neurological examination is negative
- There are no nerve tension signs

Identifying Yellow Flags

The New Zealand Acute Low Back Pain Guide describes psychosocial risk factors as being associated with yellow flags while physical risk factors are associated with red flags. Identification of red flags should lead to appropriate medical intervention, while identification of yellow flags should lead to appropriate cognitive and behavioral management. Immediate recognition of these findings is essential to successful outcomes management.

What Are Psychosocial Yellow Flags?

Yellow flags are factors that enhance the risk of developing, or perpetuating long-term disability and work loss associated with low back pain (Kendall et al, 1997). Two key outcomes were described when assessing the presence of yellow flags: (1) a decision as to whether more detailed assessment is needed (psychosocial); and (2) identification of any salient factors that can become the subject of specific intervention, thus saving time and helping to concentrate the use of resources. **Because red and yellow flags are not exclusive, a patient may require concurrent intervention of both areas.**

Why Is There a Need to Identify Psychosocial Yellow Flags?

In New Zealand, just as in the United States, there is a steady increase in the number of people who leave the workforce as a result of protracted or chronic back pain. The risk of permanent disability increases when yellow flags are present and appears to be associated with an increased proportion of patients who do not recover normal function and activity tolerance. An increased research base over the last 5 years regarding risk factors resulting in long-term work disability is inconsistent or lacking for many chronic painful conditions, except low back pain. **Because most of the known risk factors are psychosocial,** it is recommended to implement treatment approaches using the biopsychosocial model (Burton, 1995; Cherkin, 1996; Frank, 1996).

Who Is At Risk?

An individual may be considered at risk if he or she has a clinical presentation that includes one or more very strong

Table 19–4: Estimated Accuracy of History in Diagnosis of Spine Diseases Causing Low Back Problems

REFERENCES	DISEASE TO BE DETECTED	MEDICAL HISTORY RED FLAGS	TRUE-POSITIVE RATE (SENSITIVITY)	TRUE-NEGATIVE RATE (SPECIFICITY)
Deyo and Diehl (1988)	Cancer	Age ≥ to 50	.77	.71
		Previous cancer history	.31	.98
		Unexplained weight loss	.15	.94
		Failure to improve with 1 month of therapy	.31	.90
		No relief on bed rest	>.90	.46
		Duration of pain >1 month	.50	.81
		Age ≥50 or history of cancer or unexplained weight loss or failure of conservative therapy	1.00	.60
Waldvogel and Vasey (1980)	Spinal osteomyelitis	Intravenous drug abuse, UTI, or skin infection	.40	NA
Unpublished data— Deyo (1992)[a]	Compression fracture	Age ≥50	.84	.61
		Age ≥70	.22	.96
		Trauma	.30	.85
		Corticosteroid use	.06	.995
Deyo and Tsui-Wu (1987); Spangfort (1972)	Herniated disc	Sciatica	.95	.88
Turner et al (1992)	Spinal stenosis	Pseudoclaudication	.60	NA
Gran (1985)	Ankylosing spondylitis	Age ≥50	.90[b]	.70
		Positive responses 4 out of 5	.23	.82
		Age at onset ≤40	1.00	.07
		Pain not relieved in supine position	.80	.49
		Morning back stiffness	.64	.59
		Duration of pain ≥3 months	.71	.54

NA, not available; UTI, urinary tract infection.

[a] From 833 patients with back pain at a walk-in clinic as reported in Deyo, Rainville, and Kent. All received plain lumbar roentgenograms.

[b] Author's estimate.

Reprinted with permission from Bigos et al, 1994.

indicators of risk, or several less important factors that might be cumulative. Yellow flags include factors that have been found to extend resolution beyond the duration of a condition's natural history. A partial list include the following:

- A past history of prior episodes (Burton et al, 1995; Cherkin et al, 1996; Frank et al, 1996; Hazard et al, 1996)
- Severe pain intensity (Cherkin et al, 1996; Frank et al, 1996; Hazard et al, 1996)
- Duration of symptoms (Von Korff et al, 1993; Linton et al, 1998)
- Anxiety (Cherkin et al, 1996; McMahon et al, 1997)

- Locus of control (eg, ability to control pain) (Burton et al, 1995)
- Depression (Klenerman et al, 1995; Cherkin et al, 1996; Linton and Hallden, 1997)

For additional discussion of yellow flags, refer to Chapter 21. A questionnaire to help identify the presence of yellow flags is provided in Appendix I.

PROVIDE REASSURANCE AND ADVICE

As recommended by AHCPR, British Medical Guidelines, and others, offering the patient reassurance will help to alleviate unnecessary anxiety, which often accompanies acute low back pain. However, a fine line exists between offering the patient reassurance and promising a full recovery. On the one hand, anxiety may be reduced but on the other, the patient is being, in a sense, set up for poor satisfaction should a less-than-total recovery occur. Without promising the patient a cure, reassurance must address the patient realistically while avoiding an overly pessimistic tone.

PROVIDE SYMPTOMATIC RELIEF

A primary treatment goal for most patients presenting with musculoskeletal disorders is relief from pain. Other than the occasional healthy individual who presents for a "check-up" with a prospective goal of avoiding an acute low back pain episode, the majority of patients have back pain and are clearly presenting for management of their painful condition.

UTILIZE OUTCOMES MANAGEMENT

In the scheme of case management, the use of outcomes measures assures that timely clinical decision making can occur. More specifically, when outcomes management is not used, the HCP, insurer, and patient have less ability to identify endpoints in care. This can lead to protracted treatment approaches that are of less value and may influence the outcome of a case, especially if a more appropriate form of management is unnecessarily postponed. The end result is poor quality control of the case management process. The importance of this cannot be overstated, as this is the major underpinning and primary objective of this text.

To make the task of becoming outcomes based easier, a summary of the various subjective or patient-driven pen-and-paper outcomes tools can be reported on one form called an Outcomes Assessment Record. Because of the extensive normative data that exists with the SF–36 (see Chap. 5), a separate score sheet called the Health Status Questionnaire Results form is recommended (See Appendix Forms A–3 and H–4).

CLINICAL TIP 19–1
Four Steps to Becoming Outcomes Based

Four steps are necessary in order to become outcomes based. They are:

1. Become familiar with the available subjective and objective tools (see Sections II and III of this text, respectively).
2. Use and score the tools at the initial visit to establish baseline measures.
3. Repeat the instrument after a 2- to 4-week interval to track the effects of treatment changes.
4. ***Most importantly:*** Base clinical decisions on the outcome results. Only when this occurs can the benefits of outcomes management be truly appreciated.

If desired, software is available to score the outcome tools (pen-and-paper tools as well as Quantitative Functional Capacity Evaluation [QFCE]) and a percent change is calculated when the tools are repeated at reexamination time. Figure 19–1 is an example of a CareTrak report of an Oswestry Low Back Pain Disability Questionnaire. Similar reports can be generated for the Roland-Morris Questionnaire, the Neck Disability Index, the SF–36, patient satisfaction questionnaires, the QFCE, and others. These reports can be used to generate outcomes reports for:

- Marketing to other HCPs to stimulate patient referrals
- Charting documentation of patient progress
- Medico-legal documentation, depositions, and testimony
- Proving "medical necessity" in insurance appeals
- Establishing a personal profile on your own performance to facilitate marketing to groups or programs you would like to participate in

A brief report such as Figure 19–1 can be generated in less than 5 minutes for a first visit and less than 2 minutes for an established patient. More information regarding the CareTrak Software can be obtained from 1-800-393-7255. Contact information for other outcome management systems can be accessed in Chapter 23.

PROMOTE FUNCTIONAL RESTORATION

In case management, it is generally expected by third-party payers that the frequency of care will be decreased or discontinued when a point of maximum therapeutic benefit is reached, sometimes regardless of the level of recovery. The assumption is that care has been rendered and the residual effects of the injury will have to be accepted. The patient at this point is typically told that he or she will have to learn how to live with these residual "leftovers" from the original injury.

At times, of course, this may be sound advice, and "pulling the plug" and discharging the patient at a point of firm plateau is indeed appropriate as long as all treatment options have been given to the patient. Also, "medically necessary" care may include "supportive care" if failure of a condition to remain controlled in the absence of care is observed. Documentation that "proves" supportive care is required must show that the HCP gradually weaned the patient's frequency of visits after which point, the patient experienced worsening of the condition, requiring further management.

As discussed earlier in this chapter, the deconditioning that accompanies acute conditions remains long after the healing period has ended. At this point of case management, provocative tests usually fail to elicit much helpful information; physical performance tests are the most sensitive way to identify these functional deficiencies (Kishino

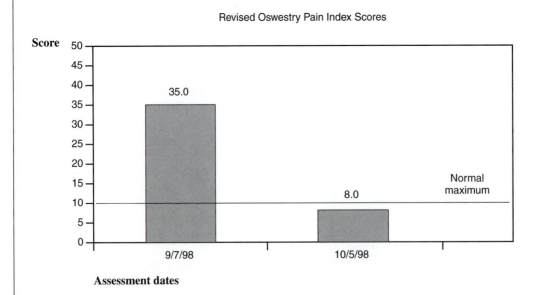

Revised Oswestry Low Back Pain Index

Date of this report: 25-Oct-98   **Site ID:** Lap-001

Last Name: Esthetic   **First Name:** Ken

Patient ID: 179   **Social Security Number:** 333-44-5555

Date First Seen: 9/7/98

Complaint: Localized low back pain

Classification: None

Diagnosis: Lumbar Sprain/Strain - 847.2

Primary Risk Factors

Duration of symptoms prior to treatment: 1 to 6 weeks

No. of prior episodes with same or similar symptoms: 4 or more

Test Results:

	Baseline	Current	Improvement
	9/7/98	10/5/98	
Oswestry Raw Scores:	35.0	8.0	77%
Percent Disability:	70%	76%	
	9/7/98	10/5/98	
Pain Severity Rating*:	83	20	76%

*Pain ratings based on a triple VAS and 100 pt. scale

Revised Oswestry Pain Index Scores

Figure 19–1. The report generated by CareTrak includes baseline and follow-up examination results. The graphic representation of the numerical data noted in the report facilitates an appreciation for the significant improvement noted in this case.

CLINICAL TIP 19–2
What Outcomes Management Has to Offer

Outcomes management is designed to establish baselines, document progress, assist in goal setting, and motivate patients. Therefore, it has something significant to offer the patient, HCP, and third-party payer.

---

et al, 1985; Curtis et al, 1994). When positive, the weak functional links identified by physical performance tests, posture, gait, and movement pattern assessments need to be specifically addressed in some form of functional restoration program (see Appendix G forms). If rehabilitation services are not part of an HCP's typical in-house approach, referral for this service is necessary to ensure that the residual deconditioning that often accompanies an injury is properly managed. Moreover, timely management of these residuals typically allows for a better outcome as postponed rehabilitation tends to reduce the beneficial effects. This recommendation has been clearly identified as a necessary step in an evidence-based management system (Bigos, 1987).

DETERMINE ENDPOINTS OF CARE

The strength of outcomes management lies in its ability to identify points of plateau or endpoints of care. This then alerts the HCP to consider additional treatment options when the objective of moving the patient beyond the plateau he or she has currently reached. The same outcomes tools previously utilized can then track the additional or new treatment plan to determine, *in a timely manner,* if the chosen treatment option(s) were appropriate to meet the goals of functional restoration. Hence, the time taken to implement outcomes into practice is well worth the effort as they act as a guide helping to identify plateaus or endpoints of care. Refer to Section II of this text for information concerning subjective outcome assessment tools. Similarly, Section III describes tools that identify endpoints of care objectively. In addition, by using Appendix Forms A–3 and H–4, the HCP's ability to recognize endpoints or plateaus is significantly enhanced as all the outcomes data are on one page and, therefore, can be easily compared between dates of assessment. Refer to Chapter 22 regarding chart organization to further enhance the implementation of outcomes management.

REPORTING AND DOCUMENTATION FOR THE EVIDENCE-BASED PRACTICE

The "gymnastics" of trying to keep track of patient data can be a significant hurdle to incorporate into practice. Recording the information into the patient file and keeping track of the information at reassessment times demands that a specific protocol be followed. This section of the chapter introduces an effective outcomes management approach with the understanding that many different approaches can apply. The information is purposely written in an outline format in order to enhance reading, comprehension, and application of the information. The forms and/or chapters that correspond to each item are also included. The required steps for becoming outcomes-oriented include:

1. Score each questionnaire using the proper methods and report the results in a separate paragraph in the **"S"** (subjective) portion of the SOAP notes and on the outcomes assessment summary page (see Appendix Form H–4).
2. Place all the physical performance tests (eg, QFCE), posture, gait, and movement pattern information under the **"O"** (objective) category of the SOAP note approach. If specific forms for documenting functional testing are desired, refer to Appendix G.
3. Describe the functional deficits (such as weak abdominals, tight hamstrings, poor proprioception, etc) in the **"A"** (assessment) portion of the SOAP note. The diagnostic classification of differentiating between red flag, nerve root, or mechanical back pain along with a checklist of yellow flags are appropriate items for inclusion in this part of the SOAP note.
4. The rehabilitation prescription is placed in the **"P"** (plan) portion of the SOAP note, as well as any passive care procedures utilized.
5. Report the appropriate questionnaire score in the **"S"** portion of the patient's chart at every re-examination. On daily visits, the HCP may repeat only a pain measure, an activity intolerance issue, and any other pertinent historical information. Repeat the other categories of questionnaires initially utilized (such as the Oswestry, Neck Disability Index, etc) at more formal times of re-examinations, such as at 2- to 4-week intervals or at times of exacerbation.
6. *Always* review the file at re-examination time and critique the outcome assessment tools to determine the quality, or outcome, from the care that was provided. If the outcome assessment tools indicate that no change or worsening of a condition has occurred, *be responsible* and consider one of the following: (a) Transition the patient from passive to active care; (b) Identify barriers to recovery and address those issues by:
   • Referral for clinical psychology/tertiary care center
   • Referral for a consult (from a specialized provider)
   • Ordering additional tests, if clinically warranted

See Chapter 20 for more detailed information regarding documentation.

CLINICAL TIP 19–4
Incorporating Supervised Rehabilitation

By the fourth week of passive care, a home exercise approach has usually been utilized. If, however, the benefits are insignificant and disability is still present, a more supervised type of rehabilitation service is required. The use of formal one-on-one, 30- to 60-minute sessions is needed for this select patient population. Once the patient has demonstrated skill with stretch, proprioception, strength and endurance exercises, the rehabilitation exercises can gradually be introduced at home. This allows for a daily exercise regimen rather than every-other-day sessions at a rehabilitation center. It also begins the process of promoting patient independence and places health management responsibility directly on the patient.

A complete discharge can often be accomplished after repeating the QFCE at the 1-month point unless many functional deficiencies persist on re-evaluation. If the latter occurs, continued persistent one-on-one training may be necessary. At discharge, however, it is very important to emphasize the need for continued self-administered rehabilitation, especially specific exercises addressing the sub-85% QFCE physical performance tests and other functional test abnormalities for an additional 3 to 6 months. This approach is necessary because of the long-term residuals of deconditioning and the need to re-educate the "pain-motor programs" (whereby abnormal movement patterns repeated often enough are learned by the cerebellum). The new programming, called an **engram,** can be inherited or secondarily acquired and this concept "is now an incontrovertible fact of contemporary neurophysiology" (Pillard, 1988).

The physiological basis behind rehabilitation is to move the patient through the following sequence: *unconscious dysfunction,* in which the patient first presents unaware of his or her dysfunction; followed by *conscious dysfunction,* in which the patient is made aware of his or her dysfunction by the HCP; followed by *conscious function,* in which the patient is taught the correct way to move and function and consciously practices it; and, finally, *unconscious function,* in which the patient no longer has to think about the correct way to move or function. When patients "catch themselves doing it right," the last step is accomplished. This process takes time and individualized training, addressing patient-specific needs.

---

6. Psychosocial tests (see Appendix Forms C–25 to C–27 and Chaps. 8, 10, and 21)
7. Disability prediction screen, Work APGAR, Vermont (VDPQ) (see Appendix Forms H–7 and H–8, respectively and Appendix I)

O. Objective: Examination
- Physical performance tests: complete as much of the QFCE as possible and start rehabilitation if not already started
- Use QFCE, qualitative tests, posture, gait and movement patterns, for rehabilitation prescription

- If rehabilitation has started, *repeat* the previously scored QFCE tests that were <85%

A. Assessment: Diagnosis (see Appendix Form H–6)
- Describe the functional deficiency (integrate with the diagnosis)
- Integrate rehabilitation treatment goals with the passive care goals
- Orient the patient to the QFCE reassessment that will occur after 4 weeks of active/rehabilitation care (stimulates compliance with rehabilitation)
- List psychosocial barriers to recovery

P. Plan (see Appendix Form H–6)
- Report any treatment changes with respective goals (must strongly consider referral/co-treatment if prior treatment was not effective)
- Consider weaning passive care (if appropriate) while increasing active care in-office and/or at home (important to avoid HCP/patient dependency)
- Work Capacity Evaluation—order from occupational therapist (OT) if the patient is still not working
- Is a tertiary pain center required? This usually includes a "quarterback," often a physiatrist (or, physical rehabilitation specialist), who directs the patient for a physical examination, and orders assessments by OT, physical therapy (PT), department of vocational rehabilitation (DVR) and clinical psychology. A course of care often including PT, work hardening, psychological consulting, and/or vocational rehabilitation is ordered for a defined time period, such as 4 weeks.
- If passive PT modalities are still utilized, describe specific goals and frequency of the modality use. Of note, passive modalities usually are not required or indicated during active care or for protracted time periods.

Third Follow-up Visit: 10 to 12 Weeks
S. Subjective: Include historical data, as well as the following information (see Table 19–5):
- Patient forms: (Use the same outcome assessment tools used initially)
  1. Triple VAS (see Appendix B)
  2. Condition-specific functional questionnaire (ie, Oswestry, Neck Disability Index, etc; see Appendix C)
  3. JDQ (see Appendix Form H–5)—should have been done by now if work factors are clinically significant
  4. Matheson's SFS (see Chap. 16—SFS and Chap. 17—Functional Capacity Evaluation)—should have been done by now if work factors are clinically significant
  5. Static Position Tolerance tests (see Appendix Form G–10)—should have been done by now if work factors are clinically significant
  6. Psychosocial tests (see Appendix Forms C–25 through C–27, and Chaps. 8, 10, and 21)
  7. Disability prediction screen Work APGAR, Ver-

CLINICAL TIP 19–5
Documenting the "Medical Necessity"
of the QFCE

Include in the records a short discussion of why a quantitative functional capacity test (QFCE) and rehabilitation approach using a one-on-one exercise training approach is "medically necessary." For example, "due to failure of a home exercise approach prescribed on _____(date) to adequately control the condition, a one-on-one exercise training approach is now 'medically necessary.' In addition, the patient demonstrated significant deconditioning during the QFCE and exercise training must be now closely supervised to ensure safety in this attempt at returning the patient to an independent, pre-injury status."

---

mont (VDPQ) (see Appendix Forms H–7 and H–8, respectively)

O. Objective: Examination
- Physical performance tests: complete as much of the QFCE as possible and start rehabilitation if not already started
- Use QFCE, qualitative tests, posture, gait and movement patterns, for rehabilitation prescription
- If rehabilitation has started, *repeat* previously scored QFCE tests that were <85%

A. Assessment: Diagnosis (see Appendix Form H–6)
- Describe the functional deficiency (integrate with the diagnosis)

- Integrate rehabilitation treatment goals with the passive care goals
- Orient the patient to the QFCE reassessment that will occur after 4 weeks of active/rehabilitation care (stimulates compliance with rehabilitation)
- List psychosocial barriers to recovery

P. Plan (see Appendix Form H–6)
- Report any treatment changes with respective goals (must strongly consider referral/co-treatment if prior treatment was not effective)
- Consider weaning passive care (if appropriate) while increasing active care in-office and/or at home (important to avoid HCP/patient dependency)
- Work Capacity Evaluation—order from OT if the patient is still not working
- Is a tertiary pain center required? This usually includes a "quarterback," often a physiatrist (or, physical rehabilitation specialist), who directs the patient for a physical examination and orders assessments by OT, PT, DVR and clinical psychology. A course of care often including PT, work hardening, psychological consulting, and/or vocational rehabilitation is ordered for a defined time period, such as 4 weeks.
- If passive physical therapy modalities are still utilized, describe specific goals and frequency of the modality use. Of note, passive modalities are usually not required or indicated during active care or for protracted time periods.

Conclusion

In this chapter, stages of healing and the difference between healing and functional restoration were emphasized. The concept of diagnostic triage and the importance of prompt identification of red and yellow flags alerts the HCP to historical and examination findings that can identify these items. The expectations of offering the patient reassurance and advice, providing symptomatic relief, utilizing outcomes management, promoting functional restoration, and determining endpoints of care were also reviewed. Finally, a time line addressing the question of "what to do when" was provided to help steer the HCP into an evidence-based model. In this time line, outcome tools of both subjective and objective varieties were included.

In order to meet the demands and requirements in a managed care setting, the evidence-based practice will have a distinct advantage as quality of care can be quantified and communicated when negotiating for contracts. The goal of this chapter is to provide the HCP with the ammunition to make the paradigm shift to an outcomes-based model of practice as smoothly and painlessly as possible in order to meet current challenges. Through collecting and tracking outcomes, the HCP will find that clinical decision making, quality of care, the ability to report to those requesting information about the care of the patient, as well as protection against malpractice will improve significantly.

REFERENCES

Bigos SJ, Battié MC. Acute care to prevent back disability: Ten years of progress. *Clin Orthop* 1987;221:121–130.

Bigos S, Bowyer O, Braen G, et al. *Acute Low Back Problems in Adults. Clinical Practice Guideline.* Rockville, MD: US Department of Health and Human Services, Public Health Service, Agency for Health Care Policy and Research; 1994.

Burton AK, Tillotson K, Main C, Hollis M. Psychosocial predictors of outcome in acute and sub-acute low back trouble. *Spine* 1995;20:722–728.

Cherkin DC, Deyo RA, Street JH, Barlow W. Predicting poor outcomes for back pain seen in primary care using patients' own criteria. *Spine* 1996;21:2900–2907.

Curtis L, Mayer T, Gatchel R. Physical progress and residual impairment quantification after functional restoration, part III: Isokinetic and isoinertial lifting capacity. *Spine* 1994;19:401–405.

Deyo RA. Early detection of cancer, infection, and inflammatory disease of the spine. *J Back Musculoskeletal Rehabil* 1991;1:69–81.

Deyo RA, Diehl AK. Cancer as a cause of back pain: Frequency, clinical presentation, and diagnostic strategies. *J Gen Intern Med* 1988;3:230–238.

Deyo RA, Rainville J, Kent DL. What can the history and physical examination tell us about low back pain? JAMA 1992;268(6):760–765.

Deyo RA, Tsui-Wu YJ. Descriptive epidemiology of low-back pain and its related medical care in the United States. *Spine* 1987;12(3):264–268.

Floman Y, Wiesel SW, Rothman RH. Cauda equina presenting as a herniated lumbar disk. *Clin Orthop* 1980;147:234–237.

Frank JW, Kerr MS, Brooker AS, et al. Disability resulting from occupational low back pain. Part 2: What do we know about secondary prevention? *Spine* 1996;21:2918–2929.

Gran JT. An epidemiology survey of the signs and symptoms of ankylosing spondylitis. *Clin Rheumatol* 1985;4(2):161–169.

Hazard RG, Haugh LD, Reid S, Preble JB, MacDonald L. Early prediction of chronic disability after occupational low back injury. *Spine* 1996;21:945–951.

Kendall NAS, Linton SJ, Main CJ. *Guide to Assessing Psychosocial Yellow Flags in Acute Low Back Pain: Risk Factors for Long-Term Disability and Work Loss.* Wellington, NZ: Accident Rehabilitation and Compensation Insurance Corporation of New Zealand and the National Health Committee; 1997.

Kishino N, Mayer T, Gatchel R, et al. Quantification of lumbar function, Part 4: Isometric and isokinetic lifting simulation in normal subjects and low back dysfunction patients. *Spine* 1985;10:921–927.

Klenerman L, Slade P, Stanley I, et al. The prediction of chronicity in patients with an acute attack of low back pain in a general practice setting. *Spine* 1995;20:478–484.

Linton SJ, Hallden K. Risk factors and the natural course of acute and recurrent musculoskeletal pain: Developing a screening instrument. In: Jensen TS, Turner JA, Wiesenfeld-Hallin Z, eds. *Proceedings of the 8th World Congress on Pain, Progress in Pain Research and Management,* Vol 8. Seattle, Wash: IASP Press; 1997.

Linton SJ, Hellsing AL, Hallden K. A population based study of spinal pain among 35–45 year olds: Prevalence, sick leave, and health care utilization. *Spine* 1998; in press.

McCarthy KA. Improving the clinician's use of orthopedic testing: An application to low back pain. *Top Clin Chiro* 1994;1(1):42–50.

McCowin PR, Borenstein D, Wiesel SW. The current approach to the medical diagnosis of low back pain. *Orthop Clin North Am* 1991;22:315–325.

McMahon MJ, Gatchel RJ, Politan, PB, Mayer TG. Early childhood abuse in chronic spinal disorder patients: A major barrier to treatment success. *Spine* 1997;22:2408–2415.

Pillard J. Posture and locomotion: Old problems and new concepts. In: Amblard B, Berthoz A, Clarac F, eds. *Posture and Gait: Development, Adaptation and Modulation.* Amsterdam: Elsevier Science Publishers; 1988:V–XII.

Selim AJ, Xinhua SR, Graeme F, et al. The importance of radiating leg pain in assessing health outcomes among patients with low back pain. *Spine* 1998;23:470–474.

Souza TA. Differentiating mechanical pain from visceral pain. *Top Clin Chiro* 1994;1(1):1–12.

Spangfort EV. The lumbar disc herniation. *Acta Orth Scand* (Suppl) 1972;142:1–95.

Turner JA, Ersek M, Herron L, Deyo R. Surgery for lumbar spinal stenosis. Attempted meta-analysis of the literature. *Spine* 1992;17:1–8.

Von Korff M, Deyo RA, Cherkin D, Barlow W. Back pain in primary care: Outcomes at 1 year. *Spine* 1993;18:855–862.

Waldvogel FA, Vasey H. Osteomyelitis: The past decade. *N Engl J Med* 1980;303:360–370.

Weinstein JN, McLain F. Primary tumors of the spine. *Spine* 1987;12:843–851.

CHAPTER 20

Integrating Outcome Assessment into Clinical Documentation and Establishing an "Outcomes-based" Practice

JEFFREY M. WILDER

INTRODUCTION

As a health care provider (HCP) reaching this point of the text, you may well be slightly overwhelmed. Clearly it is necessary to have a tracking mechanism for treatment outcomes in order to demonstrate that your patient is improving with treatment. Yet, you may have concerns that there are hundreds of different possible outcome tools, proposed by so many different authors, that the choice of which outcome assessment method to use in a given case is complicated. Similarly, you may wish to expand your clinical documentation to become more "outcome based," but are concerned that you do not have the time in your daily responsibilities with patients to turn your office into a research facility.

Fortunately, the most effective outcome assessment tools are also quite simple to administer and interpret. Most importantly, the most effective outcome assessments are those that work in conjunction with your usual clinical documentation. In many cases, the use of your usual clinical documentation can perform much of the work of an outcome assessment by carefully quantifying clinical data.

ety of electronic media now available for the storage of patient records.

c. *Pre-printed forms:* The use of prepared forms can serve as a mental checklist for areas in which the HCP wants to collect data. The use of the prepared form can also significantly reduce the amount of time spent with paperwork, or serve as a script from which a later dictation can be prepared. These forms are typically prepared by the institution, so that all HCPs within a facility are using the same forms. However, the use of proprietary forms will always be more difficult to read for persons not familiar with the format of the forms.

d. *Plain paper.* While excellent clinical records can be written entirely by hand, there are enough redundant elements of the patient record (such as the patient's name, name of the facility, name of the HCP, and date) that some sort of mechanical reproduction is nearly essential. However, the production of a quality patient record from a blank piece of paper remains the ultimate test of organization for the student interested in clinical documentation.

Patient factors can cause variability in records as well. Individual patients may or may not be reliable sources of data. The source of this potential unreliability by the patient may be:

1. Intentional, as in the case of the true malingering patient, who is seeking to deliberately deceive the HCP into believing that symptoms exist which are more severe than the patient knows to be true. The most frequent cause of this intentional misrepresentation by the patient is presumed to be the patient's pursuit of monetary settlements due to litigated claims. The frequency with which this type of fraud actually occurs is open to wide speculation.

2. Somatic amplification: Owing to a variety of psychosocial factors, patients may unwittingly exaggerate the impact of symptoms that do actually exist. In somatic amplification, the patient is not consciously attempting to deceive the HCP, but may magnify the severity of symptoms to an unbelievable level. The traditional hallmark of somatic amplification is pain that does not follow expected physiological pathways. It is possible that a quarter of the patients with nonspecific complaints, such as abdominal pain, headaches, nervousness, chest pain, and so on, are best served with a psychiatric diagnosis (Rosenthal et al, 1991). A number of tests, such as the well-known Waddell tests (Waddell et al, 1980), are designed to alert the examiner to the possibility of exaggerated responses by the patient.

3. Educational and communication difficulties: Some patients will look blankly at the HCP when asked to rate their perceived pain on a 10- or 100-point scale. These patients may simply not have the mathematics background to allow for valid or meaningful answers to the question. Language can pose another variable. Patients with poor reading skills often find the commonly used disability tools very difficult to complete. Any HCP who has attempted to interview a patient who speaks a different language through an interpreter knows the inherent frustrations in which the most important clinical questions and answers can literally be "lost in the translation." The occasional patient who is uncooperative during the interview procedure may not provide the same quality of data as the patient who thoughtfully participates in the HCP's urgings to specify the severity and location of pain.

Finally, the HCP intrinsically possesses many factors that can cause variability in records, such as the following:

1. Clinical skills and judgment: The HCP must have the requisite knowledge base to know what clinical data needs to be gathered in a given case.

2. Organizational skills: The ability of the HCP to organize various clinical data, opinions, and actions into the proper locations in the patient record is critical to the record keeping process. The clinical record that has haphazardly mixed together subjective and objective data will pose additional work when retrieving information from the record in the future.

3. Writing skills: It has often been said that the patient record should tell the story of the patient. Some HCPs are natural storytellers, and others are not. Writing skills are among the most difficult skills to teach. However, the student (or established HCP) who decides to make the effort to improve the readability of the narrative report will be rewarded with significant improvement.

4. Legibility: The burden of legibility is solely on the HCP. While we still hear jokes about the poor quality of physicians' handwriting, the HCP will seldom find humor when he or she is unable to translate that illegible record during a personal injury or malpractice trial.

5. Attention to detail: For every clinical record, there is a critical balance between unacceptable brevity and drowning in relatively insignificant information. With experience, the HCP is best able to determine the proper amount of detail to include with each case.

Bates (1991) recommends these essential criteria when deciding which information points to include and which to exclude in the patient record:

- Record all the data—both positive and negative—that contribute directly to your assessment.

- Describe specifically any pertinent negative information, such as the absence of a symptom or sign, when other portions of the physical examination suggest that an abnormality may be present.
- Data not recorded contemporaneously are data lost.
- Omit most negative findings that do not directly relate to the patient's chief complaint.
- Avoid redundancies.
- Be as objective as possible.

Methods of clinical documentation must be sufficiently flexible to allow for variations in practice methods, as well as differing complexities of individual cases. Because all patients present different challenges to the HCP, the documentation must be flexible enough to allow for variations in patient age, in the type of condition, and in the severity of the condition.

QUANTIFICATION OF SUBJECTIVE AND OBJECTIVE INFORMATION AS AN OUTCOME ASSESSMENT

The scientific method strives for increasing accuracy in the manner in which we view our world. The word *quantification* refers to the effort by an examiner to accurately measure the important characteristics of the subject being investigated. As an example, consider a simple concept such as the measurement of length. For thousands of years, humans measured length using very crude methods, even using the length of their own feet. (In the United States and Great Britain, we still measure length in "feet.") Obviously, the length of an individual's foot might vary dramatically, making for some very interesting bargaining between big- and small-footed people!

Science also demands ever-increasing precision in measurement. Until recently, in Great Britain, the English units of length were defined in terms of the imperial standard yard, which was the distance between two lines on a bronze bar made in 1845 to replace an earlier yard bar that had been destroyed by fire in 1839. In 1960 the meter was redefined in terms of wavelengths of light from a krypton-86 source. In 1983 it was again redefined as the length of the path traveled by light in a vacuum in 1/299,792,458 of a second ("Weights and Measures," 1994).

In the health sciences, the movement towards improved outcome measurement and better quality measurement of patient data is often driven by the third-party reimbursement system. Third-party payers have a legitimate need to know the reason that a patient has presented to an HCP for treatment, what symptoms were present, why a projected treatment is likely to help a patient, and that the treatment rendered was "medically necessary." Patient records can be significantly enhanced by the HCP's attempt to *quantify* the patient's clinical data. **When properly quantified, the patient's subjective complaints and objective findings can serve as quite reliable outcome assessment tools.** The use of quantified subjective complaints and objective findings as outcome assessment tools should meet the major criteria for the selection of assessment techniques for musculoskeletal clinical trials as reported by Bellamy (1993):

- The measurement process must be ethical.
- Reliability should be adequate for achieving measurement objectives.
- Validity (face, content, criterion, and construct) should be adequate for achieving measurement objectives.
- Responsiveness must be adequate (ie, the technique must be able to detect a clinically important statistically significant change in the underlying variable).

These measurements can be repeated at the HCP's discretion, and can be very useful to assess the patient's progress as treatment is administered.

SOAP: AN ORGANIZATIONAL SCHEME FOR CLINICAL DATA

The necessity for organization of the patient's clinical data into a predictable, repeatable format has been well accepted throughout the health care industry. The pre-eminent organizational format since the 1970s has been known as the SOAP (Weed, 1969, 1986) format. SOAP is a mnemonic device that represents the division of the patient information into four sections called subjective, objective, assessment, and plan. These four divisions will also form the organization of the remainder of this chapter:

- Subjective: the portion of the patient record that is derived directly from description by the patient, without the benefit of actual assessment from the examiner. The subjective portion always includes the chief complaint of the patient. The subjective portion of the record is essentially the patient history.
- Objective: the portion of the patient record that is able to be observed, measured or otherwise determined with some degree of accuracy by the HCP. The objective portion of the patient record is essentially the recording of the physical examination, plus other clinical or diagnostic observations or measurements such as radiographic, electrodiagnostic, or laboratory examination.
- Assessment: the portion of the patient record that describes the HCP's impressions of the case. This usually includes a working or final diagnostic impression. Short- and long-term goals are usually placed in this section of the clinical records. This section may also include information or opinions regarding pathogenesis of the condition, prognosis, contraindications to treatment, risk factors, alternate treatments, or other opinions by the HCP.

This section of the patient record may be thought of as the decision making associated with interpreting the data from the subjective and objective portions of the record, and synthesizing this data into the HCP's opinions on the condition of the patient.

- Plan: the portion of the patient record that deals with action by either the HCP or the patient. This may include a diagnostic plan for further objective testing, a therapeutic treatment plan, and an educational plan for the patient (Mootz, 1994). This portion of the record may be considered the result of the data from subjective and objective sections, and the opinions from the assessment, to formulate a meaningful action plan for the patient.

Each element of the SOAP format is dependent upon the quality of the information provided in the preceding element. For example, the action *plan* that is based upon an incomplete *subjective* patient history and poorly recorded *objective* physical examination is likely to be incomplete or inappropriate as well.

Various modifications of the SOAP format, such as SORE (Vernon, 1990), SNOCAMP (Larimore and Jordan, 1995), SOAPE (Christie, 1993), SOAPPR (Frank and Wakefield, 1996) and others have been forwarded by authors to meet the unique needs of various specialties. In each of these variations, the authors have expanded or made further subdivisions in the four basic elements of the SOAP record, especially the assessment or treatment plan. In each of these proposed systems, the HCP is encouraged to make entries in the appropriate category or subdivision for data, thereby leading to an organized patient record.

SUBJECTIVE ELEMENT

The subjective element of the patient record is that information obtained directly from the patient, without benefit of actual assessment by the HCP. The subjective portion of the patient history has unfairly gathered a reputation for being "soft" or unreliable when compared to more objective, HCP-determined findings. This supposed unreliability is because the source of the information is the patient. In fact, the boundaries between "hard" and "soft" findings are often quite indistinct (Deyo, 1988). Many "subjective" measures have been found to be more accurate and reproducible than many "hard" or "objective" findings (Fries and Bellamy, 1991; Deyo et al, 1994a, 1994b; Hawk, 1994).

There has been an increased emphasis in recent years on investigating the outcome of health care treatment. One definition of outcome might well be an answer to the question, "Is the patient showing improvement with treatment?" With this increased emphasis on the measurement of outcomes in treatment, there has also been an increased awareness by HCPs of the patient as a potentially reliable source of clinical information. Although some factions in health care may dispute the reliability of the patient to provide meaningful clinical information, it must be re-

membered that variability in this area can only be an issue with the patient who claims no improvement with treatment. In answer to the outcome question, "Is the patient improving with treatment?," the possible answers are "yes" or "no." For patients who claim they are not improving with treatment, the answer of "no improvement" could mean that there has been no improvement, or that there may be symptom magnification, malingering or other patient induced variables. However, for the patient who states that improvement is being shown, there would seem to be no reason to doubt the patient's validity.

The subjective portion of the patient record provides many opportunities for quantification. Depending where and when HCPs received their training, they may have learned the requisite components of the subjective part of the patient's record by various methods. However, the most common organizational scheme now in place for the subjective portion follows guidelines set by the Health Care Financing Administration, and consists of three distinct elements:

1. History of present illness (HPI)
2. Review of systems (ROS)
3. Past, family, and social history (PFSH)

History of Present Illness

The history of present illness (HPI) is a chronological description of the development of the patient's present illness from the first sign and/or symptom to the present. The Health Care Financing Administration has defined the following factors to constitute a complete history of the present illness:

- History of trauma
- Description of the chief complaint(s)
- Onset of symptomatology
- Palliative factors
- Provocative factors
- Quality of pain
- Radiation of pain
- Severity of pain frequency or timing of complaint
- Previous episodes of the chief complaint

Most of the elements of the history of the present illness can be easily remembered by the use of the mnemonic "O, P, Q, R, S, T" (Foreman and Croft, 1995).

- O = *onset* of symptoms
- P = *provocative* or *palliative* factors
- Q = *quality* of pain
- R = *radiation*
- S = *severity* of pain
- T = *timing* of pain

When using this mnemonic, many HCPs add an additional element to indicate whether the patient has experienced prior episodes of the chief complaint:

- U = previous episodes (have *you* ever had this problem before?)

Almost all of these elements can be quantitated to some degree in the patient's records. These quantitated subjective findings will serve as an important baseline to determine the patient's future progress with treatment.

Measurement of Pain

The subjective complaint of pain is the key symptom of almost every form of neuromusculoskeletal disease, but its measurement is extremely difficult (Bellamy, 1993). Pain has also been described as the most important subjective criterion that is used for assessing a patient's progress under therapeutic care (Sandoz, 1985). The most accurate measurement of pain is generally regarded to be the patient's own description of the pain (National Institutes of Health, 1986). Neither behavior nor vital signs can substitute for a self-report (Acute Pain Management Guideline Panel, 1992). The HCP may note qualitatively that the pain is described by the patient to be mild, moderate, or severe. In an effort to gain more quantitative information, the HCP may ask the patient to rate the amount of pain on a numbered scale, such as the use of a 0- to 10-point scale, or Numerical Pain Scale (NPS). Other types of simple pain quantification methods have also been shown to be valid. Jensen et al (1986) showed good correlation between the Visual Analogue Scale (VAS), 101-point numerical rating scale, 11-point numerical rating scale, and 6-point Behav-

---

CLINICAL TIP 20–1
The Benefit of a Pain Drawing

The HCP can encourage the patient to attempt to localize his or her pain more precisely, and to describe its duration, character, or other attributes. The use of a pain drawing is often very helpful to get the patient thinking in terms of communicating to the HCP regarding the exact location of the pain.

---

ioral Rating and Verbal Rating scales. Unique rating scales have been developed for the rating of children's pain (Harbeck and Peterson, 1992).

To a large degree, the choice of a pain rating scale is a matter of experience and personal preference by the HCP in anticipation of the types of cases typically seen in that practice, keeping in mind any available "gold standards." It is important that once a pain scale is chosen for use in a particular case, the use of the same pain scale should be continued throughout the case.

Consider the use of the chart notes shown in Table 20–1. For each portion of the history of present illness, a qualitative example is shown and contrasted with a preferred, quantitative version. Most of the subjective descriptors of the patient's chief complaint can be described more quantitatively by utilizing more precise descriptions as shown in the seed questions that follow:

Table 20–1: Sample Charting Notes

CLINICAL ATTRIBUTE	QUALITATIVE CHART NOTE	QUANTITATIVE CHART NOTE
Onset	The patient presented with a subacute history of lower back pain.	The patient presented with subjective complaint of lower back pain, with insidious onset 8 days ago, and reports progressively worsening symptoms.
Palliative factors	Improved with rest and use of NSAIDs.	Improved with rest after 2 hours, or with 600 mg ibuprofen after 1 hour.
Provocative factors	Increased pain is noted upon standing, sitting, driving, and lifting.	Increased pain is noted upon standing > 15 min, sitting > 30 min, driving > 45 min, or lifting > 25 pounds.
Quality	Burning, numbness, sharp, dull, tingling	Burning, numbness, sharp, dull, tingling (The *quality* of pain cannot be *quantified!*)
Radiation	Pain down R leg to mid-calf	Pain down from R lower gluteal to R posterior leg to mid calf, ranges from 3–7/10
Pain severity	The patient described moderate pain in the lower back.	The patient described pain in the lower back of 5 on a 10 point scale (5/10).
Timing	Pain in the back is intermittent.	Lower back pain over L5 area is intermittent, present approx. 50% of waking hours.
Previous episodes	Patient stated that he has had previous lower back pain, usually resolved without treatment.	Patient stated that he has periodic episodes of lower back pain, approx. 3× year, each lasting for approx. 2 weeks, with pain 3–6/10. Usually resolved without treatment.

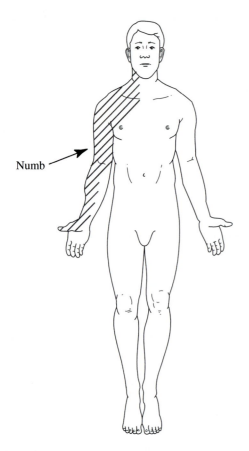

Numb

Figure 20–1. Example of a pain drawing.

A. *Onset:* When did the chief complaint start? Was the chief complaint associated with trauma, a certain activity, or insidious? Was there a definable mechanism of injury? Since the complaint began, have the symptoms generally been getting better, worse, or are they relatively unchanged?

B. *Palliative:* What specific actions improve the symptoms of the chief complaint? How long is the improvement noted? To what degree is the improvement noted? Can the patient estimate the percentage of improvement with various palliative factors?

C. *Provocative:* What specific actions aggravate the symptoms of the chief complaint? To what degree is the chief complaint aggravated? How long does the chief complaint remain aggravated after provocation?

D. *Quality:* not able to be quantified. Have the patient describe the type of pain, such as burning, throbbing, sharp, or dull. The topic of pain drawings is discussed in Chapter 6. Ask the patient to qualify the type of pain by utilizing various symbols to indicate areas of pain, numbness, burning, or throbbing.

E. *Radiation:* Describe the anatomical range of any referred or radiating pain. Consider the use of pain drawings performed by the patient, or have the HCP jot a quick sketch of the affected area (see Fig. 20–1). These methods are often more precise and more time-efficient than verbal or written descriptions of the location.

The HCP should continue to ask questions that help the patient quantify the severity of the symptoms. Is the radiating or referred pain constant or intermittent? If intermittent, what percentage of the waking hours is it noticed? How severe is the radiating or referred pain? (Use severity scales as described in paragraph F.) The HCP will also want to begin gathering data that will be helpful in the formulation of the assessment or diagnosis. From the pattern of pain displayed by the patient, does this appear to be pain radiating from a nerve root, or referred pain from other structures (sacroiliac joint, facet joints or soft tissue)?

F. *Severity:* Consider the use of a pain scale, such as an 11-point NPS, or VAS (see Chap. 6). Train the patient to use this scale consistently in the descriptions of the pain to the HCP upon each office visit or therapy session. This allows a review of the records to determine with objectivity whether the patient's perceived pain is diminishing with treatment.

G. *Timing:* What is the frequency of the chief complaint? Is the chief complaint constant or intermittent? If intermittent, have the patient estimate the percentage of waking hours that is affected. Is the chief complaint better or worse in the morning or evening? Is the complaint worse before work, during work, or after work? Is the complaint better or worse before meals or after meals? Verbal descriptions of pain frequency are common. The following definitions of pain frequency are from the AMA *Guides for the Evaluation of Permanent Impairment,* 4th edition (1993).

- Intermittent: The symptoms or signs have been documented medically to occur less than one-fourth of the time when the patient is awake.
- Occasional: The symptoms or signs have been documented medically to occur between one-fourth and one-half of the time when the patient is awake.
- Frequent: The symptoms or signs have been documented medically to occur between one-half and three-fourths of the time when the patient is awake.
- Constant: The symptoms or signs have been documented medically to occur between three-fourths and all of the time when the patient is awake.

These verbal definitions are certainly adequate if used constantly and correctly by all providers. All too often, however, common words like "frequent" are used outside the context of a strict definition. Therefore, the HCP may wish to consider utilizing actual percentages of pain frequency during a patient's waking hours as shown in Table 20–2.

H. *Past episodes:* Has the patient had the chief complaint before? How recently? How severe were the episodes? Was treatment provided? If so, for how long? Was the treatment effective?

Measurement of Disability and Other Subjective Complaints

The second most important symptom of musculoskeletal disease is disability, which is nearly as difficult to measure as

Table 20–2: Quantifying Symptom Frequency

FREQUENCY IS SAID TO BE:	WHEN SYMPTOMS ARE PRESENT BETWEEN THIS PERCENTAGE OF THE PATIENT'S WAKING HOURS:
Intermittent	0–25%
Occasional	25–50%
Frequent	50–75%
Constant	75–100%

pain (Bellamy, 1993). As it is possible to have significant pain without disability, or to have significant disability without pain, disability and pain do not necessarily correlate well (Co et al, 1993). Because of vast differences in pain sensitivity, a patient may report that he or she is unable to perform activities of daily living or work activity because of moderate pain, while another patient shows no stoppage of activities with comparable amounts of pain. Patients may report that they have difficulties with certain activities of daily living such as sitting, driving, sleeping, and so forth. It is relatively simple to quantify these activities so that patient tolerance for the various activities is described as a test of tolerance.

> *Example:* The patient notes that sitting and driving are painful.
> *Improved example:* The patient notes that sitting or driving for more than 15 minutes at a time causes pain to rise to 7/10.
> *Example:* The patient states that his sleep is disturbed.
> *Improved example:* The patient states that his sleep is disturbed approximately 3 to 4 hours per night on a nightly basis.

There are also specific questionnaires for disability, which attempt to ask the patient to quantify the disability in several specific areas. Perhaps the best known example is the Oswestry Disability Questionnaire, which is described in more detail in Chapter 7.

Review of Systems

The review of systems (ROS) is the second of the three major sections of the subjective history. The ROS is an inventory of body systems obtained through a series of questions seeking to identify signs or symptoms that the patient may be experiencing or has experienced. Contrary to common misinterpretation, the ROS is a history element, not a detailed physical examination. The Health Care Financing Administration has recommended organization of the review of systems by the following 14 bodily systems:

1. Constitutional symptoms, such as fever or weight loss
2. Eyes
3. Ears, nose, mouth, throat
4. Cardiovascular
5. Respiratory
6. Gastrointestinal
7. Genitourinary
8. Musculoskeletal
9. Integumentary (skin or breast)
10. Neurological
11. Psychiatric
12. Endocrine
13. Hematological/lymphatic
14. Allergic/immunological

Review of systems should always attempt to include the date that various prior problems were encountered, as well as a description of any treatment, whether the bodily system in question still has difficulties, and an indication of the impact the condition had on the daily activities of the patient.

Past, Family, and Social History

The third and final portion of the patient's subjective information is a review of significant events in the following three areas:

1. **Past history:** Major illness or injuries; hospitalizations; current medications; drug or food allergies; and age appropriate immunization and dietary status
2. **Family history:** Health status or cause of death of parents, siblings, and children; specific diseases related to the patient's current complaints; diseases of family members that may be hereditary or familial
3. **Social history:** Marital status; current and past employment; use of drugs, alcohol, or tobacco; level of education; sexual history or other relevant social factors

Risk Factors

Many authors have written on the prevalence of various factors that, when present, predispose the patient to increased probability for the development of a given condition. For example, Kirkaldy-Willis and Burton (1992) and Bombardier et al (1994) review a total of 22 positive associations for the development of lower back pain, including cigarette smoking, neck pain, and stomach pains (see Table 20–3).

Von Korff (1994) has recommended specific elements in the clinical workup of back pain that are described as "useful" and "mandatory" (see Table 20–4). Other authors have attempted to determine factors that may predispose individuals to future risk of developing a given condition. For example, Meeker (1990) has developed a Back Pain Risk Assessment (BPRA) which is claimed to be a valid tool in predicting future episodes of lower back pain.

Foreman and Stahl (1990) have suggested the use of the following ten "red flag" questions. These questions are designed to ascertain whether the patient has underlying health concerns in addition to (or as a possible cause of) the neuromusculoskeletal complaint.

Table 20–3: Individual Risk Factors Associated with the Development of Low Back Pain

POSITIVE ASSOCIATION	QUESTIONABLE ASSOCIATION	NO ASSOCIATION
Increasing age	Tallness	Sex
Marked scoliosis	Obesity	Body build
Poor health	Trunk strength	Increased lumbar lordosis
Lack of fitness	Intelligence	Most scolioses
Psychosocial problems	Economics	Leg lengths
Smoking		Decreased muscle strength
Drug abuse		
Headaches		
Neck pain		
Angina pectoris		
Leg discomfort		
Stomach pains		
Heavy physical work		
Non-neutral trunk postures		
Whole body vibration		
Low job satisfaction		
Monotonous work		
Poor job satisfaction		
Previous back pain		

Compiled from data in Kirkaldy-Willis and Burton, 1992, with additional factors from Bombardier et al, 1994.

1. Have you ever had cancer?
2. Does your pain ever wake you from a sound sleep?
3. Are you losing weight now without trying?
4. Are you coughing up blood or noticing it in your stools or urine?
5. Have you had any loss of bowel or bladder control?
6. Have you lost consciousness or had double vision recently?
7. Are you seeing any other doctor now for any other reason?
8. Do you have any other symptoms or health problems?
9. Are you taking any medications or over the counter drugs now?
10. Is there any chance that you are pregnant now?

Questions 1 through 4 deal with potential malignancies. Questions 5 through 6 are designed to rule out serious neurological compromise. Questions 7 through 9 are designed to elicit responses to develop a more complete patient history. Question 10 is important before any type of radiographic examination is contemplated.

Subjectively-oriented Questionnaires

In addition to the classic subjective components described previously, a number of subjective questionnaires have proven value in the assessment of various areas of clinical concern. These questionnaires are described in much more detail in Chapters 5 through 10. Several of these questionnaires have been used extensively by researchers, and have satisfactory reliability, validity and sensitivity characteristics. The following questionnaires can be recommended highly:

- General health questionnaires: SF-36
- Global pain: McGill-Melzack
- Regional disability: Oswestry Disability Index (lower back), Neck Disability Index (cervical)

These questionnaires are typically selected by the HCP for suitability to the type of case, and are administered at initial presentation (baseline) and then periodically every 2 to 4 weeks to assess the progress of the patient over time.

OBJECTIVE ELEMENT

The objective element of the patient information is the second portion of the SOAP mnemonic, and primarily details the physical examination or other areas of patient data that can be determined directly by the examiner.

Consent of the Patient

Now that the interview of the patient is completed, the objective portion of the patient workup, the physical examination, can begin. However, before the physical examination is performed, the HCP may wish to review the legal

Table 20–4: Data Relevant to Assessing the Clinical Course of Back Pain

MEASURE	ASSESS AT BASELINE	ASSESS AT FOLLOW-UP(S)
Age	Mandatory	
Sex	Mandatory	
Race/ethnicity	Mandatory	
Occupation	Useful	
Change in occupation		Useful
Employment status	Mandatory	Mandatory
Disability insurance status	Mandatory	Mandatory
Litigation status	Useful	Useful
Recency or age at first onset of back pain	Mandatory	
Recency or age when care was first sought	Mandatory	
Recency of back pain episode		Mandatory
Duration of current or most recent episode of back pain	Mandatory	Mandatory
Number of back pain days	Mandatory	Mandatory
Current pain intensity	Mandatory	Mandatory
Average pain intensity	Mandatory	Mandatory
Worst pain intensity	Useful	Useful
Ratings of interference with activities	Mandatory	Mandatory
Activity limitation days	Mandatory	Mandatory
Clinical diagnosis for this episode	Useful	Useful
Bedrest days	Useful	Useful
Work loss days	Useful	Useful
Recency of a back pain flare-up	Useful	Useful
Duration of the most recent flare-up	Useful	Useful

Compiled from data in Von Korff, 1994.

responsibilities in his or her state for obtaining the patient's consent to examine and treat him or her. While a full review of the concept of patient consent is well outside the scope of this chapter, it is essential that the prudent HCP be aware of the basic concepts of obtaining and recording patient consent.

There are basically three types of patient consent that are typically encountered in the neuromusculoskeletal practice:

1. *Consent to examination:* As the name implies, this portion of the patient consent gives the HCP the clear authority to examine the patient prior to the performance of the physical examination. The consent to examine and treat is often implied by the patient presenting for treatment. However, the prudent HCP should be aware that there have been some instances of the patient claiming that battery was committed by the HCP during the examination (Chapman-Smith and Paterson, 1994). In some jurisdictions, the assault or battery can be claimed simply because there was no evidence of consent by the patient to submit to the examina-

tion. This claim can occur in spite of the fact that the patient initiated the session with the HCP. In most cases, this unhappy situation can be avoided by asking the patient to sign a statement giving the HCP the authority to perform a physical examination. This is usually done in conjunction with the other entrance data the patient provides upon initial presentation.

2. *Consent to treat a minor child:* In nearly all jurisdictions, the HCP must have explicit written authority from a parent or legal guardian in order to examine or treat a minor child. A minor child is usually defined as less than 18 years old, but the age of majority can vary from 14 to 21 years of age in various states.

3. *Informed patient consent:* The process of obtaining informed consent by the patient requires the HCP to describe the proposed treatment plan for the condition of the patient. This treatment plan can be proposed only after the HCP has taken the subjective history, performed a physical examination, and made an assessment of the patient's condition. Therefore, a brief discussion of informed consent

will be presented in the "Treatment Plan" section later in this chapter.

The objective portion of the patient record also provides ample opportunity for increased accuracy and quantification. When the objective findings are quantified, they can be used as an outcome assessment tool in order to gauge the patient's progress during the treatment period.

For example, the HCP may determine that a provocative orthopedic test, such as the straight leg raise (SLR) test, is positive in a given patient. This test provides information that is helpful in the formulation of the diagnosis for the patient. This information can become even more useful if the HCP records the angle of the leg that reproduces the pain, the area in which pain is reproduced and the severity of pain reproduced.

In the performance of many provocative tests, such as the SLR test, this information is a vital part of the test. For example, the SLR that is positive for leg pain at 15 to 30 degrees is a reliable indicator for a lower lumbar disc lesion. The SLR that is positive for leg pain at 60 degrees is not considered clinically reliable (McCarthy, 1994). Recording this information into the patient record is a vital element of the diagnostic process and serves as a useful outcome assessment measurement tool. The degree to which a provocative orthopedic test is positive can be tracked over time to determine whether the patient is making progress with therapy.

In the same manner, most objective elements of the physical examination are very simple to quantify. When properly quantified, these objective elements yield higher quality information, which can be used as an outcome assessment tool in a given case. Consider the following possibilities for quantification in the physical examination:

Observation
Measure the size of any masses, lacerations, scars, and so forth. Measure the severity of antalgic posture in degrees using a goniometer. Measure circumferentially to determine muscle atrophy of the upper or lower extremities. Measure any leg length inequality.

Palpation
Bony tenderness has been found to be more reliable than soft tissue tenderness (McCombe et al, 1989). The use of the pressure algometer has been advocated in order to measure pain perception threshold (PPT) in trigger points. Normative values for pressure thresholds have been published by Maloney et al (1990) with a pressure algometer, and a potential link to a patient's pain perception has shown moderate correlation. Record any areas that are especially tender to palpatory touch.

Range of Motion Measurement
Range of motion can be measured using many different methods. Good inter-examiner and intra-examiner reliability has been shown using a variety of techniques and measuring tools. The most commonly described methods are:

- Active Range of Motion (AROM): The patient is asked to move the affected body part without any assistance from the examiner. This is often performed to assess muscular integrity and overall function of the body part in question.
- Passive Range of Motion (PROM): The patient is asked to allow the examiner to move the affected body part without resistance from the patient. This is often performed to assess ligamentous integrity with the voluntary muscles not playing a major role in the movement.
- Active Assisted Range of Motion (AAROM): In this type of range of motion testing, the patient provides the initial muscular effort to move the affected body part, then the examiner overstresses the joint near the end point of motion. This is often performed to gain information from both active (AROM) and passive (PROM) testing. AAROM is often notable if there is a significant difference between the active and passive portions of testing.

Range of motion testing is often used to differentiate the type of tissue involved: Pain upon resisted motion is usually considered muscular. Pain upon PROM is usually ligamentous, especially at the end point of motion. Pain upon active and passive motion is usually articular.

Range of motion can be estimated visually, or measured more accurately with the use of various mechanical aids. Range of motion measurements are usually reported with the measurement compared to the expected normal, such as "lumbar flexion of 55/90." The most common mechanical aids are:

- Goniometer: essentially a protractor with a moveable arm, this device measures angles of movement in degrees. The goniometer is available in various sizes to meet the needs of different sized body regions.
- Inclinometer, mechanical: a device that measures angles compared to gravity. Sometimes called a gravity-assisted goniometer (Mior et al, 1991).
- Inclinometer, electronic (electrogoniometer): a device that measures angles compared to the reference "zero," which is set by the operator. The electronic inclinometer allows the HCP to directly measure movements that do not begin or end at the gravitational plane without calculation.
- Measuring tape: can be used to measure lumbar flexion in fingers to floor measurement; can also be used to directly measure lumbar flexion via Schober's test (Schober, 1937)

Liebenson and Phillips (1988) reviewed varying methods of measuring trunk ROM and found the most valid methods used inclinometers, flexible rulers, spondylometers, and a modified form of the Schober test.

A simple pain scale specific to the use of ROM testing has been proposed by McKenzie (1989), which asks the HCP to note whether ROM testing causes changes in pain levels or changes in location of the pain. The pain scale consists of the following five possibilities:

1. +1P = the pain worsened with movement and peripheralization occurred
2. +1 = the pain worsened with movement
3. 0 = no change in pain with movement
4. −1 = the pain decreased with movement
5. −1C = the pain decreased with movement and centralization occurred

Example: "Lumbar flexion was tested at 55/90 +1P into the right leg from buttock to calf." This means that lumbar flexion was tested and found to be 55 degrees of an expected 90 degrees, and pain worsened with movement and moved to the periphery, in this case the right leg and buttock.

Example: "Lumbar extension was tested at 25/35 −1." This means that lumbar extension was tested and found to be 25 degrees, compared to an expected normal of 35 degrees. The pain was decreased with movement.

Provocative Orthopedic Tests

Because of the nature of "provocative" tests, it is important to note not only whether the test was positive or negative, but also the location and severity of pain that was provoked, and the amount of provocation necessary to reproduce symptomotology.

Example: Kemp's test was positive.
Improved example: Kemp's test was positive upon standing right lumbar rotation, with sharp pain noted over the ipsilateral lower lumbar facets, and peripheralization of the pain to the right lower gluteal area.
Example: The well-leg raise test (WLR) was positive.
Improved example: The WLR was positive for provocation of pain into the nonaffected leg, from the buttock to the knee, rated by the patient at 7/10.

Which provocative tests should be selected, and the reported reliability of the tests represent an area of tremendously divergent opinions. McCombe et al (1989) reviewed 62 commonly observed physical signs and orthopedic tests in conjunction with lower back pain and concluded that only 7 were reliable: pain pattern into the leg, pain on bending, pain on flexion, pain on hip flexion, leg pain on SLR, back pain on SLR, and diminished ankle jerk (see Table 20–5).

Vucetic and Svensson (1996) have reported that only three physical signs are reliable in the determination of lumbar disc herniation: ROM in the sagittal plane, Laseque's sign, and the crossed Laseque's sign (sometimes known as the well leg raising test or Fajersztajn's test; Evans, 1994). Souza (1994) has reported the following orthopedic tests to have favorable characteristics in sensitivity, specificity, and/or reliability:

Table 20–5: Reproducibility of Physical Signs in Low Back Pain

UNRELIABLE	POTENTIALLY RELIABLE	RELIABLE
Back pain pattern	Foot pain pattern	Leg pain pattern
Extension catch	Thigh pain pattern	Pain on lateral bending
Buttock tenderness	Pain on rotation	Pain on flexion
Paravertebral tenderness	Diminished rotation	Pain on hip flexion
Sacroiliac distraction	Pain on extension	SLR producing back or leg pain
Sacroiliac compression	Iliac crest tenderness	Ankle jerk
Maitland sacroiliac test	Sacroiliac tenderness	
Bowstring sign	Midline tenderness	
Buttock wasting	Pain on resisted external rotation of hip	
Toe standing	Femoral stretch test	
Heel standing	Crossed leg sciatic stretch test	
Knee jerk	SLR reproducing patient's symptoms	
Superficial tenderness (Waddell no. 1)	Muscle wasting of calf, quadriceps, hamstring, anterior compartment	
Abnormal sensory or motor disturbance (Waddell no. 1)	Lower extremity weakness (EHL, quadriceps, or hip flexors, dorsiflexors, peroneal)	
	Simulation (Waddell no. 2)	
	Distraction (Waddell no. 3)	
	Overreaction (Waddell no. 5)	

EHL, Extensor hallicus longus; SLR, straight leg raise.

Compiled from data in McCombe PF et al, 1989.

- Cervical: cervical compression, cervical distraction, shoulder abduction
- Wrist: Phalen's test, provocative pressure at the carpal tunnel to reproduce symptoms.
- Knee: Lachman's, Krawere, varus and valgus stress, pivot shift, McMurray's
- Ankle: drawer, Navicular drop test

Sensory Testing

The sensory examination is the most subjective portion of the physical examination (Hardy, 1993) and is dependent upon honest reporting by the patient. An accurate description of any anatomical areas that have sensory deficits in the patient's clinical record is critical. The HCP may wish to draw a sketch of the affected areas, which can often be both quicker and more precise than the corresponding verbiage. It is often interesting to ask the patient with a sensory deficit to describe how the affected side compares to the unaffected side. For example, when performing a pinwheel examination, ask the patient, "Can you tell me what percentage of the sharpness you no longer feel on your bad side compared to your good side?" The patient will often offer an estimate of 25%, 50%, or 75%, which can be tracked over time as the patient progresses.

Reflex Testing

Deep tendon reflex examination has generally been shown to possess good sensitivity and reliability traits. Deep tendon reflexes are performed to test the components of the reflex arc: the stimulus receptor, sensory arc neuron, synapse, motor arc neuron, and the effector organ. Asymmetrical changes in the deep tendon reflex often are pathognomonic of underlying neurological compromise. The deep tendon reflex has been called the only true objective sign in the diagnosis of disc disease, because it is not dependent upon patient effort or perception, as are the motor and sensory examinations (Hardy, 1993). In the diagnosis of lumbar disc disease, the patellar tendon reflex is diminished unilaterally in up to 60% of the patients with a herniated nucleus pulposis at L3-4 (Raaf, 1959). With a herniated nucleus pulposis at L5-S1, the Achilles reflex will be unilaterally diminished up to 89% of the time (Aronson and Dunsmore, 1963). Since 98% of all lumbar disc lesions occur at the L4-5 or L5-S1 intervertebral discs (Kelsey et al, 1990), the HCP will be rewarded by paying special attention to the depressed unilateral Achilles reflex, which is the most commonly occurring neurological deficit (McCarthy, 1994). The most commonly used scale for reporting deep tendon reflexes is the 5-point Wexler scale:

- 0: No response
- +1: Hyporeflexia
- +2: Normal
- +3: Hyperreflexia
- +4: Hyperreflexia with transient clonus
- +5: Hyperreflexia with sustained clonus

Reflexes are generally reported on a 5-point scale, such as +1/5, +2/5, +3/5, and so on. When reporting deep tendon reflexes, the use of the plus sign *before* the number helps to avoid confusion with muscle strength testing, which is also commonly reported on a five-point scale and usually puts any plus or minus signs *after* the number (such as 4+/5).

Muscle Strength Testing

Muscle strength may be tested manually or with the use of various devices. Each type of testing has its proponents. Manual muscle testers claim their methods provide speed and reliability, while each type of muscle testing machine has its own group of supporters. In the final analysis, it is up to the HCP to compare the characteristics of the various types of muscle tests, and decide what is most appropriate in terms of validity, reliability, sensitivity, and cost-effectiveness.

Manual Testing

During the epidemics of poliomyelitis of the 1950s, there was unparalleled interest in the use of manual muscle testing. With the advent of device-assisted muscle testing, there has been somewhat of a de-emphasis of this important skill in the training of some HCPs. Other writers have stressed that muscle testing is an art, which relies on the knowledge, skill, and experience of the HCP in order to be accurate and sensitive to small losses in muscle strength (Kendall et al, 1963). With manual testing, sensitivity to small differences in muscle strength has been reported as poor, while reliability and validity is good. It has been shown that decreases in muscle strength of 25% to 50% may be rated by HCPs as normal (Beasley, 1956; Watkins et al, 1984; Hislop and Montgomery, 1995).

When manually assessing muscular strength, most HCPs use a modified Lovett (Legg, 1932) scale, which assigns a number grade to the muscle strength. The most common usage of this system denotes the following muscle grades:

- Grade 5 is used to indicate "normal," or full muscle strength.
- Grades 4+, 4, and 4− are used to indicate decreasing muscle function within the "good" category, which is defined as the ability to raise the part against gravity and some resistance.
- Grades 3+, 3, and 3− are used to indicate decreasing muscle function within the "fair" category, which is defined as the ability to raise the part against gravity only.
- Grades 2+, 2, and 2− are used to indicate decreasing muscle function within the "poor" category, which is defined as the ability to raise the part only with gravity eliminated.
- Grade 1 means that the muscle contraction can be felt, but there is no joint movement. Grade 0 means no contraction is felt.

Muscle Testing in Conjunction with Functional Tests

The work of Rissanen et al (1994) showed that nondynamometric tests are still useful in clinical practice despite the development of more "accurate" (and higher cost) muscle strength evaluation methods. Yeomans and Liebenson (1996) have proposed grouping repetitive arch-up and sit-up tests with 19 other "low-tech" functional tests into a specific outcome assessment instrument called the Quantitative Functional Capacity Evaluation (QFCE). The use of muscle fatigue upon resisted manual testing has been postulated as a direct, observable outcome measure for the treatment of myofascial pain syndrome (Hsieh et al, 1992).

Decision Tree for Muscle Testing

Amundsen (1990) originally proposed the following logical sequence for assessing the skeletal muscle strength component of the patient. The six methods are arranged from simplest to most complex (and expensive):

1. *Assess activities of daily living:* Qualitative. During interview of the patient, the HCP can determine the patient's impression of his or her ability to perform necessary daily tasks.
2. *Conduct simple functional tests:* Simple quantitative. Ask the patient to demonstrate movements that are required with simple activities of daily living. The use of simple functional tasks such as step tests or lifting of small dumbbells can be helpful in the assessment of these abilities.
3. *Perform appropriate manual muscle tests.* Quantitative, to the limit of sensitivity by the examiner. These tests are often performed in sequence of spinal cord levels by the neuromusculoskeletal HCP to screen for neurological abnormalities. In addition, the potential location of any suspected lesion may be narrowed by the skillful use of manual muscle testing.
4. *Hand-held and hand grip dynamometry (or myometry):* Quantitative. These hand-held devices use springs, hydraulics, or strain gauges to measure force on a dial or a digital scale. Testing with the use of a hand held instrument may allow the examiner to detect smaller deficits of muscle strength than with manual testing alone. However, this advantage may by offset by another variable: the strength of the examiner, which is needed to hold the dynamometer in position for testing. These devices have been shown by Bohannon (1986), Riddle et al (1989), and Agre et al (1987) to have generally acceptable reliability.
5. *Isometric muscle strength testing with a fixed-load cell system:* Quantitative. Useful for measuring muscle groups in which the strength is more than can be resisted by the examiner.
6. *Dynamic muscle strength testing using isokinetic or isotonic movement:* Quantitative. Isokinetic testing is resisted exercise at a fixed speed throughout the range of motion (*iso* = same; *kinetic* = motion). Examples of common isokinetic muscle measurement tools are the Cybex or Merec machines. Isotonic testing is exercise that is resisted with equal tension throughout the range of motion (*tonic* = tension). Examples of common isotonic muscle measurement tools are the Biodex and Lido Active machines.

Objectively-oriented Outcome Assessment Measures

The HCP may consider many different types of objectively oriented outcome measures in addition to the objective portions of the examination, as listed previously. These objective tests, which are discussed in more detail in Chapters 11 through 18, provide the HCP with information regarding the patient's ability to perform certain tasks upon demand. Like their subjectively oriented cousins, these tests are typically chosen by the HCP for applicability to the specific case. The test is administered initially to form baseline data. The test is then repeated at a prescribed interval in order to document the patient's improvement. For some of these tests, normative data are available.

ASSESSMENT ELEMENT

Assessment is the third of the four elements of the SOAP format. The assessment is the section of the patient record that records the HCP's opinions concerning the case, especially the diagnostic impression. This section of the patient record may be thought of as the decision making process associated with interpreting the data from the subjective and objective portions of the record, and synthesizing this data into the HCP's opinions on the condition of the patient. Other factors that are often addressed in the assessment portion of the patient record may include:

- Initial, working, and final diagnoses
- Pathogenesis or causation of the condition
- Risk factors that may affect outcome and/or informed consent process
- Contraindications to treatment
- Alternate treatments
- Short-term goals
- Long-term goals
- Prognosis

TREATMENT PLAN ELEMENT

The treatment plan is the fourth and final section of the SOAP acronym. It is the portion of the patient record that deals with projected action by either the HCP or the patient. This may include a diagnostic plan for further objective testing, a therapeutic treatment plan, and an educational plan for the patient. This portion of the record may be considered the result of the data from subjective and objective sections, and the opinions from the assessment, to formulate a meaningful action plan for the patient. This portion of the patient record consists of the following elements:

- Informed consent
- Diagnostic plan

- Therapeutic plan
- Educational plan

Informed Consent

The patient's informed consent to accept a recommended treatment is the third type of legal consent commonly encountered in a typical neuromusculoskeletal practice. The other two types of consent are consent to examination and consent for the examination and treatment of a minor child, and are reviewed in the discussion of the "Objective Element" earlier in this chapter.

A lengthy discussion of the principles of informed consent is well outside the scope of this chapter. However, because informed consent is a very topical issue, a brief explanation at this point is appropriate. Informed consent refers to the discussion of the HCP with the patient regarding the possible risks of the proposed treatment, and the act of the patient agreeing to the proposed treatment. As is implied by the name "informed" consent, the discussion of any risks to the patient must take place *before* the treatment is provided for the first time. For this reason, informed consent is included here, at the very beginning of the treatment plan. Recommended elements (Campbell et al, 1994) of the patient's informed consent to treatment include:

- The nature of the proposed treatment
- The material or significant risks associated with the treatment
- The probability of the risks occurring
- Other treatment options that could be considered
- The risks of remaining untreated

The requirement for "informed" consent is sometimes interpreted to mean that the patient should receive more of an explanation than a preprinted form. The HCP is encouraged to report to the patient any unusual risk factors or underlying diagnostic conditions that might possibly cause a poorer outcome than an uncomplicated case. In addition, the patient should be encouraged to ask any questions prior to granting consent.

Diagnostic Plan

This portion of the treatment plan describes what steps are recommended in order to further ascertain the diagnosis of the patient's condition. For example, the HCP may list, "MRI of lumbar spine recommended at 2 weeks if lower extremity symptoms continue."

CLINICAL TIP 20–2
Legal Responsibilities and Informed Consent

It is highly recommended that the HCP review with their legal counsel the responsibilities in their jurisdiction for obtaining informed consent from their patients prior to instituting treatment.

Therapeutic Plan

This portion of the treatment plan lists the in-office treatments or therapies that are proposed for the patient.

Educational Plan

This portion of the plan describes the "home instructions" given to the patient. These instructions may be to perform at-home modalities, such as the application of ice or heat, to perform flexibility or strengthening exercises, or to perform self-directed swimming, walking, or other activities. This portion of the plan may also include information to the patient, such as advising the cessation of smoking, attendance at a back school, or general information on health and fitness.

CHART ORGANIZATION

Clinical documentation in many neuromusculoskeletal practices consists of three distinct elements: (1) initial entry, (2) daily note, and (3) progress note.

INITIAL ENTRY

As the name indicates, the initial entry is a record of the patient's first presentation to the HCP or clinic. The initial entry generally includes:

- Pertinent baseline information about the patient
- The patient's chief complaint(s)
- The results of initial physical examination and other diagnostic studies
- The HCP's assessment
- The recommended treatment plan

DAILY NOTE

The daily note represents a concise record of pertinent changes in the patient's condition and treatment on that day. A series of daily notes will show changes on a visit-to-visit basis. The daily note is often used to document ongoing or recurring treatment for a patient, such as the documentation of chiropractic, physical therapy, or rehabilitation services. The use of daily notes in this manner depends upon the performance of comprehensive charting of the initial note and subsequent progress notes to detail the bulk of the patient's subjective complaints, objective findings, clinical assessment, and treatment plan.

After the initial entry, each subsequent office visit will usually be documented by a daily note, until the next specified re-evaluation. If the initial entry clearly states the assessment and plan, it is not usually necessary to re-evaluate the patient on a daily basis or to reiterate the assessment or the treatment plan. Any significant modification of the treatment plan should be recorded in the daily note (Bronston, 1992).

Because of its brevity, the daily note will list only the most important changes in the daily presentation of the patient, and the management of the case. Therefore, the treating HCP is best qualified to decide which objective and subjective elements of the case should be recorded via the daily note.

PROGRESS NOTE

At many different points in a case, a progress note is often used to document additional patient services. These services may include:

- Re-evaluations
- Re-examinations
- Counseling
- Coordination of care

One respected author in the field of documentation (Mootz, 1994) has described the initial entry as "SOAP-ing" the patient. The progress note can be thought of as a kind of "midi-SOAP," or a somewhat abbreviated version of the original SOAP workup. This so-called "midi-SOAP" retains the same database format, yet is not necessarily as detailed as the original evaluation. The notation for a daily or routine visit is described as a "mini-SOAP," displaying the same general organizational scheme of the initial evaluation, but on a significantly smaller scale.

The National Committee for Quality Assurance (1994) has posed these questions as a self-assessment for the HCP to determine the completeness of clinical records:

1. Do all pages contain patient identification?
2. Is there biographical/personal data?
3. Is the provider identified on each entry?
4. Are all entries dated?
5. Is the record legible?
6. Is there a completed problem list?
7. Are allergies and adverse reactions to medications prominently displayed?
8. Is there an appropriate past medical history in the record?
9. Is there documentation of smoking habits and history of alcohol use or substance abuse?
10. Is there a pertinent history and physical examination?
11. Are laboratory and other studies ordered as appropriate?
12. Are working diagnoses consistent with findings?
13. Are plans of action and treatment consistent with diagnosis(es)?
14. Is there a date for return visit or other follow-up plan for each encounter?
15. Are problems from previous visits addressed?
16. Is there evidence of appropriate use of consultants?
17. Is there evidence of continuity and coordination of care between primary and specialty physicians?
18. Do consultant summaries, laboratory, and imaging study results reflect primary care physician review?
19. Does the care appear to be medically appropriate?
20. Is there a completed immunization record?
21. Are preventative services appropriately used?

PROBLEM LIST

In cases in which the patient has multiple chief complaints, especially when there are multiple chief complaints involving multiple body systems, the use of a problem list has been suggested as one possible method to help reduce confusion in the clinical records. Each complaint of the patient is numbered and briefly described, along with its date of onset or presentation and the date of resolution, if applicable (see Table 20–6).

The example shown in Table 20–6 details a patient who initially presented with a chief complaint of episodic, chronic recurring lower back pain on 04/01/98. The episode lasted approximately 6 weeks and symptoms were resolved by 05/15/98. A second episode of lower back pain was reported 07/20/98, and has not yet resolved. Additional problems of posterior leg pain, mild hypertension, and traumatic knee pain were added to the problem list as the problems were encountered. A SOAP notation can be

Table 20–6: The Problem List

DATE PROBLEM ENTERED	NUMBER	ACTIVE PROBLEMS AND ONSET	INACTIVE PROBLEMS AND DATE OF RESOLUTION
04/01/98 07/20/98	1	Lower back pain, chronic 10-year history, insidious onset	05/15/98
08/03/98	2	Mild hypertension: attempt to control with diet and exercise	
09/17/98	3	Left posterior lower extremity pain, acute onset immediately after lifting a 50# box on 09/16/98.	
11/15/98	4	Acute left medial knee pain, after slipping on wet sidewalk 11/14/98.	Symptoms resolved 12/08/98.

made for each numbered item, thereby reducing the need to repeat the nature of the complaint and the onset date. This method also helps the SOAP notation to be more organized, because each SOAP note describes only one problem, not numerous problems.

Example: Daily notes utilizing problem list format from Table 20–6

08/20/98:

#*1: LBP*

S: Diminished LBP (low back pain) over L5/L SI (sacroiliac) area to 3–4/10. Pain is now intermittent, and present approx. 50% of day. Now walking 30 min periods w/o difficulty.

O: Dejerines triad now negative. + Yeoman's test for L SI pain. SLR negative. Gait improved to near normal.

A: Chronic left SI syndrome showing early signs of resolution with treatment.

P: Continue with treatment plan (see initial note 07/20/98).

#*3: HBP*

S: None

O: 136/88.

A: Two weeks into walking program, somewhat aggravated by LBPs.

P: Continue diet/exercise modifications.

"GOLD STANDARD" FOR NEUROMUSCULOSKELETAL DOCUMENTATION

The term "gold standard" comes to us from the world of economics. In the second half of the 19th century, it became obvious that local forms of currency were not adequate to meet the needs of a more complex international economy. Great Britain was the first country to establish a standard for its paper currency in which any note could be exchanged at any time for the equivalent amount of gold. Other countries quickly followed suit, and for approximately 100 years the Western world used gold as the benchmark by which all countries' currency were valued.

In the context of health care, the "gold standard" refers to a benchmark or test that is acknowledged to be reliable and valid on a universal basis. In the clinical sciences, the quest continues for the gold standards that will be used for the measurement of meaningful clinical data. Some types of clinical data are relatively easy to measure. For example, blood pressure or pulse can be measured accurately by students with minimal training. Other types of clinical data are more resistant to accurate assessment. In the neuromusculoskeletal practice, many outcome measurements have been purported to reach this lofty standard (usually by their authors). In reality, few do.

It has been especially difficult to measure accurately some of the common factors, such as pain, which patients use to describe their complaints. It has also been difficult to measure effectively which patients are likely to improve with treatment and which patients have cases that are more prone to protraction. In lower back pain, it has been estimated by White and Gorson (1982) that a precise diagnosis probably cannot be determined in 80% of the cases. Deyo et al (1994b) acknowledge that for low back pain and radiculopathy, the true gold standard has not yet been discovered, and the honest investigator may have to settle for a "bronze" standard. Other authors (Beruskens et al, 1995) have also noted that a gold standard does not exist in many areas of neuromusculoskeletal practice, especially of the lower back. However, in another article, Deyo et al (1994a) encourages investigators to avoid "reinventing the wheel" by developing new or ad hoc measures if standardized tools are available to accomplish a similar purpose.

Conclusion

To visualize the power of an "outcomes-based" practice, take one low back pain patient from your practice, perform the documentation steps detailed in this chapter, then mix in one or two appropriate outcome measurements from the remainder of the book. For example, the patient who shows continuous positive improvement on an Oswestry Disability Questionnaire measured biweekly over an 8-week period might demonstrate graphic improvement such as the graph of disability scores shown in Figure 20–2. Conversely, the patient who is not showing improvement, and needs further workup or referral will have Oswestry scores that are obviously not showing appropriate improvement (see Fig. 20–3).

Ambrosius et al (1995) stressed the importance of using outcomes that measure our ultimate clinical goals in terms that our patients, employers, and insurers can readily understand: goals of return-to-work, increased function, and reduced pain. All of these measures can be well addressed by conscientious quantification of the HCP record and a few carefully selected outcome assessment measures. These methods must be consistently applied and the results tracked over time. When the HCP implements these methods of documentation, and uses the resulting information to make clinical decisions regarding treatment, the results are to create a truly "outcomes-based" practice.

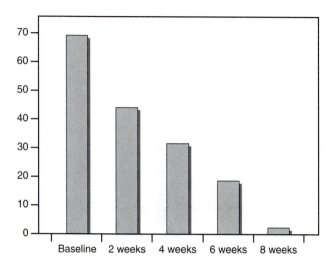

Figure 20–2. Graph of disability scores.

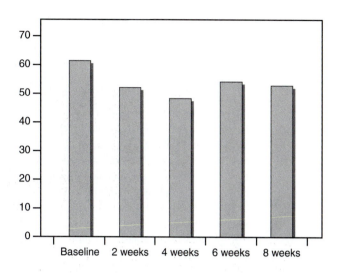

Figure 20–3. A patient whose Oswestry scores are obviously not showing appropriate improvement.

REFERENCES

Acute Pain Management Guideline Panel. *Acute Pain Management in Adults: Operative Procedures. Quick Reference Guide for Clinicians.* AHCPR Pub. No. 92-0019. Rockville, Md: Agency for Health Care Policy and Research, Public Health Service, US Department of Health and Human Services, 1992.

Agre JC, Magness JL, Huss SZ, et al. Strength testing with a portable dynamometer: reliability for upper and lower extremities. *Arch Phys Med Rehabil* 1987;68:454.

Ambrosius FM, Kremer AM, Herkner PB, DeKraker M, Bartz S. Outcome comparison of workers compensation and noncompensation low back pain in a highly structured functional restoration program. *J Orthop Sports Phys Ther* 1995;21(1):7–12.

Amundsen LR, ed. *Muscle Strength Testing: Instrumented and Non-Instrumented Systems.* New York, NY: Churchill Livingstone; 1990:1,26.

Aronson HA, Dunsmore RH. Herniated upper lumbar discs. *J Bone Joint Surg* 1963;45A:311–317.

Bates B. *A Guide to Physical Examination and History Taking,* 5th edition. Philadelphia, Pa: JB Lippincott; 1991:651–654.

Beasley W. Influence of method on estimates of normal knee extensor force among normal and postpolio children. *Phys Ther Rev* 1956;36:20–41.

Bellamy N. *Musculoskeletal Clinical Metrology.* Boston, Mass: Kluwer; 1993:4.

Beruskens AJ, de Vet HC, Koke AJ, van der Heijden GJ, Knipschild PG. Measuring the functional status of patients with low back pain. Assessment of the quality of four disease-specific questionnaires. *Spine* 1995;20(9):1017–1028.

Bohannon RW. Test retest reliability of hand-held dynamometry during single session of strength assessment. *Phys Ther* 1986;66:206.

Bombardier C, Kerr MS, Shannon HS, Frank JW. A guide to interpreting epidemiologic studies on the etiology of back pain. *Spine* 1994;19(18S):2047S–2056S.

Boorstin D. *The Discoverers.* New York, NY: Random House; 1983:340.

Bronston LJ. Record maintenance and narrative writing. In: Ferezy JS, ed. *The Chiropractic Neurological Examination.* Gaithersburg, Md: Aspen; 1992:141–156.

Campbell, L, Ladenheim CJ, Sherman R, Sportelli L. Informed consent: A search for protection. *Top Clin Chiro* 1994;1(3):55–63.

Chapman-Smith DA, Paterson RJ. Informed consent to chiropractic treatment. In: Lawrence DJ. *Advances in Chiropractic.* vol 1. St. Louis, Mo: Mosby-Year Book; 1994:193–218.

Christie J. Does the use of an assessment tool in the accident and emergency department improve the quality of care? *J Adv Nurs* 1993;18(11):1758–1771.

Co YY, Eaton S, Maxwell MW. The relationship between the St. Thomas and Oswestry disability scores and the severity of lower back pain. *J Manipulative Physiol Ther* 1993;16(1):14–18.

Deyo RA. Measuring the functional status of patients with lower back pain. *Arch Phys Med Rehabil* 1988;69:1044–1053.

Deyo RA, Andersson G, Bombardier C, Cherkin DC, Keller RB, Lee CK, Liang MH. Outcome measures for studying patients with low back pain. *Spine* 1994a;19(18S):2032S–2036S.

Deyo RA, Haselkorn J, Hoffman R, Kent DL. Designing studies of diagnostic tests for low back pain or radiculopathy. *Spine* 1994a;19(18S):2057S–2065S.

Evans RC. *Illustrated Essentials in Orthopedic Physical Assessment.* St. Louis, Mo: Mosby; 1994:276.

Foreman S, Croft A. *Whiplash Injuries: The Cervical Acceleration/Deceleration Syndrome.* 2nd ed. Baltimore, Md: Williams and Wilkins; 1995.

Foreman SM, Stahl MJ. *Medical-legal issues in chiropractic.* Baltimore, Md: Williams and Wilkins; 1990:18.

Frank RG, Wakefield, TS. Rationale for the use of a chiropractic-specific SOAP acronym in clinical documentation. *Chiro Technique* 1996;8(4):171–177.

Fries JF, Bellamy N. Introduction. In: Bellamy N, ed. *Prognosis in the Rheumatic Diseases.* Lancaster, Pa: Kluwer Academic Publishers; 1991:1–10.

Galen. *On the Natural Faculties.* Arthur John Brock, MD, trans. Cambridge, Ma: Harvard University Press; 1916.

Guides for the Evaluation of Permanent Impairment. 4th ed. Chicago, Ill: American Medical Association; 1993:316.

Harbeck C, Peterson L. Elephants dancing in my head: A developmental approach to children's concepts of specific pains. *Child Devel* 1992;63(1):138–149.

Hardy, RW, ed. *Lumbar Disc Disease.* 2nd ed. New York, NY: Raven Press; 1993:22–23.

Hawk C. Patient-centered outcome assessment. *Palmer J Res* 1994;1(2):31–34.

Hislop H, Montgomery J. *Daniels and Worthingham's Muscle Testing: Techniques of Manual Examination.* 6th ed. Philadelphia, Pa: W.B. Saunders; 1995:3.

Howse E, Baily J. Resistance to documentation—a nursing research issue. *Int J Nurs Stud* 1992;29(4):371–80.

Hsieh J, Gilbertons K, Hong J. Using muscle fatigue as an outcome measure in myofascial pain syndrome. *Proc Int Conf Spinal Manip* 1992;1:63.

Jensen MP, Koroly P, Sanford B. The measurement of clinical pain intensity: A comparison of six methods. *Pain* 1986;27:117–126.

Kelsey JL, Golden AL, Mundt DJ. Low back pain/prolapsed lumbar intervertebral disc. *Rheum Dis Clin North Am* 1990;16:699–712.

Kendall FP, MeCreary BA, Provance PG. *Muscles: Testing and Function.* 4th ed. Baltimore, Md: Williams and Wilkins; 1993:4.

Kirkaldy-Willis WH, Burton CV. *Managing Low Back Pain.* 3rd ed. New York, NY: Churchhill Livingstone; 1992:6.

Larimore WL, Jordan EV. SOAP to SNOCAMP: Improving the medical record format. *J Fam Pract* 1995;41(4):393–398.

Legg AT. Physical therapy in infantile paralysis. In: Mock, ed. *Principles and Practice of Physical Therapy.* vol. II. Hagerstown, Md: W.F. Prior; 1932:45.

Liebenson D, Phillips R. The reliability of range of motion measurements for human spine flexion: A review. *Trans Consort Chiro Res* 1988;1.

Maloney P, Petermann E, Buerger D, Robbins B, Picinich D. Pressure thresholds in the lumbar spine and their relationship to a measure of pain perception. *J Manipulative Physiol Ther* 1990;13(2):122.

McCarthy KA. Improving the clinician's use of orthopedic testing: An application to lower back pain. *Top Clin Chirop* 1994;1(1):42–50.

McCombe PF, Fairbank JCT, Cockersole BC, Pynsen, PB. Reproducibility of physical signs in low back pain. *Spine* 1989;14(9):908–919.

McKenzie RA. *The Lumbar Spine: Mechanical Diagnosis and Therapy.* Waikanae, New Zealand: Spinal Publications, Ltd; 1989.

Meeker W. Is the onset of back pain predictable? A test of epidemiological risk assessment. *J Manipulative Physiol Ther* 1990;13(1):57.

Mior SA, Gluckman J, Fournier G, Vernon H. A comparison of two objective measures in assessing cervical range of motion. *Proceedings of the 1991 International Conference on Spinal Manipulation.* Arlington, Va: Foundation for Chiropractic Education and Research; 1991:79.

Mootz RD. Maximizing the effectiveness of clinical documentation. *Top Clin Chiro* 1994;1(1):60–65.

Muller RT. Analysis and assurance of complete medical documentation. *Z Orthop Ihre Grenzgeb* 1992;130(5):367–370.

National Committee for Quality Assurance. *Reviewer Guidelines*. Washington, DC; 1994.

National Institutes of Health. The Integrated Approach to the Management of Pain. NIH Consensus Statement 1986 May 19–21;6(3):1–8.

Raaf J. Some observations regarding 905 patients operated upon for protruded lumbar intervertebral disc. *Am J Surg* 1959;97:388–397.

Riddle DL, Finucane SD, Rothstein JM, et al. Intrasession and intersession reliability of hand-held dynanometer measurements taken on brain-damaged patients. *Phys Ther* 1989;69:182.

Rissanen A, Laranta H, Sainio P, Harkonen H. Isokinetic and non-dynamometric tests in low back pain patients related to pain and disability index. *Spine* 1994;19(17):1963–1967.

Rosenthal TL, Miller S, Rosenthal R, Shadish W, Fogelman B, Dismuke E. Assessing emotional distress at the internist's office. *Behav Res Ther* 1991;29(3):249–252.

Sandoz R. The choice of appropriate clinical criteria for assessing the progress of a chiropractic case. *Ann Swiss Chiro Assn* 1985;8:53–73.

Shober von P. Lendenwibelsaule und Kruezschermenzen. *Munch Med Wochenschr* 1937;9:336–338.

Souza T. Which orthopedic tests are really necessary? In: Lawrence, DJ. *Advances in Chiropractic*. vol. 1. St. Louis, Mo: Mosby; 1994:108–150.

Vernon H. Clinical note: S-O-R-E, a record keeping system for chiropractic treatment visits. *Can Chiro Assn J* 1990;34:93.

Von Korff M. Studying the natural history of back pain. *Spine* 1994;19(18S):2041S–2046S.

Vucetic N, Svensson O. Physical signs in lumbar disc hernia. *Clin Orthop Rel Res* 1996;333:192–201.

Waddell G, McCulloch JA, Kummel E, Venner RM. Nonorganic physical signs in lower back pain. *Spine* 1980;5:117–125.

Watkins M, Harris B, Kozlowski B. Isokinetic testing in patients with hemiparesis: A pilot study. *Phys Ther* 1984;64:184–189.

Weber H. Lumbar disk herniation: A controlled prospective study with ten years of observation. *Spine* 1983;8:131–140.

Weed LL. *Medical Records, Medical Education and Patient Care*. Cleveland, Oh: Case Western Reserve University Press; 1969.

Weed LL. Medical records that guide and teach. *N Engl J Med* 1986;278:593–600,652–657.

Weights and measures. Microsoft (R) Encarta. Copyright (c) 1994 Microsoft Corporation. Copyright (c) 1994 Funk & Wagnall's Corporation.

White AA III, Gorson SL. Synopsis: Workshop on idiopathic low back pain. *Spine* 1982;7:141–149.

Yeomans SG, Liebenson C. Quantitative functional capacity evaluation: The missing link to outcomes assessment. *Top Clin Chiro* 1996;3(1):32–43.

Identif

fo

- ▶ INTRODUCTION
- ▶ RECOVERY RATE (NATURAL HISTO
- ▶ ECONOMIC FACT PAIN MANAGEME MAKING
- ▶ QUALITY ASSUR PREVENTING PER RECURRENT LOW
  Diagnostic Triage
  Identifying Yellow
  Predict a Poor

INTRODUCTIC

Quality care is needed
chronic pain and disab
able by treatment (Fra
what we do, while and
This is contrasted with
vance and, most impo
The quality and co
satisfaction, cost of ca
comes such as pain in
endurance), medicatic
the patient recovers. T
pain relief to preventi
for Health Care Polic
change the paradigm
helping patients impro

In this chapter, the problem of escalating costs for low back disability is identified along with the solution to early identification of the high-risk patient. The various definitions of what constitutes recovery are outlined and the epidemiological literature regarding the natural history of acute low back problems is reviewed. Finally, a simple, reliable, and valid way to identify risk factors of a prolonged or inadequate recovery is demonstrated.

RECOVERY RATE FOR LOW BACK PAIN (NATURAL HISTORY)

The low back pain and disability problem represents a modern epidemic. Controversy abounds regarding the recovery rate and appropriate treatment strategies. A solution to this problem is to carefully evaluate specific outcomes such as pain, activity intolerances, symptom satisfaction, or disability in patient groups receiving different types of interventions.

It is commonly stated that most disabled workers return to work within 1 month (Bigos et al, 1994; Spitzer et al, 1995; Frank et al, 1996). Data by Cheadle et al (1994) found that 62% are back at work within 1 month; 78% by 2 months; and 90% by 6 months. Reid et al (1997) concluded that there is a 95% return to work within 6 to 12 weeks.

These statistics have led to the mistaken belief that most acute back pain patients recover quickly, and therefore require minimal treatment. Many "experts" have gone as far as to contend that back pain is normal and should be tolerated. A recent random survey dispels this notion by finding that 25% of 35 to 45 year olds reported severe pain and activity intolerances due to back pain in the last year (Linton et al, 1998). These individuals had no disability at all and used their vacation days to recover.

Butler et al (1995) found that 20% to 50% of patients have recurrence of *disability* in the following year. Cherkin et al's data (1996) from 219 patients presenting to a primary care clinic showed that only 46% were *symptom-free* after 7 weeks, and 29% had poor outcomes after 1 year. This information is not new. Lloyd and Troup, in 1981, reported that 50% to 62% of patients have recurrences of *pain* in the following year (Troup et al, 1981). If we look at a relatively new outcome, *symptom satisfaction*, we find that one third of patients are satisfied with recovery after 1 week (Linton et al, 1998). The majority of patients are satisfied with recovery by the 3-week mark. However, one third of patients are dissatisfied with recovery even after 7 weeks. In this case, the question asked was, ". . . how satisfied would you be if you were to spend the rest of your life with your back and leg symptoms just the way they have been in the last 24 hours?" Von Korff and Saunders (1996) looked at the outcome of activity limitations (modified Roland Morris Questionnaire) and found 20% to 25% show substantial *activity limitations* 1 year after the initial back pain episode has resolved.

Croft et al (1998) reported that of 463 patients who had consulted a general medical practice with a new episode of low back pain, only 25% had fully recovered 12 months later. The outcomes used to determine recovery were visual analogue scale for *pain intensity* and Hanover back pain daily activity schedule for *activity limitations*.

Nonetheless, the opinion has formed amongst "experts" that the vast majority of low back pain patients recover within 1 month with or without treatment. If return-to-work is the outcome of choice, it is true that most disabled people do recover, but they also have recurrences. Furthermore, if pain relief, symptom satisfaction, or activity intolerances are utilized as outcomes, the recovery rate is far less optimistic. Many "experts" also contend that treatment has little or no influence on the natural history of spinal conditions (Frank et al, 1996). By looking at outcomes, we can question the truth of that opinion.

ECONOMIC FACTORS IN LOW BACK PAIN MANAGEMENT DECISION MAKING

Clearly, the natural history of low back pain is not as good as has been believed. Since the natural history does not tend toward resolution in the vast majority of patients, as has been touted by "experts," then **the effectiveness of management of the acute to subacute episode to influence recovery rate may not be adequate** and should be carefully reviewed.

Only a small minority of patients account for the vast majority of costs, with over 85% of the costs coming from only 7.4% of the patients (Frank et al, 1996). In fact, a surprisingly small percentage of the costs are treatment related (7%), while the vast majority are due to absenteeism and disability (93%) (van Tulder et al, 1995). Even the relatively small amount of money spent on treatment is not used on evidence-based primary care treatments. Over half of the expenses are related to hospital visits (surgery, diagnostic testing). Thus, it would seem economically advantageous to incorporate secondary prevention strategies in patients with acute or subacute low back pain to relieve pain, reduce activity intolerances, improve symptom satisfaction, reduce recurrences, and prevent the onset of chronic pain behaviors before they are established.

Simple economics suggest that if secondary prevention strategies are recommended for all low back pain patients then the treatment programs will have to be modest. **However, if at-risk individuals can be identified, a more aggressive application of limited resources can be spent on those patients.**

Economic evaluations show that an increase in secondary prevention treatment costs would result in decreased costs due to surgery and disability. Goosens and Evers (1997) reviewed 23 studies that conducted an economic analysis. They concluded that ". . . post-incidence management programs appear to produce cost savings due to reduced absenteeism" (p 15). As Burton and Cassidy (1992) state, ". . . low back pain clearly represents the single greatest and most inefficient expenditure of health care resources in our society today! The only solace evident in this is that the low back problem, once clearly identified, also represents the greatest single opportunity for productive change and cost savings."

The real question is: "At what time does the intervention take place—1 week, 7 weeks, 3 months, or later?" Do we wait for behavioral aspects of chronicity to be fully formed or can we predict those who will become chronic and take a more aggressive preventive approach? Bolton (1994) describes what has become the "holy grail" for many spinal researchers as, "Can an accurate prediction be made of a patient's prognosis early enough to take preventive action?" Early identification of those "destined for chronic disability" would allow stratification of patients into two groups, one requiring less intensive care, and the other requiring more intensive care.

QUALITY ASSURANCE METHODS IN PREVENTING PERSISTENT OR RECURRENT LOW BACK TROUBLE

Recent U.S. acute low back pain guidelines released by AHCPR suggest that diagnostic triage, reassurance, activity modification advice, and pain relief modalities (medication, manipulation) should be utilized for management of the acute pain patient (Bigos et al, 1994). **AHCPR's goal for acute care management is to change the focus of care from pain relief to activity intolerances.**

A recent evidence-based consensus study from New Zealand suggests that both "red flags" of serious disease and "yellow flags" of chronicity should be sought from the earliest possible time (Kendall et al, 1997). Patient management can then focus on de-medicalizing the problem by reassuring the patient that there is nothing seriously wrong, that "hurt" does not necessarily equal "harm," and that he or she can and should increase activities as soon as possible. Finally, pain relief with medication, manipulation, and other means should be offered to facilitate the process of re-activating the patient.

DIAGNOSTIC TRIAGE

The goal of **diagnostic triage** is to "find a needle in a haystack." History and examination can detect red flags of cancer, spinal infection, or cauda equina syndrome with over 99% sensitivity (Deyo, 1996; Waddell et al, 1996). If red flags are present or the patient does not respond to a trial of conservative care, *other tests are necessary.* Table 21–1 summarizes the most important historical and exami-

Table 21–1: Red Flags of Low Back Pain

Cancer
- History of cancer
- Unexplained weight loss
- Pain not improved with rest
- Age > 50 years
- Failure to respond to a course of conservative care (4–6 weeks)

Infection
- Prolonged use of corticosteroids
- IV drug use
- Urinary or other infection
- Immunosuppression

Spinal Fracture
- History of significant trauma
- Minor trauma in person >50 years or osteoporotic
- Age >70 years
- Prolonged use of corticosteriods

Cauda Equina
- Acute onset urinary retention or overflow incontinence
- Loss of anal sphincter tone or fecal incontinence
- Saddle anaesthesia
- Global or progressive motor weakness in lower limbs

nation features associated with red flags of serious problems.

IDENTIFYING YELLOW FLAGS: FACTORS THAT PREDICT A POOR RECOVERY

Yellow flag risk factors are reviewed in detail in Chapter 19. The yellow flags can be divided into various domains: symptom, psychosocial, functional, and disability. Much prospective evidence exists that shows that patients can be stratified into those who are likely to recover well versus those who will have persistent or recurrent trouble (see Table 21–2). Recovery is defined as resolution of symptoms and activity intolerances or disability (nonworking status). Questionnaires addressing many of the yellow flags listed in Table 21–2 can be found in Appendix Forms I–1 and I–2. Refer to Appendix Form I–3 for scoring of the questionnaire and an explanation of the use of cutoffs regarding severity indexing. The specific yellow flags addressed in the questionnaire are identified in the right-hand column of Table 21–2. A summary of some of the many studies that have investigated yellow flags can be found in Table 21–3.

ACUTE CARE (FIRST MONTH)

Frank et al (1996) state that "there is ample evidence that the prognosis for most patients with (O) LBP (who have only ordinary low back strain) is so good, even without any

Table 21–2: Yellow Flags of Low Back Pain[a]

YELLOW FLAG	REFERENCE	QUESTION
Symptoms		
Number of pain sites	Linton and Hallden, 1997, 1998	1
Duration of symptoms	Von Korff et al, 1993; Cherkin et al, 1996; Linton and Hallden, 1997, 1998	2
Duration of symptoms before the first visit	Van den Hoogen et al, 1997	
Past history of numerous episodes	Burton et al, 1995; Cherkin et al, 1996; Frank et al, 1996; Hazard et al, 1996	3
Past hospitalization or surgery for similar complaint	Lancourt and Kettelhut, 1992; Hazard et al, 1996; van den Hoogen et al, 1997	4
Severe pain intensity	Von Korff et al, 1993; Cherkin et al, 1996; Frank et al, 1996; Hazard et al, 1996	5
Frequency of painful episodes over the last 3 months	Linton and Hallden, 1997, 1998	6
Sciatica	Lancourt and Kettelhut, 1992; Burton et al, 1995; Cherkin et al, 1996; Frank et al, 1996; Selim et al, 1998	7
Psychosocial		
Anxiety	Cherkin et al, 1996	10
Locus of control	Burton et al, 1995	11
Depression	Klennerman et al, 1995; Cherkin, 1996; Linton and Hallden, 1997, 1998	12
Catastrophizing	Burton et al 1995	
Self-rated health as poor	Cherkin et al, 1996; Waddell et al, 1996	13
Heavy smoker	Cats-Baril and Frymoyer, 1991; Hazard et al, 1996; Waddell et al, 1996	14
Belief that you should not work with your current pain	Linton and Hallden, 1997, 1998	15
Job dissatisfaction	Cats-Baril and Frymoyer, 1991; Cherkin et al, 1996	22
Anticipation of trouble sitting or standing at work 6 weeks into the future	Hazard et al, 1996	23
Anticipation of disability 6 months into the future	Hazard et al, 1996	24
Function		
Does physical activity make your pain worse?	Linton and Hallden, 1997, 1998	16
Tolerance for light work	Linton and Hallden, 1997, 1998	17
Is sleep affected by your pain?	Linton and Hallden, 1997, 1998	18
Disability		
Heavy job demand	Waddell et al, 1996	19
Past disability for the same/similar complaint in prior 12 months	Hazard et al, 1996	20
Disabled at present	Hazard et al, 1996	21

[a] Four domains of yellow flags are presented, along with the respective reference(s), and the question number of Appendix Forms I–1 and I–2.

medically prescribed treatment, that only minimal investigation and treatment, together with substantial reassurance, is warranted." A number of recent studies refute this optimism regarding the natural history (Cherkin et al, 1996; Von Korff and Saunders, 1996; van den Hoogen et al, 1997; Croft et al, 1998). Nonetheless, there is good evidence that **simple advice to continue or resume normal activities is therapeutic for acute low back pain.** One

study found that advice to continue normal activities as tolerated resulted in better outcomes than patients resting 2 days or performing back mobilization exercises (Malmivaara et al, 1995).

Van den Hoogen et al (1997) reported that patients who have received physical therapy during the first 5 weeks after the initial visit had a significantly prolonged recovery (by approximately 4 weeks). Physical therapy was defined

Table 21–3: Yellow Flag Supportive Studies[a]

BURTON ET AL STUDY (1995)

Sample size: 252 low back troubled patients (initial); 74% (n = 186) at 1 year follow-up

Presentation: New occurrence of low back trouble

Outcome determining recovery: Activity intolerances determined by Roland-Morris Questionnaire

Factors that predicted 1 year recovery: Pain locus of control questionnaire: pain control $P = .007$, pain responsibility $P = .037$; catastrophizing scale of the Coping Strategies Questionnaire was about 7 times more predictive than the best of the clinical or historical variables studied in acute cases, $P = $ NA; past history of trouble (no past Hx = 94% recovered vs 66% recovered with + past Hx) $P = $ NA; sciatica $P = $ NA

HAZARD ET AL STUDY (1996)

Sample size: 163 acute patients (within 11 days of onset)

Presentation: Disabling occupational low back injury

Outcome determining recovery: Return-to-work or work status

Factors that predicted 3-month postinjury work status:

1. First episode of low back pain
2. Multiple episodes for which treatment was sought
3. Severe pain intensity
4. Anticipation of trouble sitting or standing at work 6 weeks from the present

Note: A cutoff score of .48 identified the 3-month postinjury work status with .94 sensitivity and .84 specificity. The cutoffs can be varied to meet the goals of the populations being tested.

CHERKIN ET AL STUDY (1996)

Sample size: 219 patients

Presentation: First visit for the current episode (82% less than 3 weeks since onset)

Outcome determining recovery: Symptom satisfaction (one question)

Factors that predicted 7 week recovery (7 items):

1. Younger age (under 50) ($P = .01$; odds = 1.04)
2. Depression ($P < .001$; odds = 2.1)
3. Sciatica (pain below the knee) ($P = .002$; odds = 3.6)
4. Job satisfaction in those employed (150 patients) ($P = .003$)
5. Prior treatment for back pain ($P = .004$)
6. More severe symptoms (≥ 5 on a 0–10 scale) ($P = .034$)
7. Greater back-related worry (≥ 5 on a 0–10 scale) ($P = .022$)

Factors that predicted 1 year recovery (5 items):

1. Sciatica ($P = .014$; odds = 2.4)
2. Depression ($P < .001$; odds = 2.3)
3. Female gender ($P = .005$)
4. Perceptions of being less healthy ($P = .006$)
5. Greater worry about one's back problem ($P = .007$)

VON KORFF ET AL STUDY (1993)

Sample size: 1128 patients

Presentation: Recent onset (within 6 months) vs prevalent (longer than 6 months)

Outcome determining recovery: Pain severity and activity intolerances (modified Roland-Morris Questionnaire)

Factors that predicted recovery at 1 year (based on mulitvariate analysis): Pain-related activity intolerances (Grade III odds ratio [OR] 6.14; $P < .001$) (Grade IV OR 8.1; $P < .001$) > education <12 yr (OR 3.17; $P = .004$) > days in pain over the previous 6 months (OR 4.64; $P < .001$) > female gender (OR 1.53; $P = .04$)

Pain related activity intolerances: Grade III = high pain intensity (VAS of at least 50/100) and moderate activity intolerances; Grade IV = high pain intensity and severe activity intolerances

Table 21–3: Yellow Flag Supportive Studies[a] (*continued*)

VAN DEN HOOGEN ET AL STUDY (1997)[b]

Sample size: 443 consecutive LBP patient study (389 or 88% completed first follow-up period and 269 or 60% completed the second follow-up at 1 year)

Presentation: Prospective, consecutive LBP patient study

Outcome determining recovery: Symptoms at 1 year follow-up

Factors that predicted recovery at 1 year (based on multivariate analysis):

1. Duration preceding the initial visit (number of weeks): HR = .98, LR = 25.2
2. Receiving physical therapy during the first 5 weeks after the initial visit (yes or no): HR = .62, LR = 17.9[b]
3. Pain, as an aspect of perceived health (score 0–100): HR = .99, LR = 11.6
4. History of surgery (positive or negative outcome): HR = .58; LR = 5.8

Factors that predicted relapses within 1 year (based on bivariate analysis): Daily functioning (*P* = .04)

Note: "Hazard ratio of .98 per week means that at every moment in time for each week of low back pain preceding the initial visit, patients had a 2% lower chance to recover in the following week."

CATS-BARIL AND FRYMOYER STUDY (1991)

Sample size: 5204, persons 24–70 years completed initial and final surveys (at 3 months)

Presentation: Epidemiological survey studying demographic factors to predict disability

Outcome determining recovery: Return-to-work or work status

Factors that predicted disability: 6 variables associated with disability prevalence (*P*<.05)

1. Age: 55–65 years highest (1.70% above the mean); greatest rise 45–55 years (1.33% AM)
2. Family income: <$7000 is 4× higher vs >25,000 (1.94% AM)
3. Physical activity: disabled = 27.7% IA and 18% VA; nondisabled = 16.3% IA and 29.5% VA (1.68% AM)
4. Work environment: unpleasant (*P*<.001; 1.49% AM)
5. Highest grade attended: <8th grade = 5× higher vs > 4 yrs college education (1.93% AM)
6. Marital status: highest in the divorced and widowed (1.22% AM)

LANCOURT AND KETTELHUT STUDY (1992)

Sample size: 134 patients

Presentation: Prospective, consecutive LBP patient study

Outcome determining recovery: return to work or work status

Factors that predicted return to work < or > 6 months (P values of the total sample):

1. *Personal factors/history:* Prior worker's compensation injury (yes) *P* = .008; Oswestry LBP Disability Questionnaire (≥55) = .001; history of leg pain (yes) *P* = .001
2. *Family factors:* living arrangement *P* = .000; length of living arrangement *P* = .001; relocation *P* = .012
3. *Employment information:* <26 weeks *P* = .042
4. *General stress indicators:* financial difficulty *P* = .043
5. *Nonorganic physical signs:* verbal magnification of pain (present) *P* = .001; superficial palpation *P* = NS; sciatic tension sham *P* = .001
6. *Mixed organic/nonorganic signs:* supine SLR (<100 degrees right or left) *P* = .001; lateral bending *P* = .02; gait *P* = .000; forward flexion *P* = .000; deep palpation *P* = .000
7. *Organic physical signs:* muscle atrophy (>1/4-inch loss) *P* = .025; sitting SLR (consistency of) *P* = NS

Table 21–3: Yellow Flag Supportive Studies[a] *(continued)*

LINTON AND HALLDEN (1997, 1998)

Sample size: 137 acute and subacute neck or low back patients

Presentation: Fewer than 4 months off work during past year because of pain

Outcome determining recovery: 6 month follow-up regarding accumulated sick leave—**D**; experienced pain (average pain intensity during the past 6 months multiplied by the frequency of pain—recovered = 1–16 points)—**P**; function (5 ADL questions were summed and an index of 45 equalled recovered)—**AL**

Factors that predicted 6-month accumulated sick leave—significant predictors after multivariate analysis: stress; previous sick leave; current pain intensity; light work tolerance; perceived chance of working in 6 months; belief that one should not work with current pain levels (P<.00001)—73% were correctly classified using these variables, specificity (classifying a healthy person as healthy) was 75%

Outcomes that predicted pain score after 6 months—significant predictors after mulitvariate analysis: number of pain sites first; belief that pain increases with physical activity; frequency of pain—all three together, 74% of patients are correctly classified (sensitivity = 75%; specificity = 71%) (P<.0001).

Outcomes that predicted functional score after 6 months—significant predictors after multivariate analysis: average pain during the past 3 months, sleep, number of pain sites—all three together, 73% of patients are correctly classified (sensitivity = 71%; specificity = 77%) (P<.0001).

ADL, activities of daily living; AM, above mean of 10.1%; D, disability; HR, hazard ratio; Hx, history; IA, inactive; LBP, low back pain; LR, likelihood ratio; NA, not available; NS, not significant; OR, odds ratio; P, pain; P, Pearson coefficient; SLR, straight leg raise; VA, very active.

[a] Many studies have investigated yellow flags. These summaries are only a few of the many that have been published. The authors feel that these in particular have contributed significantly to this topic.

[b] The authors stated that this surprising result may be due to ". . . it could be that patients with specific characteristics that predispose them to a less favorable course more often than others urge their general practitioners to refer them for physical therapy."

---

as, ". . . combinations of exercise therapy and modalities such as heat, cold, and massage, and advice on daily behavior." The authors describe two possible explanations. The first states that therapeutic interventions may invoke patients to consider themselves as sick or disabled which, from a behavioral viewpoint, may have a deteriorating effect. The second proposes that general practitioners may target patients for physical therapy by detecting an aspect of chronicity not detected or considered by this study.

A meta-analysis review conducted by experts working with RAND indicated that **spinal manipulation** is most effective between the second and fourth weeks, imparting a 30% improvement in rate of recovery over traditional treatments (Skekelle et al, 1992). The results are short term, but it increases patient satisfaction and can be utilized to reduce yellow flags such as anxiety and severe acute pain and facilitate reactivation (Cherkin and MacCornack, 1989). According to Great Britain's Royal College of General Practitioners (RCGP) expert consensus review of treatments for acute low back pain, the opinion that manipulation speeds recovery for acute patients was given the highest ranking (Waddell et al, 1996). The RCGP concluded that the risks of manipulation for patients with low back pain are very low, provided it is carried out by a trained therapist or practitioner (Waddell et al, 1996).

Medication is also a recommended treatment by both the RCGP and AHCPR. The RCGP summarized the benefits and risks as follows: "NSAIDs effectively reduce simple back ache . . . [but] can have serious adverse effects" (Waddell et al, 1996); muscle relaxants effectively reduce

acute back pain (Waddell et al, 1996); "muscle relaxants have significant adverse effects . . . even after relatively short courses (ie, 1 week)" (Bigos et al, 1994).

Burton et al (1995) stated, "There is good reason to suppose that a reduction in the number of nonspecific low back trouble patients progressing to chronicity may be affected by early interventions designed to promote positive coping strategies and reduce catastrophic behavior patterns." **Behaviorally based approaches have, in fact, been shown to be effective for resolving acute pain.** Fordyce et al (1986) demonstrated reduced disability 1 year later as a result of their interventions. Also, Linton et al (1993) achieved an eightfold reduction in chronicity as a result of a behaviorial approach.

SUBACUTE CARE (4 TO 12 WEEKS)

Many argue that it is best to wait until the subacute stage to treat since many patients will have resolved spontaneously (Frank et al, 1996). A study of patients with low back pain who were off work for over 8 weeks compared conventional medical treatment to a program including encouragement to perform light activities, walk with flexibility, and information about the value of activity for recovery from back pain (Indahl et al, 1995). At follow-up after 6 months, the intervention group had significantly less disability than the control group. Chiropractic treatment with *manipulation* of patients with pain over 7 weeks has demonstrated that it is more effective than traditional treatments (Triano et al, 1995). Lindstrom et al (1992) demonstrated that *rehabilitation* given to those off work for 6 weeks was more effective than a traditional treatment group.

CHRONIC CARE (AFTER 12 WEEKS)

Rehabilitation programs focusing on low-tech but specific exercise programs have been shown to be effective for groups of patients with chronic low back pain. Timm (1994) performed a randomized, controlled trial evaluating passive and active care in a large group of patients with failed back surgery (L5 laminectomy). He concluded that **low-tech exercises (stabilization and McKenzie) gave a greater benefit than high-tech exercises (Cybex), physical modalities, or joint mobilization.**

A recent randomized, controlled clinical trial evaluated the effectiveness of a specific exercise program aimed at training the transverse abdominis and multifidus muscles in chronic low back pain patients with a radiological diagnosis of spondylolysthesis (O'Sullivan et al, 1997). A total of 42 subjects were studied with a follow-up period of 3, 6, and 30 months. After the trial the *specific exercise group* (SEG) demonstrated significant decreases in pain intensity ($P < .0001$), pain descriptor scores ($P < .0001$), and Oswestry functional disability levels ($P < .0001$). Only the pain descriptor scores improved in the control group (CG) ($P = .0316$). Exercises were progressed slowly with low load. Once the patients could correctly perform the co-activation pattern without synergist substitution and hold it for 10 seconds with ten repetitions, load was added through the limbs (ie, Dead-bug). Patients were encouraged to perform the co-contractions throughout the day, "particularly in situations where they experienced or anticipated pain or felt 'unstable.' "

Frost et al (1998) recently reported successful results for a fitness program for chronic low back pain patients (ie, patients with pain lasting at least 6 months). Both groups were given a small set of specific exercises and back school. The experimental group also received fitness instruction in eight 1-hour sessions over a 4-week period. At the 2-year follow-up, there was statistically better improvement in the Oswestry disability scores of the experimental group over the control group.

There is evidence to suggest the **more challenging patients should be treated with a multi-dimensional approach, incorporating behavioral components.** Two meta-analyses of controlled trials show that such treatment returns twice as many people to work as no treatment or single modal treatment (Flor et al, 1992; Cutler et al, 1994). Treatment of the chronic, disabled patient with **multidisciplinary functional restoration** has demonstrated its cost-effectiveness. A combination of high-tech functional capacity evaluation, exercise training, and psychosocial intervention are essential to the program's success. Mayer et al (1987) used a functional restoration approach and were able to return 87% of chronically disabled people to work compared to only 41% of a comparison group. This study used a 2-year follow-up period. Hazard et al (1989) concluded after a 1-year follow-up that 81% of the treatment group returned to work compared to only 21% of the control group. Both Mayer's and Hazard's studies followed three patient groups: one getting active rehabilitation, one that dropped out from treatment, and one denied financial payment by the insurance carrier.

Frank et al's (1996) review of the literature agrees that multidimensional and functional restoration approaches get about half of the chronic patients back to work. However, they state there is "little consensus on how to *select* patients for entry into such intensive programs." Since the pivotal work of Mayer and Hazard, many other groups have also tried to show that comprehensive rehabilitation programs are effective for chronic pain patients. Sachs et al (1990) returned 73% to work compared with 38% in the control group. This approach was less costly than Mayer's or Hazard's because psychological counseling was only offered if illness behavior was documented. Alaranta et al (1994) compared a mulidisciplinary functional restoration program to a primarily passive care approach and documented improved function, pain and disability levels at a 1-year follow-up. Their approach utilized low-cost low-tech functional capacity measures rather than the Mayer, Hazard, and Sachs high-tech approaches. Burke et al (1994) found that surgical and nonsurgical patients both had higher return-to-work rates if involved in a functional restoration program. This study performed its follow-up at 6 months.

UTLIZING RISK FACTOR IDENTIFICATION IN THE CLINICAL SETTING

The bottom line is that **patients can and should be stratified into meaningful treatment groups that are appropriate for them.** The sinister back patient requires identification and referral to a specialist. Diagnostic triage is necessary to rule out sinister causes of back pain or red flags, that is, we need to find the "needle in the haystack." Simple history and examination can reduce the likelihood of malignancy to .1 or .01% (Deyo, 1996).

Acute patients without risk factors should be given reassurance and simple treatment, and should not be "medicalized" by notions of injury or disease. In other words, avoid jargon that implies injury or damage, such as "back injury" or "ruptured disc." However, acute patients with risks or subacute patients who are not recovering should be treated more intensively. Subacute patients who are not recovering should have a thorough biopsychosocial reassessment. Even with risk factor prediction, approximately 25% of patients who will become chronic will not be correctly identified (Kendall et al, 1997; Linton and Hallden, 1997, 1998). Additionally, even if correctly identified, there is not much evidence that secondary prevention of high-risk patients will be successful in preventing chronicity.

CLINICAL TIP 21–1
A Plan of Action for Low Back Pain Patients

An effective method of reporting findings to orient patients to their low back problem is to forecast only 2 weeks in advance and to promise nothing except that the back problem will not harm them (this assumes, of course, that diagnostic triage to rule out red flags has been properly exercised). Further, lay out the patient's responsibilities for each 2-week time period, such as "Centralize any radiating leg pain, rest, and use ice/anti-inflammatory therapy for the first 2 days and try not to reproduce sharp, lancing pain in your activities. Walk within the tolerance of your condition, and be aware of danger signs such as progressive neurological loss, which may include foot drop, loss of bowel and bladder control, or retention."

If the patient is unable to work, setting a return-to-work goal is very important. Lay out the overall treatment goals such as:

- *Step 1:* Reassurance that the spine is not damaged and hurt does not necessarily equal harm
- *Step 2:* Pain control, activity modification advice, and gradual resumption of activities
- *Step 3:* Development of internal locus of control with general and specific exercises for increasing mobility and activity endurance

---

tients (Cherkin et al, 1996). Most people are satisfied with their care for hypertension, cancer, and other serious medical diseases. But 20% to 25% are dissatisfied with their medical care for back and neck pain (Deyo, 1996). Chiropractic treatment has higher satisfaction (refer to Chap. 9 for more information).

Typical complaints about medical management of back pain are that the patient received inadequate explanation of the problem; the health care provider (HCP) did not understand what was wrong with the patient's back at the end of the visit; or, too little time was spent with the HCP. Solutions to these complaints include providing reassurance that severe symptoms can be caused by benign conditions; reproducing the patient's pain by movements or palpations so he or she knows that you "found it"; offering a functional explanation about how lifestyle or occupational activities cause strain; and offering activity modification advice and pain relief strategies.

Seeing into the crystal ball with new patients is extremely difficult. With respect to the prognosis for a patient's current episode, the majority of patients are satisfied with their level of recovery by the 3-week mark if they have to live with it at this level the rest of their lives (Cherkin et al, 1996). However, approximately one third of patients are satisfied after only 1 week while another one third are still dissatisfied wtih their level of recovery after 7 weeks. At 1 year, the prognosis is favorable for the majority, as 85% were satisfied with their symptoms 1 year later. However, the one third who are still having trouble at 7 weeks are just as likely as not to have trouble at the 1-year point. Therefore, making an accurate prognosis is indeed uncertain, and increasing patient satisfaction is a great challenge. Giving all patients optimistic prognoses risks creating disappointment, anxiety, and even anger among the one third still suffering at 7 weeks. On the other hand, telling patients that there is a one third chance of a slow recovery may have a negative impact on patients whose problems resolve earlier. **While it is recommended that reassurance be given to the low back pain patient, caution must be exercised when reporting the prognosis to the patient.**

Presently, chronic patients (4 to 6 months) after a brief trial of chiropractic/rehabilitation are best managed with multidisciplinary care.

Customer satisfaction is one of the most important considerations in quality assurance. Cost containment without higher customer satisfaction is not going to result in long-term sustainable changes. Obviously, predicting who is more likely to either respond or not respond quickly results in more accurate advice being given. This can reduce frustration, disappointment, and even anger in pa-

Conclusion

Capturing risk factors of chronicity influences treatment decision making. In particular, it helps avoid both over treatment of low-risk individuals and undertreatment of high-risk individuals. In measuring the effectiveness of treatment with outcomes, it is not enough to classify patients as having red flags of disease, nerve root, or mechanical problems. The presence or absence of risk factors of chronicity (including yellow flags) must be documented in order to fairly compare outcome data in different patient groups.

Prognosis takes us into uncharted waters. There is

enough evidence to **suggest** that we can do better than at present. However, there is very little evidence to **prove** that we can do better, or that we are doing better. Outcomes-based research should begin to collect data about the patient's risk factors to better determine their validity. Linton points out that we are only about 75% accurate in predicting who will not recover (van den Hoogen et al, 1997). However, the shifting of available resources toward secondary prevention for those that are identified is warranted by the evidence and simple patient stratification techniques we have.

Some risk factors can be addressed with primary (healthy individual) or secondary preventive (acute patient) strategies. The strongest proof of the validity of such risk factors will be the change in recovery rate between individuals who have had the risk factors addressed and those who have not. Obviously, some risk factors are unchangeable—such as past history. In these cases, knowledge that the risk is present will help the HCP, patient, and third-party payer understand the reason for a possibly longer than normal duration of care.

Research about risk factors of chronicity is ready for use by treating HCPs. It influences our treatment choices and education of our patients. It also influences the justification for third-party payers to either pay more or less for an individual patient's care.

The failure to document the presence of these factors compromises the decision making process in regard to choosing the most appropriate care for each patient.

REFERENCES

Alaranta H, Rytokoski U, Rissanen A, et al. Intensive physical and psychosocial training program for patients with chronic low back pain. *Spine* 1994;19:1339–1349.

Bigos S, Bowyer O, Braen G, et al. *Acute Low Back Problems in Adults. Clinical Practice Guideline.* Rockville, Md: US Department of Health and Human Services, Public Health Service, Agency for Health Care Policy and Research; 1994.

Bolton JE. Evaluation of treatment of back pain patients: Clinical outcome measures. *Eur J Chiro* 1994;42:29–40.

Burke SA, Harms-Constas CK, Aden PS. Return to work/work retention outcomes of a functional restoration program. *Spine* 1994;17;1880–1886.

Burton AK, Tillotson K, Main C, Hollis M. Psychosocial predictors of outcome in acute and sub-acute low back trouble. *Spine* 1995;20:722–728.

Burton CV, Cassidy JD. Economics, epidemiology, and risk factors. In: Kirkaldy-Willis WH, Burton CV, eds. *Managing Low Back Pain.* 3rd ed. New York, NY: Churchill-Livingstone; 1992:2.

Butler RJ, Johnson WG, Baldwin ML. Managing work disability: Why first return to work is not a measure of success. *Ind Labor Rel Rev* 1995;48(3):452–469.

Cats-Baril WL, Frymoyer JW. Demographic factors associated with the prevalence of disability in the general population: Analysis of the NHANES I database. *Spine* 1991;16:671–674.

Cheadle A, Franklin G, Wolfhagen C, et al. Factors influencing the duration of work-related disability. *Am J Public Health* 1994;84(2);190–196.

Cherkin DC, Deyo RA, Street JH, Barlow W. Predicting poor outcomes for back pain seen in primary care using patients' own criteria. *Spine* 1996;21:2900–2907.

Cherkin DC, MacCornack. Patient evaluations of low back pain care from family physicians and chiropractors. *West J Med* 1989;51:355.

Croft PR, Macfarlane GJ, Papageorgiou AC, Thomas E, Silman AJ. Outcome of low back pain in general practice: A prospective study. *BMJ* 1998;316:1356–1359.

Cutler RB, Fishbain DA, Rosomoff HL, et al. Does nonsurgical pain center treatment of chronic pain return patients to work? A review and meta-analysis of the literature. *Spine* 1994;19:643–652.

Deyo RA. Low back pain—A primary care challenge. *Spine* 1996;21:2826–2832.

Flor H, Fydrick T, Turk DC. Efficacy of multidisciplinary pain treatment centers: A meta-analytic review. *Pain* 1992;49:221–230.

Fordyce WE, Brockway JA, Bergman JA, Spengler D. Acute back pain: A control-group comparison of behavioral vs traditional management methods. *J Behav Med* 1986;9:127–140.

Frank JW, Kerr MS, Brooker AS, et al. Disability resulting from occupational low back pain. Part 2: What do we know about secondary prevention? *Spine* 1996;21:2918–2929.

Frost H, Lamb SE, Klaber Moffett JA, Fairbank JCT, Moser JS. A fitness programme for patients with chronic low back pain: 2-year follow-up of a randomized controlled trial. *Pain* 1998;75:273–279.

Goosens MEJB, Evers SMAA. Economic evaluation of back pain interventions. *J Occup Rehab* 1997;7:15–32.

Hazard RG, Fenwick JW, Kalisch SM, et al. Functional restoration with behavioral support. *Spine* 1989;14:157–161.

Hazard RG, Haugh LD, Reid S, Preble JB, MacDonald L. Early prediction of chronic disability after occupational low back injury. *Spine* 1996;21:945–951.

Indahl A, Velund L, Reikeraas O. Good prognosis for low back pain when left untampered: A randomized clinical trial. *Spine* 1995;20:473–477.

Kendall NAS, Linton SJ, Main CJ. *Guide to Assessing Psychosocial Yellow Flags in Acute Low Back Pain: Risk Factors for Long-term Disability in Work Loss*. Wellington, NZ: Accident Rehabilitation and Compensation Insurance Corporation of New Zealand and the National Health Committee; 1997.

Klenerman L, Slade P, Stanley I, et al. The prediction of chronicity in patients with an acute attack of low back pain in a general practice setting. *Spine* 1995;20:478–484.

Lancourt J, Kettelhut M. Predicting return to work for lower back pain patients receiving worker's compensation. *Spine* 1992;17:629–640.

Lindstrom A, Ohlund C, Eek C, et al. Activation of subacute low back patients. *Phys Ther* 1992;4:279–293.

Linton SJ, Hallden K. Risk factors and the natural course of acute and recurrent musculoskeletal pain: Developing a screening instrument. Jensen TS, Turner JA, Wiesenfeld-Hallin Z, eds. *Proceedings of the 8th World Congress on Pain, Progress in Pain Research and Management*. vol 8. Seattle, Wash: IASP Press; 1997.

Linton SJ, Hallden BH. Can we screen for problematic back pain? A screening questionnaire for predicting outcome in acute and subacute back pain. *Clin J Pain* 1998;14:1–7.

Linton SL, Hellsing AL, Andersson D. A controlled study of the effects of an early active intervention on acute musculoskeletal pain problems. *Pain* 1993;54:353–359.

Linton SJ, Hellsing AL, Hallden K. A population based study of spinal pain among 35–45 year olds: Prevalance, sick leave, and health care utilization. *Spine* 1998; in press.

Malmivaara A, Hakkinen U, Aro T, et al. The treatment of acute low back pain—bed rest, exercises, or ordinary activity? *N Engl J Med* 1995;332:351–355.

Mayer TG, Gatchel RJ, Mayer H, et al. A prospective two-year study of functional restoration in industrial low back injury. *JAMA* 1987;258:1763–1767.

O'Sullivan P, Twomey L, Allison G. Evaluation of specific stabilizing exercise in the treatment of chronic low back pain with radiologic diagnosis of spondylolysis or spondylolysthesis. *Spine* 1997;24:2959–2967.

Reid S, Haugh LD, Hazard RG, Tripathi M. Occupational low back pain: Recovery curves and factors associated with disability. *J Occup Rehab* 1997;7:1–14.

Sachs BL, David JF, Olimpio D, et al. Spinal rehabilitation by work tolerance based on objective physical capacity assessment of dysfunction. *Spine* 1990;15:1325–1332.

Selim AJ, Xinhau SR, Graeme F, et al. The importance of radiating leg pain in assessing health outcomes among patients with low back pain. *Spine* 1998:23:470–474.

Shekelle PG, Adams AH, Chassin MR, et al. Spinal manipulation for low-back pain. *Ann Intern Med* 1992;117:590–598.

Spitzer WO, et al. Scientific monograph of the Quebec Task Force on Whiplash-Associated Disorders. *Spine* 1995;10:8S,1S–73S.

Timm KE. A randomized-control study of active and passive treatments for chronic low back pain following L5 laminectomy. *J Orthop Sports Phys Ther* 1994;20:276–286.

Triano J, McGregor M, Hondras MA, et al. Manipulative therapy vs education program in chronic low back pain. *Spine* 1995;20:948–954.

Troup JDG, Martin JW, Lloyd DCEF. Back pain in industry: A prospective survey. *Spine* 1981;6:61–69.

van den Hoogen HJM, Koes BW, Deville W, van Eijk JTM, Bouter LM. The prognosis of low back pain in general practice. *Spine* 1997;22:1515–1521.

van Tulder MW, Koes BW, Bouter LM. A cost of illness study of back pain in The Netherlands. *Pain* 1995;62:233–240.

Von Korff M, Deyo RA, Cherkin D, Barlow W. Back pain in primary care: Outcomes at 1 year. *Spine* 1993;18:855–862.

Von Korff M, Saunders K. The course of back pain in primary care. *Spine* 1996;21:2833–2839.

Waddell G, Feder G, McIntosh A, Lewis M, Hutchinson A. *Low Back Pain Evidence Review*. London: Royal College of General Practitioners; 1996.

Practical Reality: Commonly Asked Questions Regarding Outcomes Assessment

This section opens with Chapter 22, which discusses the "how to" of implementing an outcomes-based management system into the clinical setting. This includes a process of setting up your office to effectively implement outcomes management (OM) concepts, including methodologies for staff orientation and data collection. The ultimate goal of OM is to aggregate the data and arrive at specific conclusions that can be used to educate providers, insurers, and patients as to "best practice" protocols. Chapter 23 introduces one such process whereby outcome assessment data collected from large provider-based groups can be used to establish databases across disciplines and/or diagnosis in an attempt to arrive at a "best-practice" goal. The text concludes with Chapter 24, which is intended to stimulate the health care provider to consider the future with respect to outcomes-based practice and how the utilization of these methods enhances customer service.

CHAPTER 22

Putting Outcomes-based Management into Practice

STEVEN G. YEOMANS

INTRODUCTION

Perhaps one of the most important but frequently neglected tasks of clinical practice is properly educating the office staff to concepts of outcomes management as they apply to use of questionnaires and other outcomes assessment (OA) tools. Neglecting to perform this task may ultimately cause the health care provider (HCP) to fail in becoming "outcomes based." The information that follows is based on my own experience. The importance of staff education became very clear to me when I overheard one of my front office employees agreeing with a patient who expressed displeasure when asked to fill out several different instruments. My immediate reaction was disbelief, but I soon realized that I had never educated my staff regarding the importance and objectives of using OA tools. When I asked my staff if they understood why we ask patients to complete the questionnaires, the response was an emphatic "no." This was followed by a significant amount of complaining by a number of staff people, which prompted me to hold a special office meeting to review each questionnaire, discussing how it is clinically utilized and why it is important. This discussion included an explanation of each instrument, the goals each was intended to achieve, and how the information was used to make clinical decisions. We then held a workshop to establish appropriate dialogue that could be used in preparation for the next encounter with a frustrated patient. The change in patients' responses, once the proper dialogue was established, understood, and appreciated by my staff, was totally opposite to what had been taking place. **As a result, a greater degree of compliance and effort in completing the questionnaires resulted in collection of more meaningful data.**

PREPARING THE FRONT OFFICE FOR THE EVIDENCE-BASED PRACTICE

Creating an evidence-based practice involves preparing the office for this new approach:

- Ensure that all office staff members understand the importance and purpose of OA strategies that are implemented in the office.
- Hold workshops role-playing different scenarios involving disgruntled patients. Have one staff person take the role of the patient, arguing about completing the questionnaires. Discuss the approaches used by each staff person and identify the "best" responses to implement in the clinic. Write these approaches down for periodic review and to use in educating new staff members.
- Organize questionnaires and instruments in such a way that they are accessible to all staff members. All staff members must be aware of where each instrument can be found, both in hard copy and in electronic form.

The following paragraphs provide greater detail on and specific recommendations for carrying out these steps.

FRONT DESK PREPARATION AND ORGANIZATION

Separate the forms, instruments, or questionnaires into folders that can be easily accessed when needed. A lightweight, open hanging file system on wheels works well. In this system, the folders are exposed at the top and the entire "cart" is placed next to the front desk person for easy access. In a separate folder, create "new patient packets" of forms, which may include:

1. Biographical data
2. Review of systems
3. History, past history, occupational history, social history forms
4. Outcome forms such as:
   a. Triple or Quadruple Visual Analogue Scale (VAS) and pain drawing (see Appendix Form B–1)
   b. Oswestry Low Back Pain Disability Questionnaire (see Appendix Form C–2) or Neck Disability Index (Appendix Form C–10)
   c. A general health tool such as SF-36/HSQ 2-0 (see Appendix Forms A–1 through A–3); SF-12/HSQ-12 (version 2-0) (Appendix Form A–4); Dartmouth COOP Health Charts (see Fig. 5–1)

One approach that works well is to keep separate folders or packets for patients complaining of frequently seen conditions. For example, in a spine specialty practice, separate folders/packets can be created for patients who present with cervical spine and lumbar spine problems. In this way, when office traffic is busy, the staff person only has to access one folder for all the new patient forms, which are bundled into one packet. This type of system also allows for a certain degree of flexibility. For example, when a new patient does not complain of neck or low back pain but, instead, has a shoulder complaint, the staff member can replace the neck or low back condition-specific tool with a shoulder disability questionnaire (see Appendix Forms C–17 through C–20) before handing the packet to the patient.

Because there are so many questionnaires from which to choose, Table 22–1 purposely includes only a partial list of questionnaires that I have found useful. These are forms that my staff have placed into separate folders and keep in a vertical hanging file holder at the front desk for easy access. Additional forms that may be utilized are reviewed in detail in Chapters 5 through 7 and 14 through 22. It is recommended that all staff members become familiar with the many instruments that are available. The reader should recognize that the choices listed represent my own personal biases based on utilization of these particular tools. This selection is not meant to imply that these tests are better than others. Moreover, all forms should be reviewed before making a final decision as to which tests are the best for each HCP and his or her respective needs.

COMMON PROBLEMS ASSOCIATED WITH OUTCOMES GATHERING STRATEGIES

It is important to be sure that all members of the office staff are prepared to deal with the problems that may arise in gathering outcomes data. Two general areas in which problems commonly arise include patient tolerance and HCP tolerance. The paragraphs that follow describe these potential problems in greater detail.

PATIENT TOLERANCE

Because so much of outcomes management depends on the use of pen-and-paper tools, a helpful hint in maintaining patient tolerance in the process of completing all the paperwork is to **offer the patient a clipboard** that holds all the forms. The patient should not be allowed to wait more than 15 minutes in the waiting room for the following reasons:

- A short attention span on the part of the patient; more accurate data is gathered if the collection period is spread out over time
- Time taken away from the history and examination time period (ie, the HCP falls behind schedule)

Patients can then take the clipboard of forms with them as they are transferred to the area where the history is gath-

Table 22–1: Selected Condition-specific Questionnaires For a Front-desk Filing System[a]

ANATOMICAL FOCUS	QUESTIONNAIRE
Lumbar spine	Oswestry Low Back Pain Disability Questionnaire (Form C–2)
	Roland-Morris (Form C–1)
	(See Appendix Forms C–3 to C–9 for more options)
Cervical spine	Neck Disability Index (Form C–10)
Temporomandibular joint	TMD Disability Questionnaire (Form C–15)
Headaches	Headache Disability Questionnaire (Form C–11)
	(see Forms C–12 to C–14 for dizziness, tinnitus, and hearing handicap inventories, respectively)
Shoulder	Shoulder Self-Assessment of Function (Form C–17)
	(see Forms C–18 to C–20 for more options)
Wrist	Carpal Tunnel Syndrome Questionnaire (Form C–16)
Hip	Rating of Hip Replacement Results (Form C–24)
Knee	Knee/Patellofemoral Questionnaire (Form C–21)
	Subjective Knee Score Questionnaire (Form C–22)
	Rating of Knee Replacement Results (Form C–23)
General health tools	SF-36/HSQ 2-0; Dartmouth COOP Health Charts (Fig. 5–1)

[a] It is recommended that the forms be placed in separate folders and inserted in an open hanging file holder on wheels which is placed in close proximity to the front desk person.

ered. If the HCP is behind schedule, the patient can continue to complete the questionnaires while waiting. Similarly, if x-rays or other tests are ordered, the patient can continue the paperwork while x-rays are being developed. In my experience, the majority of patients can complete the paperwork by the time they are ready to leave the office. If they have not finished all the paperwork, they can take it home and return it during the following visit. Another option is to send the patient the paperwork before his or her appointment so it can be completed at the patient's leisure and later brought back to the office. The problem with the latter approach is that the patient may fail to complete the work, forget to return it, and/or be so delayed in presenting to the clinic that the history reported is obsolete.

CLINICAL TIP 22–1
Organizing Questionnaire Files for Flexibility

Frequently, staff personnel forget to give the patient a questionnaire or give them the wrong tool. In addition, patients sometimes mention a new condition to the HCP that was not previously mentioned to the front office staff person. It is recommended that a folder containing several copies of each questionnaire, separated by dividers, be kept in the consultation/examination areas so that the HCP can easily access them when needed.

HEALTH CARE PROVIDER TOLERANCE

It can be quite frustrating for the HCP when patients identify problems in addition to those they mentioned to the front office staff person when first presenting. Because this often occurs, a folder containing several copies of each questionnaire should be kept in the consultation room so that additional forms can be easily accessed by the HCP. If a questionnaire is not available in the HCP folder, it can be ordered via the patient's route slip or some other method of communicating with the front office.

It is also very helpful to emphasize the importance of the questionnaires and to thank the patient for taking the time to complete the forms. **Point out to the patient that the information derived from the questionnaires helps to identify treatment goals by quantifying the activity intolerance.** As a result, the information helps guide the HCP through care and ensures that the patient's goals are being met. This explanation can really help the patient understand how and why the questionnaires are used clinically. Hence, compliance and effort in completing the forms is enhanced. **It is also becoming more common for some insurers, health maintenance organization (HMO) or preferred provider organization (PPO) groups, to demand the use of outcome tools. Therefore, alerting the patient that coverage may be pending if the tools are not completed can also help stimulate patient compliance.** If the patient is unable to complete the questionnaires or if enough time has not been set aside to complete them all during the initial office visit, the questionnaires may be taken home and returned upon the patient's next visit. This is not usually necessary unless additional forms are required to be completed that were given to the patient later in the initial visit.

OUTCOME TOOLS: WHICH ARE APPROPRIATE?

It is very important for the HCP to understand that in order to become outcomes based, the same questionnaires that were used initially must be repeated at a later date and the results compared to the initial findings. In general, the following categories of outcome tools and the associated questionnaire options are recommended for initial use (see Table 22–3 for additional information):

1. A general health questionnaire
   a. SF-36/HSQ 2-0 or SF-12/HSQ 12
   b. Dartmouth COOP health charts
2. A pain measuring tool
   a. Pain drawing
   b. Numerical Pain Scale (NPS)
   c. Verbal Rating Scale (VRS)
   d. Visual Analogue Scale (VAS)
   e. McGill Pain Questionnaire
3. A condition-specific tool
   a. Low Back Pain Disability Questionnaires (Oswestry or Roland-Morris)
   b. Neck Disability Index
   c. Extremity disability tools

On follow-up examinations, the same tools or questionnaires are appropriate with the exception of an entire general health questionnaire, as only some of its scales are sensitive to change over time. More specifically, of the eight scales that make up the SF-36, only three change much in a short time frame. These include: Physical Function, Bodily Pain, and Role—Physical. The remaining five scales do not change signficantly over a short time period and may be omitted in the re-examination if desired. However, I find it clinically useful to include all eight scales at the point of discharge or treatment conclusion. This may

help establish a baseline level that may be useful for comparison at the time of a future presentation. Because the titles of some of the general health scales are not the same, Table 22–2 offers a comparison of the titles; the boldface items are the most sensitive to change over time.

If a condition-specific questionnaire is available for use in assessing a specific body region that is injured, it is probably not necessary to repeat any part of the general health questionnaire again until discharge. This is because activity intolerance outcomes (numbers 1 and 2 on Table 22–2) can be captured by a more condition-specific instrument than a general health questionnaire. Similarly, bodily pain, or number 3 of Table 22–2, can be tracked using a numerical pain scale for pain, thus reducing the need for the use of the Bodily Pain scale included in the general health questionnaire. However, it must be understood that something will be lost if the tool is not readministered until discharge. Quality of life issues that are captured by a general health questionnaire will not be reassessed until case closure. Therefore, each case should be individually assessed regarding when to readminister the general health tool that the patient completed at the initial visit. Table 22–3 offers options for **when** each instrument could be performed.

The best or most applicable tool to utilize may differ significantly in different clinical settings. It has been my experience that the tools listed in Tables 22–1 and 22–3 work well in an ambulatory musculoskeletal type of practice. On the other hand, in an internal medicine practice, a general health tool may be the best and only applicable tool as a search for OA tools does not reveal any condition-specific instruments for different organic conditions. Therefore, it is important to apply the most logical tool to the individual patient as it may be quite misleading to follow a "recipe" such as that offered in Table 22–3 if the clinical setting is quite different from an ambulatory musculoskeletal practice.

CHART ORGANIZATION

Just as it is necessary to be acquainted with the outcome tools most applicable to the type of practice in which the

Table 22–2: Comparison of Scale Titles for Three Popular General Health Questionnaires[a]

SF-36	HSQ 2-0	DARTMOUTH COOP HEALTH CHARTS
1. **Physical Functioning**	**Physical Functioning**	**Physical fitness**
2. **Role—Physical**	**Role—Physical**	**Daily Activities**
3. **Bodily Pain**	**Bodily Pain**	**Pain**
4. General Health	Health Perception	Overall Health
5. Vitality	Energy/Fatigue	—
6. Social Functioning	Social Functioning	Social Activities
7. Role—Emotional	Role—Emotional	Feelings
8. Mental Health	Mental Health	Feelings

[a] Items in bold type are more sensitive to change over time compared to the others (NA = not available).

Table 22–3: Options for Use of Condition-specific Questionnaires[a]

TEST	FIRST VISIT	EACH OFFICE VISIT	RE-EXAM AT 2–4 WEEKS	EXACERBATIONS	END OF CARE
Pain	X		X	X	X
Pain drawing	a		a	a	a
VAS	b		b	b	b
NPS	c	X	c	c	c
General Health	X		Case specific		X
HSQ	a				a
COOP	b				b
Condition-Specific	X		X	X	X
Oswestry LBP Questionnaire	a		a	a	a
Neck Disability Index	b		b	b	b
Patient Satisifaction			X		X
Chiropractic Satisfaction			a		a
Visit-specific Questionnaire			b		b
Patient Satisfaction Questionnaire			c		c
Psychometric			Possibly		Possibly
Waddell's			a		a
Beck's, Zung, etc			b		b
Total	3	1	3 or 4	2	4 or 5

HSQ, health status questionnaire; LBP, low back pain; NPS, Numerical Pain Scale; VAS, Visual Analogue Scale.
[a] Options a, b, or c can be used for the main category listed (bold). It is not appropriate to administer all of the available options, only the one utilized initially. It is necessary to stay with the original choice for follow-up evaluations, as the instruments are not interchangeable.

HCP is engaged, it is also necessary to be able to access the information derived from the outcome tools in an easy manner. Chart organization can make the ability to review the outcome information easy or difficult, depending on how the patient information is set up. Table 22–4 contains recommendations for a possible method of chart organization.

The objective of chart organization is to be able to locate files quickly and efficiently. This will allow the HCP to answer questions by quickly locating documents within the file, especially the Outcomes Assessment Record (see Appendix Form H–4). The latter is particularly important as a summary of all the scores generated from the various

Table 22–4: An Optional Method of Chart Organization[a]

LEFT-HAND SIDE (FROM FRONT TO BACK)	RIGHT-HAND SIDE (FROM FRONT TO BACK)
1. Physical therapy log: allows modality details to be kept in one location (Appendix Form I–1)	1. Daily SOAP notes—handwritten (Appendix Form J–4)
2. Outcomes assessment (OA) record (Appendix Form H–4)	2. New patient history and past history forms (Appendix Forms J–5A through D)
3. General health OA record (Appendix Form A–3)	3. First color-coded tab (yellow): dictation
4. Nutritional/medication log (Appendix Form J–2)	4. Second tab (blue): X-ray report (see Appendix Form J–6 for example)
5. Biographical data: insurance card copy, name, address, phone numbers, x-ray number, SS number (can be part of Appendix Form J–3)	5. Third tab (green): referral reports/letters from outside sources (lab reports, special tests); outside patient records
6. Letters to insurance company, attorneys, etc	6. Fourth tab (red): Work restriction forms (see Appendix Form J–7)
7. Copies of records log (Appendix Form J–3)	7. Miscellaneous

[a] This approach may require significant alterations, dependent on the patient and practice type.

Table 22–6: Clinical Decision Making Arising from Various Treatment Options[a]

TREATMENT OUTCOME	MANAGEMENT OPTION
1. Condition resolved	Discharge
2. Condition improved, but not at MTB	Continue care with gradual transition into active from passive care
3. Condition improved, but has reached MTB	Wean the patient away from regimented passive care, emphasizing self-administered active care
	Consider a supervised active care program if poor activity tolerance and/or poor patient satisfaction
4. Condition unchanged	Change treatment protocols every 2 weeks for 4 weeks maximum; consider:
	• Reassess red flags
	• Identify yellow flags and institute a problem-focused treatment plan considering co-treatment or referral (see Chapters 19 and 20)
	• Obtain second-opinion
	• Discharge with coping-strategies addressed
	• Refer to a tertiary care center
5. Condition worse	• Consider referral to specialty service
	• Reassess red and yellow flags

MTB, maximum therapeutic benefit.

[a] Clinical decisions arise as a result of one of the five treatment outcomes described in the left-hand column; management options are located in the right.

CODING AND DOCUMENTATION

The use of codes when rendering services is very important so that the HCP can be properly reimbursed for the work that he or she performs. An integral step to the process of reimbursement is the use of the route slip, which is the primary form of communication between the HCP and the front desk. For example, when a patient is evaluated, the front office staff needs to obtain the following information from the HCP:

- The **evaluation and management (EM)** level of service (coding options include 99201–99205 for new patients and 99211–99215 for established patients) (ChiroCode, 1998)
- All forms of treatment rendered that visit, which are reported by **Current Procedural Terminology (CPT)** codes
- The laboratory, x-ray, or other diagnostic study completed that visit
- Any durable medical equipment such as orthotics, braces, splints, casts, and so on
- The diagnosis, which is reported in ICD-9 codes (this is often restricted to four codes due to the HCFA 1500 standard insurance form limitations)
- The date of accident/incident
- The future treatment schedule

Failure to communicate the services that were performed in a particular visit will result in improper reimbursement. Moreover, a delay in the posting of the daily business entries occurs when there are omissions or errors in communication. Therefore, the economic impact of a poor

line of communication between the HCP and the front office can be significant and can directly affect the success or failure of the practice.

Integral to the success of the communication between HCP and front office is the route slip. A route slip must be designed to allow for as many services as the HCP provides. The layout should be logical and simple, with items arranged in a manner that catches the HCP's attention so the entries are completed. The success of a route slip comes with practice: Using the form frequently leads to familiarity with the items it contains, and soon they become second nature. An example of a route slip is located in Appendix Form J–8.

Probably the most common services offered by HCPs who practice with a musculoskeletal emphasis are those described in ICD-9 and CPT coding language in the physical medicine and rehabilitation services section of the book. However, the type of practice will direct each HCP to the CPT codes that are tailored to his or her own specialty. The use of modalities is common in the physical medicine and rehabilitation practice. These modalities may include any physical agent that produces therapeutic changes to biological tissues. Examples include the use of light, thermal, mechanical, acoustic, and electrical energy. Modalities can be unsupervised (unattended) or require constant attendance. Table 22–7 includes various modalities, the associated CPT codes, and the associated relative value unit (RVU). **The RVU generally refers to the value of a service as it compares to a standard office visit fee.**

Therapeutic procedures can be described as the manner of effecting change through the application of clinical skills and/or services that attempt to improve function. These types of services require direct (one-on-one) patient contact by an HCP or therapist. Therapeutic procedures

EXAMPLE SOAP Note _____

NAME: Ken Esthetic   **Insurance:** WC   **DATE:** 4-2-98   **BD:** 1-19-55   **AGE:** 43

Dx: LBP w/o leg pain   **Test #:** ①, 2, 3, 4   **Symptom Duration:** 3 weeks

Prior Episodes: (YES)/NO (>4 prior episodes in last 12 months)

10-30-98

S. Patient presents with… *(the historical information: injury history, chief and secondary complaints using for example, the O, P, Q, R, S, T, U, approach; past history, review of systems, etc. are dictated or referenced here).* Outcomes assessment (OA) questionnaires were utilized in today's re-examination. The following OA tools and respective dates are as follows (also shown in Table 22-5):

DATE	PAIN			FUNCTION			
	VAS a. Now b. Ave. c. Range CC: LBP	Pain Drawing	Options: 1. UE 2. CTS 3. Shoulder 4. Knee	Options: 1. Headache 2. Dizziness 3. SCL-90R 4. _____	VAS & Neck Disability (NDI)	VAS & LB Disability: • Oswestry • Roland M	Patient Satisfaction
BASELINE							
8/12/98	a. 8/10 b. 7/10 c. 5–10/10	Physiological (1. Yes) 2. No	1. ____ % 2. Sx ____ % Fn ____ % 3. ____ % 4. ____ %	1. T__ ;E__ Fnctn ____ 2. T__ ;P__ F__ ;E__ 3. A__ ;D__ 4. ____	a. ____ /10 b. ____ /10 c. __-__ /10 NA %	a. 8/10 b. 7/10 a. 5–10/10 72 %	
PROGRESS							
8/26/98	a. 3/10 b. 2/10 c. 0–6/10	Physiological (1. Yes) 2. No	1. ____ % 2. Sx ____ % Fn ____ % 3. ____ % 4. ____ %	1. T__ ;E__ Fnctn ____ 2. T__ ;P__ F__ ;E__ 3. A__ ;D__ 4. ____	a. ____ /10 b. ____ /10 c. __-__ /10 NA %	a. 3/10 b. 2/10 a. 0–6/10 40 %	92%
9/18/98	a. 1/10 b. 2/10 c. 0–3/10	Physiological (1. Yes) 2. No	1. ____ % 2. Sx ____ % Fn ____ % 3. ____ % 4. ____ %	1. T__ ;E__ Fnctn ____ 2. T__ ;P__ F__ ;E__ 3. A__ ;D__ 4. ____	a. ____ /10 b. ____ /10 c. __-__ /10 NA %	a. 1/10 b. 2/10 a. 0–3/10 16 %	98%

O. Physical examination reveals: vital signs as follows… (insert height, weight, BP, pulse, respiration, temperature, age). Observation (expand), palpation (expand), auscultation (expand), ROM (expand), Ortho. (expand), Neuro. (expand) Physical performance tests (QFCE) evaluated today reveal the following (note: those tests ≤85% of "normal" are considered abnormal and are circled and highlighted in the right hand column) (time spent with patient - 97750, 3 units/45 minutes):

Figure 22–1. The inclusion of outcomes data derived from both subjective and objective sources can greatly enhance the quality of the office record. This is one example of how to implement the information effectively for ease of review (*continued*).

commonly used in a musculoskeletal type of practice are located in Table 22–8.

Other services and associated CPT codes that can be utilized by HCPs who practice with a musculoskeletal emphasis include tests and measurement procedures (Table 22–9). For example, the quantitative functional capacity

evaluation (QFCE), described in Chapter 16, utilizes physical performance tests and, therefore, can be coded specifically under the CPT code 97750, and reported in 15-minute units (4 units = 1 hour). Typically, the QFCE takes between 35 and 45 minutes to perform, and another 15 minutes to calculate the percent differences between the

TEST NAME	NORMAL	PATIENT RESULT		PERCENT OF NORMAL	
1. VAS (Pain level: 0–10 scale)	0/10	2 /10		NA	
2. Repetitive Squat*	45 / (max 50)	42 / (45)		93%	
3. ROM/Lumbar Spine					
Flexion	65°	56 °		86%	
Extension	30°	25 °		83%	
Rt. Lateral Flexion	25°	27 °		108%	
Lt. Lateral Flexion	25°	28 °		112%	
4. Waddell #1: Pain	Negative	Negative		NA	
5. Waddell #2: Simulation	Negative	Negative		NA	
6. Gastrocnemius/Ankle DF	22.5 +/– 0.7 (23)	Lt.: 21	Rt.: 24	91%	104%
7. Soleus/Ankle DF	24.9 +/– 0.8 (25)	Lt.: 23	Rt.: 26	92%	104%
8. Sitting SLR/Distraction w/ #13	LBP: YES/NO	LBP: YES/*NO*		LBP: YES/NO	
9. Waddell #4: Regional Neuro	Negative	Positive		NA	
10. Waddell #5: Exaggeration	Negative	Positive		NA	
11. ROM/Cervical					
Flexion	50°	56 °		112%	
Extension	63°	58 °		92%	
Rt. Lateral Flexion	45°	44 °		98%	
Lt. Lateral Flexion	45°	42 °		93%	
Rt. Rotation	85°	78 °		92%	
Lt. Rotation	85°	82 °		96%	
12. Modified Thomas					
Hip Extension	84°	Lt.: 76	Rt.: 64	90%	76%
13a. Waddell #3: Distraction	Negative	Positive**		NA	
13b. Straight Leg Raise*	70–90°	Lt.: 76	Rt.: 70	100%	100%
14. Repetitive Sit-Up*	34 / (max 50)	46 / (max 50)		135%	
15. Knee Flexion	147° +/– 1.6	Lt.: 126°	Rt.: 135°	86%	92%
16. Repetitive Arch-Up*	36 / (max 50)	45 / (max 50)		125%	
17. Hip Rotation ROM					
Internal Rotation ROM	41–45 (43)	Lt.: 40	Rt.: 43	93%	100%
External Rotation ROM	41–43 (42)	Lt.: 41	Rt.: 43	98%	102%
18. Static Back Endurance*	129 (max. 240 sec.)	96 seconds		74%	
19. Grip Strength*	Lt.: 47 Kg | Rt.: 49 Kg	Lt.: 52 Kg | Rt.: 58 Kg		111%	118%
20. Outcome Instrument(s)					
• Oswestry LB Disability Ques.	0/50 (0%)	NA		NA	
• Neck Disability Index	0/50 (0%)	14%		See summary chart	
• General Health					
☐ SF-36, HSQ, Rand-36 (circle)				See summary chart	
☐ Dartmouth COOP Charts				See summary chart	
☐ Other: _____				See summary chart	
21. Post-test VAS	0/10	1 /10		NA	

*Normative data is determined by age, sex and occupation (Blue vs. white collar: BC/WC) (Alaranta, et al)
**A positive test #13 (Supine SLR) and a negative sitting/distracted SLR (test #8) = +Waddell sign for Distraction

A. Lumbar sprain/strain improving, but <u>NOT</u> at a firm point of maximum therapeutic benefit. Mr. Esthetic continues to be working with restrictions and intermittent partially disabling exacerbations. He has been compliant with treatment, ergonomic modifications and home-based exercises.

Physical performance tested today due to ongoing activity intolerance, utilizing the QFCE reveals (in decreasing order of severity):
• Weakness of the low back extensor musculature (test #19) 96 sec./74% norm
• Tightness Rt. Iliopsoas muscle (modified Thomas test #12) 64°/76% norm
• Lumbar extension ROM (test #3) is limited to 25°/83% norm

Summary: Deconditioning is supported by the objective findings of weakness and poor endurance of the core extensor musculature of the trunk, tightness of the iliopsoas, and limited lumbar extension ROM. Rehabilitation of these functional deficiencies is indicated due to ongoing disabilities in spite of active and passive care.

Figure 22–1. (*Continued*).

P. Treatment plan:

OPTION 1: Treatment plan will now gradually shift from passive care to active care. Rehabilitation approaches will be performed in a one-on-one exercise training, 30 minute sessions (2 units) of functional restoration (97530). Protocols will address the functional deficiencies determined in the QFCE. Frequency of rehabilitation will be 3x/wk for 2 to 4 weeks progressively increasing the level of difficulty. Once competence is observed, the protocol will be performed at home and QFCE reassessment will be completed in approximately 4 weeks. Please refer to the rehabilitation notes for a description of the specific protocol utilized.

OPTION 2 (if a one-on-one facility is not available or clinically necessary):
Specific exercises performed with the patient today included iliopsoas muscle stretch using post-isometric relaxation self-applied, and a half sit-up from a gymnastic ball held for a count of "10". He was able to perform these exercises in my presence and was therefore instructed to perform the same at home. A gym ball was issued and the exercises will be reviewed at the time of our next visit to insure accuracy of the technique.

Passive care: today consisted of… (expand: list of all passive treatment protocols utilized if applicable). Total time spent with patient 1.5 hours.

HPC signature or initials

Figure 22–1. (*Continued*).

CTS, carpal tunnel syndrome; LBP, low back pain; NA, not applicable; SCL, Symptom Check List; Sx, symptoms; UE, upper extremity; VAS, Visual Analogue Scale.

Table 22–7: Physical Medicine and Rehabilitation Services Commonly Used in a Musculoskeletal Practice[a]

SUPERVISED MODALITIES

Code	Description	RVU
97010	Hot or cold packs	.28
97012	Traction, mechanical	.46
97014	Electrical stimulation (unattended)	.40
97016	Vasopneumatic devices	.44
97018	Paraffin bath	.30
97020	Microwave	.28
97022	Whirlpool	.38
97024	Diathermy	.28
97026	Infrared	.27
97028	Ultraviolet	.28

CONSTANT ATTENDANCE

Code	Description	RVU
97032	Electrical stimulation (manual), each 15 minutes	.41
97033	Iontophoresis, each 15 minutes	.44
97034	Contrast baths, each 15 minutes	.34
97035	Ultrasound, each 15 minutes	.35
97036	Hubbard tank, each 15 minutes	.52
97039	Unlisted attended modality (specify type and time)	.45

[a] The use of modalities in a musculoskeletal practice is common. Various attended and unattended or supervised modalities are described. The relative value units (RVUs) are located in the right-hand column.

Data compiled from ChiroCode DeskBook: The Seventh Annual Coding and Reimbursement Guide for Chiropractors. *7th ed. Phoenix, Ariz: Leavitt Crandall Institute; 1999.*

Table 22–8: Therapeutic Procedures Commonly Used in a Musculoskeletal Practice[a]

CODE	DESCRIPTION	RVU
97110	Therapeutic exercises to develop strength and endurance, range of motion, and flexibility	.62
97112	Neuromuscular re-education of movement, balance, coordination, kinesthetic sense, posture, and proprioception, each 15 minutes	.60
97113	Aquatic therapy with therapeutic exercises, each 15 minutes	.67
97116	Gait training (includes stair climbing), each 15 minutes	.54
97124	Massage, including effleurage, pertrissage, and/or tapotement (stroking, compression, percussion), each 15 minutes	.49
97139	Unlisted therapeutic procedure (specify), each 15 minutes	.39
97140	Manual therapy techniques (eg, mobilization/manipulation, manual lymphatic drainage, manual traction), one or more regions, each 15 minutes	.63
97150	Therapeutic procedure(s), group (2 or more individuals)	.49
97504	Orthotics fitting and training upper and/or lower extremities; each 15 minutes	.62
97520	Prosthetic fitting and training upper and/or lower extremities; each 15 minutes	.63
97530	Therapeutic activities, direct (one-on-one) patient contact by the provider (use of dynamic activities to improve functional performance), each 15 minutes	.63
97535	Self-care/home management training (eg, activities of daily living and compensatory training, meal preparation, safety procedures, and instructions in use of adaptive equipment) direct one-on-one contact by the provider, each 15 minutes	.64
97537	Community/work reintegration training (eg, shopping, transportation, money management, avocational activities, and/or work environment/modification analysis), work task analysis, direct one-on-one contact by the provider, each 15 minutes	.64
97542	Wheelchair management/propulsion training, each 15 minutes	.44
97545	Work hardening/conditioning; initial 2 hours	NE
97546	Each additional hour	NE

NE, not established.

[a] A listing of treatment services is found in this table with the associated CPT code number.

Data compiled from ChiroCode DeskBook: The Seventh Annual Coding and Reimbursement Guide for Chiropractors. 7th ed. Phoenix, Ariz: Leavitt Crandall Institute; 1999.

normative data and the patient's results and document the results. If a summary report is then dictated, another 15 additional minutes will be required to input the data into a template summary form. Therefore, 4 to 5 units may be recorded to complete the service at an RVU of .72. Hypothetically, if 1 RVU is $40, 4 to 5 units equal $160 to $200. Using the RVU of .72 would result in a billing of $115.20 to $144 for this service. Table 22–9 includes CPT codes associated with tests and measures as well as other procedures that fall into a "miscellaneous" type of category.

OVERVIEW OF COMMON REHABILITATION CODES AND SERVICES

It is beyond the scope of this chapter to fully discuss each of the services included in Table 22–8. However, a short description of some of the services is included, as many of these services are commonly performed in a rehabilitation setting. It is recommended that other texts be utilized that more fully address the rehabilitation techniques represented by the following codes (Liebenson, 1996; Stude, 1999).

Neuromuscular Re-education (97112)

Motor and/or sensory retraining following an **upper motor neuron (UMN)** or a **lower motor neuron (LMN)** lesion or injury are both included under the neuromuscular re-education (NMR) code, 97112: "Neuromuscular re-education of movement, balance, coordination, . . ." Examples of techniques often employed under the NMR heading include the following:

- Proprioceptive neuromuscular facilitation (PNF)
- Contract hold (CH)
- Postisometric relaxation (PIR)
- Eccentric stretch and strengthening procedures
- Concentric stretch and strengthening procedures

In UMN lesions, the goal of therapy is to retrain the motor and sensory side of the neurological loop. Additional techniques can include primitive reflex stimulation (Voita), posture retraining, and/or proprioception stimulation. Various low-tech tools that facilitate the rehabilitation process include (but are not limited to) the following:

Table 22–9: Other Services Commonly Used in a Musculoskeletal Practice[a]

TESTS AND MEASUREMENTS[b]

Code	Description	RVU
97703	Checkout for orthotic/prosthetic use, established patient, each 15 minutes	.44
97750	Physical performance test or measurement (eg, musculoskeletal, functional; capacity), with written report, each 15 minutes	.70

OTHER PROCEDURES

Code	Description	RVU
97770	Development of cognitive skills to improve attention, memory, problem solving, includes compensatory training and/or sensory integrative activities, direct (one-on-one) patient contact by the provider, each 15 minutes	.72
97780[c]	Acupuncture, one or more needles; without electrical stimulation	NE
97781[c]	With electrical stimulation	NE
97799	Unlisted physical medicine service or procedure	NE

NE, not established.

[a] When tests or measures are performed, specific CPT codes can be assigned to the service. When other services such as acupuncture are performed, CPT codes specific to those services are also available.

[b] For muscle testing, manual or electrical, joint range of motion, electromyography or nerve velocity determination, see 95831–95904.

[c] New codes (1998).

Data compiled from ChiroCode DeskBook: The Seventh Annual Coding and Reimbursement Guide for Chiropractors. 7th ed. Phoenix, Ariz: Leavitt Crandall Institute; 1998.

- Rocker/wobble board
- Tubing exercises
- Gait/posture training using wobble sandals

Modalities that can be utilized include (partial list):

- Electrical muscle stimulation (EMS; low-frequency alternating current [AC])
- High-volt
- Russian stimulation and/or interferential current (IFC)

In LMN lesions, the goal of NMR is to restore peripheral nerve function, tendon/ligament control, muscle imbalances, postural faults, loss of muscle strength, power, and endurance. Techniques may include various forms of muscle strengthening such as isometric, isotonic, and/or isokinetic; PNF and other manual resistance techniques, and balance/proprioception retraining. Tools that may be used include the following:

- Rocker/wobble board
- Tubing exercises
- Gait/posture training using wobble sandals

Modalities that can be utilized include (partial list):

- EMS (low-frequency direct or AC)
- High-volt
- Russian stimulation and/or IFC
- Microcurrent electronic nerve stimulator (MENS)

Therapeutic Activities (97530)

The therapeutic activity procedural code is reserved for use when direct one-on-one patient contact by the provider is performed in a rehabilitation setting. This procedure includes the use of dynamic activities that are specifically taught to improve the functional performance of a patient. Medical necessity is established by the documentation inclusion of abnormal physical performance findings (such as the QFCE tests; see Chap. 16) in the O (objective) portion of the SOAP note. Although each case must be considered individually prior to use of this level of service, typically a home-based exercise program has already been ordered. Despite this, however, the patient's activity intolerance and functional deficiencies may continue. Therefore, a supervised rehabilitation approach may be necessary to avoid exacerbation of the patient's condition by performance of exercises using improper technique, as well as to carefully guide the patient through specific exercise approaches that have not yet been addressed. This level of rehabilitation is usually reserved for difficult-to-manage cases in which preinjury status has not been reached and maximum therapeutic benefit is nearing. The algorithm in Figure 22–2 illustrates a clinical example of when this procedural code could be utilized. It must be emphasized, however, that each case must be individually assessed regarding "medical necessity" for rehabilitation services rather than making hard-and-fast rules that are adopted across the board. There are simply too many biological variances in presenting patients to use "recipe therapy," as different responses will require different treatment approaches.

Table 22–10: Examples of Objective Findings That Help Support "Medical Necessity" for Use of a Procedure[a]

OBJECTIVE (O)	ASSESSMENT (A)	PLAN (P)
Trigger points, muscle spasm, muscle cramp	(729.1) Myofascitis (729.82) Muscle cramp	97140 (MTT)[b] (97124) Massage (97112) NMR
Proprioception loss (one-legged stand test 3 seconds/eye closed—left)	(781.3) Lack of coordination	(97116)[b] Gait training
Weak/poor strength and endurance (repetitive squat, 22 repetitions, 46% of normal)	(728.2) Disuse atrophy and/or (728.9) weak muscle	(97110) Therapeutic exercise or (97530) therapeutic activities
Positive Phalen's test (3 seconds) and median nerve compression test in 4 seconds	(354.4) Carpal tunnel syndrome (due to repetitive motion ergonomic stressors)	(97537)[b] Work task analysis (97140)[b] MTT (active release technique)
1. Joint instability—x-ray, motion palpation 2. Painful flat fleet—TPs plantar muscle	(718.8) Instability (728.71) Plantar fascitis	(97507)[b] Orthotic fitting and training
Limited shoulder ROM	(726.0) Adhesive capsulitis	(97140)[b] Joint mobilization, or (98943) joint manipulation (CMT code; use 98943–51 if performed with spinal manipulation)
Short hamstring muscles, poor strength/endurance	(728.89) Contraction hamstring (728.9) Weak muscle	(97750)[b] Physical performance test or measurement

MTT, manual therapy techniques; NMR, neuromuscular re-education; ROM, range of motion.
[a] The presence of objective findings in a musculoskeletal complaint is needed to support "medical necessity" for the use of a procedure. Several examples of the O, A, and P portions of a SOAP note are included.
[b] Specify number of 15-minute units.

technologies. It is helpful to assume the role of a reviewer and critique your own notes periodically. An even more effective quality control technique is to obscure the name of the patient and see if you can tell who the patient is by the specific documented information. When patient identification can be ascertained by this approch, the records are typically successful in "telling a story." Other self-review issues to consider include correlating the subjective complaints with the objective findings, assessment, and treatment plan.

Make sure the billed services are included in the plan portion of the note. Also, determine the calendar of events with respect to the status of the patient at different points in time (eg, at the 2-, 4-, or 6-week points). This task helps reinforce the importance of outcomes data, as it is much easier to determine patient status when activity intolerance is quantified. Refer to Sections II and III of this text for a thorough discussion of subjective and objective outcomes measures that are practical for documentation purposes.

Conclusion

The goal of this chapter has been to offer information that can be used to facilitate the process of becoming outcomes based in a clinical setting. This text has introduced many tools that can be utilized in gathering outcomes data, and this chapter aims to help the HCP develop a method of implementing outcomes management into the clinical setting.

This process begins with the front office staff and their ability to "sell" the concept of outcomes management to the presenting patient. This step is critical, as patient attitude when completing these tools can result in a good or a poor effort, depending on whether pa-

tients feel the information is important or not. **The validity and reliability of the outcomes information pivots around the accuracy and effort the patient exerts when completing the tools.** Explaining the importance of outcomes data and its relationship to optimal care can also reduce patient anxieties as, in general, few people enjoy paperwork. The issues of patient and HCP tolerance were also discussed as well as steps required to minimize frustration centered around outcomes gathering.

Next, a review of the tools that are required for implementing outcomes data collection into a practice

Conclusion (*continued*)

setting and a time line for gathering data were included. The importance of a systematic method of organizing a chart was discussed and a method offered. The ability to quickly access information for ease of case orientation and communication was stressed with respect to chart organization, and a sample case and SOAP note example were given. The use of a route slip to enhance communication between HCP and the front office, and the importance of CPT procedural codes included on the route slip were discussed. Finally, the importance of documentation to support "medical necessity" was emphasized.

Appendix J offers forms for gathering data that can be used in the clinical setting to support the goals of meeting criteria for "medical necessity" and documentation requirements. It is highly recommended that the HCP refer to the various chapters mentioned in different sections of this chapter. The information included in those chapters will complement the implementation of outcomes management into the clinical setting.

REFERENCES

Bigos S, Bowyer O, Braen G, et al. *Acute Low Back Problems in Adults. Clinical Practice Guideline*. Rockville, Md: US Department of Health and Human Services, Public Health Service, Agency for Health Care Policy and Research; 1994.

Butler RJ, Johnson WG, Baldwin ML. Managing work disability: Why first return to work is not a measure of success. *Ind Labor Rel Rev* 1995;48(3):452–469.

Cherkin DC, Deyo RA, Street JH, Barlow W. Predicting poor outcomes for back pain seen in primary care using patients' own criteria. *Spine* 1996;21:2900–2907.

ChiroCode DeskBook: The Seventh Annual Coding and Reimbursement Guide for Chiropractors. 7th ed. Phoenix, Ariz: Leavitt Crandall Institute; 1999.

Croft PR, Macfarlane GJ, Papageorgiou AC, Thomas E, Silman AJ. Outcome of low back pain in general practice: A prospective study. *BMJ* 1998;316:1356–1359.

Liebenson C, ed. *Rehabilitation of the Spine: A Practitioner's Manual*. Philadelphia, Pa: Williams and Wilkins, 1996.

Matheson L. Evaluation of lifting. In: Liebenson C, ed. *Rehabilitation of the Spine: A Practitioner's Manual*. Philadelphia, Pa: Williams and Wilkins; 1996:145.

Stude DE. *Spinal Rehabilitation*. Stamford, Conn: Appleton and Lange, 1999.

Troup JDG, Martin JW, Lloyd DCEF. Back pain in industry: A prospective survey. *Spine* 1981;6:61–69.

Von Korff M, Saunders K. The course of back pain in primary care. *Spine* 1996;21:2833–2839.

Clinical Outcome Databases

ED DOBRZYKOWSKI

INTRODUCTION

Health care provider (HCP) systems for outcome measurement and clinical databases of patient outcomes information have originated and proliferated from the need to document and to compare the effectiveness (end result of care) and efficiency (resources and cost) of intervention. Constituents interested in this information include patients, patients' families, managed care organizations, employers, case managers, referral sources, administrators, and HCPs (Dobrzykowski, 1997). Although each constituent will have specific questions of interest, most will focus on cost, satisfaction, access to services, and clinical results. There is evidence that the public support for the release of outcomes information is increasing (Bentley and Nash, 1998).

The pertinent questions for HCPs are: What are my outcomes? How do my results compare to other HCPs with similar patients? With detailed examination of the answers to these questions, the HCP is stimulated to critically evaluate his or her treatment methods and to explore changes that may be necessary for improvement of outcomes.

Today, the rationale for measurement and management of outcomes information has expanded well beyond this original intent into the domains of continuous quality improvement and benchmarking, marketing of services, performance measurement within the context of organization accreditation, and research. Moreover, HCPs are increasingly gaining a sense of professional accountability to the public for their results. Consumers of health care services are clamoring for user-friendly information on the results of HCPs, providing a method in their selection beyond word of mouth and price.

The role of clinical outcome databases in provider practice has begun to evolve, from one of retrospective program evaluation methodology common today to a prospective, managed use of data in a "real time" environment of patient care. The purpose of this chapter is to describe some of the known outcome databases used by HCPs, and to provide examples of their applications.

DEVELOPMENT OF CLINICAL DATABASES

The development and design of an outcomes management process is a formidable task. The methodology must consider prevalent patient diagnoses, the type of constituents seeking outcomes information and their requirements, the salient outcomes of interest, and availability of outcome measures and systems (Dobrzykowski, 1997). In the creation of a clinical outcomes database, several steps are required. Very broadly, these steps include:

1. The composition and acceptance of a standard set of reliable and valid measures utilized consistently by each HCP
2. Devising methods for data collection and aggregation
3. Data analysis using appropriate statistical techniques
4. Management reporting

Many functional measures exist, particularly in medical rehabilitation (Cole et al, 1994; Lewis and McNerney, 1994). The selection of a measure for use in outcomes measurement considers:

- Identification of patient functions
- Whether data is being gathered for research or clinical purposes
- Reliability, validity, and sensitivity of the measure to change
- Conciseness and practicality of administration and scoring
- Timing of data collection
- Potential data uses
- Plans for possible publication (Dittmar and Gresham, 1997)

The essential metrics for inclusion in clinical outcome databases include measures of effectiveness (ie, patient health-related quality of life [HRQL]; patient satisfaction; functional status; employment status) and efficiency (ie, cost and resources for outcome achieved). These variables are generally collected at the initiation and conclusion of intervention, at periodic intervals, and at one or more follow-up points following patient discharge from treatment.

HCPs who have initiated an outcomes measurement process for their practice have been limited to the use of their own outcomes data, which often lacked the level of patient volume necessary to complete analyses with suffi-

cient statistical power. Also, it was difficult for many HCPs to justify the time and expense necessary for research and development of a comprehensive outcomes management system for their practice. Differences in selection of outcome measures, operational definitions, and processes for data collection, analysis, and reporting resulted in an inability to compare outcomes among HCPs. For example, patient satisfaction measurement, one of the most well-known of outcome measures, is typically comprised of myriad types of questions, scaling, and methods for data collection and analyses, which makes comparisons among HCPs and programs using different instruments difficult if not impossible. The use of patient satisfaction for comparison of HCPs and programs is compounded by a positive response tendency by consumers, and by the fact that the majority of respondents in most studies report well above average satisfaction with care received regardless of the type of service or setting (Hall and Dornan, 1988).

The use of an available clinical outcomes data collection and reporting service provides a "turn-key" solution to outcomes management; it has promulgated acceptance of a standard data set, promoted research, and may be more cost effective. Economies of scale are created in clinical database service companies with in-house expertise in measure research and design, data collection methods, statistics, risk adjustment, programming, and management reporting.

In evaluation and selection of an outcomes measurement system, several criteria should be considered:

- The number of subscribers
- The number of patients in the database
- The nature of data elements and outcome measures
- Data collection methods
- Data integrity
- Management reports
- Training and support services
- Rater reliability
- Contractual requirements
- Cost (Reynolds, 1996; Hicks, 1997)

Consideration should be made for those outcome measurement systems that have met criteria established by the Joint Commission on Accreditation of Healthcare Organizations (JCAHO) in its ORYX initiative.

Provider systems for outcome measurement and databases have developed in both the private and public sector. These include non-profit and for-profit companies, originating as "spin-offs" from research grants, products within health care information systems, government regulatory requirements, and through HCP professional associations.

Outcome databases can exist wholly as or a subset of standard clinical documentation, exemplified by the Minimum Data Set (MDS) Version 2.0 for nursing home resident assessment and care screening (Health Care Financing Administration, 1998), used as a basis for design of the Resource Utilization Groups (RUGS) and a prospective payment system for nursing homes, or the Outcome Assessment and Information Set (OASIS-B) in home care (Center for Health Services and Policy Research, 1997).

EXAMPLES OF CLINICAL DATABASES

FUNCTIONAL INDEPENDENCE MEASURE (FIM)

One of the earliest examples of an organized effort to create an outcome measurement standard and clinical database existed in inpatient rehabilitation, with the creation of the adult Functional Independence Measure (FIM) in 1983 (Granger, 1984; Granger et al, 1986). Funding was provided by a grant of the US Department of Education to the State University of New York at Buffalo. The 18 items comprising constructs of functional performance and communication/cognition in a "minimum data set" concept have proliferated in acceptance by the clinical and payer communities to the point where the FIM has become the predominant measure in inpatient rehabilitation. **The FIM is "discipline-free," with functional ratings provided by qualified occupational therapists, occupational therapy assistants, physical therapists, physical therapist assistants, registered nurses, speech language pathologists, and other members of the rehabilitation team.**

The Uniform Data System for Medical Rehabilitation (UDSMR^SM, Buffalo, NY) has available data collection and reporting services consisting of the FIM and additional measures of efficiency, and provides a national and regional comparison of effectiveness and efficacy for providers of rehabilitation services. The Adult FIM is now used in more than 700 facilities in the United States and in 15 foreign facilities. HCPs and programs participating in the database are able to determine and compare their results to hundreds of thousands of patient episodes of rehabilitation collected since 1985. With abbreviated lengths of stay for patients in inpatient rehabilitation resulting in increased levels of patient acuity in skilled nursing facilities, home care, and/or outpatient locations, the potential exists for use in these areas of the FIM and other similar measures containing constructs for basic activities of daily living. Subsequently, the Medical Rehabilitation Follow Along (MRFA) instrument (Granger et al, 1995; Baker et al, 1996) and LIFEware were created for measurement of outcomes in outpatient rehabilitation by UDSMR.

The Adult FIM has been adapted for children undergoing rehabilitation by UDSMR in a system known as the WeeFIM instrument. This instrument measures level of functional independence and dependence in children between the ages of 6 months and 7 years (and older) who exhibit delays in function primarily as the result of motor impairments (Braun, 1998).

FOCUS ON THERAPEUTIC OUTCOMES, INC. (FOTO)

The Focus On Therapeutic Outcomes, Inc. (FOTO) consortium was created in 1992 through a proprietary grant from six national rehabilitation service companies, and became a privately held database company in 1994. **FOTO sought to create a standard data set for measurement of outcomes in adult patients with musculoskeletal impairments undergoing outpatient rehabilitation,** with use primarily by physical therapists, physical therapist assistants, occupational therapists, occupational therapy assistants, and athletic trainers.

The original version of the FOTO data set contained measures of patient HRQL including the SF-36 (Medical Outcomes Trust, Boston, Mass) (McHorney et al, 1992, 1993, 1994; Ware and Sherbourne, 1992); and concurrent use of disease-specific measures including the Oswestry Low Back Pain Disability Questionnaire (Fairbanks et al, 1980) for patients with low back impairments, the Neck Disability Index (Vernon and Mior, 1991) for patients with neck impairments, and the Lysholm scale (Tegner and Lysholm, 1986) for patients with knee impairments. Measures of efficiency include number of visits, episode length, and cost, which are then correlated with outcome (ie, change in HRQL in different impairment groups). Patient satisfaction and demographic information is also collected.

As a result of multiple statistical analyses of its own database in order to eliminate measure redundancies and questions providing minimal value, revisions to the FOTO musculoskeletal version contain substantially fewer measures. Correlations were discovered with the physical domain of the SF-36 and the Oswestry and Lysholm scales (Jette and Jette, 1996a, 1996b), resulting in the elimination of the disease-specific questionnaires. Version 4.0 of the adult System A includes the health status measures of the SF-12 survey, an abbreviated version of the SF-36, which retains approximately 80% of its predictive power (Ware et al, 1996). New data collection and reporting systems have been created for comprehensive neuromuscular and cardiopulmonary rehabilitation for use in the post-acute continuum of care, which are utilized by occupational therapists, occupational therapy assistants, physical therapists, physical therapist assistants, registered nurses, licensed practical nurses, speech language pathologists, audiologists, athletic trainers, and exercise physiologists.

OUTCOME AND ASSESSMENT INFORMATION SET (OASIS)

In the public sector, the Outcome and Assessment Information Set (OASIS) was created through a grant originating from the Health Care Financing Administration

F.O.T.O., Inc.
Patient Specific Resource Predictor

Reporting Unit: Clinic A	Practice ID: 00-000-00-0
Patient ID: 123-45-6789	Date of Injury: 22–90 Days
Name: SMITH	Initial Date of Service: 12/09/1997
Initial Employment Status: Retired	

RISK ADJUSTMENT CRITERIA:

Impairment Category: Hip/Lower Extremity	Care Type: Orthopedic
Age: 70	Severity: Severe

FUNCTIONAL SCORES

	PhysFunct	Role Phys	Pain	Energy	Mental	Social
Admission	30.00	0.00	50.00	20.00	90.00	50.00
FOTO Mean	32.84	20.77	37.46	39.85	64.22	53.09

FOTO
Mean Resources Utilized (Risk Adjusted)

FOTO patients with similar functional admission scores have utilized resources as indicated below: The probability is that the patient's results will be near the mean. The number of risk adjusted patients in the FOTO database is: 1,051

Statistics:	MEANS
Visits	10.11
Duration	34.88
Dollars	$906.25
Outcome Index:	
Outcome	63.90
Value	70.51
Utilization	63.23
Satisfaction:	
Satisfaction	96.90 %
Return to Work:	
Full-time	19.49 %
Restricted	20.77 %
Still off Work	42.83 %
Other	16.92 %
Discharge	
% Non-Compliant	3.30 %
% Goals Met	67.89 %
Goals Not Met	19.28 %
Other	9.53 %

Figure 23–1. Patient Specific Resource Predictor.

(Reprinted with permission. Focus on Therapeutic Outcomes, Inc. Knoxville, Tenn.)

A process of outcomes management provides an HCP with a mechanism for differentiation of results in a market that selects providers based solely on price. Purchasers of health care primarily consider *economic* outcomes; that is, contracting with and reimbursing for services based solely on the best price, not necessarily the best value. Both HCPs and purchasers have struggled with the determination of the salient outcomes of interest to their constituents beyond cost and utilization, and how to link measures of effectiveness to their efficiency.

CASE STUDY 23-1
LINKING OUTCOMES AND COST

A physical therapy private practice organization, a well-established company of six facilities in the southeastern United States, was awarded a contract for rehabilitation services with a large self-insured employer at a price advocated by the private practice. The original request for proposal contract requirements stipulated a price reduction that would place the reimbursement for services below the practice's cost. The owners' understanding and progressive use of outcomes information brought them to a meeting fully "armed" with data. The information included several years of linked patient HRQL, patient satisfaction, cost, episode length, and utilization (visits). All information was separated into impairment groups (ie, low back, neck, shoulder) and was compared to thousands of patients in a nationally recognized outcomes database (FOTO). All data was risk-adjusted for patient age, impairment, acuity level, and severity. As a result, the practice was able to demonstrate their outcomes for a given cost, illustrate their competitiveness nationally (they ranked in the top 10 percentile of effective and efficient rehabilitation providers), and eventually was awarded a contract with the *practice's* stipulated price. At the conclusion of the meeting, one of the insurer's representatives remarked, "I would not want to be this organization's competitor."

Savvy HCPs have utilized outcomes data to counter and refute limitations on their services. For example, two visits are preauthorized by a managed care organization (MCO) for an HCP to evaluate and treat a patient regardless of the nature of an impairment. Additional visits must be approved each time by the payer, an obvious strategy to curtail utilization. An HCP's outcomes information might reveal that based on each particular patient's impairment group, severity, socioeconomic characteristics, initial health status, age, and acuity level, five visits (statistically) will optimize the patient's outcome. The MCO may be more apt to agree with the HCP who can provide this information.

ACCREDITATION

For over three decades, organizations that provide comprehensive rehabilitation services have had the option of accreditation by CARF, The Rehabilitation Accreditation Commission (Tucson, Ariz). CARF has long been an advocate of quality standards in medical rehabilitation, behavioral health, and employment and community services. Program accreditation is available in areas such as chronic pain, work hardening, brain injury, and outpatient medical rehabilitation. CARF is recognized by many payers as the de facto authority for quality in rehabilitation organizations.

An essential component to the CARF accreditation process is program evaluation, a method to assess the organization's information and outcomes management systems. CARF permits each organization to select its outcome measures of interest, and requires active measurement, monitoring, and management by the program of these outcomes over time. CARF expects that information gathered is relevant to core values and mission of an organization and needs of all stakeholders, analyzed and shared to improve performance, and allows for comparison with internal/historical data and comparable external data (CARF Medical Rehabilitation Standards Manual, 1998).

In 1997, the JCAHO (Oakbrook Terrace, Ill) began the ORYX initiative, a process to evolve performance measurement and linking of outcomes with process of care delivery into its accreditation process for hospitals, long-term care facilities, and home care. In order to accomplish this formidable task, the JCAHO solicited and evaluated vendors of outcomes data collection and reporting services, eventually approving over 200 vendors. Each measurement system contains several precise measures that may be selected by facilities and reported to JCAHO upon request of the organization. Each approved performance measurement system must comply with JCAHO attributes of conformance requirements, which include designation of performance measures, database technical capabilities, data quality and accuracy, risk adjustment/stratification, performance measure feedback, and relevance for accreditation (JCAHO, 1998).

The common goal of these accrediting organizations is to improve the quality of health care. In time, the increased cost borne by performance measurement should provide information on HCP and practice value for the consumer. The reality exists, however, that many HCPs are not required to achieve and maintain accreditation. In order for the future success of outcomes management and the ongoing proliferation of databases, there must be an increased sense of accountability and responsibility for outcomes management among all HCPs.

RESEARCH

The standardization and promotion of clinical outcome databases have begun to provide evidence for the effectiveness and efficiency of health care. Many measures have been extensively tested for their psychometric properties, and exhibit varying levels of predictive validity. The Functional Independence Measure and UDSMR database have been utilized for response to research questions pertaining to impairment groups such as stroke (Werner, 1994), and work has been completed using the FIM as the basis of a prospective payment system in rehabilitation known as Function Related Groups (Stineman, 1994; Stineman et al, 1997). The American Occupational Therapy Association (Hart and Dobrzykowski, 1998) and the American Physical Therapy Association have utilized the data set provided by FOTO to assess outcomes of occupational therapists and physical therapists, respectively. The American Speech Hearing and Language Association has utilized the data set of Medirisk, Inc., to evaluate outcomes of speech and language pathologists. These data sets are attractive for research interests because of their national scope, number of patient episodes, and variables of interest (ie, diagnoses, functional status, health status, satisfaction, utilization, cost, episode).

LIMITATIONS

There are several limitations to both the creation and applications of clinical databases. The common limitations cited include the existence of selection, response, and attribution biases; "downcoding" at admission and "upcoding" at discharge (Plant et al, 1998); lack of measure responsiveness; use of inappropriate statistical methods for analysis and quantification of outcome; quality of data; and rater reliability. Additionally, clinical database services do not generally control for the types and experience of HCPs, or the results of treatment (Hart and Dobrzykowski, 1998). Obviously, some of these limitations pertain to measure selection and use within randomized clinical trials as well. Although clinical outcome databases may compromise internal validity, the results as a whole may be more generalizable.

Conclusion

Outcomes measurement and clinical databases are proliferating and are becoming essential partners in methods of contemporary health care practice. The monitoring and management of outcomes, largely today a method of a retrospective program evaluation, is evolving to a method of prospective usage of outcomes data in a "real-time" basis. Clearly, the value of outcomes measurement and clinical databases lies with the contribution to knowledge of what works in health care and what does not, and its acceptance and incorporation by HCPs into standard practice.

The prevalence, quality, and reliance upon clinical outcomes databases should increase in the future. Clinical database development is already underway to provide links of patient outcome among HCPs in disparate practices along the continuum of care. There will be measurement and monitoring of patient outcomes from the initial acute intervention to the conclusion, albeit home or office, physician or therapist, and beyond to follow-up postdischarge.

The use of generic HRQL measures has been very promising, and their design is especially suited for utility in longitudinal measurement of outcomes in many different patient populations. In managed care organizations, HRQL measures such as the SF-36 may eventu-ally be completed by all consumers upon initial enrollment, providing a baseline measure of HRQL and a marker for comparison in the future event of compromised health. For example, the National Committee for Quality Assurance (NCQA) is currently in the midst of a demonstration project for HCFA, evaluating the Health of Seniors Survey in health maintenance organizations.

The ultimate success of clinical databases in the short term will depend on HCP acceptance, sense of professional accountability, need for accreditation, organizational leadership, and integration of critical outcome data elements into information systems for patient, HCP, and financial reporting. As data collection and reporting methods advance, respondent burden will be reduced, data input redundancy will be eliminated, and additional data elements collected will add to predictive models. In any event, the outcome measurement system and clinical database must be cost-effective and provide value for HCPs, consumers, and payers in contemporary health care delivery. There is little doubt that future HCP selection in managed health care plans will be based on value, and the ability to demonstrate improved and sustained patient outcomes. (A comprehensive listing of clinical databases can be found in Appendix Form K–1.)

REFERENCES

American College of Cardiology, Core Data Element Documentation and ACC National Cardiovascular Data Registry, Version 1.1; April 1997.

Baker JG, Granger CV, Ottenbacher KJ. Validity of a brief outpatient functional assessment measure. *Am J Phys Med Rehabil* 1996;75:356–363.

Bentley JM, Nash DB. How Pennsylvania hospitals have responded to publicly released reports on coronary artery bypass graft surgery. *Jt Comm J Qual Improv* 1998;24:40–49.

Braun S. The Functional Independence Measure for Children (WeeFIM instrument): Gateway to the WeeFIM System. *J Rehabil Outcomes Measurement* 1998;2(4):63–68.

CARF Medical Rehabilitation Standards Manual, Tucson, Arizona; 1998.

Center for Health Services and Policy Research, Denver, Colorado; 1997.

Cole B, Finch E, Gowland C, Mayo N, Basmajian J, eds. *Physical Rehabilitation Outcome Measures*. Toronto, Canada: Canadian Physiotherapy Association; 1994.

Crisler KS, Campbell BM, Shaughnessy PW. *OASIS Basics: Beginning to Use the Outcome and Assessment Information Set*. Denver, Colo: Center for Health Services and Policy Research; 1997:1.

Dittmar SS, Gresham GE. *Functional Assessment and Outcome Measures for the Rehabilitation Health Professional*. Gaithersburg, Md: Aspen; 1997.

Dobrzykowski E. The methodology of outcomes measurement. *J Rehabil Outcomes Measurement* 1997;1:1,8–17.

Fairbanks JC, Couper C, Davies JB, O'Brien JP. The Oswestry Low Back Pain Questionnaire. *Physiotherapy* 1980;66:271–273.

Frattali C, Thompson C, Holland A, Wohl C, Ferketic M. *American Speech-Language-Hearing Association Functional Assessment of Communication Skills for Adults (ASHA FACS)*. Rockville, Md: ASHA; 1995.

Granger, CV. A conceptual model for functional assessment. In: Granger CV, Gresham GE, eds. *Functional Assessment in Rehabilitation Medicine*. Baltimore, Md: Williams and Wilkins; 1984:14–25.

Granger CV, Hamilton BB, Keith RA, Zielezny M, Sherwin FS. Advances in functional assessment for medical rehabilitation. *Top Ger Rehabil* 1986;1:59–74.

Granger CV, Ottenbacher KJ, Baker JG, Sehgal A. Reliability of a brief outpatient functional outcome assessment measure. *Am J Phys Med Rehabil* 1995;74:469–475.

Hall JA, Dornan MC. Meta-analysis of satisfaction with medical care: What patients are asked about their care and how often they are asked: A meta-analysis of the literature. *Soc Sc Med* 1988;27:935–939.

Hart DL, Dobrzykowski E. Effect of clinical specialist certification on clinical outcomes: A preliminary data analysis. *J Orthop Sports Phys Ther* 1999; submitted.

Hart DL, Tepper S, Lieberman D. AOTA *Program Evaluation and Outcome Activities Forum*. Presentation AOTA Annual Conference, Baltimore, Md; 1998.

Health Care Financing Administration. Minimum Data Set Version 2.0, for Nursing Home Resident Assessment and Care Screening; 1998.

Hicks PL. Evaluating national outcomes data systems: Which one meets my needs? *J Rehabil Outcomes Measurement* 1997;1:2,38–42.

Jette DU, Jette AM. Physical therapy and health outcomes in patients with knee impairments. *Phys Ther* 1996a;76:1178–1187.

Jette DU, Jette AM. Physical therapy and health outcomes in patients with spinal impairments. *Phys Ther* 1996b;76:930–945.

Joint Commission on Accreditation of Healthcare Organizations, Oakbrook Terrace, Ill; 1998.

Lewis CB, McNerney T. *The Functional Tool Box*. Washington, DC: Learn Publications; 1994.

McHorney CA, Ware JE, Lu JFR, Sherbourne CD. The MOS 36-item short-form health survey (SF-36): III. Tests of data quality, scaling assumptions, and reliability across diverse patient groups. *Med Care* 1994;32(1):40–66.

McHorney CA, Ware JE, Raczek AE. The MOS 36-item short-form health survey (SF-36), II: Psychometric and clinical tests of validity in measuring physical and mental health constructs. *Med Care* 1993;31:247–263.

McHorney CA, Ware JE, Rogers W, et al. The validity and relative precision of MOS short- and long-form health status scales and Dartmouth COOP charts. *Med Care* 1992;30:MS253–MS265.

Mozena JP, Emerick CE, Black SC. *Clinical Guideline Development: An Algorithm Approach*. Gaithersburg, Md: Aspen; 1996.

Plant MA, Richards JS, Hansen NK. Potential for bias from functional status measures. *Arch Phys Med Rehabil* 1998;79:104–105.

Reynolds JP. Are you ready to join an outcomes database? *PT Magazine* 1996;4:10,36–42,67.

Shaugnessy PW, Crisler KS, Schlenker RE. *Medicare's OASIS: Standardized Outcome and Assessment Information Set for Home Health Care.* Center for Health Services and Policy Research, Denver, CO, 1997.

Stineman MG. Function-based classification for stroke rehabilitation and issues of reimbursement: Using person classification systems to scale payment to person complexity. *Top Stroke Rehabil* 1994;1:3,40–50.

Stineman MG, Goin JE, Granger CV, Fiedler R, Williams SV. Discharge motor FIM-function related groups. *Arch Phys Med Rehabil* 1997;78:980–985.

Tegner Y, Lysholm J. Rating system in the evaluation of knee ligament injuries. *Clin Orthop Rel Res* 1986;198:43–48.

Uniform Data System for Medical Rehabilitation. On-line: www.lifeware.org; 1998.

Vernon H, Mior S. The Neck Disability Index: A study of reliability and validity. *J Manipulative Physiol Ther* 1991;14:409–415.

Ware JE, Kosinski M, Keller SD: *SF-36 Physical and Mental Health Summary Scales: A User's Manual.* Boston, Mass: The Health Institute, New England Medical Center; 1994.

Ware JE, Kosinski M, Keller SD. A 12-item short-form health survey: Construction of scales and preliminary tests of reliability and validity. *Med Care* 1996;34:220–233.

Ware JE, Sherbourne CD. The MOS 36-item short-form health survey (SF-36), I: Conceptual framework and item selection. *Med Care* 1992;30:473–483.

Werner RA. Predicting outcome after acute stroke with the functional independence measure. *Top Stroke Rehabil* 1994;1:3,30–39.

CHAPTER 24

Positioning for the Future:
Using Outcomes Management
to Enhance Customer Service

Robert D. Mootz, Daniel T. Hansen, & Silvano Mior

INTRODUCTION

The preceding chapters have offered an extensive array of outcome assessment (OA) tools with strategies for incorporating them in practice and practical approaches for health care providers (HCPs) to use to improve delivery of care. Outcomes assessment comes in many "flavors," including general health assessment, specific functional attributes, pain and symptom assessment, psychosocial measures, and more. Measurement "instruments" range from low-tech pencil-and-paper questionnaires, filled out by patients, to high-tech functional capacity measurement equipment. Some instruments provide useful and reliable information; others are in various stages of development or may best be considered experimental.

of the HCP and patient are now firmly entrenched in managed care, health care entitlements, government regulation, and health care conglomerates (Mootz et al, 1995). Table 24–2 provides a glossary of some contemporary health care terms and concepts that can be useful for understanding the context of the changes in health care delivery. The worlds of health policy and health services research are increasingly becoming more relevant for day-to-day practice. Although mere lingo to many, the terminology of health policy is important for HCPs to understand. Marketing a practice today requires more than an experienced HCP with a caring attitude for patients. Understanding your "marketplace niche" and the expectations of consumers and purchasers of health care, not to mention the regulators, is increasingly becoming a prerequisite in order to remain competitive.

In the past, a patient was pretty much the only customer an HCP had to worry about. Today, HCPs are accountable to a wide variety of individuals and organizations, including payers, employers, clinics, and health care administrators. The reason is simple: as direct responsibility for the costs of health care expenditures shifted from the patient and their family to third-party payers, less control over spending decisions was left to the actual consumer of the service. The advent of third-party payers was originally a boon for the HCP who no longer had to deal with resistance from patients because of costs. Now, an HCP must grapple with the heavy hand of the insurance company or government agency responsible for keeping overall expenditures within budget. This changing context requires a strategic approach to meeting the needs of these "new" customers.

DEFINING THE CUSTOMERS' EXPECTATIONS

Although some of the current reporting requirements confronted by HCPs are burdensome, claim adjudicators,

Table 24–2: Health Policy Terminology

algorithms	Pathways for clinical decision making in a stepwise fashion.
appropriateness	The applicability of a method or procedure based on clinical benefit, risk, and cost.
consensus	A formal process of collapsing disagreements toward gaining agreement among a group of experts.
cost-effectiveness	To produce more benefit in health status at lower cost.
health policy	Values of the society or community in terms of how and to whom health resources are allocated.
health-related quality of life	The value assigned to duration of life as modified by the impairments, functional states, perceptions, and social opportunities that are influenced by disease, injury, treatment, or policy.
medical effectiveness evaluations	The evaluation of one or more health programs, clinical interventions, or regulatory practices to establish the magnitude of benefits, disseminate the results, and eliminate ineffective interventions.
explicit process	Use of criteria to judge scientific evidence and expert opinion in relation to attributes of care or practice.
implicit process	Use of opinions of peers and intraprofessional experts to define attributes of care or practice.
guidelines	Systematically developed statements to assist health care practitioner (HCP) and patient decisions regarding appropriate health care under specific clinical circumstances.
outcomes	The measurable status of the patient following clinical intervention.
patient-centered	Relates to clinical activities in which the patient is considered as the focus for clinically relevant decisions or issues.
practice parameters	Relates to the inventory of health care practice in general, acceptance of procedures, devices, and other attributes of practice according to available science and opinions of recognized experts.
research	Scientific or scholarly investigation.
science	A systematic approach to gaining new knowledge through observation of phenomena in order to establish a hypothesis, and challenging that hypothesis through manipulation of variables (investigation, experimentation), associated with description of the process and findings.
technology assessment	A form of policy research that evaluates technology (eg, health care technology) for providing decision makers with information on different policy options.
standards of care	Legal standards established by the trier of the fact (judge, jury) describing the conduct of HCPs that society finds acceptable.
weight of evidence	A method of summarizing quality of evidence to give greater weight to designs that are less subject to bias and error.
value	Refers to individually and socially worthwhile clinical outcomes relative to the money spent for the intervention.

From Mootz RD, Shekelle PG, Hansen DT. The politics of policy and research. Top Clin Chiro 1995;2(2):56–70. © 1995 Aspen Publishers, Inc. Reprinted with permission.

health care administrators, and others must often have clinical documentation that can withstand peer scrutiny in order to adjudicate a claim or justify reimbursement. In other words, the burden of convincing a patient of the need for a health care expenditure has evolved to a burden of also convincing a claim manager, third-party administrator, or even a personnel officer in a company of the need for the service. This must be done in a manner that individuals within the payer's hierarchy can use to defend their coverage decisions. It also must be done in a way that does not exceed the resources HCPs have to provide adequate data. Efficient, relevant, and timely information extractable from routine communications from offices and clinics can help facilitate this. But what is relevant to the new customers?

HOW THE HEALTH CARE DELIVERY SYSTEM IS CHANGING EXPECTATIONS

Even though the merits and follies of today's approaches to health care financing can be the subject of significant debate, HCPs need to find ways to minimize practices that are little more than "jumping through hoops." They must maximize procedures that are useful or essential for rendering quality care while meeting the need of a new group of customers (Raines et al, 1998). Table 24–3 outlines a number of contemporary "customers" HCPs must deal with and delineates some of their needs and expectations. By systematically considering the requirements of all who have a hand in the clinical management world these days, an HCP can help sequence and prioritize both clinical and administrative processes that optimize the ability to address the needs of the patient, HCP, and payer alike.

The concept of everyone being "the customer" is common practice in the world of business. Quality assurance (QA) and quality improvement (QI) practices implemented in the devastated post–World War II economies of Japan and Germany generated rapid rewards through modernization and growth of business and manufacturing enterprises. These strategies focused on measurement of changes in each process along the manufacturing chain. The person buying the product in the store is still the customer (indirectly), although the person at the end of your assembly line is your immediate customer.

What might this all have to do with *outcomes assessment?* Today's "customers" want more than a list of clinical findings that amount to little more than mumbo-jumbo to the average person. Although detailed reports of numbers from electrodes, exhaustive tables of ranges of motions, and force measures can help a physical medicine specialist determine what to do next, the relevance in other contexts can become cloudy.

To illustrate this point, imagine that a new drug becomes available that has been shown in randomized clinical trials to reduce cholesterol levels. Everyone knows lower cholesterol is a good thing. HCPs start prescribing it, patients start taking it, lots of serum cholesterol tests document the fact that the new drug is doing its job, and lots of insurance companies pay for it. But over time, the new drug causes renal damage. And, those individuals who suffer a myocardial infarction 3 to 5 years after taking the drug have a higher mortality rate due to renal complications.

Obviously no one wants to create such a situation; not the drug company, payer, nor HCP. The lesson is clear. A focus on the **clinical indicator** of cholesterol level may have meaning in terms of the effectiveness of the drug's physiological action; however, the consequences of such a focus could be detrimental in terms of the patient's overall health *outcome*. Although both are legitimate clinical measures, the latter may be the most relevant one.

In physical medicine, a more applicable example might involve range of motion (ROM) assessment versus return to work (RTW). ROM assessment can be helpful to HCPs in deciding how to apply exercise or manipulation (an important day-to-day clinical issue). Pre- and postintervention ROM assessment may also be valuable to determine if an intervention had a desired physiological impact. However, in terms of the ultimate social measure of intervention effectiveness, it is important that the patient be able to return to normal function. Successful RTW is an example of the kind of outcome that may have much greater relevance to "customers" beyond the HCP–patient encounter. Interestingly, however, to date there has been no formal assessment of customer expectations in injury and noninjury spine care.

HOW OUTCOMES MANAGEMENT CAN HELP HEALTH CARE PROVIDERS

The patient's HCP should be the first to know if the patient is not responding appropriately to care. It should not be the HCP down the street, the patient's employer, insurance carrier, or their malpractice attorney. It is essential to stay on top of care progress and be able to identify what has changed and to what degree. Identification of trends toward chronicity, lack of motivation, or ineffective interventions should be spotted early and appropriate resources should be brought to the problem quickly (Skogsbergh and Chapman, 1994). Outcomes management can help.

MINIMUM OUTCOMES PACKAGE

Determining which outcome measures need to be monitored requires attention to a variety of factors. **Routinely, three kinds of simple measures should be considered for establishing a baseline and assessed periodically during care: symptom outcome, function outcome, and social outcome.**

Table 24–3: Today's Health Care Customers

Patient	**Employer**
Patient	Risk managers
Worker/employee	Safety personnel
Patient's family	Supervisors
Patient advocates	Employees
Insurance carrier/managed care	**Unions**
Claims managers	Safety specialists
Medical director	Shop stewards
Quality assurance personnel	**Legal counsel**
Case managers	Plaintiff's attorneys
Billing staff	Defense attorneys
Risk managers	Paralegals
Government agencies	**Clinic/office staff**
Legal staff	Front desk personnel
Health care HCPs	Technical assistants
Attending chiropractor	QA/QI specialist
Attending primary care HCP	Transcriptionist
Ancillary therapists (PT/OT)	Partners/associate HCPs
Diagnostic specialists/facilities	Practice administrators
Treatment specialists/facilities	**Equipment/supply vendors**
In-/outpatient care facilities	Tables and instruments
Independent examiners	Durable medical equipment
Disability raters	Imaging supplies
Vocational rehabilitation	Computer hardware/software
Case managers	**Academic centers**
Training specialists	College/seminar faculty
Community health resources	Research scientists
Public health agency	Libraries/librarians
Regional health agencies	
Shelters/hospices	

Examples of Expectations (may overlap different customers)

- Access to appropriate care

- Timeliness of follow-up

- Minimal burden in pre-certification

- Completeness of records

- Definitive clinical thresholds and endpoint of care

- Clear and routine lines of communication between:

  - Different HCPs

  - HCPs and payers

  - HCPs and worksite

- Provision of appropriate, even optimal, care

- Management that enhances self-reliance

- Community-based partnerships (eg, employer–HCP–payer)

HCP, health care provider; OT, occupational therapy; PT, physical therapy; QA/QI, quality assurance/improvement.

Quantification of the Symptomatology

Any number of strategies can be employed, including visual analogue scales, pain questionnaires, or symptom diaries (eg, headache duration, distance or time walked until exacerbation). Although it is important not to only focus on symptom relief, the nature and severity of symptoms can offer insight into the impact the problem has on a patient and how care is progressing. Using a scale to document symptoms is essentially a means to quantify the "subjective" portion of SOAP (subjective, objective, assessment, plan) format chart notes.

Quantification of the Patient's Functional Ability

A variety of function questionnaires can document how the patient's problem is affecting his or her ability to perform daily activities. These questionnaires are tailored to the type of condition confronting the patient and consider specifics of how the condition affects the patient's abilities to perform particular functions. Obviously, one would expect intervention to reduce symptoms, but care should also enhance a return to normal function. It is essential to consider these kinds of issues in determining whether care is effective. A treatment may offer palliation of symptoms but not to the point that a person can return to his or her usual activities. Examples of functional OA tools include the Oswestry and Roland-Morris questionnaires, and the Neck Disability Index. Along with the usual clinical indicators HCPs track to determine next treatment steps, functional measures at periodic intervals enhance re-examination and can offer a meaningful quantification to "objective" components of chart documentation.

Quantification of the Patient's Social Outcome

Tracking something that payers and the community at large find useful should also be incorporated in a minimum outcomes management package. Although specific "outcomes" instruments per se might not be applicable, disability, employability, and chronicity need to monitored. Documenting these kinds of attributes periodically can provide ultimate insight as to how useful intervention really is. Such social outcomes are "forests" rather than "trees" and are often indirectly connected to a given specific pathology or condition (or intervention for that matter). However, psychosocial variables such as motivation, job satisfaction, and others may play strong roles here (Fordyce, 1995). HCPs need to consider the multiplicity of factors that may effect recovery. One way to do this is to regularly incorporate social goals into management programs. These kinds of issues can be readily charted in "assessment" sections of chart notes.

ENHANCED OUTCOME MEASURES

Outcome measures can also be made for general health status, patient satisfaction, and other domains. Many low-tech pencil-and-paper "instruments" exist and many more are under development. Several of the RAND short-form general health status questionnaires (eg, SF-36, SF-12) are highly validated, although somewhat tedious to score by hand (Vernon, 1996). Patient satisfaction surveys directed to specific settings (eg, chiropractic care) have been described (Coulter et al, 1994). Enhanced kinds of outcomes (beyond a basic symptom, function, and social measure) might be best used in situations where their value is clear. For example, psychological assessments (such as depression inventories) need only be considered if clinical suspicion arises. Alternatively, tools to capture information about job satisfaction may be useful to have at baseline for most patients in workers' compensation cases.

Additionally, functional and symptom measurement tools may be useful when specific clinical circumstances warrant. It should be emphasized that an awareness of the validity and reliability of the tool is also needed. One need not waste time harnessing a multitude of paperwork that may seem useful but upon further scrutiny does not validly provide the information one is seeking. Before incorporating a new outcomes instrument in practice, seek out original studies on its reliability and validity in other settings.

VALUE OF OUTCOMES IN PRACTICE

Outcomes management helps HCPs identify attributes of care that are important to all. Tracking, documenting, and reporting these outcomes can help illustrate the relevance of care to outside observers, thereby facilitating interactions with others. However, there are significant benefits for real-time patient management as well. Clinical indicators may vary over time according to factors other than pathology (eg, muscle spasm, ROM, and various orthopedic checks). There may also be intrinsic limitations in reliability impacting a measurement's usefulness as true assessment of overall progress.

Some clinical indicators, particularly in manual techniques, may be based on unverified pathological models that may or may not correlate with a patient's recovery. Tracking outcomes measures can facilitate overall clinical management regardless of what physiological rationales are optimal. For example, if range of lumbar spine motion improves over the course of care, that is often considered by HCPs in manual medicine to be indicative of effectiveness and representative of progress in a low back pain patient. However if ROM improves but capacity to engage in sitting or standing for prolonged periods (in a patient employed as a secretary or retail clerk) remains unchanged, that "progress" may be irrelevant. The HCP who touts weeks of incremental ROM improvements as significant progress without realizing that the patient is not really functioning any better may find himself or herself at a disadvantage compared to an HCP who tracked functional outcome and made appropriate early modifications in treatment.

This sort of attention to meaningful outcomes may help in the early identification of patients at risk of treatment dependency, chronicity, or dissatisfaction with care. In this era of increased competition and accountability, wasted time and care dollars can take a long-term toll on the HCP. But perhaps the overriding value of outcomes management really centers on doing the best job for the patient.

A COMMENT ON GETTING PAID

The emphasis on easy-to-administer, inexpensive questionnaires in this discussion is deliberate. At present, payers are expecting, if not requiring, more documentation and communication than ever. It is not likely that separate reimbursement, at least for simple outcomes measurement, is in the cards. The value for HCPs lies in the increased efficiency in both clinical and administrative management. Early identification of clinical progress, and appropriate rapid management and decision making offers an overall competitive edge in the marketplace at large.

Further, progress on meaningful outcomes that is readily extractable from existing clinical documentation can facilitate adjudication from those who hold the purse strings. Although there is a learning curve in modifying existing charting and reporting practices, it is not a steep one, especially when placed in the perspective of increasing pressures for accountability and greater marketplace competition.

HOW AN OUTCOMES EMPHASIS CAN HELP YOUR PROFESSION

Clinical management and documentation aimed solely at justifying continued care is easy to spot and reflects poorly on individual HCPs and their respective professions. An emphasis on determining and monitoring both clinically and socially relevant outcomes helps HCPs to focus on care quality in all its manifestations. Professions and specialties that work toward a quality and appropriateness of care focus (rather than a special-, or self-interest one) seem more likely to become the resources the system turns to time and again.

Outcomes assessments are increasingly being used in research on the comparative effectiveness of different treatments. Hence, HCPs addressing outcome measures that are well-established in published studies may have additional benefits. HCPs and professional societies that use and encourage monitoring of care for outcomes that science and society have deemed useful, valid, and reliable

can more readily find literature support to help document clinical necessity and effectiveness.

COMMUNICATING RELEVANT OUTCOMES INFORMATION

Raw outcomes scores by themselves are typically of little use. By nature and design, most outcome instruments are geared toward assessing change over time within the same individual. Hence, in many instances, the magnitude of the change may be more significant than an absolute value. **In communicating and reporting outcome instrument results, the interpretation of the result should be emphasized, not the scores themselves.** Although raw scores may be a part of a patient's total chart, it can be most useful to comment about the percent change in the assessment section of a progress note entry, or include an annotation regarding the trend of several outcome variables.

Just as a learning curve can be present for HCPs who are learning to use and interpret various outcome instruments, peer reviewers and adjudicators may not be aware of outcomes management issues and types of instruments used to track progress. When reports or letters are written conveying outcomes information, it may be best to outline the results in general categories. For example, stating that "limitations in performing activities of daily living due to their back problem have improved 30% as measured by the Oswestry Back Pain Disability index" is more meaningful than simply reporting the pre- and post-treatment scores.

PERSPECTIVES ON COMPETITION AND MARKET POSITIONING

Optimizing clinical practice for the future seems to have become a continuous process these days. As outcomes management increasingly becomes the norm, increased quantification of various quality attributes will become routine. However, incorporating measurement and quantification into clinical domains that have previously been considered qualitative and reflect the "art" of practice, by implication, will initiate a new series of expectations and standards (Enzmann, 1997).

Setting up one's own clinical performance standards as a course of business now can place you ahead of the curve later. For example, tracking the total cost of your care as well as duration of treatment times for the most common conditions seen in your practice is often done actuarially by payers based on billing records, yet HCPs rarely track this information themselves for quality improvement purposes. Referral rates to specialists by condition, magnetic resonance imaging (MRI) ordering rates, clinical laboratory testing, and plain film imaging are other performance measures that might be useful to track.

Perhaps the biggest "paradigm-shift" regarding a quality and outcomes focus, centers around routinely making

CLINICAL TIP 24–3
Tracking Performance Measures

Tracking the following performance measures will be very helpful to improving your practice:

- Total cost of care
- Duration of treatment times (for most common conditions seen in your practice; include both the duration of care and the total number of visits)
- Referral rates to specialists (by condition)
- Co-management with other service: occupational therapy, physical therapy, allopathic, osteopathic, acupuncture, other)
- Magnetic resonance imaging and other special test ordering rates (keep track of each type of test separately)
- Clinical laboratory testing
- Plain film imaging

such information available to consumers, patients, payers, and regulators. Enzmann (1997) suggests that viewing data as the province of only the clinical professionals is "elitist" and points out that the more the "customer" knows, the more the HCP's skills will be appreciated. Despite debates about how quantifiable measurements of quality and clinical value really are, they are a modern reality (Hansen, 1994; Hansen and Vernon, 1997). **Making better information available to consumers and regulators upon which to make quality of care judgments is essential.** Incorporating outcomes management strategies can help.

Care for expensive conditions such low back pain and carpal tunnel syndrome is coming under greater scrutiny. As Enzmann (1997) points out, a simple Pareto analysis performed by any health plan or HCP in a risk-bearing capitation agreement illustrates the issue well (Table 24–4). In the United States, the surgery rate for low back pain is ten times greater than in other industrialized nations and studies have documented that 80% to 90% of low back pain patients will get better in 4 to 6 weeks without care or under conservative management (Andersson, 1991; Bigos, 1994). Add to that the results of a study comparing treatment of low back pain patients by chiropractors, primary care HCPs, and orthopedists, which showed similar clinical outcomes (Carey et al, 1995). Interestingly,

the only differences seen were in patient satisfaction, total cost, and system resources that were used.

WHAT DO POLICY MAKERS AND REGULATORS THINK?

Setting aside one's own professional preferences, consider what policy makers and health plans might do with the following kinds of data from a couple of recent reports (Bigos, 1994; Cherkin et al, 1994; Carey et al, 1995).

- Chiropractors and orthopedists used plain x-rays two to three times more frequently than primary care HCPs while non-HMO primary care HCPs and orthopedists use advanced imaging more frequently.
- While orthopedists use computed tomography (CT) or MRI on 18% of patients, neurologists use it on 60% of patients.
- Chiropractors spent the most time with patients (seeing patients three to four times more often than primary care HCPs or orthopedists).
- HCPs frequently used corticosteroid and lidocaine injection procedures of trigger points and facet joints that are not recommended by federal guidelines.
- Overall cost was lowest for the health maintenance organization (HMO)-based primary care HCPs and highest for orthopedists.
- Chiropractic care costs were surprisingly high, apparently due to high visit frequency and heavy use of x-rays (however, the study did not include chiropractors in any form of managed care).
- Overall, functional outcomes were similar but practice patterns showed a great deal of variability.

What should a health plan do? Managed primary care HCPs cost the least, but customer satisfaction was highest with chiropractors. Consider what kinds of competitive issues would evolve if chiropractors systematically incorporated outcomes management strategies driven by successful functional measures. Alternatively, if family HCPs incorporated more hands-on approaches, such as manipulation, in lieu of "scientific" injections or just telling patients to wait until they improve, what could happen to their satis-

Table 24–4: Low Back Patient Outcomes

CATEGORY	COST ($)	X-RAY (%)	CT/MRI (%)	VISITS (NO.)	SATISFACTION (%)
PCP, non-HMO	510	28	10	4.5	
PCP, HMO	365	19	6	3.1	26, excellent
Orthopedist	809	72	17	5.5	
Chiropractor (urban)	809	67	8	15	42, excellent

CT, computed tomography; HMO, health maintenance organization; MRI, magnetic resonance imaging; PCP, primary care provider.

Chapter 5: General Health Questionnaires

FORM A–1. HEALTH STATUS QUESTIONNAIRE (HSQ-36): DECODED VERSION*

NAME_____ AGE_____ DATE_____ DATE OF INJURY_____

DECODED KEY: SEE INFORMATION ON LAST PAGE FOR SCORING

HEALTH STATUS QUESTIONNAIRE (HSQ-36)

---

1. In general, would you say your health is:

	(circle one number)	Decode
Excellent	1	100
Very Good	2	85
Good	3	60
Fair	4	25
Poor	5	0

2. Compared to one year ago, how would you rate your health in general now?

	(circle one number)	
Much better now than one year ago	1	none
Somewhat better now than one year ago	2	
About the same	3	
Somewhat worse now than one year ago	4	
Much worse now than one year ago	5	

The following items are about activities you might do during a typical day. Does your health now limit you in these activities? If so, how much?

	Yes, limited a lot	Yes, limited a little	No, not limited at all	Decode
	(circle one number on each line)			
3. Vigorous activities, such as running, lifting heavy objects, participating in strenuous sports	1	2	3	0, 50, 100
4. Moderate activities, such as moving a table, pushing a vacuum cleaner, bowling, or playing golf	1	2	3	0, 50, 100
5. Lifting or carrying groceries	1	2	3	0, 50, 100
6. Climbing several flights of stairs	1	2	3	0, 50, 100
7. Climbing one flight of stairs	1	2	3	0, 50, 100
8. Bending, kneeling or stooping	1	2	3	0, 50, 100
9. Walking more than a mile	1	2	3	0, 50, 100
10. Walking several blocks	1	2	3	0, 50, 100
11. Walking one block	1	2	3	0, 50, 100
12. Bathing or dressing yourself	1	2	3	0, 50, 100

During the past 4 weeks, have you had any of the following problems with your work or other regular daily activities as a result of your physical health?

	(circle one number on each line)		Decode
	Yes	No	
13. Cut down the amount of time you spent on work or other activities	1	2	0, 100
14. Accomplished less than you would like	1	2	0, 100
15. Were limited in the kind of work or other activities	1	2	0, 100
16. Had difficulty performing the work or other activities (for example, it took extra effort)	1	2	0, 100

During the past 4 weeks, have you had any of the following problems with your work or other regular daily activities as a result of any emotional problems (such as feeling depressed or anxious)?

	(circle one number on each line)		
17. Cut down the amount of time you spent on work or other acitivities	1	2	0, 100
18. Accomplished less than you would like	1	2	0, 100
19. Didn't do work or other activities as carefully as usual	1	2	0, 100

20. During the past 4 weeks, to what extent has your physical health or emotional problems interfered with your normal social activities with family, friends, neighbors, or groups?

(circle one number)		
Not at all	1	100
Slightly	2	75
Moderately	3	50
Quite a bit	4	25
Extremely	5	0

21. How much bodily pain have you had during the past 4 weeks?

(circle one number)		
None	1	100
Very mild	2	80
Mild	3	60
Moderate	4	40
Severe	5	20
Very severe	6	0

22. During the past 4 weeks how much did pain interfere with your normal work (including both work outside the home and housework)?

(circle one number)		Decode
None at all	1	100
A little bit	2	75
Moderately	3	50
Quite a bit	4	25
Extremely	5	0

These questions are about how you feel and how things have been with you during the past 4 weeks. For each question, please give the one answer that comes closest to the way you have been feeling.

How much of the time during the past 4 weeks . . .

	All of the time	Most of the time	A good bit of the time	Some of the time	Little	None	
23. Did you feel full of pep?	1	2	3	4	5	6	100, 80, 60, 40, 20, 0
24. Have you been a very nervous person?	1	2	3	4	5	6	0, 20, 40, 60, 80, 100

25. Have you felt so down in the dumps that nothing could cheer you up?	1	2	3	4	5	6	0, 20, 40, 60, 80, 100
26. Have you felt calm and peaceful?	1	2	3	4	5	6	100, 80, 60, 40, 20, 0
27. Did you have a lot of energy?	1	2	3	4	5	6	100, 80, 60, 40, 20, 0
28. Have you felt downhearted and blue?	1	2	3	4	5	6	0, 20, 40, 60, 80, 100
29. Did you feel worn out?	1	2	3	4	5	6	0, 20, 40, 60, 80, 100
30. Have you been a happy person?	1	2	3	4	5	6	100, 80, 60, 40, 20, 0
31. Did you feel tired?	1	2	3	4	5	6	0, 20, 40, 60, 80, 100

32. During the past 4 weeks, how much of the time has your physical health or emotional health problems interfered with your social activities (like visiting with friends, relatives, etc.)?

	(circle one number)	
All of the time	1	0
Most of the time	2	25
Some of the time	3	50
A little of the time	4	75
None of the time	5	100

How TRUE or FALSE is *each* of the following statements for you?

	Definitely true	Mostly true	Don't know	Mostly false	Definitely false	Decode
33. I seem to get sick a little easier than other people	1	2	3	4	5	0, 25, 50, 75, 100
34. I am as healthy as anybody I know	1	2	3	4	5	100, 75, 50, 25, 0
35. I expect my health to get worse	1	2	3	4	5	0, 25, 50, 75, 100
36. My health is excellent	1	2	3	4	5	100, 75, 50, 25, 0

Please answer YES or NO for each question by circling "1" or "2" on each line.

	Yes	No	(No decode)
37. In the past year, have you had 2 weeks or more during which you felt sad, blue or depressed; or when you lost all interest or pleasure in things that you usually cared about or enjoyed?	1	2	
38. Have you had 2 years or more in your life when you felt depressed or sad most days, even if you felt okay sometimes?	1	2	
39. Have you felt depressed or sad much of the time in the past year?	1	2	

SECOND STEP—COMPUTING SCALE SCORES

Scale	No. of Items	Scale Items	Minimum No. of Items Needed to Compute a Score
Health Perception	5	1, 33, 34, 35, 36	3
Physical Functioning	10	3, 4, 5, 6, 7, 8, 9, 10, 11, 12	5
Role Limitations due to Physical Health	4	13, 14, 15, 16	2
Role Limitations due to Emotional Problems	3	17, 18, 19	2
Social Functioning	2	20, 32	1
Mental Health	5	24, 25, 26, 28, 30	3
Bodily Pain	2	21, 22	1
Energy/Fatigue	4	23, 27, 29, 31	2

Formula: $\dfrac{HSQ24 + HSQ25 + HSQ26 + HSQ28 + HSQ30}{5}$ = Mental Health Score

LAST STEP: The average for each of the 8 categories is calculated and then transferred to the summary page.

EXAMPLE:	NO. OF ITEMS	QUESTION NO'S	SCORES	TOTAL	AVERAGE
1. Health Perception	n = 5:	1, 33, 34, 35, 36	85 + 75 + 75 + 75 + 50 =	360/5 =	72
2. Physical Function:	n = 10:	3–12	50 + 50 + 100 + 100 + 100 + 50 + 50 + 50 + 100 + 100 =	750/10 =	75
↓	↓	↓	↓	↓	↓
8. Role—Energy Fatigue:	n = 4:	23, 27, 29, 31	80 + 80 + 100 + 80 =	340/4 =	85

* Use for scoring.

**Transfer scores to Form A–3 (p. 500). See "Rules" on p. 503.

FORM A–2. HEALTH STATUS QUESTIONNAIRE (HSQ-36)

NAME_____ AGE_____ DATE_____ DATE OF INJURY_____

HEALTH STATUS QUESTIONNAIRE (HSQ-36)

1. In general, would you say your health is:

   (circle one number)

Excellent	1
Very Good	2
Good	3
Fair	4
Poor	5

2. Compared to one year ago, how would you rate your health in general now?

   (circle one number)

Much better now than one year ago	1
Somewhat better now than one year ago	2
About the same	3
Somewhat worse now than one year ago	4
Much worse now than one year ago	5

The following items are about activities you might do during a typical day. Does your health now limit you in these activities? If so, how much?

(circle one number on each line)

	Yes, limited a lot	Yes, limited a little	No, not limited at all
3. Vigorous activities, such as running, lifting heavy objects, participating in strenuous sports	1	2	3
4. Moderate activities, such as moving a table, pushing a vacuum cleaner, bowling, or playing golf	1	2	3
5. Lifting or carrying groceries	1	2	3
6. Climbing several flights of stairs	1	2	3
7. Climbing one flight of stairs	1	2	3
8. Bending, kneeling or stooping	1	2	3
9. Walking more than a mile	1	2	3
10. Walking several blocks	1	2	3
11. Walking one block	1	2	3
12. Bathing or dressing yourself	1	2	3

During the past 4 weeks, have you had any of the following problems with your work or other regular daily activities as a result of your physical health?

(circle one number on each line)

	Yes	No
13. Cut down the amount of time you spent on work or other activities	1	2
14. Accomplished less than you would like	1	2
15. Were limited in the kind of work or other activities	1	2
16. Had difficulty performing the work or other activities (for example, it took extra effort)	1	2

During the past 4 weeks, have you had any of the following problems with your work or other regular daily activities as a result of any emotional problems (such as feeling depressed or anxious)?

(circle one number on each line)

	Yes	No
17. Cut down the amount of time you spent on work or other activities	1	2
18. Accomplished less than you would like	1	2
19. Didn't do work or other activities as carefully as usual	1	2

20. During the past 4 weeks, to what extent has your physical health or emotional problems interfered with your normal social activities with family, friends, neighbors, or groups?

(circle one number)

Not at all	1
Slightly	2
Moderately	3
Quite a bit	4
Extremely	5

21. How much bodily pain have you had during the past 4 weeks?

(circle one number)

None	1
Very mild	2
Mild	3
Moderate	4
Severe	5
Very severe	6

22. During the past 4 weeks how much did pain interfere with your normal work (including both work outside the home and housework)?

(circle one number)

None at all	1
A little bit	2
Moderately	3
Quite a bit	4
Extremely	5

These questions are about how you feel and how things have been with you during the past 4 weeks. For each question, please give the one answer that comes closest to the way you have been feeling.

How much of the time during the past 4 weeks . . .

(circle one number on each line)

	All of the time	Most of the time	A good bit of the time	Some of the time	Little of the time	None of the time
23. Did you feel full of pep?	1	2	3	4	5	6
24. Have you been a very nervous person?	1	2	3	4	5	6
25. Have you felt so down in the dumps that nothing could cheer you up?	1	2	3	4	5	6
26. Have you felt calm and peaceful?	1	2	3	4	5	6
27. Did you have a lot of energy?	1	2	3	4	5	6
28. Have you felt downhearted and blue?	1	2	3	4	5	6
29. Did you feel worn out?	1	2	3	4	5	6
30. Have you been a happy person?	1	2	3	4	5	6
31. Did you feel tired?	1	2	3	4	5	6

LAST STEP: The average for each of the 8 categories is calculated and t

Example	No. of Items	Question No's
1. Physical Function	n = 3	2–4
2. Role-Physical	n = 1	5
↓	↓	↓
8. Mental Health	n = 3	9, 11, 12

RULES:

1. Step 1: Recode the response values from the instrument (use the recoding

2. Step 2: Calculate the average of the recoded response values for the multi

3. The higher the score, the better the health status.

4. Scoring may be completed manually with a calculator or with a standard d
   SPSS, FoxPro, dBASE). It is more efficient and reliable to enter the numb
   spreadsheet or data entry package, allowing the computer to process the n

5. Missing responses for scales 1 and 8 can be estimated by averaging the 2 co
   the 2 into the missing 1 question slot). When a missing response from a sin

* Use for scoring.

**Transfer scores to Form A–6 (p. 506)

FORM A–

NAME

DECODED KE

HEALTH STATU

1. In general, w

The following ite
much?

2. Lifting or carr
3. Climbing sev
4. Walking sev
5. During the **pa**
   health? (*circle*

6. During the **pas**
   result of emoti

7. During the **past**
   with family, frie

32. During the past 4 weeks, how much of the time has your physical health or emotional health problems interfered with you social activities (like visiting with friends, relatives, etc.)?

   (circle one number)

All of the time	1
Most of the time	2
Some of the time	3
A little of the time	4
None of the time	5

How TRUE or FALSE is *each* of the following statements for you?

	Definitely true	Mostly true	Don't know	Mostly false	Definitely false
33. I seem to get sick a little easier than other people	1	2	3	4	5
34. I am as healthy as anybody I know	1	2	3	4	5
35. I expect my health to get worse	1	2	3	4	5
36. My health is excellent	1	2	3	4	5

Please answer YES or NO for each question by circling "1" or "2" on each line.

	Yes	No
37. In the past year, have you had 2 weeks or more during which you felt sad, blue or depressed; or when you lost all interest or pleasure in things that you usually care about or enjoyed?	1	2
38. Have you had 2 years or more in your life when you felt depressed or sad most days, even if you felt okay sometimes?	1	2
39. Have you felt depressed or sad much of the time in the past year?	1	2

FORM A–3. S

NAME_____

SCALE
1. HEALTH PE
2. PHYSICAL I
3. ROLE—PHY
4. ROLE—EMC
5. SOCIAL FUI
6. BODILY PAI
7. MENTAL HI
8. ENERGY FA
9. MAJOR DEI
10. DYSTHEMI.
11. BOTH 9 & 1

◯ CIRCLE SU

SIGNED_____

8. How much bodily pain have you had during the past 4 weeks?

These questions are about how you feel and how things have been with you duri
one answer that comes closest to the way you have been feeling.

How much of the time during the **past 4 weeks** . . .

(circle one number o

	All of the time	Most of the time	A good bit of the time
9. Have you felt calm and peaceful?	1	2	3
10. Did you have a lot of energy?	1	2	3
11. Have you felt downhearted and blue?	1	2	3
12. Have you been a happy person?	1	2	3

SECOND STEP—HSQ-12 SCORING ALGORITHMS/SECOND STEP—CO

Scale	No. of Items	Scal
Physical Functioning	3	2
Role Limitations Attributable to: Physical Health (Role—Physical)	1	
Bodily Pain	1	
Health Perception	1	
Energy/Fatigue	1	
Social Functioning	1	
Role Limitations Attributable to: Mental Health (Role—Mental)	1	
Mental Health	3	9,

SCORING THE HSQ-12

Formula: $\dfrac{\text{Sum of Recoded Scale Iter}}{\text{Number of Completed Scale I}}$

$$\frac{HSQ9 + HSQ11 + HSQ12}{3} =$$

FORM A–6. SF-12 HEALTH STATUS SUMMARY

NAME_____ DATE_____ AGE_____ DOB_____ SEX M/F_____

Scale	SF-12 Mean[a]	Initial Baseline	1st Re-Exam	2nd Re-Exam	3rd Re-Exam
1. HEALTH PERCEPTION	72				
2. PHYSICAL FUNCTION	84				
3. ROLE—PHYSICAL	81				
4. ROLE—EMOTIONAL	81				
5. SOCIAL FUNCTIONING	83				
6. BODILY PAIN	75				
7. MENTAL HEALTH	75				
8. ENERGY FATIGUE	61				

[a] Not yet established (1996); the mean scores are those derived from the HSQ-2.0 (36-item questionnaire)

◯ CIRCLE SUB-MEAN SCORES

SIGNED_____ DATE_____

FORM A–7. DARTMOUTH COOP CHARTS

PHYSICAL FITNESS

During the past 4 weeks . . .
What was the hardest physical activity
you could do for at least 2 minutes ?

Very heavy, (for example) •Run, fast pace •Carry a heavy load upstairs or uphill (25 lbs/10 kgs)		1
Heavy, (for example) •Jog, slow pace •Climb stairs or a hill moderate pace		2
Moderate, (for example) •Walk, medium pace •Carry a heavy load level ground (25 lbs/10 kgs)		3
Light, (for example) •Walk, medium pace •Carry light load on level ground (10 lbs/5kgs)		4
Very light, (for example) •Walk, slow pace •Wash dishes		5

FEELINGS

During the past 4 weeks . . .
How much have you been bothered by
emotional problems such as feeling anxious,
depressed, irritable or downhearted and blue ?

Not at all		1
Slightly		2
Moderately		3
Quite a bit		4
Extremely		5

DAILY ACTIVITIES

During the past 4 weeks . . .
How much difficulty have you had doing your usual
activities or task, both inside and outside the house
because of your physical and emotional health ?

No difficulty at all		1
A little bit of difficulty		2
Some difficulty		3
Much difficulty		4
Could not do		5

SOCIAL ACTIVITIES

During the past 4 weeks . . .
Has your physical and emotional health limited
your social activities with family, friends,
neighbors or groups ?

Not at all		1
Slightly		2
Moderately		3
Quite a bit		4
Extremely		5

Source: Copyright © Tr

FORM I

INSTRUCT
NOTE: If yo
each compla
EXAMPLE:

no pain

1. What is

no pain

2. What is

no pain

3. What is

no pain

What pe

4. What is

no pain

What pe

NAME

SCORE: #1

Compiled from

During t
How r
gener

No pain
Very mild pain
Mild pain
Moderate pain
Severe pain

O

During the past
How would y

Excellent
Very good
Good
Fair
Poor

FORM A–8

SCALE

FUNCTION

1. Physical fitn

2. Feelings

3. Daily activit

4. Social activi

OVERALL HI

5. Pain

6. Change in h

7. Overall heal

QUALITY OI

8. Social supp

9. Quality of li

Scale range 1 to

COMMENTS:

_____
_____
_____
_____

NAME_____

SECTION 9—Traveling

A I get no pain while traveling.

B I get some pain while traveling, but none of my usual forms of travel make it any worse.

C I get extra pain while traveling, but it does not compel me to seek alternative forms of travel.

D I get extra pain while traveling which compels me to seek alternative forms of travel.

E Pain restricts all forms of travel.

F Pain prevents all forms of travel except that done lying down.

SECTION 10—Changing Degree of Pain

A My pain is rapidly getting better.

B My pain fluctuates, but overall is definitely getting better.

C My pain seems to be getting better, but improvement is slow at present.

D My pain is neither getting better nor worse.

E My pain is gradually worsening.

F My pain is rapidly worsening.

COMMENTS:_____

NAME:_____ DATE:_____ SCORE:_____

From Fairbank J, Davies J, et al. The Oswestry Low Back Pain Disability Questionnaire. *Physiotherapy* 1980;66(18):271–273.

FORM C–3. THE QUEBEC BACK PAIN DISABILITY SCALE

Name_____ Age_____ Date_____ Score_____

This questionnaire is about the way your back pain is affecting your life. People with back problems may find it difficult to perform some of their daily activities. We would like to know if you find it difficult to perform any of the activities listed below, because of your back. For each activity there is a scale of 0 to 5 (0 = normal; 5 = severe. Please choose one response option for each activity (do not skip any activities) and check the corresponding box.

Today, do you find it difficult to perform the following activities because of your back?	0	1	2	3	4	5
1. Get out of bed.						
2. Sleep through the night (sleep at least 6 hours).						
3. Turn over in bed.						
4. Ride in a car (travel 1 hour in a car).						
5. Stand up for 20–30 minutes.						
6. Sit for 4 hours in a chair.						
7. Climb one flight of stairs.						
8. Walk a few blocks (300–400 m).						
9. Walk several miles.						
10. Reach up to high shelves.						
11. Throw a ball.						
12. Run two blocks (about 200 m).						
13. Take food out of the refrigerator.						
14. Make your bed.						
15. Put on socks (panty hose).						
16. Bend over a sink for 10 minutes.						
17. Move a chair.						
18. Pull or push heavy doors.						
19. Carry two bags of groceries.						
20. Lift and carry a heavy suitcase (or 40 pounds).						
SUB-TOTAL						
TOTAL SCORE						

Comments: _____

_____

_____

_____

_____

Scored by:_____ SCORE:_____ Date:_____

From Kopec JA, Esdaile JM, Abrahamowicz M, Abenhaim L, Wood-Dauphinee S, Lamping DL. The Quebec Back Pain Disability Scale: Measurement properties. *Spine* 1995;20:341–352.

FORM C–4. NORTH AMERICAN SPINE SOCIETY LOW BACK PAIN OUTCOME INSTRUMENT

Baseline
A. Personal Information
B. Medical History, Expectations and Outcomes
C. Employment History and Work Status

Dear Program Participant:

The following questions will help us tell how your back is doing and will allow us to track your progress in treatment. Please take 15–20 minutes to fill out this questionnaire today. Please answer all questions to the best of your ability.

If you have any questions, please ask the receptionist for help. You may give the questionnaire back to the receptionist when you are done.

Thank you!

HISTORY

Chief Complaint:

_____

_____

_____

_____

Onset of symptoms_____

_____

_____

Have you had spine surgery in the past? [ ] Yes [ ] No

If yes, state when and what area of your spine:

_____

_____

_____

Physician who performed surgery:_____

ARE YOU NOW HAVING, OR HAVE YOU EVER HAD:

	Weakness	Numbness	Tingling	N/A
Arms	[ ]	[ ]	[ ]	[ ]
Face	[ ]	[ ]	[ ]	[ ]
Hands	[ ]	[ ]	[ ]	[ ]
Fingers	[ ]	[ ]	[ ]	[ ]
Legs	[ ]	[ ]	[ ]	[ ]
Feet	[ ]	[ ]	[ ]	[ ]

ARE YOU NOW, OR HAVE YOU EVER EXPERIENCED ANY OF THE FOLLOWING:

	Present	Past	N/A
Difficulty eating	[ ]	[ ]	[ ]
Difficulty talking	[ ]	[ ]	[ ]
Spotty vision	[ ]	[ ]	[ ]
Tunnel vision	[ ]	[ ]	[ ]
Temporary confusion or loss of consciousness	[ ]	[ ]	[ ]
Blurred vision or temporary loss of vision	[ ]	[ ]	[ ]
Seeing double	[ ]	[ ]	[ ]
Dizziness	[ ]	[ ]	[ ]
Ringing in your ears	[ ]	[ ]	[ ]
Loss of hearing	[ ]	[ ]	[ ]

Medical History:

	Yes	No		Yes	No
Hypertension	[ ]	[ ]	Kidney disease	[ ]	[ ]
Diabetes mellitus	[ ]	[ ]	Major surgery	[ ]	[ ]
Heart disease	[ ]	[ ]	Type/date:_____
Cancer	[ ]	[ ]	_____
			_____

CURRENT MEDICATIONS AND DOSAGE:

_____

_____

_____

_____

Are you currently seeing another doctor(s) for treatment of this spine pain?   [ ] Yes   [ ] No

Name:_____

Name:_____

Name:_____

Name:_____

Name:_____

Are you presently using oral contraceptives:	[ ] Yes	[ ] No	[ ] N/A
Is there a history of stroke in your family:	[ ] Yes	[ ] No	
Is there a history of high blood pressure?	[ ] Yes	[ ] No	
Are you diabetic?	[ ] Yes	[ ] No	

_____

Patient's signature

ID#_____

A. PERSONAL INFORMATION (CIRCLE ALL THAT APPLY):

1. Your gender:

1   Male

2   Female

2. Your race

1   White

2   Black or African-American

3   Hispanic

4   Asian or Pacific Islander

5   Native American Indian

6   Other, please specify:_____

3. How much schooling have you completed?

1   Completed less than high school

2   Graduated from high school

3   Completed 1 to 3 years of college

4   Graduated from a 2-year associate degree program or technical school

5   Graduated from college (Bachelors degree or equivalent)

6   Completed post-graduate or professional degree

4. What is your current marital situation?

1   Married/Living with significant other

2   Divorced/Separated

3   Widowed

4   Single (never married)

B. MEDICAL HISTORY, EXPECTATIONS AND OUTCOMES

1. How long ago did your *current* episode begin?

1   Less than two weeks ago

2   Two weeks to less than eight weeks ago

3   Eight weeks to less than three months ago

4   Three months to less than six months ago

5   Six to twelve months ago

6   More than twelve months ago

2. How did your *current* episode begin?

1   Suddenly

2   Gradually

3. Have you had back symptoms before your current episode?

1   No (IF NO, GO TO QUESTION 6)

2   Yes, one episode

3   Yes, two or more episodes

QUESTIONS 4 AND 5 ARE ABOUT YOUR **PAST** BACK SYMPTOMS

4. Did you receive Workers' Compensation for your *past* back symptoms?

1   No

2   Yes

5. How much work did you miss because of your worst prior episode?

1   None

2   1 day to 2 weeks

3   More than 2 weeks to 4 weeks

4   More than 4 weeks to 12 weeks

5   More than 12 weeks to 24 weeks

6   More than 24 weeks

6. Have you had previous back surgery?

1   No (if no, go to question 9)

2   Yes. How many surgeries?_____

QUESTIONS 7 AND 8 ARE ABOUT YOUR *PAST* BACK SURGERIES

7. After your most recent surgery, did you return to work?

1   No

2   Yes, with limitations

3   Yes, with no limitations

4   Never stopped working

5   Did not work: A. Homemaker

B. Student

C. Retired

D. Other

8. After your most recent surgery, did you return to full function?

1   No

2   Yes

THERE WILL BE SEVERAL QUESTIONS ABOUT LEG AND BACK PAIN IN THIS QUESTIONNAIRE. WHEN WE SAY LEG, WE MEAN YOUR THIGH, CALF, ANKLE, AND FOOT. WHEN WE SAY BACK, WE MEAN YOUR LOW BACK AND BUTTOCKS.

9. Which hurts you more, your legs or back?

1   Legs hurt much more

2   Legs hurt somewhat more

3   Legs and back hurt about the same

4   Back hurts somewhat more

5   Back hurts much more

PLEASE ANSWER EVERY QUESTION IN THE BOX BELOW

In the *past week*, how often have you suffered:	None of the time	A little of the time	Some of the time	A good bit of the time	Most of the time	All of the time
10. Low back and/or buttock pain	1	2	3	4	5	6
11. Leg pain	1	2	3	4	5	6
12. Numbness or tingling in leg and/ or foot	1	2	3	4	5	6
13. Weakness in leg and/or foot (such as difficulty lifting foot)	1	2	3	4	5	6

PLEASE ANSWER EVERY QUESTION IN THE BOX BELOW

In the *past week*, how bothersome have these symptoms been?	Not at all bothersome	Slightly bothersome	Somewhat bothersome	Moderately bothersome	Very bothersome	Extremely bothersome
10. Low back and/or buttock pain	1	2	3	4	5	6
11. Leg pain	1	2	3	4	5	6
12. Numbness or tingling in leg and/or foot	1	2	3	4	5	6
13. Weakness in leg and/or foot (such as difficulty lifting foot)	1	2	3	4	5	6

33. During the *last week,* how often have you taken non-narcotic medication such as aspirin, Motrin, or Tylenol for your back and/or leg pain?

    1   3 or more times a day

    2   Once or twice a day

    3   Once every couple of days

    4   Once a week

    5   Not at all

34. Have you used alcoholic beverages (beer, wine, liquor) to relieve your current back or leg pain?

    1   No

    2   Yes, once in a while

    3   Yes, often

35. If you had to spend the rest of your life with your *back condition as it is right now,* how would you feel about it?

    1   Extremely dissatisfied

    2   Very dissatisfied

    3   Somewhat dissatisfied

    4   Neutral

    5   Somewhat satisfied

    6   Very satisfied

    7   Extremely satisfied

WHAT EXPECTATIONS DO YOU HAVE FOR YOUR TREATMENT AT THIS OFFICE?

As a result of my treatment, I expect . . .	Not likely	Slightly likely	Somewhat likely	Very likely	Extremely likely
36. Complete pain relief	1	2	3	4	5
37. Moderate pain relief	1	2	3	4	5
38. To be able to do more everyday household or yard activities	1	2	3	4	5
39. To be able to sleep more comfortably	1	2	3	4	5
40. To be able to go back to my usual job	1	2	3	4	5
41. To be able to do more sports, go biking, or go for long walks	1	2	3	4	5

42. What other results do you expect from your treatment? Please describe:

_____

_____

_____

_____

HOW IMPORTANT ARE THE FOLLOWING TREATMENT OUTCOMES FOR YOU?

How important is . . .	Not Important	Slightly Important	Somewhat Important	Very Important	Extremely Important
43. Pain relief	1	2	3	4	5
44. To be able to do more everyday household or yard activities.	1	2	3	4	5
45. To be able to sleep more comfortably.	1	2	3	4	5
46. To be able to go back to my usual job.	1	2	3	4	5
47. To be able to do more sports, go biking, or go for long walks.	1	2	3	4	5
48. Other (See your answer to #42 above):_____ _____	1	2	3	4	5

FOLLOWING ARE SOME QUESTIONS ABOUT YOUR GENERAL HEALTH.

49. In general, would you say your health is:

1 Excellent
2 Very good
3 Good
4 Fair
5 Poor
6 Terrible

50. Have you ever had any of the following conditions? (CIRCLE ALL THAT APPLY)

1 Diabetes
2 Heart Disease
3 Stroke
4 Arthritis or other pain in your back
5 Asthma or other lung disease
6 Depression
7 High Blood Pressure (Hypertension)
8 Colitis
9 Psoriasis
10 None of the above

51. Do you currently smoke cigarrettes?

1 I have never smoked
2 Yes
3 No, I quit in the last six months
4 No, I quit more than six months ago

THE FOLLOWING QUESTIONS ARE ABOUT HOW YOU FEEL AND HOW THINGS HAVE BEEN WITH YOU *DURING THE LAST WEEK.* FOR EACH QUESTION, PLEASE INDICATE THE ONE ANSWER THAT COMES CLOSEST TO THE WAY YOU HAVE BEEN FEELING. **PLEASE CIRCLE ONE ANSWER ON EACH LINE.**

How much of the time during the last week	All of the time	Most of the time	A good bit of time	Some of the time	Little of the time	None of the time
52. Have you been a very nervous person?	1	2	3	4	5	6
53. Have you felt so down in the dumps nothing could cheer you up?	1	2	3	4	5	6
54. Have you felt calm and peaceful?	1	2	3	4	5	6
55. Have you felt down-hearted and blue?	1	2	3	4	5	6
56. Have you been a happy person?	1	2	3	4	5	6

C. EMPLOYMENT HISTORY AND WORK STATUS

PLEASE CIRCLE YOUR RESPONSES TO THE FOLLOWING QUESTIONS:

1. How many jobs have you had in the last 3 years?

    1   None

    2   One or two

    3   Three or more

2. Which statements describe your current employment situation? (CIRCLE ALL THAT APPLY)

    1   Currently working

    2   On paid leave

    3   On unpaid leave

    4   Unemployed

    5   Homemaker

    6   Student

    7   Retired (Not due to health)

    8   Disabled and/or retired because of my back problems

    9   Disabled due to a health problem not related to my back

    10   Other, please specify_____

3. Are you self-employed?

    1   No

    2   Yes

4. If not working now, how long has it been since you stopped?

    1   Less than one week ago

    2   One week to less than three months ago

    3   Three months to less than six months ago

    4   Six months to less than twelve months ago

    5   One to two years ago

    6   More than two years ago

    7   Currently working

    8   Never employed

5. What is your primary occupation? If you are not working now, what was your primary occupation? (PLEASE BE AS SPECIFIC AS POSSIBLE)

Occupation:_____

6. Is your current job the same one you had when your current back symptoms started?

1   Yes, exact same job

2   Yes, but job was modified or hours reduced because of my back

3   No, I have changed jobs because of my back symptoms

4   No, I have changed jobs but for reasons unrelated to my back

5   Not working now

7. How long have you worked at your current job?

1   Less than six months

2   Six to twelve months

3   More than twelve months

4   Not working now

PLEASE ANSWER EACH OF THE FOLLOWING QUESTIONS ABOUT YOUR CURRENT JOB (OR THE ONE YOU PLAN TO GO BACK TO IF ON LEAVE). **CIRCLE ONE ANSWER ON EACH LINE.**

	All of the time	Most of the time	A good bit of the time	Some of the time	Little of the time	None of the time
8. How much sitting does your work involve?	1	2	3	4	5	6
9. How much standing or walking does your work involve?	1	2	3	4	5	6
10. How often do you lift 25 lbs. on the job?	1	2	3	4	5	6
11. How often do you lift 50 lbs. on the job?	1	2	3	4	5	6

PLEASE ANSWER EACH OF THE FOLLOWING QUESTIONS ABOUT YOUR **CURRENT JOB (OR** THE ONE YOU PLAN TO GO BACK TO IF ON LEAVE)

	Extremely	Very much	Quite a bit	Somewhat	A little	Not at all
12. Is your current work physically demanding?	1	2	3	4	5	6
13. Is your work stressful to you?	1	2	3	4	5	6
14. How much do you like your job?	1	2	3	4	5	6
15. How much do you like your co-workers?	1	2	3	4	5	6
16. How much do you like your supervisor?	1	2	3	4	5	6

17. Other than your salary, what other sources of income does your household receive? (CIRCLE ALL THAT APPLY)

1   Another person's salary

2   State support

3   Social Security

4   Disability

5   Other (Investments, retirement plan, etc.)

6   No other source of income

FORM C–5B. CURTIN BACK SCREENING QUESTIONNAIRE

NAME:_____ AGE:_____ DATE:_____ SCORE:_____

	Total
1. On average, how severe is your back pain? No pain Mild Moderate Severe pain	
2. How many good days do you have in a week? 6–7 days 4–5 days 2–3 days 0–1 days	
3. Since your injury do you take longer to do things? Same as usual Slightly longer Longer Much longer than usual	
4. Since your injury how much difficulty do you have doing your housework, shopping and other general household duties? No difficulty Light Moderate Extreme difficulty	
5. Since your injury do you find it difficult to do things with your children and family (or with close friends if no family)? No, not at all No more than usual More than usual Much more than usual	
6. Since your injury, are you feeling socially isolated or left out? Not at all Sometimes More than usual Much more than usual	
7. Since your injury do you take part in physical or outdoor activities for shorter periods of time? Same time as usual Shorter Much shorter Unable to participate	
8. Since your injury have you been taking longer over the things you do? No, not at all No more than usual Longer than usual Much longer than usual	
TOTAL SCREENING SCORE	

From Harper AC, Harper DA, Lambert LJ, et al. Development and validation of the Curtin Back Screening Questionnaire (CBSQ). *Pain* 1995;6:73–81.

FORM C–6. ACTIVITIES DISCOMFORT SCALE

For each of the following activities, please place a check in the one column that best describes how much pain the activity presently causes, on the average (does not include unusual or prolonged activity).

Activity	Doesn't Hurt At All	Hurts A Little	Hurts Very Much	Almost Unbearable	Unbearable Pain Prevents Activity
1. Walking					
2. Sitting					
3. Bending					
4. Standing					
5. Sleeping					
6. Lifting					
7. Running or jogging					
8. Climbing stairs					
9. Carrying					
10. Pushing and pulling					
11. Driving					
12. Dressing					
13. Reading					
14. Watching TV					
15. Household chores					
16. Gardening					
17. Sports					
18. Employment					
TOTAL					

COMMENTS:_____

_____

_____

_____

_____

NAME:_____ DATE:_____ SCORE:_____

From Turner JA, Robinson J, McCreary CP. Chronic low back pain: Predicting response to nonsurgical treatment. *Arch Phys Med Rehabil* 1983;64:560–563.

FORM C–7. LOW BACK OUTCOME SCALE: SCORING TEMPLATE

NAME:_____ DATE:_____ SCORE:_____

		Scores
Factors Scoring 9 points		
Current pain (visual analogue scale)	7–10	0
	5–6	3
	3–4	6
	0–2	9
Employment (housewives related to previous abilities)	Unemployed	0
	Part-time	3
	Full-time, lighter	6
	Full-time, orginial	9
Domestic chores or "odd jobs"	None	0
	A few but not many	3
	Most, or all but more slowly	6
	Normally	9
Sport/active social (dancing)	None	0
	Some—much less than before	3
	Back to previous level	9
Factors scoring 6 points		
Resting	Resting more than half the day	0
	Little rest needed, occasionally	4
	No need to rest	6
Treatment or consultation	More than once per month	0
	About once per month	2
	Rarely	4
	Never	6
Analgesia	Several times each day	0
	Almost every day	2
	Occasionally	4
	Never	6
Sex life	Severely affected, impossible	0
	Moderately affected, difficult	2
	Mildly affected	4
	Unaffected	6
Factors scoring 3 points		
Sleeping, walking, sitting, traveling, dressing	Severely affected, impossible	0
	Moderately affected, difficult	1
	Mildly affected	2
	Unaffected	3

Modified from Greenough CG, Fraser RD. Assessment of outcome in patients with low back pain. *Spine* 992;17:36–41.

FORM C–8. CLINICAL BACK PAIN QUESTIONNAIRE

NAME:_____ AGE:_____ DATE:_____ SCORE:_____

1. In the last two weeks, for how many days did you suffer pain in the back or leg(s)? (Please check one)

   None at all____ Between 1 and 5 days____ Between 1 and 10 days____ For more than 10 days____

2. On the worst day during the last two weeks, how many pain killing tablets did you take? (Please check one)

   None at all____ Less than 4 tablets____ Between 4 & 8 tablets____ Between 9 & 12 tablets____ More than 12____

3. Is the pain made worse by any of the following? (Please check all that apply to you)

   Coughing____ Sneezing____ Sitting____ Standing____ Bending____ Walking____

4. Do any of the following movements ease the pain? (Please check all that apply to you)

   Lying down____ Sitting down____ Standing____ Walking____

5. In your right leg, do you have any pain in the following areas? (Please check all that apply to you)

   Pain in the buttock____ Pain in the thigh____ Pain in the shin/calf____ Pain in the foot/ankle____

6. In your left leg, do you have any pain in the following areas? (Please check all that apply to you)

   Pain in the buttock____ Pain in the thigh____ Pain in the shin/calf____ Pain in the foot/ankle____

7. Do you have any loss of feeling in your legs? (Please check one)

   No____ Yes, just one leg____ Yes, both legs____

8. In your right leg, do you have any weakness or loss of power in the following areas? (Please check all that apply to you)

   The hip____ The knee____ The ankle____ The foot____

9. In your left leg, do you have any weakness or loss of power in the following areas? (Please check all that apply to you)

   The hip____ The knee____ The ankle____ The foot____

10. If you were to try and bend forwards *without bending your knees*, how far down do you think you could bend before the pain stopped you? (Please check one)

    I could touch the floor____ I could touch my ankles with the tips of my fingers____
    I could touch my thighs with the tips of my fingers____ I couldn't bend forward at all____

11. On the worst night during the last two weeks, how badly was your sleep affected by pain? (Please check one)

    Not affected at all____ I didn't lose any sleep but needed tablets____ It prevented me from sleeping but I slept for more than four hours____ I only had 2–4 hours of sleep____ I had less than 2 hours of sleep____

12. On the worst day during the last two weeks, did the pain interfere with your ability to sit down? (Please check one)

    I was able to sit in any chair as long as I liked____ I could only sit in my favorite chair as long as I liked____
    Pain prevented me from sitting more than 1 hour____ Pain prevented me from sitting more than 30 minutes____
    Pain prevented me from sitting more than 15 minutes____ Pain prevented me from sitting at all____

13. On the worst day during the last two weeks, did the pain interfere with your ability to stand? (Please check one)

    I could stand as long as I wanted without extra pain____ I could stand as long as I wanted but it gave me extra pain____
    Pain prevented me from standing for more than 1 hour____ Pain prevented me from standing for more than 30 minutes____
    Pain prevented me from standing for more than 15 minutes____ Pain prevented me from standing at all____

14. On the worst day during the last two weeks, did the pain interfere with your ability to walk? (Please check one)

    Pain did not prevent me walking any distance____ Pain prevented me walking more than 1 mile____
    Pain prevented me walking more than 1/2 mile____ Pain prevented me walking more than 1/4 mile____
    I can walk but less than 1/4 mile____ I was unable to walk at all____

15. In the last two weeks, did the pain prevent you from carrying out your work/housework and other daily activities? (Please check one)

    No, not at all____ I could continue with my work, but my work suffered____ Yes, for one day____
    Yes, for 2–6 days____ Yes, for more than 7 days____

16. In the last two weeks, for how many days have you had to stay in bed because of the pain? (Please check one)

Not at all____ Between 1 and 5 days____ Between 6 and 10 days____ For more than 10 days____

17. In the last two weeks, has your sex life been affected by your pain? (Please check one)

Not affected by the pain____ Mildly affected by the pain____ Moderately affected by the pain____
Pain prevents any sex life at all____ Does not apply____

18. In the last two weeks, have your leisure activities been affected by your pain (including sports, hobbies and social life)? (Please check one)

Not affected by the pain____ Mildly affected by the pain____ Moderately affected by the pain____
Severely affected by the pain____ Pain prevents any social life at all____

19. In the last 2 weeks, has the pain interfered with your ability to look after yourself, eg. washing, dressing, etc? (Please check one)

Not at all____ Because of the pain, I needed some help looking after myself____
Because of the pain, I needed a lot of help looking after myself____ Because of the pain, I could not look after myself at all____

COMMENTS:_____
_____
_____

From Ruta DA, Garratt AM, Wardlaw D, Russell IT. Developing a valid and reliable measure of health outcome for patients with low back pain. *Spine* 1994;19:1887–1896.

FORM C—9. SPINAL STENOSIS TREATMENT OUTCOME QUESTIONNAIRE

SYMPTOM SEVERITY SCALE

In the *LAST MONTH,* how would you describe:	1	2	3	4	5
1. The pain you have had on average including pain in your back, buttocks and pain that goes down the legs?	NONE	MILD	MODERATE	SEVERE	VERY SEVERE
2. How often have you had back, buttock, or leg pain?	< once a week	At least once a week	Every day, for at least a few minutes.	Every day, for most of the day.	Every day, every minute of the day.
3. The pain in your back or buttocks?	NONE	MILD	MODERATE	SEVERE	VERY SEVERE
4. The pain in your legs or feet?	NONE	MILD	MODERATE	SEVERE	VERY SEVERE
5. Numbness or tingling in your legs or feet?	NONE	MILD	MODERATE	SEVERE	VERY SEVERE
6. Weakness in your legs or feet?	NONE	MILD	MODERATE	SEVERE	VERY SEVERE
7. Problems with your balance?	NONE		SOMETIMES balance is off, less sure footed		OFTEN balance is off and not sure footed

PHYSICAL FUNCTION SCALE

In the *LAST MONTH,* on a typical day:	1	2	3	4
1. How far have you been able to walk?	> 2 miles	> 2 blocks but < 2 miles	> 50 feet but < 2 blocks	Less than 50 feet
2. Have you taken walks outdoors or in malls for pleasure?	Yes, comfortably	Yes, but sometimes with pain	Yes, but always with pain	No
3. Have you been shopping for groceries or other items?	Yes, comfortably	Yes, but sometimes with pain	Yes, but always with pain	No
4. Have you walked around the different rooms in your house or apartment?	Yes, comfortably	Yes, but sometimes with pain	Yes, but always with pain	No
5. Have you walked from your bedroom to the bathroom?	Yes, comfortably	Yes, but sometimes with pain	Yes, but always with pain	No

FORM C–12. DIZZINESS HANDICAP INVENTORY

NAME:_____ DATE:_____ AGE:_____ Score Totals:_____; E____; F____; P____
                                                                                    (100)   (36)   (36)   (28)

INSTRUCTIONS: Please CIRCLE the correct response:

1. I have dizziness/unsteadiness: [1] 1 per month   [2] > 1 but < 4 per month   [3] more than one per week
2. My dizziness/unsteadiness is: [1] mild   [2] moderate   [3] severe

INSTRUCTIONS: (Please read carefully): The purpose of the scale is to identify difficulties that you may be experiencing because of your dizziness or unsteadiness. Please answer "YES," "SOMETIMES," or "NO" to each question. Answer each question as it pertains to your dizziness or unsteadiness problem only.

	YES	SOMETIMES	NO
P1. Does looking up increase your problem?	☐	☐	☐
E2. Because of your problem, do you feel frustrated?	☐	☐	☐
F3. Because of your problem, do you restrict your travel for business or recreation?	☐	☐	☐
P4. Does walking down the aisle of a supermarket increase your problem?	☐	☐	☐
F5. Because of your problem, do you have difficulty getting into or out of bed?	☐	☐	☐
F6. Does your problem significantly restrict your participation in social activities such as going out to dinner, going to movies, dancing, or to parties?	☐	☐	☐
F7. Because of your problem, do you have difficulty reading?	☐	☐	☐
P8. Does performing more ambitious activities like sports, dancing, household chores such as sweeping or putting dishes away increase your problem?	☐	☐	☐
E9. Because of your problem, are you afraid to leave your home without someone accompanying you?	☐	☐	☐
E10. Because of your problem, have you been embarrassed in front of others?	☐	☐	☐
P11. Do quick movements of your head increase your problem?	☐	☐	☐
F12. Because of your problem, do you avoid heights?	☐	☐	☐
P13. Does turning over in bed increase your problem?	☐	☐	☐
F14. Because of your problem, is it difficult for you to do strenuous house work or yard work?	☐	☐	☐
E15. Because of your problem, are you afraid people may think you are intoxicated?	☐	☐	☐
F16. Because of your problem, is it difficult for you to go for a walk by yourself?	☐	☐	☐
P17. Does walking down a sidewalk increase your problem?	☐	☐	☐
E18. Because of your problem, is it difficult for you to concentrate?	☐	☐	☐
F19. Because of your problem, is it difficult for you to walk around your house in the dark?	☐	☐	☐
E20. Because of your problem, are you afraid to stay home alone?	☐	☐	☐
E21. Because of your problem, do you feel handicapped?	☐	☐	☐
E22. Has your problem placed stress on your relationships with members of your family or friends?	☐	☐	☐
E23. Because of your problem, are you depressed?	☐	☐	☐
F24. Does your problem interfere with your job or household responsibilities?	☐	☐	☐
P25. Does bending over increase your problem?	☐	☐	☐

From Jacobson GP, Newman CW. The development of the dizziness handicap inventory. *Arch Otolarngol Head Neck Surg* 1990;116:424–427.

FORM C–13. TINNITUS HANDICAP INVENTORY

NAME:_____ DATE:_____ AGE:_____ Score Totals:_____; E____; F____; P____
                                                                          (100)   (36)   (44) (20)

INSTRUCTIONS: Please CIRCLE the correct response:

On a scale from 0 to 10. . . .

1. . . . rate the loudness of your tinnitus: (None) 0 1 2 3 4 5 6 7 8 9 10 (Extreme)

2. . . . rate the pitch of your tinnitus: (Low) 0 1 2 3 4 5 6 7 8 9 10 (Very high)

INSTRUCTIONS: (Please read carefully): The purpose of the scale is to identify difficulties that you may be experiencing because of your tinnitus. Please answer "YES," "SOMETIMES," or "NO" to each question. Please do not skip any questions.

	YES	SOMETIMES	NO
F1. Because of your tinnitus, is it difficult for you to concentrate?	☐	☐	☐
F2. Does the loudness of your tinnitus make it difficult for you to hear?	☐	☐	☐
E3. Does your tinnitus make you angry?	☐	☐	☐
F4. Does your tinnitus make you feel confused?	☐	☐	☐
C5. Because of your tinnitus, do you feel desperate?	☐	☐	☐
E6. Do you complain a great deal about your tinnitus?	☐	☐	☐
F7. Because of your tinnitus, do you have trouble falling to sleep at night?	☐	☐	☐
C8. Do you feel as though you cannot escape your tinnitus?	☐	☐	☐
F9. Does your tinnitus interfere with your ability to enjoy your social activities (such as going out to dinner, to the movies, etc)?	☐	☐	☐
E10. Because of your tinnitus, do you feel frustrated?	☐	☐	☐
C11. Because of your tinnitus, do you feel that you have a terrible disease?	☐	☐	☐
F12. Does your tinnitus make it difficult for you to enjoy life?	☐	☐	☐
F13. Does your tinnitus interfere with your job or household responsibilities?	☐	☐	☐
E14. Because of your tinnitus do you find that you are often irritable?	☐	☐	☐
F15. Because of your tinnitus, is it difficult for you to read?	☐	☐	☐
E16. Does your tinnitus make you upset?	☐	☐	☐
E17. Do you feel that your tinnitus problem has placed stress on your relationships with members of your family and friends?	☐	☐	☐
F18. Do you find it difficult to focus your attention away from your tinnitus and on other things?	☐	☐	☐
C19. Do you feel that you have no control over your tinnitus?	☐	☐	☐
F20. Because of your tinnitus, do you often feel tired?	☐	☐	☐
E21. Because of your tinnitus, do you feel depressed?	☐	☐	☐
E22. Does your tinnitus make you feel anxious?	☐	☐	☐
C23. Do you feel that you can no longer cope with your tinnitus?	☐	☐	☐
F24. Does your tinnitus get worse when you are under stress?	☐	☐	☐
E25. Does your tinnitus make you feel insecure?	☐	☐	☐

From Newman CW, Jacobson GP, Spitzer JB. Development of the tinnitus handicap inventory. *Arch Otolaryngol Head Neck Surg* 1996;122:143–148.

FORM C–14. HEARING HANDICAP INVENTORY FOR ADULTS

NAME:_____ DATE:_____ AGE:_____ Score Total:_____; E____; S____
(100)   (52)   (48)

INSTRUCTIONS: (Please read carefully): The purpose of the scale is to identify the problems your hearing loss may be causing you. Please answer "YES," "SOMETIMES," or "NO" to each question. Do not skip a question if you avoid a situation because of a hearing problem.

	YES	SOMETIMES	NO
S1. Does a hearing problem cause you to use the phone less often than you would like?	☐	☐	☐
E2. Does a hearing problem cause you to feel embarrassed when meeting new people?	☐	☐	☐
S3. Does a hearing problem cause you to avoid groups of people?	☐	☐	☐
E4. Does a hearing problem make you irritable?	☐	☐	☐
E5. Does a hearing problem cause you to feel frustrated when talking to members of your family?	☐	☐	☐
S6. Does a hearing problem cause you difficulty when attending a party?	☐	☐	☐
S7. Does a hearing problem cause you difficulty hearing/understanding coworkers, clients, or customers?	☐	☐	☐
E8. Do you feel handicapped by a hearing problem?	☐	☐	☐
S9. Does a hearing problem cause you difficulty when visiting friends, relatives, or neighbors?	☐	☐	☐
E10. Does a hearing problem cause you to feel frustrated when talking to coworkers, clients, or customers?	☐	☐	☐
S11. Does a hearing problem cause you difficulty in the movies or theater?	☐	☐	☐
E12. Does a hearing problem cause you to be nervous?	☐	☐	☐
S13. Does a hearing problem cause you to visit friends or relatives less often than you would like?	☐	☐	☐
E14. Does a hearing problem cause you to have arguments with family members?	☐	☐	☐
S15. Does a hearing problem cause you difficulty when listening to TV or radio?	☐	☐	☐
S16. Does a hearing problem cause you to go shopping less often than you would like?	☐	☐	☐
E17. Does any problem or difficulty with your hearing upset you at all?	☐	☐	☐
E18. Does a hearing problem cause you to want to be by yourself?	☐	☐	☐
S19. Does a hearing problem cause you to talk to family members less often than you would like?	☐	☐	☐
E20. Do you feel that any difficulty with your hearing limits or hampers your personal or social life?	☐	☐	☐
S21. Does a hearing problem cause you difficulty when in a restaurant with relatives or friends?	☐	☐	☐
E22. Does a hearing problem cause you to feel depressed?	☐	☐	☐
S23. Does a hearing problem cause you to listen to TV or radio less often than you would like?	☐	☐	☐
E24. Does a hearing problem cause you to feel uncomfortable when talking to friends?	☐	☐	☐
E25. Does a hearing problem cause you to feel left out when you are with a group of people?	☐	☐	☐

From Newman CW, Weinstein BE, Jacobson GP, Hug GA. Test-retest reliability of the hearing handicap Inventory for Adults. *Arch Otolaryngol Head Neck Surg.* 1991;12:355–357.

FORM C–15A. TMD DISABILITY INDEX

NAME_____ M/F_____ AGE_____ DATE_____ SCORE_____

Please check the one statement that best pertains to you (not necessarily exactly) in each of the following categories.

1. **Communication (talking).**

   ( ) I can talk as much as I want without pain, fatigue or discomfort.

   ( ) I talk as much as I want, but it causes some pain, fatigue and/or discomfort.

   ( ) I can't talk as much as I want because of pain, fatigue and/or discomfort.

   ( ) I can't talk much at all because of pain, fatigue and/or discomfort.

   ( ) Pain prevents me from talking at all.

2. **Normal living activities (brushing teeth/flossing).**

   ( ) I am able to care for my teeth and gums in a normal fashion without restriction, and without pain, fatigue or discomfort.

   ( ) I am able to care for all my teeth and gums, but I must be slow and careful, otherwise pain/discomfort, jaw tiredness results.

   ( ) I do manage to care for my teeth and gums in a normal fashion, but it usually causes some pain/discomfort, jaw tiredness no matter how slow and careful I am.

   ( ) I am unable to properly clean all my teeth and gums because of restricted opening and/or pain.

   ( ) I am unable to care for most of my teeth and gums because of restricted opening and/or pain.

3. **Normal living activities (eating, chewing).**

   ( ) I can eat and chew as much of anything I want without pain/discomfort or jaw tiredness.

   ( ) I can eat and chew most anything I want, but it sometimes causes pain/discomfort and/or jaw tiredness.

   ( ) I can't eat much of anything I want, because it often causes pain/discomfort, jaw tiredness or because of restricted opening.

   ( ) I must eat only soft foods (consistency of scrambled eggs or less) because of pain/discomfort, jaw fatigue and/or restricted opening.

   ( ) I must stay on a liquid diet because of pain and/or restricted opening.

4. **Social/recreational activities (singing, playing musical instruments, cheering, laughing, social activities, playing amateur sports/hobbies, and recreation, etc).**

   ( ) I am enjoying a normal social life and/or recreational activities without restriction.

   ( ) I participate in normal social life and/or recreational activities but pain/discomfort is increased.

   ( ) The presence of pain and/or fear of likely aggravation only limits the more energetic components of my social life (sports, exercising, dancing, playing musical instruments, singing).

   ( ) I have restrictions socially, as I can't even sing, shout, cheer, play and/or laugh expressively because of increased pain/discomfort.

   ( ) I have practically no social life because of pain.

5. **Non-specialized jaw activities (yawning, mouth opening and opening my mouth wide).**

   ( ) I can yawn in a normal fashion, painlessly.

   ( ) I can yawn and open my mouth fully wide open, but sometimes there is discomfort.

   ( ) I can yawn and open my mouth wide in a normal fashion, but it almost always causes discomfort.

   ( ) Yawning and opening my mouth wide are somewhat restricted by pain.

   ( ) I cannot yawn or open my mouth more than two finger widths (2.8–3.2 cm) or, if I can, it always causes greater than moderate pain.

6. **Sexual function (including kissing, hugging and any and all sexual activities to which you are accustomed).**

   ( ) I am able to engage in all my customary sexual activities and expressions without limitation and/or causing headache, face or jaw pain.

   ( ) I am able to engage in all my customary sexual activities and expression, but it sometimes causes some headache, face, or jaw pain, or jaw fatigue.

   ( ) I am able to engage in all my customary sexual activities and expression, but it usually causes enough headache, face or jaw pain to markedly interfere with my enjoyment, willingness and satisfaction.

   ( ) I must limit my customary sexual expression and activities because of headache, face or jaw pain or limited mouth opening.

   ( ) I abstain from almost all sexual activities and expression because of the head, face or jaw pain it causes.

FORM C–15C. SCORING METHOD FOR THE TMD DISABILITY INDEX

Example:

Score	Question
	1. Communication (talking)
0	( ) a. I can talk as much as I want without pain, fatigue or discomfort.
1	( ) b. I talk as much as I want, but it causes some pain, fatigue and/or discomfort.
2	( ) c. I can't talk as much as I want because of pain, fatigue and/or discomfort.
3	( ) d. I can't talk much at all because of pain, fatigue and/or discomfort.
4	( ) e. Pain prevents me from talking at all.

If the patient chooses "c" a score of 2 is calculated for this first of 10 questions. The total points from the 10 questions are added together and is divided by the total number possible. If all 10 sections are completed, the maximum score possible is 40.

Formula:

- Pt Score/Maximum Score Possible × 100 = _____%

Example:

- 31 (Patient's score)/40 (Total score possible) × 100 = 77.5%

TMD SYMPTOM INTENSITY SCALE

1. Jaw pain	No pain	0 1 2 3 4 5 6 7 8 9 10	Most intense pain
2. Painful jaw clicking	No pain	0 1 2 3 4 5 6 7 8 9 10	Most intense pain
3. Jaw locking	No pain to open mouth	0 1 2 3 4 5 6 7 8 9 10	Can barely open mouth
4. Headaches	No pain	0 1 2 3 4 5 6 7 8 9 10	Most intense pain
5. Neck and/or upper shoulder muscle pain	No pain	0 1 2 3 4 5 6 7 8 9 10	Most intense pain
6. Dizziness	No dizziness	0 1 2 3 4 5 6 7 8 9 10	Most intense dizziness
7. Ringing in the ears	No ringing	0 1 2 3 4 5 6 7 8 9 10	Most intense ringing

- **Total possible (denominator)** = 7 sections times maximum score of 10 = 70.
- **Formula:** Total Patient score/maximum score possible (70 if all 7 sections are completed) × 100 = *Final Score (calculate the same way for the "usual" and the "maximum" scores).*
- **Example:** 2 scores ("usual" score) 33/70 × 100 = 47%; ("maximum" score) 62/70 × 100 = 89%

TMD SYMPTOM FREQUENCY SCALE is scored the same way but there is only one score (since there is no "usual" or "maximum" score to calculate). Example: (Pt score/max possible × 100) 36/70 × 100 = 51%

FORM C–16. CARPAL TUNNEL SYNDROME QUESTIONNAIRE (CTSQ)

The following questions refer to your symptoms for a typical twenty-four hour period during the past two weeks (circle one answer to each question).

SEVERITY SCALE: 0 = None or Never; 1 = Mild; 2 = Moderate; 3 = Severe; 4 = Very severe

SYMPTOM SEVERITY SCALE

Question Severity Score 0 = None; 4 = Severe	0	1	2	3	4
1. How severe is the hand or wrist pain that you have at night?	0	1	2	3	4
2. How often did hand or wrist pain wake you up during a typical night in the past two weeks (times/night)?	0	1	2–3	4–5	5+
3. Do you typically have pain in your hand or wrist during the daytime?	0	1	2	3	4
4. How often do you have hand or wrist pain during the daytime (times/day)?	0	1–2	3–5	5+	constant
5. How long, on average, does an episode of pain last during the daytime (minutes)?	0	<10	10–60	>60	constant
6. Do you have numbness (loss of sensation) in your hand?	0	1	2	3	4
7. Do you have weakness in your hand or wrist?	0	1	2	3	4
8. Do you have tingling sensations in your hand?	0	1	2	3	4
9. How severe is numbness (loss of sensation) or tingling at night?	0	1	2	3	4
10. How often did hand numbness or tingling wake you up during a typical night during the past two weeks?	0	1	2–3	4–5	5+
11. Do you have difficulty with the grasping and use of small objects such as keys or pens?	0	1	2	3	4

FUNCTIONAL STATUS SCALE

Question Severity Score 0 = None; 4 = Severe	0	1	2	3	4
1. Writing	0	1	2	3	4
2. Buttoning of clothes	0	1	2	3	4
3. Holding a book while reading	0	1	2	3	4
4. Gripping of a telephone handle	0	1	2	3	4
5. Opening of jars	0	1	2	3	4
6. Household chores	0	1	2	3	4
7. Carrying of grocery bags	0	1	2	3	4
8. Bathing and dressing	0	1	2	3	4

COMMENTS:_____

_____

_____

_____

NAME_____ M/F_____ AGE_____ DATE_____ DOB_____

From Levine DW, Simmons HP, Koris MJ, et al. A self-administered questionnaire for the assessment of severity of symptoms and functional status in carpal tunnel syndrome. *J Bone Joint Surg* 1993;75A:1585–1592.

FORM C–17A. SHOULDER EVALUATION FORM (American Shoulder and Elbow Surgeons)

NAME_____ M/F_____ AGE_____ DATE_____ SCORE_____

I. **PAIN:** (5 = None; 4 = slight; 3 = after unusual activity; 2 = moderate; 1 = marked; 0 = complete disability; NA = not available) _____

II. **MOTION:**

   A. Patient sitting

      1. Active total elevation of arm (FFL): _____ degrees*

      2. Passive internal rotation:

          (Circle segment of posterior anatomy reached by thumb)

          (Indicate if reach is restricted by limited elbow flexion)

1 = less than trochanter	5 = L5	9 = L1	13 = T9	17 = T5
2 = trochanter	6 = L4	10 = T12	14 = T8	18 = T4
3 = gluteal	7 = L3	11 = T11	15 = T7	19 = T3
4 = sacrum	8 = L2	12 = T10	16 = T6	20 = T2

      1. Active external rotation with arm at side: _____ degrees

      2. Active external rotation at 90° abduction: _____ degrees

   B. Patient supine

      1. Passive total elevation of arm: _____ degrees*

      2. Passive external rotation with arm at side: _____ degrees

III. **STRENGTH:** (5 = normal; 4 = good; 3 = fair; 2 = poor; 1 = trace; 0 = paralysis)

   A. Anterior deltoid _____   C. External rotation _____

   B. Middle deltoid _____   D. Internal rotation _____

IV. **STABILITY:** (5 = normal; 4 = apprehension; 3 = rare subluxation; 2 = recurrent subluxation; 1 = recurrent dislocation; NA = not available)

   A. Anterior _____   B. Posterior _____   C. Inferior _____

V. **FUNCTION:** (4 = normal; 3 = mild compromise; 2 = difficulty; 1 = with aid; 0 = unable, NA = not available)

Activity	Score	Activity	Score
1. Use back pocket		9. Sleep on the affected side	
2. Perineal care		10. Pulling	
3. Wash opposite underarm		11. Use hand overhead	
4. Eat with utensil		12. Throwing	
5. Comb hair		13. Lifting	
6. Use hand with arm at shoulder level		14. Do usual work	
7. Carry 10 to 15 lbs with arm at side		15. Do usual sport	
8. Dress		**TOTAL**	

* Total elevation of the arm measured by viewing patient from the side and using a goniometer to determine the angle between the arm and the thorax.

(Reproduced with permission from Barrett WP, Franklin JL, Jackins SE, et al. Total shoulder arthroplasty. *J Bone Joint Surg* 1987;69A:865–872.

FORM C–17B. SHOULDER INJURY SELF-ASSESSMENT OF FUNCTION

Please rate your ability to do the following common tasks as they relate to your injured shoulder by placing a "✓" mark in the appropriate box.

	0	1	2	3	4	
	Normal	Mild Compromise	Difficult	Very Difficult (with aid)	Unable	Other/ Cannot Say
1. Use back pocket						
2. Wipe after bowel movement						
3. Wash opposite underarm						
4. Eat with fork or spoon						
5. Comb hair						
6. Use hand with arm at shoulder level						
7. Carry 10–15 pounds with arm at side						
8. Dress						
9. Sleep on affected side						
10. Pulling						
11. Use hand overhead						
12. Throwing						
13. Lifting						
14. Do usual work						
15. Do usual sport						

NAME_____ DATE_____ AGE_____ SCORE_____

Modified from Rowe CR. Evaluation of the shoulder. In Rowe CR (ed): *The Shoulder*. New York: Churchill Livingstone; 1987:633. Courtesy of the American Shoulder and Elbow Surgeons.

FORM C–18. RATING SCALE OF THE AMERICAN SHOULDER AND ELBOW SURGEONS

NAME_____ DATE_____ AGE_____ SCORE_____

PAIN: (5 = none; 4 = slight; 3 = after unusual activity; 2 = moderate; 1 = marked; 0 = complete disability: _____)

FUNCTION: (4 = normal; 3 = mild compromise; 2 = difficulty; 1 = with aid; 0 = unable, NA = not available)

Activity	Score	Activity	Score
1. Use back pocket		7. Carry 10 to 15 lbs with arm at side	
2. Reach behind back, fasten brassiere		8. Dress	
3. Wash opposite underarm		9. Sleep on the affected side	
4. Eat with utensil		10. Pulling	
5. Comb hair		11. Use hand overhead	
6. Use hand with arm at shoulder level		12. Lifting	
		TOTAL	

SPORTS:

	Points
Same overhead sport, equal performance (normal)	4
Same non-overhead sport, equal performance (mild compromise)	3
Same sport, decreased performance (difficult)	2
Different sport (with aid)	1
Sports not possible (unable)	0

Modified from Gartsman GM. Arthroplastic acromioplasty for lesions of the rotator cuff. *J Bone Joint Surg* 1990;72A:169–180.

FORM C–19. SIMPLE SHOULDER TEST QUESTIONNAIRE

NAME_____ DATE_____ AGE_____ SCORE_____

OCCUPATION:_____ Dominant Hand: Right/Left/Ambidextrous; Shoulder eval. L/R

Answer each question below by checking "Yes" or "No"

	Yes	No
1. Is your shoulder comfortable with your arm at rest by your side?		
2. Does your shoulder allow you to sleep comfortably?		
3. Can you reach the small of your back to tuck in your shirt with your hand?		
4. Can you place your hand behind your head with the elbow straight out to the side?		
5. Can you place a coin on a shelf at the level of your shoulder without bending your elbow?		
6. Can you lift one pound (a full pint container) to the level of your shoulder without bending your elbow?		
7. Can you lift eight pounds (a full gallon container) to the level of your shoulder without bending your elbow?		
8. Can you carry twenty pounds at your side with the affected extremity?		
9. Do you think you can toss a softball under-hand ten yards with the affected extremity?		
10. Do you think you can toss a softball over-hand twenty yards with the affected extremity?		
11. Can you wash the back of your opposite shoulder with the affected extremity?		
12. Would your shoulder allow you to work full-time at your regular job?		
TOTALS		

Office Use Only

Diagnosis: DJD, RA AVN, IMP RCT FS, TUBS AMBRII, Other:_____

Dx Confirmed?_____ Pt #_____ Physician_____

SST: Initial/Pre-op/Follow-up: 6 mon 1 yr 18 mon 2 yr 3 yr 4 yr 5 yr Other:_____

Initial SST Date: ____/____/____ Rx:_____ Surgery date:____/____/____

From Matsen FA III, Ziegler DW, BeBartolo SE. Patient self-assessment of health status and function in glenohumeral degenerative joint disease. *J Shoulder Elbow Surg* 1995;4:345–351.

FORM C–22. SUBJECTIVE KNEE SCORE QUESTIONNAIRE

NAME_____ SCORE_____ DATE_____ DOB_____ AGE_____

PLEASE CHECK THE STATEMENT THAT BEST DESCRIBES THE CONDITION OF YOUR KNEE

PAIN

20____ I experience no pain in my knee.

16____ I have occasional pain with strenuous sports or heavy work. I don't think that my knee is entirely normal. Limitations are mild and tolerable.

12____ There is occasional pain in my knee with light recreational sports or moderate work.

8____ I have pain brought on by sports, light recreational activities, or moderate work. Occasional pain is brought on by daily activities such as standing or kneeling.

4____ The pain I have in my knee is a significant problem with activities as simple as walking. The pain is relieved by rest. I can't participate in sports.

0____ I have pain in my knee at all times, even during walking, standing, or light work.

Intensity:	A [ ] Mild	B [ ] Moderate	C [ ] Severe
Frequency:	A [ ] Constant	B [ ] Intermittent	
Location:	A [ ] Medial (inner side)	B [ ] Lateral (outer side)	C [ ] Anterior (front)
	D [ ] Posterior (back)	E [ ] Diffuse (all over)	
Occurs:	A [ ] Kneel	B [ ] Stand	C [ ] Sit	D [ ] Stairs
Type:	A [ ] Sharp	B [ ] Aching	C [ ] Throbbing	D [ ] Burning

SWELLING

10____ I experience no swelling in my knees.

8____ I have occasional swelling in my knee with strenuous sports or heavy work.

6____ There is occasional swelling with light recreational activities or moderate work.

4____ Swelling limits my participation in sports and moderate work. Occurs infrequently with simple walking or light work. Occasionally with simple walking or light work—about 3 times a year.

2____ My knee swells after simple walking activities and light work. Rest relieves the swelling.

0____ I have severe swelling with simple walking activities. Rest does not relieve the swelling.

STABILITY

20____ My knee does not give out.

16____ My knee gives out only with strenuous sports or heavy work.

12____ My knee gives out occasionally with light recreational activities or moderate work; it limits my vigorous activities, sports, or heavy labor.

8____ Because my knee gives out, it limits all sports and moderate work. It occasionally gives out with walking or light work.

4____ My knee gives out frequently with simple activities such as walking. I must guard my knee at all times.

0____ I have severe problems with my knee giving out. I can't turn or twist without my knee giving out.

Stiffness:	A [ ] None	B [ ] Occasional	C [ ] Frequent	D [ ] Constant
Grinding:	A [ ] None	B [ ] Mild	C [ ] Moderate	D [ ] Severe
Locking:	A [ ] None	B [ ] Occasional	C [ ] Frequent	D [ ] Constant

OVERALL ACTIVITY LEVEL

20____ No limitations. I have a normal knee, and I am able to do everything including strenuous sports and/or heavy labor.

16____ I can partake in sports including strenuous ones but at a lower level. I must guard my knee and limit the amount of heavy labor or sports.

12____ Light recreational activities are possible with RARE symptoms. I am limited to light work.

8____ No sports or recreational activities are possible. Walking activities are possible with RARE symptoms. I am limited to light work.

4____   Walking activities and daily living cause moderate problems and persistent symptoms.

0____   Walking and other daily activities cause severe problems.

WALKING

10____   Normal, unlimited.

8____   Slight, mild problems.

6____   Moderate problem, flat surface up to half a mile.

4____   Severe problems, only 2–3 blocks.

2____   Severe problems, need cane or crutches.

STAIRS

5____   Normal, unlimited.

4____   Slight, mild problems.

3____   Moderate problems, only 10–15 steps possible.

2____   Severe problems, require banister for support.

1____   Severe problems, only 1–5 steps without support.

RUNNING

10____   Normal, unlimited, fully competitive.

8____   Slight, mild problems, run at half speed.

6____   Moderate problems, only 1–2 miles possible.

4____   Severe problems, only 1–3 blocks possible.

2____   Severe problems, only a few steps.

JUMPING AND TWISTING

5____   Normal, unlimited, fully competitive.

4____   Slight, mild problems, some guarding.

3____   Moderate problems, gave up strenuous sports.

2____   Severe problems, affects all sports, always guarding.

1____   Severe problems, only light activity possible (pool/swim).

COMMENTS:_____

_____

_____

_____

_____

_____

_____

_____

_____

Modified with permission from Noyes FR, et al. Functional disability in the anterior cruciate insufficient knee syndrome. Review of knee rating systems and project risk factors in determining treatment. *Sports Med* 1984;1:278–302. Copyright © Adis International, Inc.

FORM C–23. RATING OF KNEE REPLACEMENT RESULTS[a]

Category	Number of Points
PAIN	
None	50
Mild or occasional	45
Stairs only	40
Walking and stairs	30
Moderate	
Occasional	20
Continual	10
Severe	0
RANGE OF MOTION	
Add 1 point per 5 degrees	25
STABILITY (maximum movement in any position)	
Anteroposterior	
<5 mm	10
5–9 mm	5
>9 mm	0
Mediolateral	
5°	15
6°–9°	10
10°–14°	5
≥15°	0
Subtotal	
Deductions (minus)	
Flexion contracture	
5°–9°	2
10°–15°	5
16°–20°	10
>20°	20
Extension lag	
<10°	5
10°–20°	10
>20°	15
Alignment	
0°–4°	0 points
5°–10°	3 points per degree
11°–15°	3 points per degree
>15°	20
Deductions subtotal (points)	
TOTAL	

[a] The point total for estimating knee replacement results is the sum of the points in categories a, b, and c minus the sum of the points in categories d, e, and f.

Modified from Insall JN, Dorr LD, Scott RD. Rationale of the Knee Society clinical rating system. *Clin Orthop* 1989;248:14. See p. 596 for complete version.

NAME_____ SCORE_____ DATE_____ DOB_____ AGE_____

Impairment Rating Calculation (only report if requested and the condition is stabilized and unlikely to change).

Result	Points	Impairment: Whole Person (lower extremity) %
Good result	85–100 points	15 (37)
Fair result	50–84 points	20 (50)
Poor result	Less than 50 points	30 (75)

Modified from *Guides to the Evaluation of Permanent Impairment*, 4th ed. Chicago, IL: American Medical Association; 1993:85.

FORM C–24. RATING OF HIP REPLACEMENT RESULTS[a]

Category	Number of Points
PAIN	
None	44
Slight	40
Moderate	
Occasional	30
Continual	20
Marked	10
FUNCTION	
Limp	
None	11
Slight	8
Moderate	5
Severe	0
Support device	
None	11
Cane for long walks	7
Cane	5
One crutch	3
Two canes	2
Two crutches	0
Distance walked	
Unlimited	11
Six blocks	8
Three blocks	5
Indoors	2
In bed or chair	0
ACTIVITIES	
Stairs climbing	
Normal	4
Using railing	2
Cannot climb readily	1
Unable to climb	0
Putting on shoes and socks	
With ease	4
With difficulty	2
Unable to do	0
Sitting	
Any chair, 1 hour	4
High chair	2
Unable to sit comfortably	0
Public transportation	
Able to use	1
Unable to use	0

DEFORMITY	
Fixed adduction	
<10°	1
> or = 10°	0
Fixed internal rotation	
<10°	1
> or = 10°	0
Fixed external rotation	
<10°	1
> or = 10°	0
Fixed contracture	
<10°	1
> or = 10°	0
Leg length discrepancy	
<1.5 cm	1
> or = 1.5 cm	0
RANGE OF MOTION	
Flexion	
<90°	1
> or = 90°	0
Abduction	
<15°	1
> or = 15°	0
Adduction	
<15°	1
> or = 15°	0
External rotation	
<30°	1
> or = 30°	0
Internal rotation	
<15°	1
> or = 15°	0
TOTAL	

[a] Add the points from categories a, b, c, d, and e to determine the total and characterize the result of replacement.

Source: Compiled from data in Callaghan JJ, Dysart SH, Savory CF, Hopkinson WJ. Assessing the results of hip replacement: A comparison of five different rating systems. *J Bone Joint Surg Br.* 1990;72B:1008–1009.

NAME_____ SCORE_____ DATE_____ DOB_____ AGE_____

Impairment Rating Calculation (only report if requested and the condition is stabilized and unlikely to change).

Result	Points	Impairment: Whole Person (lower extremity) %
Good result	85–100 points	15 (37)
Fair result	50–84 points	20 (50)
Poor result	Less than 50 points	30 (75)

Modified from *Guides to the Evaluation of Permanent Impairment*, 4th ed. Chicago, IL: American Medical Association; 1993:85.

FORM C–27. MODIFIED ZUNG DEPRESSION INDEX

NAME:_____ DATE:_____ SCORE:_____

Please indicate for each of these questions which answer best describes how you have been feeling recently.

	Rarely or none of the time (less than 1 day per week)	Some or little of the time (1–2 days per week)	A moderate amount of time (3–4 days per week)	Most of the time (5–7 days per week)
1. I feel downhearted and sad.	0	1	2	3
2. Morning is when I feel best.	3	2	1	0
3. I have crying spells or feel like it.	0	1	2	3
4. I have trouble getting to sleep at night.	0	1	2	3
5. I feel that nobody cares.	0	1	2	3
6. I eat as much as I used to.	3	2	1	0
7. I still enjoy sex.	3	2	1	0
8. I notice I am losing weight.	0	1	2	3
9. I have trouble with constipation.	0	1	2	3
10. My heart beats faster than usual.	0	1	2	3
11. I get tired for no reason.	0	1	2	3
12. My mind is as clear as it used to be.	3	2	1	0
13. I tend to wake up too early.	0	1	2	3
14. I find it easy to do the things I used to.	3	2	1	0
15. I am restless and can't keep still.	0	1	2	3
16. I feel hopeful about the future.	3	2	1	0
17. I am more irritable than usual.	0	1	2	3
18. I find it easy to make a decision.	3	2	1	0
19. I feel quite guilty.	0	1	2	3
20. I feel that I am useful and needed.	3	2	1	0
21. My life is pretty full.	3	2	1	0
22. I feel that others would be better off if I were dead.	0	1	2	3
23. I am still able to enjoy the things I used to.	3	2	1	0

Reproduced with permission from the publisher, from Main CJ, Waddell G. The detection of psychological abnormality in chronic low-back pain using four simple scales. *Curr Concepts Pain* 1984;2:10–15.

Note: Forms C–26 and C–27 are used together to make up the DRAM.

Chapter 9: Patient Satisfaction and Experience

FORM D–1. EXAMPLE OF A CLIENT EXPERIENCE SURVEY

Name (Optional):   **Date:**

_____ _____

Please help us to evaluate our program by answering some questions about the evaluation in which you participated. We are interested in your honest opinions, regardless of whether they may be positive or negative. Please answer the questions below by circling the answer that best describes your answer. Please feel free to write in any explanations below the answers.

• The Center was easy to find and well marked	Yes	No	NA
• The parking lot was open and accessible	Yes	No	NA
• The receptionist was courteous when I arrived	Yes	No	NA
• The receptionist was expecting me	Yes	No	NA
• My appointment started on time	Yes	No	NA
• The inside of the building was neat and clean	Yes	No	NA
• The room temperature was comfortable	Yes	No	NA
• The clinical staff members were courteous	Yes	No	NA
• All testing procedures were fully explained	Yes	No	NA
• The reason for meeting with various professionals was fully explained to me	Yes	No	NA
• Clinical staff members seemed concerned about my problem	Yes	No	NA
• Contact with clinical staff members was smooth and organized	Yes	No	NA
• There was an opportunity to discuss my problem	Yes	No	NA
• The visit today addressed all the problems for which I was referred	Yes	No	NA
• Following today's services, I know how the information gathered will be used	Yes	No	NA

✓ **Overall, the services you received today at the Occupational Rehabilitation and Ergonomics Center were:**

Please put a check in the box that best reflects your answer.

Excellent	Good			Fair			Poor			Unacceptable
A	A–	B+	B	B–	C+	C	C–	D+	D	F
☐	☐	☐	☐	☐	☐	☐	☐	☐	☐	☐

Other comments:

_____

_____

Anything else you wanted or needed?

_____

_____

THANK YOU VERY MUCH FOR YOUR HELP!
Please return the completed survey to the receptionist in the envelope provided.

FORM D–2. THE CHIROPRACTIC SATISFACTION QUESTIONNAIRE

NAME:_____ DATE:_____ DOB:_____

Here are some questions about the visit you just had. In terms of your satisfaction, how would you rate each of the following? (Circle one number on each line.)

	Very good	Poor	Fair	Good	Very good	Excellent	The best
1. The amount of privacy you were given	1	2	3	4	5	6	7
2. Interest shown in you as a person	1	2	3	4	5	6	7
3. Friendliness, warmth, and personal manner of the chiropractor who treated you	1	2	3	4	5	6	7
4. Explanations of treatment	1	2	3	4	5	6	7
5. Willingness to listen to what you had to say	1	2	3	4	5	6	7
6. Understanding of your health problem	1	2	3	4	5	6	7
7. Answers given to your questions	1	2	3	4	5	6	7
8. Amount of time spent with you	1	2	3	4	5	6	7
9. Cost of the care to you	1	2	3	4	5	6	7
10. Skill and ability of the chiropractor	1	2	3	4	5	6	7
11. Advice about ways to avoid illness and stay healthy	1	2	3	4	5	6	7
12. Ability of the chiropractor to put you at ease	1	2	3	4	5	6	7
13. Courtesy, politeness, and respect shown by the chiropractor	1	2	3	4	5	6	7
14. Care received overall	1	2	3	4	5	6	7

Note: To score the questionnaire, first average responses to each item to obtain a score ranging between 1 and 7. Next, subtract 1 from the average. Then divide the result by 6. Finally, multiply by 100.

Editor's note: A median score of approximately 90 was obtained in California from 486 patients of 44 chiropractors using this survey. Until further research is completed, chiropractic physicians may wish to interpret scores from their patients as below average, average, or above average relative to this score. This instrument may also be useful for identifying specific areas of care for quality improvement efforts.

From The Chiropractic Satisfaction Questionnaire. *Top Clin Chiro* 1994;1(4):79. © Aspen Publishers, Inc. Reprinted with permission.

Chapter 14: Spinal Range of Motion

FORM E–1. MCKENZIE EXAMINATION FORM

NAME_____ DATE_____ DOB_____ DOI_____

	Date:_____	Date:_____	Date:_____	Date:_____
TESTS *Standing*	**INITIAL**	**1ST RE-EXAM**	**2ND RE-EXAM**	**3RD RE-EXAM**
Pre-test VAS	_____/10	_____/10	_____/10	_____/10
1. Flexion in Standing (FIS) Single movement: 1 rep. (McK. #3) (a. pain; b. syndrome; c. lat shift)	a. Pain: +1, 0, −1 b. Syndrome: Fl/Ext c. Lat. shift: Y/N	a. Pain: +1, 0, −1 b. Syndrome: Fl/Ext c. Lat. shift: Y/N	a. Pain: +1, 0, −1 b. Syndrome: Fl/Ext c. Lat. shift: Y/N	a. Pain: +1, 0, −1 b. Syndrome: Fl/Ext c. Lat. shift: Y/N
2. Extension in Standing (EIS) Single movement: 1 rep. (McK. #2) (a. pain; b. syndrome; c. lat shift)	a. Pain: +1, 0, −1 b. Syndrome: Fl/Ext c. Lat. shift: Y/N	a. Pain: +1, 0, −1 b. Syndrome: Fl/Ext c. Lat. shift: Y/N	a. Pain: +1, 0, −1 b. Syndrome: Fl/Ext c. Lat. shift: Y/N	a. Pain: +1, 0, −1 b. Syndrome: Fl/Ext c. Lat. shift: Y/N

3. Side Gliding (McK. #1)
Repeated movement: 10 reps.
a. Pain: +1, 0, −1
b. Limited: L = Left; R = Right
c. Blocked: L = Left; R = Right

	L	R	L	R	L	R	L	R
	a. +1,0,−1 b. L-L/R c. B-L/R	a. +1,0,−1 b. L-L/R c. B-L/R	a. +1,0,−1 b. L-L/R c. B-L/R	a. +1,0,−1 b. L-L/R c. B-L/R	a. +1,0,−1 b. L-L/R c. B-L/R	a. +1,0,−1 b. L-L/R c. B-L/R	a. +1,0,−1 b. L-L/R c. B-L/R	a. +1,0,−1 b. L-L/R c. B-L/R

Supine	L	R	L	R	L	R	L	R
4. Flexion Supine (McK#4) Repeat 1 rep.	1 rep: +1,0,−1 • Centralization • Peripheralization		1 rep: +1,0,−1 • Centralization • Peripheralization		1 rep: +1,0,−1 • Centralization • Peripheralization		1 rep: +1,0,−1 • Centralization • Peripheralization	
5. Flexion Supine (McK#5) Repeat 10 reps.	10 rep: +1,0,−1 • Centralization • Peripheralization		10 rep: +1,0,−1 • Centralization • Peripheralization		10 rep: +1,0,−1 • Centralization • Peripheralization		10 rep: +1,0,−1 • Centralization • Peripheralization	
6. Flexion Supine (McK#6) Sustain last rep. 10 seconds	1 sus rep: +1,0,−1 • Centralization • Peripheralization		1 sus rep: +1,0,−1 • Centralization • Peripheralization		1 sus rep: +1,0,−1 • Centralization • Peripheralization		1 sus rep: +1,0,−1 • Centralization • Peripheralization	

Prone	L	R	L	R	L	R	L	R
7. Single Ext. in Lying (SEL) (McK #7) (a. pain; b. syndrome; c. lat shift)	a. Pain: +1,0,−1 b. Syndrome: Fl/Ext c. Lat. shift: Y/N		a. Pain: +1,0,−1 b. Syndrome: Fl/Ext c. Lat. shift: Y/N		a. Pain: +1,0,−1 b. Syndrome: Fl/Ext c. Lat. shift: Y/N		a. Pain: +1,0,−1 b. Syndrome: Fl/Ext c. Lat. shift: Y/N	
8. Repeated Ext. in Lying (RE) (McK. #8) (a. pain; b. syndrome; c. lat shift)	a. Pain: +1,0,−1 b. Syndrome: Fl/Ext c. Lat. shift: Y/N d. # reps _____/10		a. Pain: +1,0,−1 b. Syndrome: Fl/Ext c. Lat. shift: Y/N d. # reps _____/10		a. Pain: +1,0,−1 b. Syndrome: Fl/Ext c. Lat. shift: Y/N d. # reps _____/10		a. Pain: +1,0,−1 b. Syndrome: Fl/Ext c. Lat. shift: Y/N d. # reps _____/10	
9. Sustained Ext. in Lying (SusEI) (McK. #9) (a. pain; b. syndrome; c. lat shift)	a. Pain: +1,0,−1 b. Syndrome: Fl/Ext c. Lat. shift: Y/N d. # Sec. _____/10		a. Pain: +1,0,−1 b. Syndrome: Fl/Ext c. Lat. shift: Y/N d. # Sec. _____/10		a. Pain: +1,0,−1 b. Syndrome: Fl/Ext c. Lat. shift: Y/N d. # Sec. _____/10		a. Pain: +1,0,−1 b. Syndrome: Fl/Ext c. Lat. shift: Y/N d. # Sec. _____/10	
Post-test VAS	_____/10		_____/10		_____/10		_____/10	

NUMERICAL PAIN SCALE	DEFINITION
+1	Increase or periphealrization of pain
0	No pain
−1	Decrease or centralization of pain

Definitions and References for McKenzie Tests appear in Appendix G–8 (pp. 625 to 632), as follows:

1. Flexion in Standing   *See* Form G–8, Test 4
2. Extension in Standing   *See* Form G–8, Test 3
3. Side Gliding   *See* Form G–8, Test 6
4. to 6. Flexion Supine   *See* Form G–8, Tests 17 to 19
7. Single Extension in Lying   *See* Form G–8, Test 23
8. Repeated Extension in Lying   *See* Form G–8, Test 24
9. Sustained Extension in Lying   *See* Form G–8, Test 25

McKenzie R A. *The Lumbar Spine: Mechanical Diagnosis and Therapy.* Waikanae, NZ: Spinal Publications, 1981. Reprinted 1989.

Chapter 15: Outcome Measures
for the Upper and Lower Extremities

FORM F–1. CONSTANT SCALE

NAME:_____ DATE:_____ DOB:_____

Pain (max = 15)

15 = none
10 = mild
 5 = moderate
 0 = severe

Activities of daily living (max = 20)

   Activity level (max = 10)

Full work = 4
Full recreation/sport = 4
Unaffected sleep = 2

   Positioning (max = 10)

Up to waist = 2
Up to xiphoid = 4
Up to neck = 6
Up to top of head = 8
Above head = 10

Range of motion (max = 40)

   Forward (max = 10) and lateral elevation (max = 10)

0–30° = 0
31–60° = 2
61–90° = 4
91–120° = 6
121–150° = 8
151–180° = 10

   External rotation (max = 10), hand position:

Behind head, elbow forward = 2
Behind head, elbow back = 2
Top of head, elbow forward = 2
Top of head, elbow back = 2
Full elevation, from top of head = 2

   Internal rotation (max = 10), position of dorsum of hand:

Lateral thigh = 0
Buttock = 2
Lumbosacral region = 4
Waist (L3 vertebra) = 6
T12 vertebra = 8
Interscapular (T7 vertebra) = 10

Muscle strength (lb), max = 25

From Constant CR, Murley AHG. A clinical method of functional assessment of the shoulder. *Clin Orthop* 1987;214:160–164.

FORM F–2. HOSPITAL FOR SPECIAL SURGERY SCORE SHEET FOR TOTAL SHOULDER REPLACEMENT

Dominant arm_____

Involved arm_____

	Score	Pre	6M	1Y	2Y	3Y	4Y	5Y	Pre	6M	1Y	2Y	3Y	4Y	5Y
Pain on motion (15 points—circle one)															
None:	15														
Mild: occasional, no compromise in activity	10														
Moderate: Tolerable, makes concession, uses ASA	5														
Severe: Serious limitations, disabling, uses Codeine, etc	0														
Pain at rest (15 points—circle one)															
None: Ignores	15														
Mild: Occasional, no medication, no affect on sleep	10														
Moderate: Uses ASA, night pain	5														
Severe: Marked, medication stronger than ASA	0														
Function (20 points—circle all appropriate)															
Comb hair	5														
Lie on shoulder	5														
Hook brassiere (back)	5														
Toilet	5														
Lift weight in pounds 1–10 1 point per pound—maximum 10 pts None															
Muscle strength (15 pts—rate each) (Normal = 3, Good = 2, Fair = 1, Poor = 0) Forward flexion Abduction Adduction Internal rotation External rotation															
Range of motion (25 pts—1 point per 20° of motion) Forward flexion (max 8) Abduction (max 7) Adduction (max 2) Internal rotation (max 5) External rotation (max 3)															
Record range of motion (no pts) Backward extension Glenohumeral abduction (scapula fixed)															
Total															

Patient name_____ Date_____ DOB_____

ASA, acetylsalicylic acid.

From Warren RF, Ranawat CS, Inglis AE: Total shoulder replacement indications and results of the Neer nonconstrained prosthesis. In: Inglis AE, ed. *The American Academy of Orthopedic Surgeons Symposium on Total Joint Replacement of the Upper Extremity.* St. Louis, Mo: Mosby; 1982:56–57.

FORM F–3. SHOULDER FUNCTION ASSESSMENT SCALE

Pain on VAS, cm, max = 20

No pain for each VAS = 10
    Pain on motion = 10; pain at rest = 10

Activities of daily living, max = 20

Dress = 5
Comb hair = 5
Wash opposite axilla = 5
Use toilet = 5
For all items: 5 = without difficulty, 3 = with little difficulty,
    2 = with much difficulty, 1 = with aid, 0 = impossible

Range of motion, max = 20
    Active total abduction, 1 point per 10° of motion, max = 18

6 = possible
3 = partly possible
0 = impossible

    Combined movement

Hand on top of head with elbow back = 6
Hand on top of head, elbow forward = 6

VAS, visual analogue scale.

From van Den Ende CH, Rozing PM, Dijkmans BA, Verhoef JA, Voogt-van der Harst EM, Hazes JM. Assessment of shoulder function in rheumatoid arthritis. *J Rheumatol* 1996;23(12):2043–2048.

FORM F–4. CROFT'S MEASUREMENT OF SHOULDER-RELATED DISABILITY

NAME:_____ DATE:_____ DOB:_____

When your shoulder hurts, you may find it difficult to do some of the things you normally do. This list contains some sentences that people have used to describe themselves when they have trouble with their shoulder. When you read them, you may find that some stand out because they describe you TODAY. As you read them, think of yourself TODAY.

When you read a sentence that describes you today, please tick the 'YES' box. If the sentence does not describe you, then please tick the 'NO' box and go on to the next one. Please only tick the 'YES' box for a sentence if you are sure that it describes you today.

	YES	NO
1. Because of pain in my shoulder, I move my arm or hand with some difficulty.	☐	☐
2. I do not bathe myself completely because of my shoulder.	☐	☐
3. Because of my shoulder trouble, I get dressed with help from someone else.	☐	☐
4. I get dressed more slowly than usual because of my shoulder.	☐	☐
5. Because of my shoulder trouble, I fasten my clothing with some difficulty (eg, buttons, shoelaces, ties, zips or bra)	☐	☐
6. I have trouble putting on a jersey, coat, shirt, blouse or jacket because of my shoulder problem.	☐	☐
7. Because of my shoulder problem I change position frequently in bed at night.	☐	☐
8. I cannot lie on my right side at night because of my shoulder.	☐	☐
9. I cannot lie on my left side at night because of my shoulder.	☐	☐
10. I stay at home most of the time because of my shoulder problem.	☐	☐
11. Because of my shoulder problem I do less of the daily household jobs than I would usually do.	☐	☐
12. I avoid heavy jobs around the house because of my shoulder trouble.	☐	☐
13. Because of my shoulder I do not carry any shopping.	☐	☐
14. Because of my shoulder trouble, I am cutting down on some of my usual sports or more active pastimes.	☐	☐
15. Because of my shoulder trouble, I am not doing any of my usual physical recreation or more active pastimes.	☐	☐
16. Because of my shoulder, I try to get other people to do things for me.	☐	☐
17. My shoulder makes me more irritable and bad tempered with people than usual.	☐	☐
18. Because of my shoulder, I have more minor accidents (eg, dropping things).	☐	☐
19. I sleep less well because of my shoulder.	☐	☐
20. Because of my shoulder, I rest more often during the day.	☐	☐
21. My appetite is not very good because of my shoulder problem.	☐	☐
22. Because of my shoulder, I have trouble writing or typing.	☐	☐

Reprinted with kind permission of BMJ Publications Group. From Croft P, Pope D, Zonca M, O'Neill T, Silman A. Measurement of shoulder related disability: Results of a validation study. *Ann Rheum Dis*. 1994;53(8):525–528.

FORM F–5. WOLFGANG'S ASSESSMENT OF ROTATOR CUFF INJURY

NAME:_____ DATE:_____ DOB:_____

Criteria for Rating Results

Pain

4 Absent regardless of activity

3 Mild with vigorous activity

2 Moderate, restricting some activity

1 Moderate, restricting most activity

0 Severe, constant, disabling

Motion (abduction)

4 More than 150 degrees

3 120 to 149 degrees

2 90 to 119 degrees

1 10 to 89 degrees

0 Less than 10 degrees

Strength

4 Normal

3 Mild weakness (against resistance)

2 Moderate weakness (against gravity)

1 Severe weakness (gravity eliminated)

0 Absent

Function

4 No impairment

3 Restricts strenuous work

2 Restricts all working

1 Prevents most common usage

0 No functional value

Satisfaction

1 Pleased

0 Not pleased*

Total points	Overall rating:
15–17	Excellent
11–14	Good
8–10	Fair
1–7	Poor

*1 implies that one point will be subtracted from the overall point total in computing the overall rating.

From Wolfgang GL. Surgical repair of tears of the rotator cuff of the shoulder. *J Bone Joint Surg,* 1994;56A:15–26.

FORM F–6. SHOULDER PAIN AND DISABILITY INDEX (SPADI)

NAME:_____ DATE:_____ DOB:_____

Pain scale: 0–10 numeric, where 0 = "no pain at all," and 10 = "worst pain imaginable"

How severe is your pain:

1. At its worst?
2. When lying on the involved side?
3. Reaching for something on a high shelf?
4. Touching the back of your neck?
5. Pushing with the involved arm?

Disability scale: 0–10 numeric where 0 = "no difficulty," and 10 = "so difficult it required help"

How much difficulty do you have

1. Washing your hair?
2. Washing your back?
3. Putting on an undershirt or pullover sweater?
4. Putting on a shirt that buttons down the front?
5. Putting on your pants?
6. Placing an object on a high shelf?
7. Carrying a heavy object of 10 pounds?
8. Removing something from your back pocket?

From Williams JW Jr, Holleman DR Jr, Simel DL. Measuring shoulder function with the Shoulder Pain and Disability Index. *J Rheumatol* 1995;22(4):727–732.

FORM F–7. SHOULDER RATING QUESTIONNAIRE (SRQ)

NAME:_____ DATE:_____ DOB:_____

Which is your dominant arm?

　　Left　　Right

For which shoulder(s) have you been evaluated or treated?

　　Left　　Right　　Both

Please answer the following questions regarding the shoulder for which you have been evaluated or treated. If a question does not apply to you, leave that question blank.

If you indicated that both shoulders have been evaluated or treated, please complete a separate questionnaire for each shoulder and mark the corresponding side (Left or Right) at the top of each form.

1. Considering all the ways that your shoulder affects you, mark X on the scale below for how well you are doing.

   Very poorly_____Very well

The following questions refer to pain.

2. During the past month, how would you describe the usual pain in your shoulder at rest?

   A) Very severe
   B) Severe
   C) Moderate
   D) Mild
   E) None

3. During the past month, how would you describe the usual pain in your shoulder <u>during activities</u>?

   A) Very severe
   B) Severe
   C) Moderate
   D) Mild
   E) None

4. During the past month, how often did the pain in your shoulder make it <u>difficult for you to sleep</u> at night?

   A) Every day
   B) Several days per week
   C) One day per week
   D) Less than one day per week
   E) Never

5. During the past month, how often have you had <u>severe pain</u> in your shoulder?

   A) Every day
   B) Several days per week
   C) One day per week
   D) Less than one day per week
   E) Never

The following questions refer to <u>daily activities</u>.

6. Considering all the ways you use your shoulder during <u>daily personal and household activities</u> (ie, dressing, washing, driving, household chores, etc), how would you describe your ability to use your shoulder?

   A) Very severe limitation; unable
   B) Severe limitation
   C) Moderate limitation
   D) Mild limitation
   E) No limitation

Questions 7–11: During the past month, how much difficulty have you had in each of the following activities <u>due to your shoulder</u>?

7. Putting on or removing a pullover sweater or shirt.

   A) Unable
   B) Severe difficulty
   C) Moderate difficulty
   D) Mild difficulty
   E) No difficulty

8. Combing or brushing your hair.

   A) Unable
   B) Severe difficulty
   C) Moderate difficulty
   D) Mild difficulty
   E) No difficulty

9. Reaching shelves that are above your head.

   A) Unable
   B) Severe difficulty
   C) Moderate difficulty
   D) Mild difficulty
   E) No difficulty

10. Scratching or washing your lower back with your hand.

    A) Unable
    B) Severe difficulty
    C) Moderate difficulty
    D) Mild difficulty
    E) No difficulty

11. Lifting or carrying a full bag of groceries (5 to 10 pounds [3.6 to 4.5 kilograms]).

    A) Unable
    B) Severe difficulty
    C) Moderate difficulty
    D) Mild difficulty
    E) No difficulty

The following questions refer to <u>recreational or athletic activities</u>.

12. Considering all the ways you use your shoulder during <u>recreational or athletic activities</u> (ie, baseball, golf, aerobics, gardening, etc), how would you describe the function of your shoulder?

    A) Very severe limitation; unable
    B) Severe limitation
    C) Moderate limitation
    D) Mild limitation
    E) No limitation

13. During the past month, how much difficulty have you had <u>throwing a ball overhand or serving tennis</u> due to your shoulder?

    A) Unable
    B) Severe difficulty
    C) Moderate difficulty
    D) Mild difficulty
    E) No difficulty

14. List one activity (recreational or athletic) that you particularly enjoy and then select the degree of limitation you have, if any, <u>due to your shoulder</u>.

    Activity_____

    A) Unable
    B) Severe limitation
    C) Moderate limitation
    D) Mild limitation
    E) No limitation

FORM F–13. PATIENT RATED WRIST EVALUATION

NAME:_____ DA

*The questions below will help us understand how n
with your wrist in the past week. You will be descr
symptoms __over the past week__ on a scale of 0-10. I*
**ALL questions. If you did not perform an activ
pain or difficulty you would expect. If you have
you may leave it blank.**

1. PAIN

*Rate the average amount of pain in your wrist over
that best describes your pain on a scale from 0-10. A zero
pain and a ten (10) means that you had the worst pain you
could not do the activity because of pain.*

Sample scale ➔   0   1
No Pain

RATE YOUR PAIN:

At rest	0 1
When doing a task with a repeated wrist movement	0 1
When lifting a heavy object	0 1
When it is at its worst	0 1

How often do you have pain?	0 1
	Never

FORM

NAME:____

Function	
Pain	
Motion	
Stability	
Function	
Total	

From Morrey BF. T

FC
US

NAM

Durir

1. F

2. F

3. F
(

4. I

5. (

6.

7.

8.

The following questions refer to <u>work</u>.

15. During the past month, what has been your main form of work?
   A) Paid work (list type)_____
   B) Housework
   C) Schoolwork
   D) Unemployed
   E) Disabled due to your shoulder
   F) Disabled secondary to other causes
   G) Retired

If you answered D, E, F, or G to the above question, please skip questions 16–19 and go on to question 20.

16. During the past month, how often were you <u>unable</u> to do <u>any</u> of your usual work because of your shoulder?
   A) All days
   B) Several days per week
   C) One day per week
   D) Less than one day per week
   E) Never

17. During the past month, on the days that you did work, how often were you unable to do your work as <u>carefully</u> or as <u>efficiently</u> as you would like because of your shoulder?
   A) All days
   B) Several days per week
   C) One day per week
   D) Less than one day per week
   E) Never

18. During the past month, on the days that you did work, how often did you work a <u>shorter day</u> because of your shoulder?
   A) All days
   B) Several days per week
   C) One day per week
   D) Less than one day per week
   E) Never

19. During the past month, on the days that you did work, how often did you have to <u>change</u> the way that your <u>usual work</u> is done because of your shoulder?
   A) All days
   B) Several days per week
   C) One day per week
   D) Less than one day per week
   E) Never

The following questions refer to <u>satisfaction</u> and <u>areas for improvement</u>.

20. During the past month, how would you rate your overall degree of satisfaction with your shoulder?
   A) Poor
   B) Fair
   C) Good
   D) Very good
   E) Excellent

21. Please rank the two areas in which you would most like to see <u>improvement</u> (place a 1 for the most important, a 2 for the second most important).
   Pain_____
   Daily personal and household activities_____
   Recreational or athletic activities_____
   Work_____

This is the end of the Shoulder Rating Questionnaire. Thank you for your cooperation.

From L'Insalata JC, Warren RF, Cohen SB, Altchek DW, Peterson MG. A self-administered questionnaire for assessment of symptoms and function of the shoulder. *J Bone Joint Surg* 1997;79A(5):738–748.

FORM

9. Could you

Name:___

Please an

1. Is yo
2. Does
3. Can
4. Can
5. Can
6. Can
7. Can
8. Can
9. Do y
10. Do y
11. Can
12. Wou

Are the

Previous
Previous
Previous

How ma
Previous

Are the
Any fan

From Ma

10. Have you be

11. How much ha

12. Have you been

From Dawson J, Fitzpat

FORM F–12. ELBOW FUNCTIONAL RATING INDEX

NAME:_____ DATE:____

Motion
  Degree of flexion (0.2 × arc) (*Example: 0.2 × 60° flexion = 12 points*)
  Degree of pronation (0.1 × arc)
  Degree of supination (0.1 × arc)

Strength
  Normal
  Mild loss (appreciated but not limiting, 80% of opposite side)
  Moderate loss (limits some activity, 50% of opposite side)
  Severe loss (limits everyday tasks, disabling)

Stability
  Normal
  Mild loss (perceived by patients, no limitation)
  Moderate loss (limits some activity)
  Severe loss (limits everyday tasks)

Pain
  None
  Mild (with activity, no medication)
  Moderate (with or after activity)
  Severe (at rest, constant medication, disabling)

From Broberg MA, Morrey BF. Results of delayed excision of the radial head after fracture. *J Bone*

FORM F–17. WESTERN ONTARIO AND MCMASTER UNIVERSITIES (WOMAC) OSTEOARTHRITIS INDEX

NAME:_____ DATE:_____ DOB:_____

INSTRUCTIONS TO PATIENTS

In Sections A, B and C questions will be asked in the following format and you should give your answers by putting an "X" on the horizontal line.

NOTE:

1. If you put your "X" at the left-hand end of the line, i.e.

  NO PAIN |——X—————————————————| EXTREME PAIN

  then you are indicating that you have no pain.

2. If you place your "X" at the right-hand end of the line, i.e.

  NO PAIN |—————————————————X——| EXTREME PAIN

  then you are indicating that your pain is extreme.

3. Please Note:
  a) that the further to the right-hand end you place your "X" the **more** pain you are experiencing.
  b) that the further to the left-hand end you place your "X" the **less** pain you are experiencing.
  c) **Please do not** place your "X" outside the end markers.

You will be asked to indicate on this type of scale the amount of pain, stiffness, or disability you are experiencing. Please remember the further you place your "X" to the right, the more pain, stiffness or disability you are indicating that you experience.

Section A
INSTRUCTIONS TO PATIENTS

The following questions concern the amount of pain you are currently experiencing due to arthritis in your hips and/or knees. For each situation please enter the amount of pain recently experienced. (Please mark your answers with an "X").

QUESTION: How much pain do you have?

1. Walking on a flat surface.

  NO PAIN |—————————————————————| EXTREME PAIN

2. Going up or down stairs.

  NO PAIN |—————————————————————| EXTREME PAIN

3. At night while in bed.

  NO PAIN |—————————————————————| EXTREME PAIN

4. Sitting or lying.

  NO PAIN |—————————————————————| EXTREME PAIN

5. Standing upright.

  NO PAIN |—————————————————————| EXTREME PAIN

Section B
INSTRUCTIONS TO PATIENTS

The following questions concern the amount of joint stiffness (not pain) you are currently experiencing in your hips and/or knees. Stiffness is a sensation of restriction or slowness in the ease with which you move your joints. (Please mark your answers with an "X").

1. How **severe** is your stiffness **after first wakening** in the morning?

    NO STIFFNESS |————————————————————| EXTREME STIFFNESS

2. How **severe** is your stiffness after sitting, lying or resting **later in the day?**

    NO STIFFNESS |————————————————————| EXTREME STIFFNESS

Section C
INSTRUCTIONS TO PATIENTS

The following questions concern your physical function. By this we mean your ability to move around and to look after yourself. For each of the following activities, please indicate the degree of difficulty you are currently experiencing due to arthritis in your hips and/or knees. (Please mark your answers with an "X").

QUESTION: What degree of difficulty do you have with

1. Descending stairs.

    NO DIFFICULTY |————————————————————| EXTREME DIFFICULTY

2. Ascending stairs.

    NO DIFFICULTY |————————————————————| EXTREME DIFFICULTY

3. Rising from sitting.

    NO DIFFICULTY |————————————————————| EXTREME DIFFICULTY

4. Standing.

    NO DIFFICULTY |————————————————————| EXTREME DIFFICULTY

5. Bending to floor.

    NO DIFFICULTY |————————————————————| EXTREME DIFFICULTY

6. Walking on flat surface.

    NO DIFFICULTY |————————————————————| EXTREME DIFFICULTY

7. Getting in/out of car.

    NO DIFFICULTY |————————————————————| EXTREME DIFFICULTY

8. Going shopping.

    NO DIFFICULTY |————————————————————| EXTREME DIFFICULTY

9. Putting on socks/stockings.

    NO DIFFICULTY |————————————————————| EXTREME DIFFICULTY

10. Rising from bed.

    NO DIFFICULTY |————————————————————| EXTREME DIFFICULTY

11. Taking off socks/stockings.

    NO DIFFICULTY |————————————————————| EXTREME DIFFICULTY

12. Lying in bed.

NO | _____ | EXTREME
DIFFICULTY | | DIFFICULTY

13. Getting in/out of bath.

NO | _____ | EXTREME
DIFFICULTY | | DIFFICULTY

14. Sitting.

NO | _____ | EXTREME
DIFFICULTY | | DIFFICULTY

15. Getting on/off toilet.

NO | _____ | EXTREME
DIFFICULTY | | DIFFICULTY

16. Heavy domestic duties.

NO | _____ | EXTREME
DIFFICULTY | | DIFFICULTY

17. Light domestic duties.

NO | _____ | EXTREME
DIFFICULTY | | DIFFICULTY

From Bellamy N, Buchanan WW, Goldsmith CH, Campbell J, Stitt LW. Validation study of WOMAC: A health status instrument for measuring clinically important patient relevant outcomes to antirheumatic drug therapy in patients with osteoarthritis of the hip or knee. *J Rheumatol* 1988;15(12):1833–1840. Contact Dr. Nicholas Bellamy, Division of Rheumatology, Victoria Hospital, P.O. Box 5375, London, Ontario, Canada N6A 4G5. Telephone: 519-667-6815. Fax: 519-667-6687.

FORM F–18. INDEX OF SEVERITY FOR HIP OSTEOARTHRITIS

NAME:_____ DATE:_____ DOB:_____

Pain or Discomfort	Points
During nocturnal bedrest	
None or insignificant	0
Only on movement or in certain positions	1
With no movement	2
Morning stiffness or regressive pain after rising	
1 minute or less	0
More than 1 but less than 15 minutes	1
15 minutes or more	2
After standing for 30 minutes	0 or 1
While ambulating	
None	0
Only after ambulating some distance	1
After initial ambulation and increasingly with continued ambulation	2
With prolonged sitting (2 hours)	0 or 1

Maximum Distance Walked (may walk with pain)	
Unlimited	0
More than 1 km, but limited	1
About 1 km (0.6 mi), (in about 15 min)	2
From 500 to 900 m (1,640–2,952 ft or 0.31–0.56 mi), (in about 8–15 min)	3
From 300 to 500 m (984–1,640 ft)	4
From 100 to 300 m (328–984 ft)	5
Less than 100 m (328 ft)	6
With one walking stick or crutch	1
With two walking sticks or crutches	2

Activities of Daily Living[a]	
Put on socks by bending forward	0 to 2
Pick up an object from the floor	0 to 2
Climb up and down a standard flight of stairs	0 to 2
Can get into and out of a car	0 to 2
Sexual Activity (in sexually active women when considering hip prosthesis)[a]	0 to 2

_____

TOTAL SCORE _____

[a] Without difficulty: 0; with some difficulty: 0.5; moderate: 1; important difficulty: 1.5; unable: 2.

From Lequesne M. Indices of severity and disease activity for osteoarthritis. *Semin Arthritis Rheum* 1991;20(6 suppl 2):48–54.

FORM F–19. INTERNATIONAL KNEE DOCUMENTATION COMMITTEE ASSESSMENT FORM

NAME:_____ DATE:_____ DOB:_____

The Seven Groups	The Four Grades				Group Grades			
	A: Normal	**B:** Nearly Normal	**C:** Abnormal	**D:** Sev Abnormal	A	B	C	D
PATIENT SUBJECTIVE ASSESSMENT								
On a scale of 0 to 3 how did you rate your pre-injury activity level?	☐ 0	☐ 1	☐ 2	☐ 3	☐	☐	☐	☐
On a scale of 0 to 3 how did you rate your current activity level?	☐ 0	☐ 1	☐ 2	☐ 3				
If your normal knee performs 100%, what percentage does your operated knee perform?	_____%				☐	☐	☐	☐
SYMPTOMS	I	II	III	IV				
(Grade at highest activity level known by patient)	Strenuous Activities	Moderate Activities	ADL/Light Activities	ADL Problems				
Pain	☐	☐	☐	☐				
Swelling	☐	☐	☐	☐				
Partial giving away	☐	☐	☐	☐				
Full giving away	☐	☐	☐	☐	☐	☐	☐	☐
RANGE OF MOTION								
Flexion/Ext: Index side:								
Opposite side:								
Lack of extension (from zero degrees)	☐ <3°	☐ 3–5°	☐ 6–10°	☐ > 10°				
Δ Lack of flexion	☐ 0–5°	☐ 6–15°	☐ 16–25°	☐ >25°	☐	☐	☐	☐
LIGAMENT EXAMINATION								
Δ Lachman (25° flex.) (manual, instrumented, x-ray)	☐ 1 to 2 mm	☐ 3 to 5 mm	☐ 6 to 10 mm	☐ >10 mm				
Endpoint: ☐ firm ☐ soft	☐ firm		☐ soft					
Total a.p. transl (70° flex)	☐ 0 to 2 mm	☐ 3 to 5 mm	☐ 6 to 10 mm	☐ >10 mm				
Post. Sag in 70° flex	☐ 0 to 2 mm	☐ 3 to 5 mm	☐ 6 to 10 mm	☐ >10 mm				
Med. joint opening (valgus rotation)	☐ 0 to 2 mm	☐ 3 to 5 mm	☐ 6 to 10 mm	☐ >10 mm				
Lat. joint opening (varus rotation)	☐ 0 to 2 mm	☐ 3 to 5 mm	☐ 6 to 10 mm	☐ >10 mm				
Pivot shift	☐ neg.	☐ + (glide).	☐ ++ (clunk).	☐ +++ gross				
Reversed pivot shift	☐ equal	☐ glide	☐ marked	☐ gross	☐	☐	☐	☐
COMPARTMENTAL FINDINGS								
Crepitus patellofemoral	☐ none		☐ moderate	☐ severe				
Crepitus medial compartment	☐ none		☐ moderate	☐ severe				
Crepitus lateral compartment	☐ none		☐ moderate	☐ severe	☐	☐	☐	☐
			(palpable & audible)					

X-RAY FINDINGS								
Med joint space narrowing	☐ none		☐ < 50%	☐ > 50%				
Lat joint space narrowing	☐ none		☐ < 50%	☐ > 50%				
Patellofemoral joint space narrowing	☐ none		☐ < 50%	☐ > 50%	☐	☐	☐	☐
FUNCTIONAL TEST								
One leg hop (% of opposite side)	☐ 100–90%	☐ 90–76%	☐ 75–50%	☐ < 50%	☐	☐	☐	☐
FINAL EVALUATION					☐	☐	☐	☐

Footnotes:
- Group grade: The lowest grade within a group determines the group grade.
- Final evaluation: The worst group determines the final evaluation.
- In a final evaluation all 7 groups are to be evaluated, for a quick knee profile the evaluation of groups 1–4 are sufficient.
- IKDC = International Knee Documentation Committee.

From Insall JN, Dorr LD, Scott RD, Scott WN. Rationale of the Knee Society clincial rating system. *Clin Orthop* 1989;248:13–14.

FORM F–20. AMERICAN KNEE SOCIETY'S ASSESSMENT SYSTEM

NAME:_____ DATE:_____ DOB:_____

Pain	Points	Function	Points
None	50	Walking	
Mild or occasional	45	Unlimited	50
Stairs only	40	> 10 blocks	40
Walking and stairs	30	5–10 blocks	30
Moderate		< 5 blocks	20
Occasional	20	Household	10
Continual	10	Unable	0
Severe	0	Stairs	
Range of motion (5° = 1 point)	25	Normal up and down	50
Stability (maximum movement in any position)		Normal up; down with rail	
			40
Anteroposterior (mm)		Up and down with rail	30
< 5	10	Up with rail; unable down	15
5–10	5	Unable	0
10	0	*Subtotal*	—
Mediolateral (degrees)		Deductions (minus)	
< 5	15	Cane	5
6–9	10	Two canes	10
10–14	5	Crutches or walker	20
15	0		
Subtotal	—	*Total deductions*	—
Deductions (minus)			
Flexion contracture (degrees)		*Final score*	—
5–10	2		
10–15	5		
16–20	10		
> 20	15		
Extension lag (degrees)			
< 10	5		
10–20	10		
> 15	15		

Alignment (degrees)			
5–10	0		
0–4	3 points each °		
11–15	3 points each °		
Other	20		
Total deductions	—		
Knee score	—		

(If total is a minus number, score is 0).

A. Unilateral or bilateral (opposite knee successfully replaced)
B. Unilateral, other knee symptomatic
C. Multiple arthritis or medical infirmity

From Insall JN, Dorr LD, Scott RD, Scott WN. Rationale of Knee Society clinical rating system. *Clin Orthop* 1989;248:13–14.

FORM F–21. ANTERIOR KNEE PAIN QUESTIONNAIRE

ANTERIOR KNEE PAIN (Sheet code:_____)

Name: _____ Date:_____ Age: _____

Knee: Left/Right

Duration of symptoms: _____years _____months

For each question, circle the latest choice (letter) which corresponds to your knee symptoms.

1. Limp
   (a) None (5)
   (b) Slight or periodical (3)
   (c) Constant (0)
2. Support
   (a) Full support without pain (5)
   (b) Painful (3)
   (c) Weight bearing impossible (0)
3. Walking
   (a) Unlimited (5)
   (b) More than 2 km (3)
   (c) 1–2 km (2)
   (d) Unable (0)
4. Stairs
   (a) No difficulty (10)
   (b) Slight pain with descending (8)
   (c) Pain both when descending and ascending (5)
   (d) Unable (0)
5. Squatting
   (a) No difficulty (5)
   (b) Repeated squatting painful (4)
   (c) Painful each time (3)
   (d) Possible with partial weight bearing (2)
   (e) Unable (0)
6. Running
   (a) No difficulty (10)
   (b) Pain after more than 2 km (8)
   (c) Slight pain from start (6)
   (d) Severe pain (3)
   (e) Unable (0)
7. Jumping
   (a) No difficulty (10)
   (b) Slight difficulty (7)
   (c) Constant pain (2)
   (d) Unable (0)
8. Prolonged sitting with knees flexed
   (a) No difficulty (10)
   (b) Pain after exercise (8)
   (c) Constant pain (6)
   (d) Pain forces to extend knees temporarily (4)
   (e) Unable (0)

9. Pain
    (a) None (10)
    (b) After severe exertion (8)
    (c) Interferes with sleep (6)
    (d) Occasionally severe (3)
    (e) Constant and severe (0)
10. Swelling
    (a) None (10)
    (b) After severe exertion (8)
    (c) After daily activities (6)
    (d) Every evening (4)
    (e) Constant (0)
11. Abnormal painful kneecap (patellar movements subluxations)
    (a) None (10)
    (b) Occasionally in sports activities (6)
    (c) Occasionally in daily activities (4)
    (d) At least one documented dislocation (2)
    (e) More than two dislocations (0)
12. Atrophy of thigh
    (a) None (5)
    (b) Slight (3)
    (c) Severe (0)
13. Flexion deficiency
    (a) None (5)
    (b) Slight (3)
    (c) Severe (0)

From Kujala UM, Jaakkola LH, Koskinen SK, Taimela S, Hurme M, Nelimarkka O. Scoring of patellofemoral disorders. *Arthroscopy* 1993;9(2):159–163.

FORM F–22. HARRISON'S PATELLOFEMORAL PAIN SYNDROME SCALE

NAME:_____ DATE:_____ DOB:_____

1. How much pain do you have in your knee:

    a. At its worst?

    |——————————————————————————————————|
    No pain   Pain as severe
    as it could be

    b. At its least?

    c. As it usually feels?

2. How often do you have pain in your knee?

3. How long does the pain in your knee last?

4. How does the pain in your knee affect your lifestyle?

5. Has the pain in your knee changed since your first visit to the clinic?

6. Do you have any problems or any discomfort in your knee with the following activities?

    a. walking a short distance (about a city block)

    b. running a short distance, say 100 meters (about a city block)

    c. climbing up 4 flights of stairs (about 32 steps)

    d. sitting for prolonged periods with your knees bent in one position

    e. kneeling

    f. squatting

    g. climbing up 2 flights of stairs (about 16 steps)

    h. walking as far as a mile

    i. jumping

    j. sitting for a short period with your knees bent in one position

    k. walking down 1 flight of stairs

    l. running as far as a mile

7. How does your knee affect your normal activities?

8. What was your sports or physical activity level before your knee condition?

9. At the present time, what is your level of sports or recreational activity?

10. Has your sports or recreational activity level changed due to your knee condition?

11. Does your knee condition affect your performance in sport activities?

12. Has your performance at work changed due to your knee condition?

From Harrison E, Magee D, Quinney H. Development of a clinical tool and patient questionnaire for evaluation of patellofemoral pain syndrome patients. *Clin J Sport Med* 1996;6(3):163–170.

FORM F–23. INDEX OF SEVERITY FOR KNEE OSTEOARTHRITIS

NAME:_____ DATE:_____ DOB:_____

	POINTS
Pain or Discomfort	
During nocturnal bedrest	
None or insignificant	0
Only on movement or in certain positions	1
With no movement	2
Morning stiffness or regressive pain after rising	
1 minute or less	0
More than 1 but less than 15 minutes	1
15 minutes or more	2
After standing for 30 minutes	0 or 1
While ambulating	
None	0
Only after ambulating some distance	1
After initial ambulation and increasingly with continued ambulation	2
After getting up from sitting without the help of arms	0 or 1
Maximum Distance Walked (may walk with pain)	
Unlimited	0
More than 1 km, but limited	1
About 1 km (0.6 mi), (in about 15 min)	2
From 500 to 900 m (1,640–2,952 ft or 0.31–0.56 mi), (in about 8–15 min)	3
From 300 to 500 m (984–1,640 ft)	4
From 100 to 300 m (328–984 ft)	5
Less than 100 m (328 ft)	6
With one walking stick or crutch	1
With two walking sticks or crutches	2
Activities of Daily Living[a]	
Able to climb up a standard flight of stairs?	0 to 2
Able to climb down a standard flight of stairs?	0 to 2
Able to squat or bend on the knees?	0 to 2
Able to walk on uneven ground?	0 to 2
	_____

TOTAL SCORE

[a] Without difficulty: 0; with some difficulty: 0.5; moderate: 1; important difficulty: 1.5; unable: 2.

From Lequesne M. Indices of severity and disease activity for osteoarthritis. *Semin Arthritis Rheum* 1991;20(6 suppl 2):48–54.

FORM F–24. SCORING SYSTEM OF SUBJECTIVE CLINICAL EVALUATION (ANKLE)

NAME:_____ DATE:_____ DOB:_____

SCORE	SUBJECTIVE CLINICAL RESULT
4	No pain; normal ankle
3	Pain is noted only after severe and prolonged stress; participation in sports and ability to walk or work not limited
2	Pain is moderately incapacitating, but no cane or other walking aid is used; mild analgesics are occasionally required; walking is restricted, but patient is able to walk more than five blocks; patient may have changed occupations due to painful ankle but works full-time and has no reduction in pay
1	Pain is severe and may require use of a brace or cane and daily analgesics; walking is restricted to less than five blocks; patient is unemployable on a full-time basis due to the ankle but is able to care for himself
0	Pain is constant and incapacitating; patient is unable to walk sufficiently to care for himself and desires fusion of the ankle

From Joy G, Patzakis MJ, Harvey JP Jr. Precise evaluation of the reduction of severe ankle fractures. *J Bone Joint Surg* 1974;56A(5):979–993.

FORM F–25. OLERUD AND MOLANDER SCORING SYSTEM (ANKLE)

NAME:_____ DATE:_____ DOB:_____

PARAMETER	DEGREE	SCORE
I. Pain	None	25
	While walking on uneven surface	20
	While walking on even surface outdoors	10
	While walking indoors	5
	Constant and severe	0
II. Stiffness	None	10
	Stiffness	0
III. Swelling	None	10
	Only evenings	5
IV. Stair-climbing	No problems	10
	Impaired	5
	Impossible	0
V. Running	Possible	5
	Impossible	0
IV. Jumping	Possible	5
	Impossible	0
VII. Squatting	No problems	5
	Impossible	0
VIII. Supports	None	10
	Taping, wrapping	5
	Stick or crutch	0
IX. Work, activities of daily life	Same as before injury	20
	Loss of tempo	15
	Change to a simpler job/part-time work	10
	Severely impaired work capacity	0

From Olerud C, Molander H. A scoring system for symptom evaluation after ankle fracture. *Arch Orthop Trauma Surg* 1984;103(3):190–194.

FORM F–26. ANKLE CLINICAL SCORING SYSTEM

NAME:_____ DATE:_____ DOB:_____

Subjective (80 points)

Pain (54 points)

Always alter any activity	0
Prolonged after mild activity	10
Transient after mild activity	20
Prolonged after heavy activity	35
Transient after heavy activity	40
None	50
Requires medication for pain regularly	0
Requires medication occasionally	2
Requires no medication	4

Function (26 points)

Unable to climb stairs	0
Uses normal foot first	1
Requires aid of banister	2
Climbs normally	3
Unable to descend stairs	0
Uses normal foot first	1
Requires aid of banister	2
Descends normally	3
Walks <1 block	0
Walks <5 blocks	2
Walks <10 blocks	3
Walks >10 blocks	5
Walks unlimited distances	6
Recreational activities limited	0
No activities limited	3
Requires walker	0
Requires crutches	1
Requires one crutch	2
Requires cane	4
Requires no aids	8
Dissatisfied	0
Moderately satisfied	2
Very satisfied	3

Objective (20 points)

Gait (6 points)

Antalgic limp	0
External rotation gait	3
Normal gait	6

Range of motion: difference from normal side (14 points)

Dorsiflexion

Difference >20 degrees	0
Difference 10–20 degrees	2
Difference <10 degrees	4
No difference	7

Plantar flexion

Difference >20 degrees	0
Difference <20 degrees	2
No difference	3

Supination

Difference >0 degrees	0
No difference	2

Pronation

Difference >0 degrees	0
No difference	2

From Phillips WA, Schwartz HS, Keller CS, et al. A prospective, randomized study of the management of severe ankle fractures. *J Bone Joint Surg* 1985;67A(1):67–78.

FORM F–27. ANKLE GRADING SYSTEM

NAME:_____ DATE:_____ DOB:_____

Pain

None, or patient ignores it	50
Slight when going up or down stairs or walking long distances (no restriction of activities of daily living)	45
Moderate when going up or down stairs or walking long distances; none during level gait; occasional non-narcotic medication needed	40
During level gait, with more pain on stairs; none at rest; daily medication used	25
At rest or at night in addition to during walking; narcotic medication required	10
Continuous, regardless of activity	0
Disabled because of pain	0

Total _____

Function

Limp, antalgic

None	6
Slight	4
Moderate	2
Marked	0

Total _____

Distance

Unlimited	6
4–6 blocks	4
1–3 blocks	2
Indoors only	1
Bed-chair	0
Unable to walk	0

Total _____

Support

None	6
Cane, long walks only	5
Cane, full time	3
2 canes or crutches	1
Walker required or unable to walk	0

Total _____

Hills (up)

Climbs normally	3
Climbs with foot externally rotated	2
Climbs on toes or by side-stepping	1
Unable to climb hills	0

Total _____

Hills (down)

Descends normally	3
Descends with foot externally rotated	2
Descends on toes or by side-stepping	1
Unable to descend	0

Total _____

Stairs (up)

    Climbs normally   3

    Needs banister   2

    Steps up with normal foot only   1

    Unable to climb stairs   0

            Total _____

Stairs (down)

    Descends normally   3

    Needs banister   2

    Steps down with normal foot only   1

    Unable to descend stairs   0

            Total _____

Ability to rise on toes (stability)

    Able to rise on toes × 10 repetitions   5

    Able to rise on toes × 5 repetitions   3

    Able to rise on toes × 1 repetition   1

    Unable to rise on toes   0

            Total _____

Running

    Able to run as much as desired   5

    Able to run but limited   3

    Unable to run   0

            Total _____

Range of motion

    Dorsiflexion beyond neutral

        40 degrees   5

        30 degrees   4

        20 degrees   3

        10 degrees   2

        5 degrees   1

        0 degrees   0

            Total _____

Plantar flexion

    40 degrees   5

    30 degrees   4

    20 degrees   3

    10 degrees   2

    5 degrees   1

    0 degrees   0

            Total _____

From Mazur JM, Schwartz E, Simon SR. Ankle arthrodesis. Long-term follow-up with gait analysis. *J Bone Joint Surg* 1979;61A(7):964–975.

FORM F–28. A PERFORMANCE TEST PROTOCOL AND SCORING SCALE FOR THE EVALUATION OF ANKLE INJURIES

NAME:_____ DATE:_____ DOB:_____

I	Subjective assessment of the injured ankle	
	No symptoms of any kind[a]	15
	Mild symptoms	10
	Moderate symptoms	5
	Severe symptoms	0
II	Can you walk normally?	
	Yes	15
	No	0
III	Can you run normally?	
	Yes	10
	No	0
IV	Climbing down stairs[b]	
	Under 18 seconds	10
	18–20 seconds	5
	Over 20 seconds	0
V	Rising on heels with injured leg	
	Over 40 times	10
	30–39 times	5
	Under 30 times	0
VI	Rising on toes with injured leg	
	Over 40 times	10
	30–39 times	5
	Under 30 times	0
VII	Single-limbed stance with injured leg	
	Over 55 seconds	10
	50–55 seconds	5
	Under 50 seconds	0
VII	Laxity of the ankle joint (ADS)	
	Stable (≤ 5 mm)	10
	Moderate instability (6–10 mm)	5
	Severe instability (>10 mm)	0
IX	Dorsiflexion range of motion, injured leg	
	≥10°	10
	5°–9°	5
	<5°	0

Total score: 100–85 = excellent; 80–70 = good; 65–55 = fair; ≤ 50 = poor.

[a] Pain, swelling, stiffness, tenderness of giving way during activities (mild, only one symptom is present; moderate two to three of these symptoms are present; severe four or more of these symptoms are present).

[b] Two levels of staircase (length, 12 m) with 44 steps (height, 18 cm; depth 22 cm).

From Kaikkonen A, Kannus P, Jarvinen M. A performance test protocol and scoring scale for the evaluation of ankle injuries. *Am J Sports Med* 1994;22(4):462–469.

Chapter 16: Measuring
Physical Performance

FORM G–1. HEALTH-RELATED FITNESS TEST BATTERY FOR ADULTS

NAME_____ DATE_____ AGE_____ BD_____ M/F_____

4: EO, EC, Hd Turn Rt Hd Turn Lt	1. **One-leg balance** (eyes open, closed, head turning): Sport shoes; heel of opposite foot by med. knee of bal. Leg w/ER hip rot outwards, arms hanging at side. Time start before eyes closed, hd turns (50 b/m metr.). Pt chooses leg most comfortable w/, *count seconds* until loose foot-to-knee contact or change position of supporting leg; 60 sec max EO (2 trials) and 30 sec EC+ hd turns (L and R); (2–3 trials). **Leg: R L (Circle)** SCORE: EO _____ sec. (Max. 60 sec.); EC _____ sec. (Max. 30 sec.); Head turn _____ sec. (Max. 30 sec.)
3: Scores 0, 1, 2	2. **Shoulder-neck mobility:** *Visual obsv;* 1.5 feet lengths from wall, lean butt/back/shoulders on wall; arms over hd, elbows straight next to ears; back of hands flat on wall. SCORE scale: (circle) 0 = severe restriction; 1 = moderate restriction of ROM (only fingers reach wall); 2 = no restriction of ROM (whole dorsal side hands on wall)
3: N°, LLF RLF	3. **Side-bending:** Feet 15 cm apart next to wall; scap/butt on wall; arms straight at sides; mark tip D3 on lat thigh at N° and at max LF (no trunk/pelvis rotation allowed); *measure* cloth tape and ave. the 2 readings SCORE: RLF _____cm; LLF _____cm; AVERAGE: _____cm
4: Prone clap hands; PU; PU touch back of hand; Prone	4. **Modified push-up:** Prone on mat; each cycle begins by clapping hands behind back; straight-leg push-up/lock elbows; touch top of 1 hand with other to standardize the up posi.; return to prone posi = 1 cycle; *count* max. # reps in 40 sec. SCORE: _____total # of push-ups
2: Set-up in up-posi; Lean back posi.	5. **Isometric sit-up:** Knees fl ~90°/feet flat on floor, unsupported, straight back sit-up; arms at side/finger tips gently touch mat; no L-spine Fl allowed; lean back to 90° thigh-trunk angle/hold max. 240 sec./verbals q 30 sec. (1 sec. or less = 0); record total # of sec. SCORE: _____seconds (max. 240)
3: Pre-test Mg mark; Semi-squat posi, Max jump	6. **Jump and reach test:** Lat to wall, arm up mark wall w/Mg Powdered D3; may swing arms to facilitate jump-may bend knees but not move feet; meas cm dif between Mg chalk marks; 2 trials, record best (1 practice) SCORE: Trial 1 _____cm; Trial 2 _____cm (Use the greater of the 2)
3: 2-Leg squat; lunge w/wts—L and R	7. **One-leg squat test** (lunge): 1st 2-leg squat to 90° (pre-1 leg trials); 1st: body wt; 2nd: 10% body wt (weight belt used to add extra wts) each × up to 30% body wt; test ends when can't lunge w/wts. (Circle scale score) SCORE: 0 = unable 2 legs; 1 = able 2 legs; 2 = 1 leg—body wt (BW) only; 3 = 1 leg—10% BW; 4 = 20%; 5 = 30% of BW

COMMENTS_____

_____

_____

_____

_____

FORM G–2. PRONE PRESS-UP EXAMINATION FORM

NAME_____ **DATE**_____ **DOB**_____ **DOI**_____

A. Pain

Location of complaint	☐ Back ☐ Right leg ☐ Left leg	
Before Initiation	☐	
Symptoms at Initiation	☐	
Symptoms at termination	☐	Time to Onset_____ sec.
Symptoms after termination	☐	Time to Onset_____ sec., min., hrs, days (circle)

B. Paresthesia

Location of complaint	☐ Back ☐ Right leg ☐ Left leg	
Before Initiation	☐	
Symptoms at Initiation	☐	
Symptoms at termination	☐	Time to Onset_____ sec.
Symptoms after termination	☐	Time to Onset_____ sec., min., hrs, days (circle)

Comments:

_____
_____
_____
_____
_____
_____
_____
_____
_____
_____
_____
_____
_____
_____
_____
_____
_____

Signed _____ **Date scored**_____

From Moffroid MT, Haugh LD, Henry SM, Short B. Distinguishable groups of musculoskeletal low back pain patients and asymptomatic control subjects based on physical measures of the NIOSH low back atlas. *Spine* 1994;19:1350–1358. Moffroid MT: personal communication 3-11-97; 5-18-98.

FORM G–3. NIOSH DISTINGUISHING LBP TESTS

NAME_____ DATE_____ DOB_____ Gender: M/F_____

SYMMETRY Pelvic height	1. Iliac Crest Height: standing (posterior) 2. PSIS standing	Even: Yes/No (Low: L/R) Even: Yes/No (Low: L/R)

STRENGTH	3. Upper Abdominal Muscle Strength
	   Pt supine, hips straight or sl. flex
	   Raise head and shoulders "curling" the trunk
		Grading Scheme:
		A: Scapulae off table with hands locked behind head (Best)
		B: Scapulae off table with arms across chest
		C: Scapulae off table with arms at sides
		D: Cannot complete the procedure (Worst)

PASSIVE MOBILITY	4. Hip rotation (single gravity goniometer)
	   (L & R sides)
	   Internal
	   External
		LEFT RIGHT
		
		IR_____ _____
		ER_____ _____

DYNAMIC MOBILITY Angle difference	1. Forward flexion: Dual inclinometers 2. Single straight leg raise	Flexion_____ SLR_____/_____° Left Right
Presence of *pain* Prone press-up (PPU)	3. Whether PPU had any effect Pain at initiation of PPU	Centralize/No change/Peripheralize Yes/No

Abbreviations: L, left; PSIS, posterior superior iliac spine; PPU, prone press up; R, right; SLR, straight leg raise.

COMMENTS_____
_____
_____
_____
_____
_____
_____

Signed_____ Date scored_____

From Moffroid MT, Haugh LD, Henry SM, Short B. Distinguishable groups of musculoskeletal low back pain patients and asymptomatic control subjects based on physical measures of the NIOSH low back atlas. *Spine* 1994;19:1350–1358.

FORM G–4. SACROI...

NAME_____

TESTS *Standing*
Pre-test VAS
1. Standing Flexion Test

Sitting
2. PSIS Sitting (PSISSI)

Supine
3. Supine to Long Sitting

Prone
4. Prone Knee Flexion Test
Post-test VAS

PAIN (Key): +1 = ↑pain and/or peri...

Definitions and References for Sacroi...

1. PSIS Flexion in Standing   *See Form...*
2. PSIS Sitting   *See Form...*
3. Supine to Long Sitting   *See Form...*
4. Prone Knee Flexion   *See Form...*

From Delitto A, Cibulka MT, Erhard RE, et al...
tion pilot study. *Phys Ther* 1993:73;216–228.

FORM G–6. QUANTITATIVE FUNCTIONAL CAPACITY EVALUATION

NAME_____ DATE_____ DOB_____ DOI_____

Dx:_____

TESTS	INITIAL Date: ____/10		1ST RE-EXAM Date: ____/10		2ND RE-EXAM Date: ____/10		3RD RE-EXAM Date: ____/10	
1. Pre-Test VAS								
2. Rep. Squat (feet 15 cm apart) Thigh horizontal, 1 rep./2–3 sec., note # of reps; max. reps 50	____# of reps.		____# of reps.		____# of reps.		____# of reps.	
3. ROM: Lumbar Extremity (L/R) Flexion (Forw. Flex.) Extension (Backward Ext.) Rt. Lat. Flex. (Abduction) Lt. Lat. Flex. (Adduction)	FL ___ +2,1,0,–1,2[a] EXT ___ +2,1,0,–1,2 RLF ___ +2,1,0,–1,2 LLF ___ +2,1,0,–1,2		FL ___ +2,1,0,–1,2 EXT ___ +2,1,0,–1,2 RLF ___ +2,1,0,–1,2 LLF ___ +2,1,0,–1,2		FL ___ +2,1,0,–1,2 EXT ___ +2,1,0,–1,2 RLF ___ +2,1,0,–1,2 LLF ___ +2,1,0,–1,2		FL ___ +2,1,0,–1,2 EXT ___ +2,1,0,–1,2 RLF ___ +2,1,0,–1,2 LLF ___ +2,1,0,–1,2	
4. PAIN (Superficial): Waddell #1	+/–		+/–		+/–		+/–	
5. SIMULATION: Waddell #2	+/–		+/–		+/–		+/–	
a. Trunk Rotation	+/–		+/–		+/–		+/–	
b. Axial Compression (5 kg)	+/–		+/–		+/–		+/–	
TESTS	L	R	L	R	L	R	L	R
6. Gastroc/Ankle DF (Knee extd)	___°	___°	___°	___°	___°	___°	___°	___°
7. Soleus/Ankle DF (Knee flexed)	___°	___°	___°	___°	___°	___°	___°	___°
7a. One-Leg Stand (eyes open)[a]	___Sec.	___Sec.	___Sec.	___Sec.	___Sec.	___Sec.	___Sec.	___Sec.
7b. One-Leg Stand (eyes closed)[a]	___Sec.	___Sec.	___Sec.	___Sec.	___Sec.	___Sec.	___Sec.	___Sec.
7c. CERVICAL STRENGTH— mm Hg[a]	Fl___ RLF___ Ext___ LLF___		Fl___ RLF___ Ext___ LLF___		Fl___ RLF___ Ext___ LLF___		Fl___ RLF___ Ext___ LLF___	

TESTS *Seated*	L	R	L	R	L	R	L	R
8. Sitting SLR/DISTRACTION (Waddell #3; see #13) ↑ LBP: (circle)	↑ LBP: yes/no	↑ LBP: yes/no	↑ LBP: yes/no	↑ LBP: yes/no	↑ LBP: yes/no	↑ LBP: yes/no	↑ LBP: yes/no	↑ LBP: yes/no
9. Regional Neuro. (Waddell #4)	+/–	+/–	+/–	+/–	+/–	+/–	+/–	+/–
10. Exaggeration (Waddell #5)	+/–		+/–		+/–		+/–	
11. ROM: Cervical Extremity (L/R) Flexion (Forw. Flex.) Extension (Backward Ext.) Rt. Lat. Flex. (Abduction) Lt. Lat. Flex. (Adduction) Rt. Rotation (Ext. Rot.) Lt. Rotation (Int. Rot.)	FL ____ +2,1,0,–1,2[a] EXT ____ +2,1,0,–1,2 RLF ____ +2,1,0,–1,2 LLF ____ +2,1,0,–1,2 RR ____ +2,1,0,–1,2 LR ____ +2,1,0,–1,2		FL ____ +2,1,0,–1,2 EXT ____ +2,1,0,–1,2 RLF ____ +2,1,0,–1,2 LLF ____ +2,1,0,–1,2 RR ____ +2,1,0,–1,2 LR ____ +2,1,0,–1,2		FL ____ +2,1,0,–1,2 EXT ____ +2,1,0,–1,2 RLF ____ +2,1,0,–1,2 LLF ____ +2,1,0,–1,2 RR ____ +2,1,0,–1,2 LR ____ +2,1,0,–1,2		FL ____ +2,1,0,–1,2 EXT ____ +2,1,0,–1,2 RLF ____ +2,1,0,–1,2 LLF ____ +2,1,0,–1,2 RR ____ +2,1,0,–1,2 LR ____ +2,1,0,–1,2	

[a]PAIN SCALE: –2 = centralization; –1 = decreased pain; 0 = no change in pain; +1 = increased pain; +2 = peripheralization.

COMMENTS_____
_____
_____
_____
_____

NAME:_____ DATE:_____ DOB:_____

TESTS *Supine*	L	R	L	R	L	R	L	R
12. Hip Flexion Test/Modified Thomas Measure: Passive hip extension (psoas tension)	a. ____°	a. ____°	a. ____°	a. ____°	a. ____°	a. ____°	a. ____°	a. ____°
13. Hip Flexion/Supine SLR **a. Waddell #3:** supine + vs. sit—SLR **b. Measure angle:** at point of knee flexion	a. +/– b. ____°	a. +/– b. ____°	a. +/– b. ____°	a. +/– b. ____°	a. +/– b. ____°	a. +/– b. ____°	a. +/– b. ____°	a. +/– b. ____°
14. Repetitive Sit-up Test Sit-up, knees 90°, feet anchored, 1 rep./2–3 sec, touch thenar to patella, curl back down; max. 50 reps.	*Endurance* reps. _____/50		*Endurance* reps. _____/50		*Endurance* reps. _____/50		*Endurance* reps. _____/50	
14a. Double Leg Lowering (maintain pelvic tilt <60°)	_____°		_____°		_____°		_____°	
TESTS *Prone*	L	R	L	R	L	R	L	R
15. Repetitive Arch Up Test Waist at table's edge fixed at ankle flexed 45° raises up to horizontal; 1 rep./2–3 seconds; max. 50 reps.	reps. _____/50		reps. _____/50		reps. _____/50		reps. _____/50	
16. Knee Flexion Test/Modified Nachlas Test	____°	____°	____°	____°	____°	____°	____°	____°
17. Hip ROM Internal Rotation External Rotation	IR ____° ER ____°	IR ____° ER ____°	IR ____° ER ____°	IR ____° ER ____°	IR ____° ER ____°	IR ____° ER ____°	IR ____° ER ____°	IR ____° ER ____°

TESTS	L	R	L	R	L	R	L	R
18. Grip Dynamometry 　　**Dominant: Left/Right (circle)** 　　Use Jamar 　　Use position 1 or 2 　　Three trials (average)	1.____ 2.____ 3.____ ave	1.____ 2.____ 3.____ ave	1.____ 2.____ 3.____ ave	1.____ 2.____ 3.____ ave	1.____ 2.____ 3.____ ave	1.____ 2.____ 3.____ ave	1.____ 2.____ 3.____ ave	1.____ 2.____ 3.____ ave
19. Static Back Endurance 　　Static Back Endurance: Pt 　　holds trunk horizontal up 　　to max. of 240 sec.	Static Time____/240 sec.		Static Time____/240 sec.		Static Time____/240 sec.		Static Time____/240 sec.	
20. Outcomes Instruments: 　　**a. Oswestry LB Disabil. Q.** 　　**b. Neck Disability Index** 　　**c. Gen. Health (separate report)**	a.____% b.____%		a.____% b.____%		a.____% b.____%		a.____% b.____%	
21. Post-Test VAS	____/10		____/10		____/10		____/10	

COMMENTS_____

_____

_____

_____

_____

SIGNED_____ DATE_____ TIME OUT_____

SIGNED_____ DATE_____ TIME OUT_____

SIGNED_____ DATE_____ TIME OUT_____

SIGNED_____ DATE_____ TIME OUT_____

FORM G–7. QUANTITATIVE FUNCTIONAL CAPACITY RESULTS

NAME:_____ Occupation: <u>WC/BC</u>[a] DATE:_____ BD:_____ AGE:_____

Dx:_____ Test #:<u>1, 2, 3, 4</u> Symptom Duration:_____ Prior Episodes: <u>YES/NO</u>

TEST NAME	NORMAL		PATIENT RESULT		PERCENT OF NORMAL	
1. VAS	0/10		_____/10		%	
2. Repetitive Squat[a]	_____/(max. 50)		_____/( )		%	
3. ROM/Lumbar Spine						
Flexion	65°		_____°		%	
Extension	30°		_____°		%	
Rt. Lateral Flexion	25°		_____°		%	
Lt. Lateral Flexion	25°		_____°		%	
4. Waddell #1: Pain	Negative		Positive/Negative		NA	
5. Waddell #2: Stimulation	Negative		Positive/Negative		NA	
6. Gastrocnemius/Ankle DF	23°		Lt:	Rt:	%	%
7. Soleus/Ankle DF	25°		Lt:	Rt:	%	%
8. Sitting SLR/Distraction w/#13	LBP: YES/NO		LBP: YES/NO		NA	
9. Waddell #4: Regional Neuro	Negative		Positive/Negative		NA	
10. Waddell #5: Exaggeration	Negative		Positive/Negative		NA	
11. ROM/Cervical						
Flexion	50°		_____°		%	
Extension	63°		_____°		%	
Rt. Lateral Flexion	45°		_____°		%	
Lt. Lateral Flexion	45°		_____°		%	
Rt. Rotation	85°		_____°		%	
Lt. Rotation	85°		_____°		%	
12. Modified Thomas						
Iliopsoas	84°		Lt:	Rt:	%	%
13a. Waddell #3: Distraction[b]	Negative		Positive/Negative		NA	
13b. Straight Leg Raise[a]	80°		Lt:	Rt:	%	%
14. Repetitive Sit-up[a]	_____ (max. 50)		_____/( )			%
15. Repetitive Arch-up[a]	_____ (max. 50)		_____/( )			%
16. Knee Flexion	147 +/– 1.6		Lt:	Rt:	%	%
17. Hip Rotation ROM						
Internal Rotation ROM	41–45 (43)		Lt:	Rt:	%	%
External Rotation ROM	41–43 (42)		Lt:	Rt:	%	%
18. Grip Strength[a]	Lt: Kg	Rt: Kg	Lt: Kg	Rt: Kg	%	%

19.	Static Back Endurance[a]	_____ (max. 240 sec.)	_____ seconds	%
20.	Outcome Instrument(s)			
	Oswestry LB Disability Ques.	0/50 (0%)	%	%
	Neck Disability Index	0/50 (0%)	%	%
21.	Post-test VAS	0/10	_____/10	%
22.	One leg standing test	EO ____sec/EC____	L___/___ R___/___	L___/___ R___/___
23.	Cervical spine strength	NOT ESTABLISHED	Fl____ RLF____ Ext____ LLF____	Fl____ RLF____ Ext____ LLF____
24.	Double leg lowering	<65° w/pelvic tilt	_____°	_____%

	AGE (years)	EYES OPEN (seconds)	EYES CLOSED (seconds)
Normative data for one leg standing test (test #23)	20–59	29–30	21–28.8 (25 sec. ave.)
	60–69	22.5 ave	10
	70–79	14.2	4.3

[a]Normative data is determined by age, sex and occupation (Blue vs. white collar: BC/WC)

[b]A positive test #13 (supine SLR) and a negative sitting/distracted SLR (test #8) = +Waddell sign for Distraction

SIGNED_____ DATE_____

FORM G–8. QUALITATIVE FUNCTIONAL TESTS

NAME_____ DATE_____ DOB_____ DOI_____

TESTS *Standing*	INITIAL Date:	1ST RE-EXAM Date:	2ND RE-EXAM Date:	3RD RE-EXAM Date:			
Pre-test VAS	_____/10	_____/10	_____/10	_____/10			
1. **Rep. Squat (feet 15 cm apart)** a. Knee flex 90°; 1 rep./2–3 sec. b. No. reps. when: LB lordosis ↑ or ↓ c. Observe for: heel raise	a. Pass/Fail b. ____ # reps. when lordosis ↑ or ↓ c. Heel raise Y/N	a. Pass/Fail b. ____ # reps. when lordosis ↑ or ↓ c. Heel raise Y/N	a. Pass/Fail b. ____ # reps. when lordosis ↑ or ↓ c. Heel raise Y/N	a. Pass/Fail b. ____ # reps. when lordosis ↑ or ↓ c. Heel raise Y/N			
2. **Lunge-Kneel** Note if patient can perform lunge to kneeling position and return w/o lumbar kyphosis	Pass_____ Fail_____ Trunk Flex Y/N	Pass_____ Fail_____ Trunk Flex Y/N	Pass_____ Fail_____ Trunk Flex Y/N	Pass_____ Fail_____ Trunk Flex Y/N			
3. **Extension in Standing (EIS)** Single movement: 1 rep. (McK. #2) (a. pain; b. syndrome; c. lat shift)	a. Pain: +1, 0, −1 b. Syndrome: Fl/Ext c. Lat. shift: Y/N	a. Pain: +1, 0, −1 b. Syndrome: Fl/Ext c. Lat. shift: Y/N	a. Pain: +1, 0, −1 b. Syndrome: Fl/Ext c. Lat. shift: Y/N	a. Pain: +1, 0, −1 b. Syndrome: Fl/Ext c. Lat. shift: Y/N			
4. **Flexion in Standing (FIS)** Single movement: 1 rep. (McK. #3) (a. pain; b. syndrome; c. lat shift)	a. Pain: +1, 0, −1 b. Syndrome: Fl/Ext c. Lat. shift: Y/N	a. Pain: +1, 0, −1 b. Syndrome: Fl/Ext c. Lat. shift: Y/N	a. Pain: +1, 0, −1 b. Syndrome: Fl/Ext c. Lat. shift: Y/N	a. Pain: +1, 0, −1 b. Syndrome: Fl/Ext c. Lat. shift: Y/N			
5. **Standing Flexion Test (SIJ #1)**	a. + = ↑Rt/Lt; b. − = even hts.	a. + = ↑Rt/Lt; b. − = even hts.	a. + = ↑Rt/Lt; b. − = even hts.	a. + = ↑Rt/Lt; b. − = even hts.			
6. **Side Gliding (McK. #1)** Repeated movement: 10 reps. a. Pain: +1, 0, −1 b. Limited: L = Left; R = Right c. Blocked; L = Left; R = Right	L a. +1,0,−1 b. L-L/R c. B-L/R	R a. +1,0,−1 b. L-L/R c. B-L/R	L a. +1,0,−1 b. L-L/R c. B-L/R	R a. +1,0,−1 b. L-L/R c. B-L/R	L a. +1,0,−1 b. L-L/R c. B-L/R	R a. +1,0,−1 b. L-L/R c. B-L/R	L a. +1,0,−1 b. L-L/R c. B-L/R

TESTS *Sitting*	INITIAL Date:	1ST RE-EXAM Date:	2ND RE-EXAM Date:	3RD RE-EXAM Date:
7. **PSIS Sitting (PSISSI) (SIJ #2)** (Circle appropriate response)	a. + = ↑Rt/Lt; b. − = even hts.	a. + = ↑Rt/Lt; b. − = even hts.	a. + = ↑Rt/Lt; b. − = even hts.	a. + = ↑Rt/Lt; b. − = even hts.
8. **ASIS SITTING (ASISSI)**	a. + = ↑Rt/Lt; b. − = even hts.	a. + = ↑Rt/Lt; b. − = even hts.	a. + = ↑Rt/Lt; b. − = even hts.	a. + = ↑Rt/Lt; b. − = even hts.
9. **PSIS FL in Sitting (PSISSI)**	a. + = ↑Rt/Lt; b. − = even hts.	a. + = ↑Rt/Lt; b. − = even hts.	a. + = ↑Rt/Lt; b. − = even hts.	a. + = ↑Rt/Lt; b. − = even hts.

NUMERICAL PAIN SCALE	DEFINITION
+1	Increase or peripheralization of pain
0	No pain
−1	Decrease or centralization of pain

NAME:_____ DATE:_____ DOB:_____

TESTS *Seated*	L	R	L	R	L	R	L	R
10. T/L ROTATION (goniometer) a. Measure b. ✓ for asymmetry c. Circle increased R/L (↑R/L)	a. ____° b. Y/N c. ↑R/L	a. ____° b. Y/N c. ↑R/L	a. ____° b. Y/N c. ↑R/L	a. ____° b. Y/N c. ↑R/L	a. ____° b. Y/N c. ↑R/L	a. ____° b. Y/N c. ↑R/L	a. ____° b. Y/N c. ↑R/L	a. ____° b. Y/N c. ↑R/L
11. Shoulder Abduction Coordination & Endurance Scapular-humeral rhythm: ABd. UEs 90° record pt of contraction of upper traps (N = 30 – 60°) Time point UEs fall below horizontal when making small circle	Upper Trap. contract _____° (30 – 60 = N) Time____	Upper Trap. contract _____° (30 – 60 = N) Time____	Upper Trap. contract _____° (30 – 60 = N) Time____	Upper Trap. contract _____° (30 – 60 = N) Time____	Upper Trap. contract _____° (30 – 60 = N) Time____	Upper Trap. contract _____° (30 – 60 = N) Time____	Upper Trap. contract _____° (30 – 60 = N) Time____	Upper Trap. contract _____° (30 – 60 = N) Time____

TESTS *Supine*	L	R	L	R	L	R	L	R
12. HIP ADDUCTORS (Measure w/ goniometer) (a. 1-joint; b. 2-joint)	a.____° b.____°	a.____° b.____°	a.____° b.____°	a.____° b.____°	a.____° b.____°	a.____° b.____°	a.____° b.____°	a.____° b.____°
13. Supine to Long Sitting (SIJ #3)	+/–		+/–		+/–		+/–	
14. Pelvic Tilt Coordination (supine hook lying) a. a/p tilt (w/ knees flexed) b. Maintain a/p tilt and ext. legs c. Maintain a/p tilt and 2 leg raise (2–3 sec. hold)	Grade 1_____ (A–C normal) Grade 2_____ (A, B) Grade 3_____ (A only) can't do a Pel. Tlt___		Grade 1_____ (A–C normal) Grade 2_____ (A, B) Grade 3_____ (A only) can't do a Pel. Tlt___		Grade 1_____ (A–C normal) Grade 2_____ (A, B) Grade 3_____ (A only) can't do a Pel. Tlt___		Grade 1_____ (A–C normal) Grade 2_____ (A, B) Grade 3_____ (A only) can't do a Pel. Tlt___	
15. Trunk Flex. Coord/Endur. Janda Coordination	*Coord* lordosis ↑Y/N feet press dwn *Y/N* no scap. raised *Y/N*		*Coord* lordosis ↑Y/N feet press dwn *Y/N* no scap. raised *Y/N*		*Coord* lordosis ↑Y/N feet press dwn *Y/N* no scap. raised *Y/N*		*Coord* lordosis ↑Y/N feet press dwn *Y/N* no scap. raised *Y/N*	
16. Head/Neck Endur/Coord. (Tuck chin raise head 1 cm off table. Patient holds. +test if chin pokes or head drifts forward).	Chin poke Y/N Head forward Y/N		Chin poke Y/N Head forward Y/N		Chin poke Y/N Head forward Y/N		Chin poke Y/N Head forward Y/N	
17. Flexion Supine (McK #4) Repeat 1 rep.	1 rep: +1, 0, –1 • Centralization • Peripheralization		1 rep: +1, 0, –1 • Centralization • Peripheralization		1 rep: +1, 0, –1 • Centralization • Peripheralization		1 rep: +1, 0, –1 • Centralization • Peripheralization	
18. Flexion Supine (McK #5) Repeat 10 reps	10 rep: +1, 0, –1 • Centralization • Peripheralization		10 rep: +1, 0, –1 • Centralization • Peripheralization		10 rep: +1, 0, –1 • Centralization • Peripheralization		10 rep: +1, 0, –1 • Centralization • Peripheralization	
19. Flexion Supine (McK #6) Sustain last rep. 10 seconds	1 sus rep: +1, 0, –1 • Centralization • Peripheralization		1 sus rep: +1, 0, –1 • Centralization • Peripheralization		1 sus rep: +1, 0, –1 • Centralization • Peripheralization		1 sus rep: +1, 0, –1 • Centralization • Peripheralization	
20. Respiratory Synkinesis a. Excessive lat. chest excursion b. Chest raises > abdomen c. Scalene muscles active	Normal: Y/N a. Y/N b. Y/N c. Y/N		Normal: Y/N a. Y/N b. Y/N c. Y/N		Normal: Y/N a. Y/N b. Y/N c. Y/N		Normal: Y/N a. Y/N b. Y/N c. Y/N	

NAME:_____ DATE:_____ DOB:_____

TESTS *Side Lying*	L	R	L	R	L	R	L	R
21. Hib Abd. Coordination **3 Steps:**								
1. Measure AROM w/inclinometer 2. Perform actively (pass/fail = P/F) 3. If passes, pre-position and observe	1.____° P/F	1.____° P/F	1.____° P/F	1.____° P/F	1.____° P/F	1.____° P/F	1.____° P/F	1.____° P/F
3a. Hip flexion	P/F	P/F	P/F	P/F	P/F	P/F	P/F	P/F
3b. Hip external rotation	P/F	P/F	P/F	P/F	P/F	P/F	P/F	P/F
3c. Pelvic rotation	P/F	P/F	P/F	P/F	P/F	P/F	P/F	P/F
3d. Hip hiking	P/F	P/F	P/F	P/F	P/F	P/F	P/F	P/F

TESTS *Prone*	L	R	L	R	L	R	L	R
22. Hip Extension Coordination *Record the order each contracts:*	Pass____ Fail____	Pass____ Fail____	Pass____ Fail____	Pass____ Fail____	Pass____ Fail____	Pass____ Fail____	Pass____ Fail____	Pass____ Fail____
1. Hamstrings	1,2,3,4,5	1,2,3,4,5	1,2,3,4,5	1,2,3,4,5	1,2,3,4,5	1,2,3,4,5	1,2,3,4,5	1,2,3,4,5
2. Gluteus maximus	1,2,3,4,5	1,2,3,4,5	1,2,3,4,5	1,2,3,4,5	1,2,3,4,5	1,2,3,4,5	1,2,3,4,5	1,2,3,4,5
3. Contralat. erector spinae	1,2,3,4,5	1,2,3,4,5	1,2,3,4,5	1,2,3,4,5	1,2,3,4,5	1,2,3,4,5	1,2,3,4,5	1,2,3,4,5
4. Ipsilat. erector spinae	1,2,3,4,5	1,2,3,4,5	1,2,3,4,5	1,2,3,4,5	1,2,3,4,5	1,2,3,4,5	1,2,3,4,5	1,2,3,4,5
5. Contralat. shoulder/neck	1,2,3,4,5	1,2,3,4,5	1,2,3,4,5	1,2,3,4,5	1,2,3,4,5	1,2,3,4,5	1,2,3,4,5	1,2,3,4,5

TESTS *Prone* (cont.)				
23. Single Ext. in Lying (SEL) **(McK. #7)** (a. pain; b. syndrome; c. lat shift)	a. Pain: +1, 0, −1 b. Syndrome: Fl/Ext c. Lat. shift: Y/N	a. Pain: +1, 0, −1 b. Syndrome: Fl/Ext c. Lat. shift: Y/N	a. Pain: +1, 0, −1 b. Syndrome: Fl/Ext c. Lat. shift: Y/N	a. Pain: +1, 0, −1 b. Syndrome: Fl/Ext c. Lat. shift: Y/N
24. Repeated Ext. in Lying (REIL) (McK. #8) (a. pain; b. syndrome; c. lat shift)	a. Pain: +1, 0, −1 b. Syndrome: Fl/Ext c. Lat. shift: Y/N d. # reps ____/10	a. Pain: +1, 0, −1 b. Syndrome: Fl/Ext c. Lat. shift: Y/N d. # reps ____/10	a. Pain: +1, 0, −1 b. Syndrome: Fl/Ext c. Lat. shift: Y/N d. # reps ____/10	a. Pain: +1, 0, −1 b. Syndrome: Fl/Ext c. Lat. shift: Y/N d. # reps ____/10
25. Sustained Ext. in Lying (SusEIL) (McK. #9) (a. pain; b. syndrome; c. lat shift)	a. Pain: +1, 0, −1 b. Syndrome: Fl/Ext c. Lat. shift: Y/N d. # Sec. ____/10	a. Pain: +1, 0, −1 b. Syndrome: Fl/Ext c. Lat. shift: Y/N d. # Sec. ____/10	a. Pain: +1, 0, −1 b. Syndrome: Fl/Ext c. Lat. shift: Y/N d. # Sec. ____/10	a. Pain: +1, 0, −1 b. Syndrome: Fl/Ext c. Lat. shift: Y/N d. # Sec. ____/10
26. Prone Knee Flexion Test (SIJ #4)	+/−	+/−	+/−	+/−
27. Push Up Janda: Scapular winging Maximum reps.	Scap. wing: Y/N Reps._____	Scap. wing: Y/N Reps._____	Scap. wing: Y/N Reps._____	Scap. wing: Y/N Reps._____
28. Sit to Stand Test	Pass/Fail (circle)	Pass/Fail (circle)	Pass/Fail (circle)	Pass/Fail (circle)
Post-test VAS	____/10	____/10	____/10	____/10

COMMENTS:_____

_____

_____

_____

_____

_____

SIGNED_____ DATE_____ TIME IN/OUT_____

DEFINITION AND REFERENCES FOR QUALITATIVE TESTS

1. SQUAT COORDINATION (REPETITIVE SQUAT) TEST

Patient Position:

- Patient stands with feet about shoulder width apart and is instructed to perform a squat.
- Patient should do a deep knee bend with the back straight to about 90 degrees of knee flexion.

Dr. Position: In front of patient, observing.

Quantification: None.

Qualification:

- Pass/Fail (Circle the appropriate answer).
- + test if patient flexed the trunk or cannot reach 90 degrees knee flexion.

Note: If heels raise off floor (soleus tightness).

Purpose: Qualifiable test for balance, coordination, quadriceps strength, and soleus flexibility.

2. STAND TO KNEEL (LUNGE–KNEEL COORDINATION) TEST

Patient Position:

- Patient stands with feet about shoulder width apart.
- Patient is instructed to perform a lunge to the kneeling position.
- One foot steps forward with knee flexing to 90 degrees and back knee just touches the floor.
- The back should remain straight with arms at the side.

Dr. Position: At patient's side.

Quantification: None, except with Chattanooga lumbar motion monitor.

Qualification:

- Pass/Fail.
- + test if patient flexes the trunk while performing test.

Also note:

- Balance of forward foot.
- Strength of quadriceps.
- Mobility of hip joint and flexibility of hip flexors of back leg.

Purpose: Qualifiable test for balance, coordination, hip extension mobility, and quadriceps strength.

3. EXTENSION IN STANDING (EIS) (Delitto, 1992)

Patient Position: Standing; patient reports the amplitude, location, and if radiation of symptoms occurs before and 30 seconds after the test.

Dr. Position: Behind patient, observing the patient extending backward and returning to the neutral, starting position (1 rep.).

Quantification: None.

Qualification:

Patient reports:

1. Increase in pain or peripheralization (+1)
2. No change in symptoms (0)
3. Decrease in pain or centralization (−1)

Lateral shifting of the trunk.

Purpose:

- To classify a patient as flexion or extension bias (into a category of extension or flexion syndrome, respectively).
- To direct the type of exercise protocol (ie, flexion/William's, or extension/McKenzie exercises).

3a. REPEATED EXTENSION IN STANDING (RES) (Delitto, 1992)

Patient Position: Standing; patient reports the amplitude, location, and if radiation of symptoms occurs before and 30 seconds after the test.

Dr. Position: Behind patient, observing the patient extending backward and returning to the neutral, starting position (10 reps.).

Quantification: Record the number of reps. short of 10 (+ test).

Qualification:

Patient reports:

1. Increase in pain or peripheralization (+1)

2. No change in symptoms (0)

3. Decrease in pain or centralization (−1)

Lateral shifting of the trunk.

Purpose:

- To classify a patient as flexion or extension bias (into a category of extension or flexion syndrome, respectively).

- To direct the type of exercise protocol (ie, flexion/William's, or extension/McKenzie exercises).

3b. SUSTAINED EXTENSION IN STANDING (SustEIS) (Delitto, 1992)

Patient Position: Standing; patient reports the amplitude, location, and if radiation of symptoms occurs before and 30 seconds after the test.

Dr. Position: Behind patient, observing as the patient extends backward, holds 10 seconds, and returns to the neutral, starting position.

Quantification: Record the number of seconds short of 10 (+ test).

Qualification:

Patient reports:

1. Increase in pain or peripheralization (+1)

2. No change in symptoms (0)

3. Decrease in pain or centralization (−1)

Lateral shifting of the trunk.

Purpose:

- To classify a patient as flexion or extension bias (into a category of extension or flexion syndrome, respectively).

- To direct the type of exercise protocol (ie, flexion/William's, or extension/McKenzie exercises).

4. FLEXION IN STANDING (FIS) (McKenzie, 1989; Delitto, 1992)

Patient Position: Standing; patient reports the amplitude, location, and if radiation of symptoms occurs before and 30 seconds after the test.

Dr. Position: Behind patient, observing the patient bend forward and return to the neutral, starting position (1 rep.).

Quantification: None.

Qualification:

Patient reports:

1. Increase in pain or peripheralization (+1)

2. No change in symptoms (0)

3. Decrease in pain or centralization (−1)

Lateral shifting of the trunk.

Purpose:

- To classify a patient as flexion or extension bias (into a category of extension or flexion syndrome, respectively).

- To direct the type of exercise protocol (ie, flexion/William's, or extension/McKenzie exercises).

4a. REPEATED FLEXION IN STANDING (RFS) (Delitto, 1992)

Patient Position: Standing; patient reports the amplitude, location, and if radiation of symptoms occurs before and 30 seconds after the test.

Dr. Position: Behind patient, observing the patient bend forward and return to the neutral, starting position (10 reps.).

Quantification: Record the number of reps. short of 10 (+ test).

Qualification:

Patient reports:

1. Increase in pain or peripheralization (+1)

2. No change in symptoms (0)

3. Decrease in pain or centralization (−1)

Lateral shift of the trunk.

Purpose:

- To classify a patient as flexion or extension bias (into a category of extension or flexion syndrome, respectively).

- To direct the type of exercise protocol (ie, flexion/William's, or extension/McKenzie exercises).

4b. SUSTAINED FLEXION IN STANDING (SustFIS) (Delitto, 1992)

Patient Position: Standing; patient reports the amplitude, location, and if radiation of symptoms occurs before and 30 seconds after the test.

Dr. Position: Behind patient, observing as the patient bends forward, holds 10 seconds, and returns to the neutral, starting position.

Quantification: Record the number of seconds short of 10 (+ test).

Qualification:

Patient reports:

1. Increase in pain or peripheralization (+1)

2. No change in symptoms (0)

3. Decrease in pain or centralization (−1)

Lateral shifting of the trunk.

Purpose:

• To classify a patient as flexion or extension bias (into a category of extension or flexion syndrome, respectively).

• To direct the type of exercise protocol (ie, flexion/William's, or extension/McKenzie exercises).

5a. ILIAC CREST HEIGHT STANDING (ICHS) (Delitto, 1992)

Patient Position: Standing.

Dr. Position: Behind patient, palpating the iliac crest heights.

Quantification: None

Qualification:

Reporting (+):

1. High right

2. High left

Reporting (−):

1. Equal

Purpose:

• To classify a patient as a candidate for manipulation (a + test).

• To direct the type of exercise protocol and in-office care.

5b. POSTERIOR SUPERIOR ILIAC SPINE STANDING (PSISST) (Delitto, 1992)

Patient Position: Standing.

Dr. Position: Behind patient, palpating the PSIS heights.

Quantification: None.

Qualification:

Reporting (+):

1. High right

2. High left

Reporting (−):

1. Equal

Purpose:

• To classify a patient as a candidate for manipulation (a + test).

• To direct the type of exercise protocol and in-office care.

5c. PSIS FLEXION IN STANDING (PSISFLST) (Delitto, 1992)

Patient Position: Standing.

Dr. Position: Behind patient, palpating the PSIS heights at full forward flexion.

Quantification: None.

Qualification:

Reporting (+):

1. High right

2. High left

Reporting (−):

1. Equal

Purpose:

- To classify a patient as a candidate for manipulation (a + test).
- To direct the type of exercise protocol and in-office care.

6. **SIDE GLIDING TEST (McKenzie test)** (McKenzie, 1989; Delitto, 1992, 1993; Erhard, 1994)

Patient Position: Standing; patient shifts shoulders and hips in opposite directions (keeping shoulders parallel to floor) for 10 reps., wait 30 seconds and record pain (+1, 0, −1).

Quantification: None.

Qualification:

Patient may exhibit pain:

1. Grade +1 = increased localized pain and/or peripheralization
2. Grade 0 = no increase or peripheralization in pain
3. Grade −1 = reduction and/or centralization of pain

Watch for limitation ("L") in ROM comparing L to R; quite common for unilateral losses.

Watch for a blocked ("B") = movement pattern; quite common in antalgic presentations.

Note: Defined as a combination of lateral flexion and rotation.

PATIENT SEATED

7. **PSIS SITTING (PSISSI) (SIJ #2)** (Delitto, 1992)

Patient Position: Sitting.

Dr. Position: Behind patient, palpating the PSIS heights at neutral.

Quantification: None.

Qualification:

Reporting (+):

1. High right
2. High left

Reporting (−):

1. Equal

Purpose:

- To classify a patient as a candidate for manipulation (a + test).
- To direct the type of exercise protocol and in-office care.

8. **ANTERIOR SUPERIOR ILIAC SPINE SITTING (ASISSI)** (Delitto, 1992)

Patient Position: Sitting.

Dr. Position: Behind or in front of patient, palpating the ASIS heights at full forward flexion.

Quantification: None.

Qualification:

Reporting (+):

1. High right
2. High left

Reporting (−):

1. Equal

Purpose:

- To classify a patient as a candidate for manipulation (a + test).
- To direct the type of exercise protocol and in-office care.

9. **PSIS FLEXION IN SITTING (PSISSI)** (Delitto, 1992)

Patient Position: Sitting.

Dr. Position: Behind seated patient, palpating the PSIS heights at full forward flexion.

Quantification: None.

Qualification:

Reporting (+):

1. High right
2. High left

Reporting (−):

1. Equal

Purpose:

- To classify a patient as a candidate for manipulation (a + test).
- To direct the type of exercise protocol and in-office care.
- When 3 of the 4 tests are + (tests include numbers 5, 7, 13, and 26), this supports "SIJ regional pain" and qualified patients to be placed in a manipulation category.

10. THORACOLUMBAR ROTATION

Patient Position: Sitting; keep legs fixed (only the trunk is allowed to rotate).

Dr. Position: Behind seated patient.

Quantification: Measure the angle with goniometer between the horizontal (seat backrest) and thorax at scapulae level.

Qualification:

- Check spine and thorax for symmetry. Report as right increased or left increased ("↑ R/L").
- Report as yes ("Y") and indicate the side of increase ("↑ R/L") by circling the R or L.
- Circle the no ("N") if symmetrically equal.

Purpose:

- To determine side of hypertonicity.
- To direct the type of exercise protocol and in-office care.

11. SHOULDER ABDUCTION COORDINATION TEST (Lewit, 1991)

Patient Position:

- Patient is seated with elbow flexed to 90 degrees to limit unwanted rotation.
- Patient is instructed to slowly abduct the arm.

Dr. Position: Behind patient observing scapulohumeral rhythm.

Quantification: With dynamic electromyogram or with inclinometer. Endurance is measured by timing the duration to the point of arms dropping when small circular motions are made with the arms abducted 90°.

Qualification:

- Pass/Fail.
- + test if scapular elevation or rotation (laterally) occurs in first 30 to 60 degrees.
- A false + can occur if scapulae is already elevated and laterally rotated with arms at side.

Purpose:

- Identify loss of normal glenohumeral rhythm due to overactivity of the upper trapezius and/or levator scapulae muscles.
- To determine the endurance capacity of shoulder abduction.
- To direct the type of exercise protocol and in-office care.

SUPINE TESTS

12. HIP ADDUCTORS

Patient Position: Supine.

Dr. Position: To the side of the patient.

Quantification: Measure the angle produced by adduction, first with the knee flexed (1 joint assessment) and second, with knee straight (2 joint assessment).

Qualification: Is + when there is a shift anterior of the leg when the knee is extended.

Purpose: To direct the type of exercise protocol and in-office care.

13. SUPINE TO LONG SITTING (SIJ #3) (Delitto, 1992)

Patient Position: Supine.

Dr. Position: At the foot of the table checking the relative leg length at the inferior aspect of the medial malleoli; measurement is repeated after the patient sits up and the two compared.

Quantification: None.

Qualification:

- + or −.
- Is + when there is a change in the leg lengths from the neutral supine position to the flexion position.
- Is − when there is no change in the leg lengths.

Purpose: When 3 of the 4 tests are + (tests include numbers 5, 7, 13, and 26), this supports "SIJ regional pain" and qualified patients to be placed in a manipulation category.

14. **PELVIC TILT COORDINATION (Supine Hook Lying)** (Reid, 1987)

Patient Position: Patient is supine with knees bent.

Dr. Position:

- Health care provider (HCP) places hand under lumbar spine and instructs patient to first arch, then flatten low back without raising buttocks off the table.
- HCP may cue movement or offer counter-resistance to facilitate coordination.
- Patient is next asked to hold back flat (posterior pelvic tilt) while sliding legs to extended position.
- Patient is then asked to raise both legs while holding back flat (legs should be held for 2–3 seconds).

Quantification: None.

Qualification:

- Grade I able to perform A, B, and C.
- Grade II able to perform A and B.
- Grade III able to perform only A.
- Grade IV cannot do a pelvic tilt (A, B, or C).

Purpose:

- Evaluate lumbopelvic coordination and control.
- Lower abdominal strength test.

15. **TRUNK FLEXION COORDINATION/STRENGTH** (Lewit, 1991; Nelson, 1988)

Patient Position: Patient is supine with knees bent, arms across chest, and feet flat on the table.

Dr. Position:

- HCP may either contact patient's heels or place under small of the back.
- Patient is instructed to perform posterior pelvic tilt and raise trunk up until scapulae are off the table and then hold for 2 seconds.
- Patient should hold the pelvic tilt while lowering back to the table.
- Patient is asked to perform 10 repetitions; the last repetition is held for 30 seconds.
- + test if heels rise up or patient loses posterior pelvic tilt.
- Fewer false negatives (more sensitive) if HCP places hands under heels than if HCP merely watches if feet lift up.

Note:

- If heels rise off table (+ test).
- If posterior pelvic tilt cannot be maintained (+ test).
- If excessive shaking occurs.
- If head is markedly forward of trunk.
- If curl up is performed segmentally or as mass movement at the hip joint.

Quantification:

- With dynamic electromyogram.

Qualification:

- Pass/Fail.
- Fail if heels rise up or lumbar spine arches before 10 repetitions and a 30-second hold can be accomplished.

Purpose: Quantify rectus abdominus strength/endurance and coordination.

16. **HEAD-NECK FLEXION COORDINATION TEST** (Lewit, 1991)

Patient Position: Patient is supine and is instructed to bring chin to chest

Dr. Position:

- To side of patient.
- Over-pressure may be added at end point.
- More sensitive test (fewer false negatives) if patient's neck is pre-positioned in chin tuck and raised 1 cm off table.

Observe:

- If chin juts forward during movement.
- If there is shaking during movement.
- If there is chin jutting or shaking with over-pressure added.
- If head elevates from 1-cm position (this indicates a change in the center of mass of the head).

Quantification: With strain gauge.

Qualification:

- Pass/Fail.
- Fail if chin juts forward during movement.

Purpose:

- To identify if neck flexor weakness or incoordination is present.
- In particular to identify if deep neck flexors are weak and the sternocleidomastoid is tight or overactive.

17–19. FLEXION SUPINE (Delitto A, personal conversation March 2, 1995)

Patient Position: Supine, raising the knees to the chest.

Dr. Position: At side of patient, observing the patient perform 1 rep. and return to the neutral, starting position.

Quantification: None.

Qualification:

Patient reports:

1. Increase in pain or peripheralization (+1): *DON'T* do more than 1 rep. if pain peripheralizes (proceed with 10 reps. with last rep. sustained 10 seconds if pain increases remain localized).
2. No change in symptoms (0): Proceed with 10 reps, sustaining the last for 10 seconds.
3. Decrease in pain or centralization (−1): Proceed with 10 reps., sustaining the last for 10 seconds.

Purpose:

- To classify a patient as flexion or extension bias (into a category of extension or flexion syndrome, respectively).
- To direct the type of exercise protocol (ie, flexion/William's, or extension/McKenzie exercises).

20. RESPIRATION COORDINATION TEST (Lewit, 1991)

Patient Position: Supine patient is asked to take in a deep breath.

Dr. Position: To side of patient (try different positions if needed).

Observation:

- Excessive chest breathing.
- Lateral chest excursion.
- If scalene muscles are visibly active during respiration.

Quantification: None.

Qualification:

- Pass/Fail.
- Fail if chest raises more than the abdomen.

Purpose: To identify if paradoxical breathing (chest breathing predominates over diaphragm) is present.

21. HIP ABDUCTION (Gluteus Medius, TFL, QL, Piriformis) COORDINATION TEST (Lewit, 1991)

- Patient side lying with lower knee flexed and upper leg extended.
- Pelvis is placed in a slightly untucked position.

a. Concentric Test

- Upper leg is raised into abduction and held for 2 seconds.
- + test if any pelvic movement occurs:
  1. Hip hiking (QL)
  2. Posterior rotation of the ilium
- + test if hip external rotation occurs (piriformis).
- + test if hip flexion occurs (TFL).

Observation:

- If patient can raise leg.
- Shaking or twisting.
- Any hip flexion or hip external rotation.
- Excessive hip hiking.
- Posterior rotation of upper ilium.

Quantification: Only with dynamic electromyogram.

Qualification:

- Pass/Fail.
- Fail if cannot abduct leg without hip flexion, if foot raises less than 6 inches, if hip externally rotates, pelvis rotates or hip hiking occurs.

b. Isometric Test: Pre-position leg in abduction without flexion and ask patient to hold leg for 5 seconds. Support may be suddenly removed to increase the difficulty.

Observation:

- If shaking occurs.
- Hip flexion, external rotation, pelvic rotation, or hip hiking (+ test).

Quantification: None.

Qualification: Pass/Fail.

Purpose:

- To identify coordination of hip abduction.
- To identify tightness/overactivity of quadratus lumborum (hip hiking), tensor fascia latae (hip flexion and external rotation), thigh adductors (limited abduction range), piriformis (external rotation), psoas (hip flexion).
- To identify poor hip joint mobility (decreased extension).
- To identify weakness of gluteus medius.

22. **HIP EXTENSION COORDINATION/STRENGTH** (Lewit, 1991)

Patient Position: Prone; patient attempts to raise leg into extension with knee held in extended position.

Dr. Position: To side of the patient.

Observation:

- + test if erector spinae musculature contracts before gluteus maximus.
- HCP should observe the activation sequence of hamstrings and gluteus maximus (1st), contralateral lumbar erector spinae (2nd), and ipsilateral erector spinae (3rd).
- Palpation should only be used to confirm the results.

Quantification: With dynamic electromyogram.

Qualification:

- Pass/Fail.
- Fail if erector spinae contracts before gluteus maximus.
- Record activation sequence or firing order of gluteus maximus, hamstrings, lumbar erector spinae, thoracolumbar erector spinae (ipsilateral and contralateral).
- Note if contralateral shoulder/neck musculature contracts.

Purpose:

- To identify incoordination of hip extension.
- To determine if gluteus maximus is weak or inhibited.
- To determine if erector spinae is overactive.
- To determine if hamstring is overactive.
- To determine if hip joint has reduced extension mobility or if psoas is shortened.

FORM G–9. POSTURE, GAIT, AND MOVEMENT PATTERN ASSESSMENT

NAME_____ DATE_____ DOB_____ DOI_____

GAIT ANALYSIS

	SIGN	FUNCTIONAL PATHOLOGY
☐	1. Hyperpronation during swing phase	1. Forefoot instability
☐	2. Hip hiking during gait	2. QL over-activity, glut. medius weakness or inhibition

CHECKLIST FOR POSTURE

	SIGN: *Anterior to Posterior*	FUNCTIONAL PATHOLOGY
☐	1. Hypertrophied SCM	1. Overactive SCM
☐	2. Gothic shoulders	2. Shortened upper trapezius
☐	3. UE internal rotation/round shoulders	3. Shortened pectorals
☐	4. Prominence of the iliotibial tract	4. Shortened TFL and ITB
☐	5. Lateral deviation of the patellae	5. Shortened TFL or ITB and/or lengthened vastus medialis
	SIGN: *Posterior to Anterior*	**FUNCTIONAL PATHOLOGY**
☐	6. Flattening Sup./Lat. buttock quadrant	6. Weak glutei
☐	7. Hypertrophied T-L erector spinae m.	7. Overactive T-L erector spinea muscle
☐	8. Scapula winging	8. Lengthened serratus anterior
☐	9. Medial rotated scapula	9. Shortened upper trapezius or lev. scap. and/or lengthened lower and middle trapezius
	SIGN: *Lateral*	**FUNCTIONAL PATHOLOGY**
☐	10. Protruding abdomen	10. Lengthened rectus abdominus
☐	11. Forward head carriage	11. Lengthened deep neck flexors and/or shortened suboccipitals

MOVEMENT PATTERNS

TEST	FINDING	TREATMENT (Tx)
☐ Postural exam and palpation	Weak gluteus maximus	Ball-Bridge w/downward heel press
☐ Trunk flexion test	Weak rectus abdominus	Ball—abdominal crunch (2 ways)
☐ Modified Thomas test	Tight/short illiopsoas	Office and home stretch of psoas muscle
☐ Hip extension test	Weak G. max. and/or hamstr., short QL	Bridge, hamstr. Wall PNF, ball stretches
☐ One leg stand	Poor proprioception	Balance board or shoes, "small foot"
☐ Posture and gait assessment	Leg length, ankle pron./SubT instabil	Heel, sole, arch lifts, "small foot"
☐ Hip abduction test	Weak gluteus medius	Facilitate gluteus medius, inhibit adductors

Comments

_____

_____

_____

_____

_____

_____

_____

_____

Signed_____ **Date scored**_____

Abbreviations: G, gluteus; ITB, iliotibial band; lev, levator; med, medius; max, maximus; PNF, proprioceptive neuromuscular facilitation; scap, scapulae; SCM, sternocleidomastoid; TFL, tensor fascia lata.

FORM G–10. STATIC POSITION TOLERANCE TESTS

NAME_____ DATE_____ BD/AGE_____ SEX: M/F_____

1. Measures "anthropometric" ROM—Uses the evaluee's own stature as a frame of reference.

2. The process begins by explaining the purpose of the test to the evaluee.

3. Method: The evaluee stands in front of a solid wall, at a distance with arms outstretched, lightly touching the wall, feet shoulder width apart.

INSTRUCTIONS (the following text may vary to suit the evaluee's needs):

    1. This is a test of your ability to reach with both hands to various heights while standing, stooping, crouching and kneeling.

    2. I will be asking you to maintain each of these postures for fifteen seconds.

    3. As we go through this test, I will be interested in any symptoms that you may have. Please let me know.

    4. Do you have any questions?

4. Questions are addressed, and the evaluee is asked if they understand what is wanted and, with an affirmative answer, the test is carried out.

5. The evaluee is instructed to move from a standing position to each posture and to return to a standing position according to the heights listed below:

    HEIGHT/POSTURE: Patient reaches to Shoulder Level, Eye Level, **from** a stand posture; and, Knee Level, **from** a stoop, crouch, and kneel postures, respectively.

6. Up to a one-minute standing rest is allowed between postures. The evaluator counts down 15 seconds for the evaluee on each of the five postures.

SCORE CHOICES (see middle column of below chart)

1. **ABLE:**	Able to perform the task with no restrictions.	
2. **SLIGHTLY RESTRICTED:**	Able to perform the tasks with slight restrictions.	
	Can hold the hands at the designated level for 15 seconds.	
3. **MODERATELY RESTRICTED:**	Able to assume the proper position, but is unable to maintain the position for 15 seconds (but greater than 5).	
4. **VERY RESTRICTED:**	Able to assume the position, but only up to five seconds (max.).	
5. **UNABLE:**	Unable to assume the position.	

TEST (Reach to–From)	SCORE (See Above for Definition of 1 = Able; 5 = Unable)	COMMENTS (See Below for Definition of the Quality Grade)	PAIN BEHAVIOR
Shoulder—Stand	1 2 3 4 5	Held for ____seconds. Posture quality is 1 2 3 4 5	1 2 3 4
Eye—Stand	1 2 3 4 5	Held for ____seconds. Posture quality is 1 2 3 4 5	1 2 3 4
Knee—Stoop	1 2 3 4 5	Held for ____seconds. Posture quality is 1 2 3 4 5	1 2 3 4
Knee—Crouch	1 2 3 4 5	Held for ____seconds. Posture quality is 1 2 3 4 5	1 2 3 4
Knee—Kneel	1 2 3 4 5	Held for ____seconds. Posture quality is 1 2 3 4 5	1 2 3 4

POSTURE QUALITY CHOICES (see "COMMENTS" above)[a]

1.	Excellent	No signs of difficulty maintaining the position
2.	Good	Mild signs of strain
3.	Fair	Moderate signs of strain with or without compensatory posture shifting
4.	Poor	Significant signs of strain with compensatory posture shifting
5.	Zero	Can't assume the position

PAIN BEHAVIOR (see "PAIN BEHAVIOR" above, right hand column)[a]

1.	None	No observable pain behavior
2.	Mild	Some signs of pain behavior and complaints only when asked
3.	Moderate	May include volunteered verbal complaints, facial grimace, position shift
4.	Excessive	May include declining of the test &/or excessive/outward exaggerated behavior

[a] Posture and pain behavior were not included in the original SPTT—these were added by this author.

Data compiled with permission from Leonard N. Matheson, PhD, CRC. *The Cal-FCP Manual.* Copyright © Employment Improvement Corporation, 1451 Ridgetree Trails Drive, Wildwood, MO 63021.

Chapter 19: Case Management
in an Evidence-based Practice

FORM H–1. CARETRAK CHECKLIST: LOW BACK CLASSIFICATION

NAME:_____ DATE:_____ DOB:_____

Findings based on history

Cauda Equina Syndrome - Emergency referral

	YES			YES
Saddle anesthesia	0	Loss of sexual function		0
Recent onset bladder dysfunction (urinary retension, incontinence, increased frequency)				0
Severe progressive neurological deficit (lower extremity, widespread neurology)				0

Red Flags for potentially serious conditions – (constant, progressive pain, no relief with bed rest)

Tumor or Infection

	YES			YES
> 50 or < 20 years old	0	Constant pain unrelated to movement		0
History of cancer	0	History of unexplained weight loss (> 10 lbs. or 4.5 kg.)		0
Night pain unrelated to movement	0			

		YES
History of malaise (appears acutely ill or generalized weakness)		0
History of fever or chills (abdominal pain, hematuria, rectal bleeding or urethral discharge)		0

Red Flags for potentially serious conditions – (constant, progressive pain, no relief with bed rest)

Tumor or Infection

	YES
Recent bacterial infection (such as urinary tract infection)	0
IV drug abuse	0
Immunosuppression (chronic steroid use, transplant, or HIV)	0

Possible fracture

	YES
Major trauma (motor vehical accident, fall from a height, or blunt trauma)	0
Minor trauma or even strenuous lifting (in older or potentially osteoporotic patient)	0
History of prolonged steroid use	0
Over 70 years of age	0
Osteoporosis	0

Possible Nerve Root Problem

	YES
Lower leg pain > back pain	0
Pain radiates to lower leg	0
Dermatomal numbness and paresthesia	0
Other 0 Describe _____	

Mechanical / Simple Low Back Pain

	YES
Low back, buttocks and/or thigh pain	0
"Mechanical" LBP (pain that varies with posture and movement)	0

Risk factors for chronic pain, prolonged recovery.	YES	(Data entered in Patient Data form, see Mercy, CSAG Lists)	YES
Personal problems - marital, financial	0	Pre-existing structural pathology or skeletal anomaly directly related to new injury or condition - such as spondylolesthesis	0
Adversarial medico-legal problems	0		

NAME:_____

Findings bas

| Spinal Cord Co |
| Upper motor neu |
| Pathological refle |

Red Flags for p
Tumor or Infec

Temperature > 1

BP > 160/90 mr

Pulse > 100 bpr

Respiration > 2£

Nerve root

Segmental moto

Dermatomal nui

Diminished or lc

Circumferential
with motor or se

Mechanical / C

Cervical, shoulc

Positive Orth

1. _____
2. _____
3. _____

Diagnosis (I(

Planned Tre:

Payment So

NAME:_____ DATE:_____ DOB:_____

Findings based on physical examination

	YES
Cauda Equina Syndrome - Emergency referral	
Unexpected laxity of the anal sphincter	0
Perianal / perineal sensory loss	0
Major motor weakness – knee extension weakness, ankle plantar flexors, evertors, dorsiflexors (foot drop)	0

Red Flags - Urgent referral (< 3 weeks) (constant, progressive pain, no relief with bed rest)
Possible serious pathology (tumor or infection)

Vital signs	YES		YES
Temperature > 100	0	Respiration > 25 bpm	0
BP > 160/90 mm/Hg	0	Blood/Urine tests show pathology	0
Pulse > 100 bpm	0	X-Ray evidence of pathology/fracture	0

Possible Nerve Root Problem	YES		YES
Segmental motor paresis	0	Circumferential mensuration > 2 cm difference (consistent with motor or sensory loss)	0
Dermatomal numbness and paresthesia	0		
Diminished or loss of deep tendon reflex	0	Positive nerve tension tests (SLR); well leg raise pain, foot dorsiflexion, hip internal rotation	0

Mechanical / Simple Low Back Pain	YES
Lumbar, SI, or buttocks pain which varies with different movements or positions	0

Illness Behavior (Waddell Signs)	YES		YES
Pain/tenderness to superficial stimulation (nonanatomical/superficial pain response)	0	Distraction (sitting straight leg raise)	0
Lower back pain to simulation (axial compression)	0	Inconsistent, nonanatomical neurological findings (regional neurology)	0
Lower back pain to simulation (trunk rotation)	0	Exaggeration or overreaction	0

Positive Orthopedic/Neurological Tests/Findings:

1. _____   4. _____
2. _____   5. _____
3. _____   6. _____

Diagnosis (ICD-9 Code):

_____

Planned Treatment Protocol If known _____

Payment Source _____

FORM H–3. CAI

FORM

NAME:_____

Findings base

Spinal Cord Cor

Progressive neuro

Recent onset blad

Red Flags for p
Tumor or Infecti

> 50 or < 20 year

History of cancer

Night pain unrela

Constant pain un

Red Flags for p
Tumor or Infect

Bilateral upper e

Polyarthralgia

Dysphagia

Nuchal rigidity, e

Cranial neurolog

Pain related to g

Possible fractu

Major trauma (m

Minor trauma or

History of prolor

Over 70 years o

Possible Nerve

Arm pain > neck

Pain radiates to

Mechanical / C

Neck, scapular

"Mechanical" C

Other Cervical

Neck complaint

Risk factors fo

Personal proble

Adversarial mec

Name____

Job Title_

1. How

2. Worl

— Si

— St

— W

— W

3. How

NO
(

4. How

NO
(

5. How

NO
(

6. How

NO
(

7. Do

NO
(

8. On

10
20
50
Mo

9. On

10
20
50
Mo

PROCEDURES

PASSIVE CARE:

- ☐ CMT _____
- ☐ PT _____
- ☐ MFR _____
- ☐ PNF/NMR (MRT's) _____
- ☐ Manual Traction_____
- ☐ Hot/Cold_____
- ☐ Vibration_____
- ☐ Other _____

ACTIVE CARE:

Kinetic Activity
Home exercise

- ☐ Williams _____
- ☐ McKenzie _____
- ☐ PNF_____
- ☐ Tubing/Band _____
- ☐ Other _____

Pelvic stabilization

- ☐ Gym Ball_____
- ☐ Floor _____
- ☐ Other _____

Proprioceptive retraining

- ☐ Gym Ball_____
- ☐ Balance Shoes_____
- ☐ Balance Board_____
- ☐ Rocker Board _____
- ☐ Other _____

FUNCTIONAL CAPACITY EVALUATION

- ☐ Spinal Function Sort
- ☐ QFCE
- ☐ Static Position Tolerance Tests
- ☐ Lift/Carry tests (ie, EPIC, PILE)

REFERRAL/CO-TREATMENT/MONITOR/DISCHARGE

FORM H–7. MODIFIED WORK APGAR

Name_____ Date_____ Age/BD_____

	0	1	2
	Almost Always	Some of the Time	Hardly Ever
1. I am satisfied that I can turn to a fellow worker for help when something is troubling me.			
2. I am satisfied with the way my fellow workers talk things over with me and share problems with me.			
3. I am satisfied with the way my fellow workers accept and support my new ideas or thoughts.			
4. I am satisfied with the way my fellow workers respond to my emotions, such as anger, sorrow, or laughter.			
5. I am satisfied with the way my fellow workers and I share time together.			
6. I enjoy the tasks involved in my job.			
7. Please check the column that indicates how well you get along with your closest or immediate supervisor.			

COMMENTS:_____

_____

_____

_____

_____

_____

_____

_____

_____

_____

_____

Signed by_____ DATE_____

Modified with permission from Bigos SJ, Battie MC, Spengler DM, et al. A prospective study of work perceptions and psychosocial factors affecting the report of back injury. *Spine* 1991;16:2, Fig. 1.

FORM H–8. VERMONT DISABILITY PREDICTION QUESTIONNAIRE

1. Have you ever had back problems before this injury?

   ☐ Yes (Continue with Question 2)   ☐ No (Skip to Question 5)

2. How many times have you visited a medical doctor in the past for back problems?

   ☐ Never   ☐ 6 to 10 times   ☐ More than 20 times

   ☐ 1 to 5 times   ☐ 11 to 20 times

3. How many times have you been hospitalized for low back pain?

   ☐ Never   ☐ One   ☐ Two   ☐ Three or more times

4. How many times have you had surgery for low back pain?

   ☐ Never   ☐ One   ☐ Two   ☐ Three or more times

5. Who or what do you think is to blame for your back problem?

   ☐ Work   ☐ Yourself   ☐ No one   ☐ Something else

6. How many times have you been married?

   ☐ Zero   ☐ One   ☐ Two   ☐ Three

7. On a scale of 0 to 10, how much pain in your back do you have RIGHT NOW? Think of 0 as meaning *NO PAIN AT ALL* and 10 as meaning the *WORST PAIN POSSIBLE*.

   NO PAIN AT ALL   0   1   2   3   4   5   6   7   8   9   10   WORST PAIN POSSIBLE

8. On a scale of 0 to 10, how physically demanding is your present job? Think of 0 as meaning *NOT AT ALL DEMANDING* and 10 as meaning *VERY DEMANDING*.

   NO TROUBLE AT ALL   0   1   2   3   4   5   6   7   8   9   10   VERY DEMANDING

9. On a scale of 0 to 10, how much trouble do you think you will have sitting or standing long enough to do your job, six weeks from now. Think of 0 as meaning *NO TROUBLE AT ALL SITTING OR STANDING*, and 10 as meaning *SO MUCH TROUBLE SITTING AND STANDING THAT YOU WON'T BE ABLE TO DO YOUR JOB AT ALL.*

   NO TROUBLE AT ALL   0   1   2   3   4   5   6   7   8   9   10   SO MUCH TROUBLE I
                                                                                                      WON'T BE ABLE TO DO
                                                                                                      MY JOB AT ALL

10. On a scale of 0 to 10, how well do you get along with your co-workers? Think of 0 as meaning you *DON'T GET ALONG WELL AT ALL* and 10 as meaning you *GET ALONG VERY WELL*.

    DON'T GET   GET ALONG
    ALONG WELL AT ALL   0   1   2   3   4   5   6   7   8   9   10   VERY WELL

11. On a scale of 0 to 10, how certain are you that you will be working in six months? Think of 0 as meaning *NOT AT ALL CERTAIN* and 10 as meaning *VERY CERTAIN*.

    NOT AT ALL CERTAIN   0   1   2   3   4   5   6   7   8   9   10   VERY CERTAIN

NAME_____ DATE_____ TOTAL SCORE:_____

VERMONT DISABILITY PREDICTION QUESTIONNAIRE (VDPQ) SCORING METHOD

1. Simply add the score of each question to obtain the sum.
2. The score cut-off can be moved to suit the needs of individuals and agencies who may want to use the VDPQ for different purposes.
   a. **Example 1:** Occupational Health Officer
      1. Objective: to identify those who are at high risk for becoming chronically disabled and enroll them into an intensive/expensive treatment program.
      2. In this case, since a lot of dollars and high patient demands are required, setting the cut-off relatively high (sacrifice sensitivity for increased specificity) would be wise.
   b. **Example 2:** Government agency
      1. Screening brochures mailed trying to prevent disability by encouraging people to return to work ASAP.
      2. In this case, setting the cut-off low to achieve maximum sensitivity so a higher number of people could be "caught" by the instrument to optimize benefits from the screen would be wise.
   c. **Example 3:** Resources required for a given intervention strategy were only sufficient for 23% of the current sample, a cut-off score of 0.48 would be appropriate as shown in the table below.

VDPQ Score Cut-off	kappa	Sensitivity	Specificity	% Predicted to be Disabled
0.34	0.315	1.00	0.70	37
0.48	0.484	0.94	0.84	23
0.50	0.492	0.88	0.86	21
0.60	0.496	0.75	0.90	17
0.65	0.449	0.62	0.91	18

VDPQ = Vermont Disability Prediction Questionnaire

Reprinted with permission from Hazard RG, Haugh LD, Reid S, Preble JB, MacDonald L. Early prediction of chronic disability after occupational low back injury. *Spine* 1996;21:945–951.

Chapter 21: Identification of the Patient at Risk for Low Back Trouble

FORM I–1. RISK FACTOR ASSESSMENT: STANDARD QUESTIONNAIRE

STANDARD FORM: Primary complaint—*Please circle:* Low back/leg *or* Neck/arm

Name_____ DATE_____ BD_____ SC_____

1. Where do you have pain? Place a ✓ for all appropriate sites. (2x)

   ☐ neck ☐ shoulders ☐ upper back ☐ lower back ☐ leg

2. How long ago did your *current* episode begin? (2x)

   1. ☐ Less than 2 weeks ago
   2. ☐ 2 weeks to <8 weeks ago
   3. ☐ 8 weeks to <3 months ago
   4. ☐ 3 months to < six months ago
   5. ☐ >6 months ago

3. How many previous episodes required treatment? (2x)

   ☐ None ☐ 1 ☐ 2 ☐ 3 ☐ 4 or more

4. Have you been hospitalized or had surgery for the same or similar complaint before? Y/N

5. Please indicate your usual level of pain during the past week:

   No pain   0 1 2 3 4 5 6 7 8 9 10   Worst possible pain

6. How often would you say that you have experienced pain episodes, on average during the past 3 months? (Circle one number)

   Never   0 1 2 3 4 5 6 7 8 9 10   Always

7. Does pain, numbness, tingling or weakness *extend* into your leg (from the low back) and/or arm (from the neck)?

   None of the time   0 1 2 3 4 5 6 7 8 9 10   All of the time

8. During the *last week*, how often have you taken medication (such as aspirin, Motrin, Tylenol, or prescription medication) for your pain complaint?

   Not at all   0 1 2 3 4 5 6 7 8 9 10   3 or more times a day

9. If you had to spend the rest of your life with your *condition as it is right now,* how would you feel about it?

   Delighted   0 1 2 3 4 5 6 7 8 9 10   Terrible

10. How anxious (eg, tense, uptight, irritable, fearful, difficulty in concentrating/relaxing) you have been feeling during the past week:

    Not at all   0 1 2 3 4 5 6 7 8 9 10   Extremely anxious

11. How much you have been able to control (ie, reduce/help) your pain/complaint on your own during the past week:

    I can reduce it   0 1 2 3 4 5 6 7 8 9 10   I can't reduce it at all

12. Please indicate how depressed (eg, down-in-the-dumps, sad, downhearted, in low spirits, pessimistic, feelings of hopelessness) you have been feeling in the past week:

    Not depressed at all   0 1 2 3 4 5 6 7 8 9 10   Extremely depressed

13. How would you rate your general health? (10–X)

    Poor   0 1 2 3 4 5 6 7 8 9 10   Excellent

14. Do you smoke tobacco a pack a day or more? Y/N

15. An increase in pain is an indication that I should stop what I am doing until the pain decreases. (10–X)

    Completely agree   0 1 2 3 4 5 6 7 8 9 10   Completely disagree

16. Physical activity makes my pain worse?

    Completely disagree   0   1   2   3   4   5   6   7   8   9   10   Completely agree

17. I can do light work for an hour? (10–X)

    Can't do it because   0   1   2   3   4   5   6   7   8   9   10   Can do it without
    of pain problem   pain being a problem

18. I can sleep at night. (10–X)

    Can't do it because   0   1   2   3   4   5   6   7   8   9   10   Can do it without
    of pain problem   pain being a problem

19. How physically demanding is your job—include housework if not employed outside the home?

    Not at all   0   1   2   3   4   5   6   7   8   9   10   Very demanding
    demanding

20. Have you been *disabled* due to the same or similar pain/complaint in the last 12 months? Y/N

21. I should not do my normal work with my present pain.

    Completely   0   1   2   3   4   5   6   7   8   9   10   Completely agree
    disagree

    If you are currently disabled from work, when did your disability start? Date_____

22. How well do you like your work? (10–X)

    Not at all   0   1   2   3   4   5   6   7   8   9   10   Very much

23. What kind of trouble at work do you think you will have sitting or standing *6 weeks from now*?

    No trouble   0   1   2   3   4   5   6   7   8   9   10   Extreme trouble

24. On a scale of 0 to 10, how certain are you that you will be working in *6 months*?

    Very certain   0   1   2   3   4   5   6   7   8   9   10   Not certain at all

Chapter 22: Putting Outcomes-based Management Into Practice

FORM J–1. PHYSICAL THERAPY LOG

NAME_____ PHYSICAL THERAPY_____

DATE	THERAPY		AREA/SETTING/NOTES	DATE	THERAPY		AREA/SETTING/NOTES
	HOT COLD LA-TX IS-TX	IFC US GALV MSTIM			HOT COLD LA-TX IS-TX	IFC US GALV MSTIM	
	HOT COLD LA-TX IS-TX	IFC US GALV MSTIM			HOT COLD LA-TX IS-TX	IFC US GALV MSTIM	
	HOT COLD LA-TX IS-TX	IFC US GALV MSTIM			HOT COLD LA-TX IS-TX	IFC US GALV MSTIM	
	HOT COLD LA-TX IS-TX	IFC US GALV MSTIM			HOT COLD LA-TX IS-TX	IFC US GALV MSTIM	
	HOT COLD LA-TX IS-TX	IFC US GALV MSTIM			HOT COLD LA-TX IS-TX	IFC US GALV MSTIM	
	HOT COLD LA-TX IS-TX	IFC US GALV MSTIM			HOT COLD LA-TX IS-TX	IFC US GALV MSTIM	
	HOT COLD LA-TX IS-TX	IFC US GALV MSTIM			HOT COLD LA-TX IS-TX	IFC US GALV MSTIM	
	HOT COLD LA-TX IS-TX	IFC US GALV MSTIM			HOT COLD LA-TX IS-TX	IFC US GALV MSTIM	

FORM J–3. PHOTOCOPY LOG

NAME:_____

DATE	COPIED FOR:	

HOT IFC COLD US LA-TX GALV IS-TX MSTIM			HOT IFC COLD US LA-TX GALV IS-TX MSTIM	
HOT IFC COLD US LA-TX GALV IS-TX MSTIM			HOT IFC COLD US LA-TX GALV IS-TX MSTIM	
HOT IFC COLD US LA-TX GALV IS-TX MSTIM			HOT IFC COLD US LA-TX GALV IS-TX MSTIM	
HOT IFC COLD US LA-TX GALV IS-TX MSTIM			HOT IFC COLD US LA-TX GALV IS-TX MSTIM	
HOT IFC COLD US LA-TX GALV IS-TX MSTIM			HOT IFC COLD US LA-TX GALV IS-TX MSTIM	
HOT IFC COLD US LA-TX GALV IS-TX MSTIM			HOT IFC COLD US LA-TX GALV IS-TX MSTIM	
HOT IFC COLD US LA-TX GALV IS-TX MSTIM			HOT IFC COLD US LA-TX GALV IS-TX MSTIM	

FORM J–2. NUTRITION/MEDICATION/BRACE–ORTH

NAME:_____

Name/Address:	Phone #'s: Daytime: Evening:
	Fax:
X-ray #:	SS#:

INSURANCE CARD PHOTOCOPY

DATE	NUTRITION/ MEDICATION/ BRACE-ORTHOTIC	DOSE/RECOMMENDATIONS	DA

FORM J–4. DAILY SOAP NOTES

Name_____ Age_____ BD_____ Injury Date_____ 1st visit_____

Dx: C-, T-, L, SI- Spr/str, IVDS, other: _____

Rx: Spinal C, T, L, S, P; Levels: O/1 C / T →/←; T- T/L Ant/PA; L- ; SI/L/R; NMR: Psoas, hamstring MFR: _____

_____

Complicating Factors: 1. Illness behavior; 2. Job dis.; 3. Past Hx of >4 episodes; 4. Symptoms > 1 wk;
  5. Severe pain intensity; 6. New condition/injury related to pre-existing structural pathology or skeletal anomaly

DATE___/___/___   VISIT #____   Ins.: WC; P; PI; HMO_____; PPO_____

S. ( ) Improved   ( ) No change   ( ) Worse   Osw.____% NDI_____

  ( ) Exacerbation   % Improvement_____%   Pain Scale: Now: ____/10; Ave.:___/10; R:___-___/10

Comments:_____

_____

_____

_____

_____

_____

_____

O. ( ) Observation_____ ( ) Palpation Pain/spasm_____

C-/TL-ROM: Fl___ ____/4 Ext____ ____/4 RLF___ ____/4 LLF___ ____/4 RR___ ____/4 LR___ ____/4 LOC_____

Ortho.:_____

Neuro.:_____

992 11, 12, 13, 14, 15:_____

A. See above Dx ( ) S/O improved   ( ) S/O no change   ( ) S/O worse   L/S Goal #_____met   Time w/patient _____m

_____

P. See Rx at top of page; Lab, X-ray: <u>C, T, L, 2, 3, 5, 7</u> **NMR-PNF/MFR:** CH, PIR, RI, Conc., eccen., Spr/Str.: C, T, L, Hamst, Psoas,___

PT: IFC, LA-TX, ISTX, Man. Tx, Hot, Cold, Kin.Act., Vib, **Active Care:** Ice/Heat; LB-/C-exer.; Proprio: Ball, WB, 1LS, BS, FCE, _____

989-40, -41, -42;C:____ T:____ L:____ P:____ S:____ Non SP 98943-51:____ _____

_____ (Dr:_____)

DATE___/___/___   **VISIT #**_____

S. ( ) Improved   ( ) No change   ( ) Worse   Osw.____% NDI_____

   ( ) Exacerbation   % Improvement_____%   Pain Scale: Now:___/10; Ave.:___/10; R:___-___/1

Comments:_____

_____

_____

_____

_____

_____

O. ( ) Observation_____ ( ) Palpation Pain/spasm_____

C-/TL-ROM: Fl___ ___/4 Ext___ ___/4 RLF___ ___/4 LLF___ ___/4 RR___ ___/4 LR___ ___/4 LOC_____

Ortho.:_____

Neuro.:_____

992 11, 12, 13, 14, 15:_____

A. See above Dx ( ) S/O improved   ( ) S/O no change   ( ) S/O worse   L/S Goal #____met   Time w/patient _____m

_____

P. See Rx at top of page; Lab, X-ray: <u>C, T, L, 2, 3, 5, 7</u> **NMR-PNF/MFR:** CH, PIR, RI, Conc., eccen., Spr/Str.: C, T, L, Hamst, Psoas,___

PT: IFC, LA-TX, ISTX, Man. Tx, Hot, Cold, Kin.Act., Vib, **Active Care:** Ice/Heat; LB-/C-exer.; Proprio: Ball, WB, 1LS, BS, FCE,_____

989-40, -41, -42;C:____ T:____ L:____ P:____ S:____ Non SP 98943-51:____ _____

_____ (Dr:_____

FORM J–5B. PAST HISTORY

NAME:_____ DATE:_____ DOB:_____

PREVIOUS INJURIES (MVA, WC, etc.)_____
_____

PREVIOUS TREATMENT HISTORY

DATE	DR/HOSP	TREATMENT	RESPONSE (G, NG, NChnge)	TREATMENT DURATION	TEST(S)	TEST RESULT

PAST HOSPITALIZATIONS / ILLNESS_____
SURGICAL HISTORY_____
GENERAL STATE OF HEALTH_____
MEDICATIONS/VITAMINS_____
ALLERGIES_____
IMMUNIZATIONS _____

FAMILY HISTORY   [1. FATHER, 2. MOTHER, 3. SISTER (a, b, etc), 4. BROTHER (a, b, etc.)]
CANCER (   )_____**DIABETES** (   )_____; **CARDIAC** (   )_____;
CVA (   )_____; **BP** (   )_____; **EPILEPSY** (   )_____; **TB** (   )_____
OTHER_____

PSYCHO-SOCIAL HISTORY
OCCUPATIONAL

DATE	OCCUPATION	WC CLAIMS	DISABILITIES	ENJOYED

Activities of Daily Living (Changes as a result of injury: _____
RECREATIONAL/EXERCISE: Type: _____ **Freq.** ____/wk; **Duration** _____ **Min. / Hrs;**_____

SOCIAL HISTORY
MARITAL STATUS (Circle): Single, Married, Divorced, Widowed
EDUCATIONAL LEVEL: ☐ < High School; ☐ H.S. Grad.; ☐ College (yrs:___) Degree: _____; Tech. (yrs___) Dipl.: ____
SOCIAL HABITS (Please circle appropriate responses and fill in the blank)
TOBACCO: ___ pk / ___day, wk, for ___ yrs; Chew ___ yrs; Pipe___ yrs **CAFFEINE (SODA, COFFEE, TEA)** _____/ day
ALCOHOL ____ glasses of wine, beer, mixed dr. / day, wk, mo.; **SLEEP INTERRUPTED?** ____ x's / night for ____ mo, yrs

WORK ROUTINE	ABLE	RESTRICTED		UNABLE		
Sit in office chair	1	2	3	4	5	
Stand concrete	1	2	3	4	5	
Climb steps / stairs	1	2	3	4	5	
Stoop to retrieve	1	2	3	4	5	
Crouch to retrieve	1	2	3	4	5	
Kneel to retrieve	1	2	3	4	5	
Reach overhead	1	2	3	4	5	
Lift waist to shoulder	1	2	3	4	5	
Carry 100 feet	1	2	3	4	5	
Push	1	2	3	4	5	
Pull	1	2	3	4	5	
Balance	1	2	3	4	5	
Crawl	1	2	3	4	5	
Reach	1	2	3	4	5	
Handling	1	2	3	4	5	
Fingering	1	2	3	4	5	

FORM J–5C. REVIEW OF SYSTEMS (ROS)

NAME:_____ DATE:_____ DOB:_____

Please write in a number: 1. PRESENTLY HAVE; 2. PREVIOUSLY HAD; 3. RELATED TO ACCIDENT (Date: _____)

GENERAL
___Allergy
___Chills
___Convulsions
___Dizziness
___Fainting
___Fatigue
___Fever
___Headache
___Sleep loss
___Weight loss
___Nervousness/depression
___Neuralgia
___Numbness
___Sweats
___Tremors

EYES, EARS, NOSE, THROAT
___Asthma
___Colds
___Sore throat
___Deafness
___Dental decay
___Earache/noises
___Ear discharge
___Sinus infection
___Enlarged glands
___Enlarged thyroid
___Nose bleeds
___Failing vision
___Far sighted
___Gum trouble
___Hay fever
___Hoarseness
___Nasal obstruction
___Near sighted

MUSCULOSKELETAL
___Arthritis
___Bursitis
___Foot Trouble
___Hernia
___Low back pain
___Lumbago
___Neck pain/stiffness
___Shoulder blade pain
Pain or numbness in:
___ Shoulders
___ Arms
___ Elbows
___ Hands
___ Hips
___ Legs
___ Knees
___ Feet
___Painful tailbone
___Poor posture
___Sciatica
___Spinal curvature

GENITO-URINARY
___Bedwetting
___Blood in urine
___Frequent urination
___Inability to control bladder
___Kidney infection or stones
___Painful urination
___Prostate trouble
___Pus in urine
___Painful menstruation
___Hot flashes
___Irregular cycle
___Lumps in breasts

CARDIOVASCULAR
___Hardening of arteries
___High blood pressure
___Low blood pressure
___Pain over heart
___Poor circulation
___Rapid heart beat
___Slow heart beat
___Swelling of ankles

RESPIRATORY
___Chest pain
___Chronic cough
___Difficult breathing
___Spitting up blood
___Spitting up phlegm
___Wheezing

GASTROINTESTINAL
___Belching or gas
___Colitis
___Colon trouble
___Constipation
___Diarrhea
___Difficult digestion
___Distention of abdomen
___Excessive hunger
___Gall bladder trouble
___Hemorrhoids
___Intestinal worms
___Jaundice
___Liver trouble
___Nausea
___Pain over stomach
___Poor appetite
___Vomiting
___Vomiting blood

OTHER:_____
_____
_____
_____
_____
_____
_____
_____
_____
_____
_____
_____

FORM J–5D. CERVICAL SPINE AND LUMBAR SPINE EXAMINATION FORMS

CERVICAL SPINE PHYSICAL EXAM

Name_____ **Date**_____ **DOI**_____ **(LEFT/RIGHT)**

L ◯ R ◯

1. VITAL SIGNS
Brachial B.P: Lt_____/_____ Rt_____/_____ Pulse_____ Respirations _____
Height_____ Weight_____ Temperature_____ Age_____

2. OBSERVATION
Posture_____ Gait_____(Pronated; Supinated) Other_____
_____

3. PALPATION
Spasm,TP's, Pain: Cerv_____Dors_____
Lum_____SIJ (L/R)_____
Temp_____Mankopf: Pulse _____ to _____ b/m @ TP _____ ___/4
Abdomen Murphy's, R / L UQ; R / L LQ: _____Rectal_____Chest/Breast_____
Other (masses, thyroid, lymph nodes, pulses, capillary filling, trophic changes) _____

4. ROM (active, active assisted and/or passive) (visual, inclinometer, other:_____)

Cervical	Exam	Pain (0–4 Grade)	Location/ / ↑ pain = +1; ↓ pain = -1 Peripheralize = +2; Centralize = -2	Quality
Flexion	/ 50	0-1-2-3-4		sharp / dull / pull
Extension	/ 63	0-1-2-3-4		sharp / dull / pull
L Lat Flex	/ 45	0-1-2-3-4		sharp / dull / pull
R Lat Flex	/ 45	0-1-2-3-4		sharp / dull / pull
L Rot.	/ 85	0-1-2-3-4		sharp / dull / pull
R Rot.	/ 85	0-1-2-3-4		sharp / dull / pull

5. ORTHOPEDIC EXAMINATION

Cervical	L	R	Findings		L	R	Findings
Cerv. Distraction				TOS: Adson			
Max. Cerv. Rot.Comp.				Rev.Adson			
Vert./Basiler Insuff.				Costoclav.			
Shoulder Depression				Wright			
Drop Arm				Wrist: Tinel's			
Ext. Rot. (P.A.R.)				Phalen			
Int. Rot. (P.A.R.)				Rev Phalen			
Mill / Cozen				Med.N.Tether t.			
Pron.T. (Compr/Tinel)				DeQuervain			
Radial T (Compr/Tinel)				CT Compression			
Cubital T (Compr/Tinel)				Bakody's Sign			

6. NEUROLOGICAL EXAMINATION

Level	Motor test, [cord level, nerve]	Motor x/5 +/-		Reflex [cord level]	DTR Wexler		Sensation	Exam (1.Pin; 2.2-Pt; 3.Vib; 4.Semmes-W)	
		L	R		L	R		L	R
C5	Deltoid [C5 axillary n.]	__/5	__/5	Biceps [C5, C6]			C5 / Axillary n.		
	Biceps [C5,6 musculocutaneous n]	__/5	__/5		/5	/5			
C6	Biceps [C5,6 musculocutaneous n]	__/5	__/5	Brachioradialis [C6]			C6 / Musculocut. n.		
	Wrist Extensors [C6,7 radial n]*rad=C6 uln=C7*	__/5	__/5		__/5	__/5			
C7	Triceps [C7 radial n.]	__/5	__/5	Triceps [C7]			C7 / Digit 3, palmar [variable]		
	Wrist Flexors [C7 median/ulnar n]	__/5	__/5		__/5	__/5			
	Finger Extenders [C7 radial n]	__/5	__/5						
C8	Finger Flexors [C8,T1 median/ulnar n]	/5	/5	Wrst(C7,8); Uln(C8,1)	/5	/5	C8 / Med antebr cut n.		
T1	Finger Abd/Add [T1 ulnar n]	/5	/5	Ulnar (C8, T1)	/5	/5	T1 / Med antebr cut n.		

CN II-XII ☐ wnl	II: Fundus, acuity, fields	III, IV, VI: "H", diplopia, ptosis, PERRLA	V: Corneal, light touch, mastication VII: Facial expression & Taste	VIII: Rinne, Weber, nystagmus IX: Dysphagia	X: Soft palate elev, larynx XI: SCM, upper trap XII: Tongue Dev./Strength

Vestibular: ☐ wnl	Cerebellum: ☐ wnl	D.Columns: ☐ wnl	Cerebrum: ☐ wnl; S O M A	Labrinth: ☐ wnl

Pathological	Babinski (Corticospinal tract) / UMN /	Clonus (L / R elb / knee)	Spastic / flaccid Paralysis L / R UE / LE

Grip / Pinch Strength Dominant L/R (Circle)	Right hand: (Pain induced Y / N) 1st ____ kg/lbs; 2nd ____ kg/lbs; 3rd ____ kg lbs	Left hand: (Pain induced Y / N) 1st ____ kg/lbs; 2nd ____ kg/lbs; 3rd ____ kg/lbs

Circumference	Upp Ext.: Brach. ____ in. / cm (___ " above elbow)	AnteBr. ____ in. / cm (___ " below elbow)
Chest: Insp ____ Exp ____ (___ ICS)	Low Ext.: Thigh ____ in. / cm (___ " above Patella)	Calf ____ in. / cm (___ " below patella)

NAME   DATE

Shoulder	Abd	Add	Flex	Ext	IR	ER	Scap Ele	Scap Pro	Scap Ret	Painful arc
Normal	180	75	180	60	90	90				
Left										
Right										
MM	Mid Delt, SS	PecMaj, Lat	Delt, Coracobr	Lat, TeresMaj	IS,TeresMin	Subscap, Pect	Trap, LevSc	SerrAnt	Rhom [2]	

Shoulder Test	Exam	Finding	Test	Exam	Finding
SS Tendonitis	/	SS tendonitis	Yergason's/Speed's	/	Bicipital tendonitis
Apley Scratch t.	/	Rot cuff tendonitis, ss	Drawer, apprehension	/	Recurrent dislocation
Drop Arm test	/	Rotator cuff tear	Dawburns	/	Sub-AC bursitis

Elbow	Flex		Ext	Sup		Pro
Normal	150		10	90		90
Left						
Right						
MM	Brachialis, Biceps C5, 6		Triceps C7	Biceps C5, 6 supinator C6		Pronator teres C6 , Pronator quad C8-T1

Elbow Test	Exam	Finding	Test	Exam	Finding
Tinel (Ulnar T,PT)	/	Neuroma / N. compression	Ligamentous instability	/	Med or lat collateral damage
Cozen's t.	/	Lat. epicondylitis	Golfer's elbow t.	/	Med. epicondylitis
Mill's t.	/	Lat. epicondylitis	Rev. Cozen's t.	/	Med. epicondylitis
Med.N.Comp. t.	/	Pron. Teres L: sec. / R: sec.	Radial Tunnel Compr. t.	/	Radial Nerve L: sec. / R: sec.
Palp: Lat. / Med Epi., Rad Head , Olecranon ,			Cubital Tunnel Compr.t	/	Ulnar Nerve L: sec. / R: sec.

Wrist	Flexion	Extension	Ulnar Deviation	Radial Deviation
Normal	80	70	30	20
Left				
Right				
MM	FCR, FCU	ECRL, ECRB, ECU	FCU, ECU	ECRB, ECRL, APL, EPB

Wrist Test	Exam	Finding	Test	Exam	Finding
Phalen's	/	CTS L: sec. / R: sec.	Tinel's	/	L = 1 2 3 4; R = 1 2 3 4 (Severity)
Rev. Phalen's	/	CTS L: sec. / R: sec.	Finkelstein's	/	Sten. tenosynovitis APL, EPB; Crepitus /
Med.N.Comp. t.	/	CTS L: sec. / R: sec.	Allen's	/	Radial, ulnar a. occlusion
Med.N.Tether t.	/	Stenosing tenosynovitis Flexor tendons	Grip: L R Dominant L / / R / /		(lbs / kg)

Assessment: (Circle: Mechanical, Nerve root, Pathology); C-disc @ C-____ w/ o radiation above / below elbow; C-sprain / strain / myofascitis / myositis; Nerve root tether C-____; Torticollis L / R; Other: _____
DD:_____

Complicating Factors: 1. Abnormal illness behavior; 2. Job dissatisfaction; 3. Past Hx of >4 episodes; 4. Symptoms > 1 wk;
   5. Severe pain intensity; 6. New condition / injury related to pre-existing structural pathology or skeletal anomaly

Goal Setting: Short-term Goals: Long-term Goals:
   1. Decrease pain _____% in _____ days.   1. Functional restoration.
   2. Increase ROM _____% in _____ days.   2. Initiate Active / Home care.
   3. Decrease spasm in _____ days.   3. Rehabilitation / Strengthening.
   4. Return to work in _____ days.   4. Education / "Back school".
   5._____   5. _____

Plan:

	Therapy	Frequency	Remarks
☐	Chiro. manipulative therapy	____ x/week x ____ weeks; Other	
☐	Ice/heat	15 minute rotations: on / off / on x 3 (= 1.25 hr / session)	
☐	Interferential mm. stim.	Acute: 80-100 cps / 10 min.; Chronic: 0-10 cps / 15 min.	
☐	Traction ☐ Cerv. long axis ☐ Lumb. long axis ☐ Intersegmental	Office: _____ Pounds / _____ minutes Home: _____ Pounds / _____ minutes	
☐	Exercises ☐ Flexion ☐ Extension ☐ QFCE _____ (date) ☐ Work hardening	Acute: Isometric w/in pain boundaries Subacute: Isotonic, passive ROM to boundary, Initiate proprioception retraining Chronic: Evaluate functional status (QFCE) Initiate isokinetic, progressive resistance	
☐	MRI / CT / Bone scan		
☐	X-R	Lumbar, Thoracic, Cervical: Davis, 5-, 3-, 2-views	
☐	Lab	Blood Test _____; Urine Test: UA, Culture, ___	
☐	Restrict activities: ☐ Work ☐ ADL's	Work: Regular duty Light duty Total temporary disability: ____ days, weeks, month	
☐	Reeval for RTW	days, weeks	
☐	Progress reeval	1, 2, 3, 4, 6, weeks	
☐	Referral to:		
☐	Disability / impairment rating		

LUMBAR SPINE PHYSICAL EXAM

Name_____ **Date**_____ **DOA**_____ (**LEFT/RIGHT**)

L ⬡ R ⬡ ⬡

1. VITAL SIGNS
Brachial B.P: Lt_____ / _____ Rt_____ / _____ Pulse_____ Respirations_____
Height_____ Weight_____ Temperature_____ Age_____

2. OBSERVATION
Posture_____ Gait_____ (Pronated; Supinated) Other_____
_____

3. PALPATION
Spasm, **TP**'s, **P**ain: Cerv_____Dors_____
Lum_____SIJ (L/R)_____
         Temp_____Mankopf: Pulse _____ to _____ b/m @ TP_____

Abdomen Murphy's, R / L UQ; R / L LQ: _____ Rectal_____ Chest/Breast_____
Other (masses, thyroid, lymph nodes, pulses, capillary filling, trophic changes) _____

4. ROM (active, active assisted and/or passive) (visual, inclinometer, other: _____)

Lumbar	Range of Motion (degrees) Location of complnt	Pain (0-4 Grade)	McKenzie Tests ↑ pain = +1; ↓ pain = -1 Peripheralize = +2; No Change = 0; Centralize = -2	Quality
Flexion	___ / 65	0 1 2 3 4	FIS: 1 Rep: +2 +1, 0, -1 -2; 10 reps: +2 +1, 0, -1 -2	sharp / dull / pull
Extension	___ / 30	0 1 2 3 4	EIS: 1 Rep: +2 +1, 0, -1 -2; 10 reps: +2 +1, 0, -1 -2	sharp / dull / pull
L Lat Flex	___ / 25	0 1 2 3 4	Side Gliding: +2,+1, 0,-1,-2; Limited Y / N; Blocked Y / N	sharp / dull / pull
R Lat Flex	___ / 25	0 1 2 3 4	Side Gliding: +2,+1, 0,-1,-2; Limited Y / N; Blocked Y / N	sharp / dull / pull

5. ORTHOPEDIC EXAM (Pain Scale 0-4; Centralize -1; Peripheralize = +1); OBJECTIVE: DD Mechanical LBP from Nerve Root

Lumbar	L	R	Findings	Test	L	R	Findings
Facet:				**Nerve Tension:**	- / +	- / +	
Kemp	0 1 2 3 4	0 1 2 3 4		Chin to chest= LBP	0 1 2 3 4	0 1 2 3 4	
Double SLR	0 1 2 3 4	0 1 2 3 4		Supine SLR (A P)	0 1 2 3 4	0 1 2 3 4	___ / (70)
Sacroiliac:				Foot DF + SLR	0 1 2 3 4	0 1 2 3 4	
Yeoman	0 1 2 3 4	0 1 2 3 4		Hip IR + SLR	0 1 2 3 4	0 1 2 3 4	
Hibb	0 1 2 3 4	0 1 2 3 4		Well-leg Raise	0 1 2 3 4	0 1 2 3 4	
Motion palp.	0 1 2 3 4	0 1 2 3 4		Sitting SLR	0 1 2 3 4	0 1 2 3 4	
Gaenslin's	0 1 2 3 4	0 1 2 3 4		Bow String	0 1 2 3 4	0 1 2 3 4	
Delitto (3 of 4 = +)	1. Standing Flexion PSIS 2. Sitting PSIS 3. Supine to Long Sitting 4. Prone Knee Flexion			Slump Test	0 1 2 3 4	0 1 2 3 4	
Compr. / Distrac.	0 1 2 3 4	0 1 2 3 4		Jugular vv compress.	0 1 2 3 4	0 1 2 3 4	
Hip: Ext. Coord.	LB >G.Max	LB >G.Max		Janda Trunk Flex	1.Incr. Lord. Y/N; 2.Foot press Dn: Y/N; 3.Scap Raise Y/N		
Hip Abduction	Pass/Fail	Pass/Fail	___ /	Int. Rot (A P)	0 1 2 3 4	0 1 2 3 4	___ / (45)
P. Fabere	0 1 2 3 4	0 1 2 3 4		Ext. Rot (A P)	0 1 2 3 4	0 1 2 3 4	___ / (43)

Waddell Non-organic LBP signs: Score ___ / 5	☐ 3. Distraction: + "flip sign"
☐ 1. Superficial Pain	☐ 4. Regional Neurology.
☐ 2. Simulation Tests: ☐ Axial Cmpr; ☐ Trunk Rotation	☐ 5. Exaggeration

6. NEUROLOGICAL EXAMINATION: *Red Flag:* Rule out Nerve Root lesion

Level	Motor test: [cord level, nerve]	Motor √5 +/- L	Motor √5 +/- R	Reflex [cord level]	DTR (Wexler) L	DTR (Wexler) R	Sensation	Exam (1.Pin; 2.2-pt 3.Vib; 4.Semmes-W) L	Exam R
T12-L3	Iliopsoas -Hip Flexion [T12-L3]	___/5;	___/5	Cremasteric (L1,2)	P / A	P / A	T12-L3 derm.		
L2-L4	Quadriceps - Knee Ext. [L3,4 femoral n.] Hip adductors [L2-4 obturator n.]	___/5;	___/5	Patellar [L2,L3, L4]			L2-L4 dermatome		
L4	Tibialis Anterior [L4, deep peroneal n.]	___/5;	___/5	Patellar [L2,L3, L4]	___/5;	___/5	L4 dermatome		
L5	Ext Hall Long [L5, deep peroneal n.] Ext Dig Long/Brev [L5, deep peroneal n.] Gluteus Medius [L5, supr glut.n.]	___/5;	___/5	Hamstring / (semitendinosis) [L4 L5, S1, 2]	___/5;	___/5	L5 dermatome		
S1	Peroneus Lng/Brev [L5,S1 sup peroneal n] Gastrocnemius-soleus [S1, inf glut. n.]	___/5;	___/5	Achilles [S1]	___/5;	___/5	S1 dermatome		

CN II-XII	II: Fundus, acuity, fields	III, IV, VI: "H", diplopia, ptosis, PERRLA	V: Corneal, light touch, mastication VII: Facial expression & Taste	VIII: Rinne, Weber, nystagmus IX: Dysphagia	X: Soft palate elev., larynx XI: SCM, upper trap XII: Tongue Dev./Strength
☐ wnl					

Vestibular: ☐ wnl	Cerebellum: ☐ wnl	D.Columns: ☐ wnl	Cerebrum: ☐ wnl; S O M A	Labrinth: ☐ wnl
Pathological	Babinski (Corticospinal tract) / UMN ___ /	Clonus (L / R elb / knee)	Spastic / flaccid Paralysis L / R UE / LE	
Grip / Pinch Strength Dominant L/R (Circle)	Right hand: (Pain induced Y / N) 1st ___ kg/lbs; 2nd ___ kg/lbs; 3rd ___ kg lbs		Left hand: (Pain induced Y / N) 1st ___ kg/lbs; 2nd ___ kg/lbs; 3rd ___ kg/lbs	
Circumference	Upp Ext.: Brach. ___ in. / cm (___ " above elbow)		AnteBr. ___ in. / cm (___ " below elbow)	
Chest: Insp ___ Exp ___ (___ ICS)	Low Ext.: Thigh ___ in. / cm (___ " above Patella)		Calf ___ in. / cm (___ " below patella)	

NAME_____DATE_____ (Pg. 2 L-spine Exam)

Hip	Abduction	Adduction	Flexion	Extention	Internal Rotation	External Rotation
Normal	50	30	135	30	40	60
Left						
Right						
MM	Glut medius	Adductor longus	Iliopsoas	Glut Max	Adductor longus, brevis	Glut max, obt. ext.

Hip Test	Exam	Finding	Test	Exam	Finding
Fabere	/	Inflammatory hip	Ober's t	/	TFL or tibial band contracture
Trendelenberg	/	Glut med weakness [contralateral]	Thomas t.	/	Hip flexor contracture
Hibb's	/	SI vs. hip	Psoas Contracture	/	Tight hip flexors

Knee	Flex		Ext		IR		ER
Normal	135		0		10		10
Left							
Right							
MM	Semimemb/tend/biceps		Quad		cannot be isolated		cannot be isolated

Knee Test	Exam	Finding	Test	Exam	Finding
McMurray	/	Posterior meniscus tear	Varus/Valgus stress	/	Lat/med collateral lig
Apley Distraction	/	Meniscus vs ligamentous lesion	Ant/post draw signs	/	Ant/post cruciate lig
Apley Compression	/	Medial vs. lateral meniscus tear	Bounce home	/	Meniscus
Patellar grinding	/	Chondromalacia pat/retropatellar OA	Patella Battotement	/	Edema

Ankle	Dorsiflexion	Plantar flexion	Inversion	Eversion
Normal	20	50	35	15
Left				
Right				
MM	Tibialis ant, EDL, EHL	Gastroc, Soleus, Plantaris	Tibialis post, FDL, FHL	Peronius, long, brev, tertius

Ankle Test	Exam	Finding	Test	Exam	Finding
Ant/post Drawer	/	Ant/post talofibular lig	Med Lat stability t.	/	Ant talofibular/calcaneofibular lig
Pronation / Pes Pl.	/	(w/ w/o metatarsalgia / loss)	Supination	/	
Tinel's	/	Ant. Tarsal Tunnel / Deep Peroneal n.	Tinel's	/	Post. Tarsal Tunnel / Tibial n.

Assessment: (Circle: Mechanical, Nerve root, Pathology); L-disc @ L-____ w/o radiation above / below knee; L-sprain / strain / myofascitis / myositis; SIJ sprain L / R; Hip - synovitis, arthritis, bursitis. _____ Other: _____

DD:_____

Complicating Factors: 1. Abnormal illness behavior; 2. Job dissatisfaction; 3. Past Hx of >4 episodes; 4. Symptoms > 1 wk; 5. Severe pain intensity; 6. New condition / injury related to pre-existing structural pathology or skeletal anomaly

Goal Setting: **Short-term Goals:**

1. Decrease pain _____% in _____ days.
2. Increase ROM _____% in _____ days.
3. Decrease spasm in _____ days.
4. Return to work in _____ days.
5._____

Long-term Goals:

1. Functional restoration.
2. Initiate Active / Home care.
3. Rehabilitation / Strengthening.
4. Education / "Back school".
5._____

Plan:

	Therapy	Frequency	Remarks
☐	Chiro. manipulative therapy	x/week x ____ weeks; Other	
☐	Ice/heat	15 minute rotations: on / off / on x 3 (= 1.25 hr session)	
☐	Interferential mm. stim.	Acute: 80-100 cps / 10 min.; Chronic: 0-10 cps / 15 min.	
☐	Traction ☐ Cerv. long axis ☐ Lumb. long axis ☐ Intersegmental	Office: _____ Pounds _____ minutes Home: _____ Pounds _____ minutes	
☐	Exercises ☐ Flexion ☐ Extension ☐ QFCE ____ (date) ☐ Work hardening	Acute: Isometric w/in pain boundaries Subacute: Isotonic, passive ROM to boundary. Initiate proprioception retraining Chronic: Evaluate functional status (QFCE) Initiate isokinetic, progressive resistance	
☐	MRI / CT / Bone scan		
☐	X-R	Lumbar, Thoracic, Cervical: Davis, 5-Series, 3-series, 2-series	
☐	Lab	Blood Test ____, Urine Test, U.A. Culture,	

☐	Restrict activities: ☐ Work ☐ ADL's	Work: Regular duty Light duty Total temporary disability: ____ days, weeks, month	
☐	Reeval for RTW	____ days, weeks	
☐	Progress reeval	1, 2, 3, 4, 6, ____ weeks	
☐	Referral to:		
☐	Disability / impairment rating		

FORM J–6. SAMPLE X-RAY REPORT

(Include only if the x-rays are not read by a certified radiologist with accompanying report)

_____

Date:

Patient's name, birth date/age

X-ray study information: x-ray #, views included, date of x-ray, location x-rays taken, comparison views from past.

Dx and clinical information:

Findings reveal:

Impressions: (list numerically the highlights of the findings)

Signed by Dr._____

EXAMPLE:

June 30, 1999

Patient: Sample Patient

BD: 2-26-59   Age: 39

X-ray taken 6-29-99

X-ray #7537

AP, lateral lumbar

Dx: Acute onset, lumbar sprain/strain without radiculopathy

Findings reveal:

Elevation right hemipelvis with 7-mm left leg length deficiency, with a compensatory 6-degree sacral base unleveling inferior left. There is a 3-degree right lateral flexion malposition of T11 resulting in a 9-degree levorotoscoliosis, grade 1 pedicular drift, apexing left at L2. The sacral base angle is accentuated at 50 degrees and there is a marked, 5-cm anterior shift in the weight-bearing line, supporting the presence of significant facet overload preponderance at the lumbosacral junction. The IVD/IVF spacings are patent and free of clutter. There is no signficant hip or SI joint pathology noted and the pubic symphysis is well aligned. There are no signs of fracture, dislocation and bone density appears normal.

Impressions:

1. Pelvic obliquity is quite significant with a 7-mm left leg length deficiency, compensatory 6-degree sacral base unleveling to the left, setting up a T11 and S1, 9-degree levorotoscoliosis, grade 1 pedicular drift, apexing left at L3.
2. Accentuated sacral base angle at 50 degrees, and a 5-cm anterior shift in the weight-bearing line is supportive of facet overloading at the lumbosacral junction.
3. IVD/IVF spacings are patent and free of clutter.
4. There are no signs of fracture, dislocation. Bone density appears adequate.

FORM J–7. ATTENDING PHYSICIAN'S RETURN TO WORK RECOMMENDATIONS[a]

Employer:_____

Employee Name:_____

TO BE COMPLETED BY ATTENDING PHYSICIAN:

Diagnosis:_____

Injury or Illness:_____ Work or Non-work related?_____

I saw and treated this employee on (date)_____ and:

1._____Recommended his/her return to work with no limitations on (date)_____

2._____He/She may return to work capable of performing the degree of work checked below with the following limitations.

DEGREE	LIMITATIONS
_____ **Sedentary Work.** Lifting 10 pounds maximum and occasionally lift and/or carrying such articles as dockets, ledgers and small tools. Although a sedentary job is defined as one which involves sitting, a certain amount of walking and standing is often necessary in carrying out job duties. Jobs are sedentary if walking and standing are required only occasionally and other sedentary criteria are met.	1. In a 10 hour work day patient may: a. Stand/Walk ____None ____4–6 Hours ____1–4 Hours ____6–10 Hours b. Sit ____1–3 Hours ____3–5 Hours ____5–10 Hours

2. Patient may use hands for repetitive actions such as:

	Simple Grasping	Firm Grasping	Fine Manipulating
Right:	___Yes___No	___Yes___No	___Yes___No
Left:	___Yes___No	___Yes___No	___Yes___No

_____ **Light Work.** Lifting 20 pounds maximum with frequent lifting and/or carrying of objects weighing up to 10 pounds. Even though the weight lifted may be only a neglible amount, a job is in this category when it requires walking or standing to a significant degree or when it involves sitting most of the time with a degree of pushing and pulling of arm and/or leg controls.

3. Patient may use feet for repetitive movement as in operating foot controls: ____Yes ____No

_____ **Medium Light Work.** Lifting 35 pounds maxium with frequent lifting and/or carrying of objects weighing up to 30 pounds.

_____ **Medium Work.** Lifting 50 pounds maximum with frequent lifting and/or carrying of objects weighing up to 35 pounds.

_____ **Heavy Work.** Lifting 75 pounds maximum with frequent lifting and/or carrying of objects weighing up to 50 pounds.

_____ **Very Heavy Work.** Lifting objects in excess of 100 pounds with frequent lifting and/or carrying of objects weighing 75 pounds or more

4. During work day, patient is unable to:

	67–100%	34–66%	1–33%	0%
a. Bend	____	____	____	____
b. Squat	____	____	____	____
c. Climb	____	____	____	____
d. Twist Body	____	____	____	____
e. Push	____	____	____	____
f. Pull	____	____	____	____
g. Balance	____	____	____	____
h. Kneel	____	____	____	____
i. Crawl	____	____	____	____
j. Grasp	____	____	____	____
k. Reach	____	____	____	____

Other restrictions and/or limitations_____

_____

3. These restrictions are in effect until (date)_____ or until employee is re-evaluated on (date)_____.

4. He/She is totally incapicitated at this time. Employee will be re-evaluated on (date)_____.

PHYSICIAN'S SIGNATURE_____ DATE:_____
(No rubber stamp, please)

[a] Complete Form H–5(p. 646), Job Demands Questionnaire when work is restricted.

FORM J–8. ROUTE SLIP

_____ Patient   _____ Date   _____ Account #

$_____ $_____ $_____   _____

Previous Balance   Total Charges   Payment   Injury Date

		SCHEDULE:	REV:	REHAB:	EXERCISES:	REFERRAL TO RMC:
☐ Work Comp	☐ U-Care	M T W Th F____	NDI	QFCE	Neck	MRI, CT, Bone Scan
☐ Auto Accident	☐ WEA/WPCN	2x____	Oswestry	Floor	LBK	Other_____
☐ United Health	☐ Medical Assist.	3x____	SF-12/SCL-90R	Ball	Shoulder	Area_____
☐ Network Health	☐ Medicare	____wks	Severity Index			
			Comp Health Q			
			Other_____			

NEW PATIENT - modifier - 25

99201 208 193	Focused History/Exam	_____
99202 209 194	Focused History/Exam	_____
99203 210 195	Detailed History/Exam	_____
99204 211 196	Comp. History/Exam	_____
99205 212 197	Comp. History/Exam	_____
99455	Disability Exam	_____

ESTABLISHED PATIENT - modifier - 25

99211 213 198	O.V./Eval.	_____
99212 214 199	Focused History/Exam	_____
99213 215 200	Focused History/Exam	_____
99214 216 201	Detailed History/Exam	_____
99215 217 202	Comp. History/Exam	_____
99401 (15 min)	Prevent. Med. Counsel.	_____
99402 (30 min)	Prevent. Med. Counsel.	_____

TREATMENT

			MC
98940 218	CMT Spinal 1–2 regions	_____	_____
98941 219	CMT Spinal 3–4 regions	_____	_____
98942 220	CMT Spinal 5 regions	_____	_____
98943	207 CMT extra-sp 1+	_____	
98943-51	206 CMT extra-sp 1+	_____	
W9010	116 Spinal Adjustment/ Manipulation E.D.S.	_____	

PHYSIOTHERAPY TREATMENT

97010	100 Hot/Cold Pack	_____
97012	101 Interseg. Traction	_____
97014	102 Electrical Stimulation	_____
A4556	190 Electrodes	_____
97012	120 Traction	
97112	154 PMT, Neuromuscular	_____
97530	175 Therapeutic activities, direct (one on one) patient contact by the provider (use of dynamic activities to improve functional performance), each 15 minutes.	_____
97750	186 FCE, Rehab screen ($_____/15 min. testing)	_____
97140	(15 min. units):mobil, manip, manual trac, lymphatic drainage	_____
97504	Orthotic Fitting	_____
97535	Self-care/home mgmt. training (ADLs) (ea/15 min.)	_____

LABORATORY SERVICE

49	Chem. Screen 26	_____
50	CBC With Differential	_____
51	Arthritic Profile	_____
52	Urinalysis	_____
53	Glucose	_____
56	Sedimentation Rate	_____
57	TMA	_____
58	Thyroxine (T-4)	_____
61	HDL	_____
63	Beta Strep	_____
118	Lymes	_____
127	Lab Handling	_____
182	Executive Panel	_____
_____		_____

RADIOLOGY (-22 Additional x-ray)
(-52 One Less x-ray)

72040	178	Cervical Spine AP/LAT	_____
72040	18	Cervical Spine AP/LAT/OM	_____
72050	19	Cervical Spine 5 Views	_____
		Flex/ext	
		Obliques	
72052	20	Davis Series Complete	_____
72050	21	Stress C-Spine 3 Views	_____
72070	22	Thoracic Spine 2 Views	_____
72100	23	Lumbosacral 2 Views	_____
72110	24	Lumbosacral Com./6 Views	_____
72170	25	Pelvis A/P	_____
73564	27	Knee 4 Views	_____
73030	28	Shoulder 2 Views	____
73630	29	Foot 3 Views	_____
73610	30	Ankle 3 Views	_____
73520	36	Hip 3 Views	_____
76140	47	Exam of Films/Report	_____
72020	40	X-Ray, Single View	_____
72200	230	Sacroiliac joints, 1–2 views	_____
		_____	_____
		_____	_____

SUPPORTIVE THERAPY (plus TAX)

82	Cervical Pillow	_____
87	C-Traction	_____
88	Ice Pack	_____
91	Heel Lift	_____
93	Prescription Foot Orthotics	_____
98	Nutritional Supplementation	_____
183	Gym Ball	_____
184	Balance Board	_____
	Theratube	_____
188	Intracell	_____
191	Foam Roll	_____
191	1/2 Roll	_____
_____		_____

ORTHOPEDIC APPLIANCES

_____   _____

Chapter 23: Clinical Outcome Databases

CLINICAL DATABASES

ACC National Cardiovascular Data Registry™
American College of Cardiology
9111 Old Georgetown Road
Bethesda, MD 20814-1699
Ph: (800) 253-4636

American Society of Hand Therapists
401 North Michigan Avenue
Chicago, IL 60611-4267
Ph: (312) 321-6866
http://www.asht.org

Bio* Analysis Systems
408-B Bayview Drive, P.O. Box 4805
Frisco, CO 80443
Ph: (970) 668-8593

Focus On Therapeutic Outcomes, Inc. (FOTO,™ Inc.)
P.O. Box 11444
Knoxville, TN 37939
Ph: (800) 482-3686, (423) 450-9699
Fax: (423) 450-9484
http://www.fotoinc.com

Medirisk, Inc.
155 N. Wacker Drive, Suite 725
Chicago, IL 60606
Ph: (312) 849-4200
Fax: (312) 849-3060
http://www.medirisk.com

MODEMS™
American Academy of Orthopedic Surgeons
6300 N. River Road
Rosemont, IL 60018
Ph: (800) 288-0018
Fax: (847) 823-8027
http://www.modems.org

Therapeutic Associates, Inc.
10700 SW Beaverton-Hillsdale Hwy.
Suite 622
Beaverton, OR 97005
Ph: (503) 626-7724

Uniform Data System for Medical Rehabilitation (UDSMR)
82 Farber Hall
SUNY—Main St.
Buffalo, NY 14212
Ph: (716) 829-2076
Fax: (716) 829-2080
http://www.udsmr.org
http://www.lifeware.org

OUTCOMES SOFTWARE VENDORS

Assist Technologies
3295 North Civic Center Boulevard
Scottsdale, AZ 85251
Ph: (602) 874-9400
http://www.outcomes-analyzer.com

CareTrak
Synergy Solutions, Inc.
P.O. Box 5103
Grand Rapids, MN 55744-5103
Ph: (218) 326-0437
http://www.caretrak-outcomes.com

Focus On Therapeutic Outcomes, Inc (FOTO,™ Inc.)
P.O. Box 11444
Knoxville, TN 37939
Ph: (800) 482-3686, (423) 450-9699
Fax: (423) 450-9484
http://www.fotoinc.com

Medirisk, Inc.
155 N. Wacker Drive, Suite 725
Chicago, IL 60606
Ph: (312) 849-4200
Fax: (312) 849-3060
http://www.medirisk.com

Outcomes Today
101 Diecks Drive
Elizabethtown, KY 42701
Ph: (502) 737-1731

Point-of-View Survey Systems, Inc.
1380 Lawrence, Suite 820
Denver, CO 80204
Ph: (303) 534-3044

Symphony Rehabilitation Services
11215 Knott Avenue, Suite A
Cypress, CA 90630
Ph: (714) 896-9644

Uniform Data System For Medical Rehabilitation (UDSMR)
82 Farber Hall
SUNY—Main St.
Buffalo, NY 14212
Ph: (716) 829-2076
Fax: (716) 829-2080
http://www.udsmr.org
http://www.lifeware.org

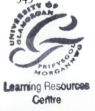